OCCUPATIONAL THERAPY CONSULTATION

Theory, Principles, and Practice

Evelyn G. Jaffe, M.P.H., O.T.R., F.A.O.T.A.
Cynthia F. Epstein, M.A., O.T.R., F.A.O.T.A.

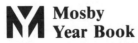
Mosby Year Book

St. Louis   Baltimore   Boston   Chicago   London   Philadelphia
Sydney   Toronto

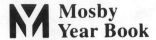
Mosby
Year Book

Dedicated to Publishing Excellence

Sponsoring Editor: David K. Marshall
Assistant Editor: Julie Tryboski
Associate Managing Editor, Manuscript Services: Deborah Thorp
Production Supervisor: Karen Halm

Mosby-Year Book, Inc.
11830 Westline Industrial Drive
St. Louis, MO 63146

1 2 3 4 5 6 7 8 9 0 SP MV 96 95 94 93 92

Library of Congress Cataloging-in-Publication Data

Jaffe, Evelyn.
    Occupational therapy consultation : theory, principles, and
practice / Evelyn Jaffe, Cynthia Epstein.
        p.   cm.
    Includes bibliographical references and index.
    ISBN 0-8016-6204-4
    1. Occupational therapy—Practice.   2. Medical consultation.
I. Epstein, Cynthia F.   II. Title.
    [DNLM: 1. Occupational Therapy.   2. Referral and Consultation.
WB 555 J23o]
RM735.4.J24   1991   91-28050
615.8'515—dc20   CIP
DNLM/DLC
for Library of Congress

Contributors

Susan Bachner, M.A., O.T.R./L., F.A.O.T.A.
Self-Employed Consultant and Practitioner
Greenwich, Connecticut

Beverly K. Bain, Ed.D., O.T.R., F.A.O.T.A.
Coordinator of RSA Technology Grant
New York University
New York, New York

Rondell S. Berkeland, M.P.H., O.T.R.
Director, Program in Occupational Therapy
University of Minnesota
Minncapolis, Minncsota

Christine Chang, M.P.H., M.P.A., O.T.R.
Senior Policy Analyst
New York State Council on Children and Families
Albany, New York

Richelle N. Cunninghis, M.Ed., O.T.R.
Executive Director
Geriatric Educational Consultants
Willingboro, New Jersey

Elizabeth B. Devereaux, M.S.W., A.C.S.W./L., O.T.R./L., F.A.O.T.A.
Associate Professor
Department of Psychiatry
Director, Division of Occupational Thcrapy
Marshall University School of Medicine
Huntington, West Virginia

Georgette DuFresne, M.P.A., O.T.R.
Lead Occupational Therapist
Dominican Hospital
Santa Cruz, California

Winnie Dunn, Ph.D., O.T.R., F.A.O.T.A.
Professor and Chairman
Occupational Therapy Education
University of Kansas Medical Center
Kansas City, Kansas

Melanie T. Ellexson, M.B.A., O.T.R., F.A.O.T.A.
Assistant Vice President
Executive Director
Schwab Rehabilitation Center's STEPS Rehabilitation Clinics
Chicago, Illinois

Cynthia F. Epstein, M.A., O.T.R., F.A.O.T.A.
Executive Director
Occupational Therapy Consultants, Inc.
Bridgewater, New Jersey

Diane Gibson, M.S., O.T.R./L.
Director Rehabilitation Services (Retired)
Sheppard Pratt Hospital
Baltimore, Maryland

Gordon Muir Giles, DipCOT., O.T.R.
Director of Occupational Therapy
Guardian Foundation
Berkeley, California

Elnora M. Gilfoyle, D.Sc., O.T.R., F.A.O.T.A.
Provost-Academic Vice President
Colorado State University
Fort Collins, Colorado

Ann P. Grady, M.A., O.T.R., F.A.O.T.A.
Director of Access Ability Resource Center
The Children's Hospital
Denver, Colorado

Ruth A. Hansen, Ph.D., O.T.R., F.A.O.T.A.
Graduate Coordinator
Associate Professor
Eastern Michigan University
Ypsilanti, Michigan

Satoru Izutsu, Ph.D., O.T.R., F.A.O.T.A., F.A.A.M.D.
Professor of Public Health and Psychiatry
John A. Burns School of Medicine
University of Hawaii
Honolulu, Hawaii

Karen Jacobs, M.S., O.T.R./L., F.A.O.T.A.
Assistant Professor
Boston University
Boston, Massachusetts

Evelyn G. Jaffe, M.P.H., O.T.R., F.A.O.T.A.
Consultant
Private Practice
Tiburon, California

Sylvia Harlock Kauffman, Ph.D., O.T.R., F.A.O.T.A.
Auxillary Faculty Appointment at the University of Washington
Administrator, Rehabilitation Center
St. Joseph Hospital and Health Care Center
Tacoma, Washington

Elayne Klasson, Ph.D., M.P.H., O.T.R.
Lecturer, Department of Occupational Therapy
San Jose State University
San Jose, California

Barbara L. Kornblau, J.D., O.T.R., C.I.R.S.
Attorney at Law
Occupational Therapist
Adjunct Professor
Florida International University
ADA Consultants, Incorporated
Miami, Florida

Susan Lang, M.B.A., O.T.R., A.T.R.
Private Practice
San Francisco, California

Sandra L. Jacobson Lerner, O.T.R./L.
Executive Director
Comprehensive Therapeutics, Limited
Northbrook, Illinois

Lela A. Llorens, Ph.D., O.T.R., F.A.O.T.A.
Professor, Chairman, and Graduate Coordinator
Department of Occupational Therapy
Co-Director, Division of Health Professions
San Jose State University
San Jose, California

Katherine M. Post, M.S., O.T.R./L.
Assistant Professor of Occupational Therapy
Springfield College
Springfield, Massachusetts

Joan C. Rogers, Ph.D., O.T.R., F.A.O.T.A.
Professor of Occupational Therapy
University of Pittsburgh
Director of Occupational Therapy—Geriatrics
Western Psychiatric Institute and Clinic
Pittsburgh, Pennsylvania

Jane Davis Rourk, O.T.R/L., F.A.O.T.A.
Clinical Associate Professor
Division of Occupational Therapy
University of North Carolina
Chapel Hill, North Carolina

Louise Samson, O.T.R./L., F.A.O.T.A.
Private Practice
Sarasota, Florida

Karen C. Spencer, M.A., O.T.R.
Assistant Professor
Department of Occupational Therapy
Colorado State University
Fort Collins, Colorado

Diane R. Weiss, M.A., O.T.R.
Associate Director
Occupational Therapy Consultants, Inc.
Bridgewater, New Jersey

Donna Weiss, M.A., O.T.R/L.
Assistant Professor
Department of Occupational Therapy
Temple University
Philadelphia, Pennsylvania

Wilma L. West, M.A., O.T.R., F.A.O.T.A.
President Emerita
American Occupational Therapy Foundation
Reston, Virginia

Wendy Wood, M.A., O.T.R.
Jane Goodall Fellow for Doctoral Studies in Occupational Science
University of Southern California
Los Angeles, California

Rhona Reiss Zukas, M.O.T., O.T.R., F.A.O.T.A.
Assistant Dean
Texas Woman's University School of Occupational Therapy
Duncanville, Texas

Dedication

To Bob Jaffe and Alan Epstein,
to Joseph Epstein,
and to Aliya Joy Jaffe Whitney, whose winsome smile brings true joy to all who
meet her

Acknowledgments

The completion of this book is a celebration of professional development. It could never have been conceived and arrived at fruition without the encouragement and support of many people.

We owe much to those who fostered our professional growth and gave direction to our ideas. Willis West's mentorship and broad vision of occupational therapy's role in the health care system, particularly relative to prevention and consultation, fostered the growth and development of concepts that have guided Evie Jaffe's professional practice and Cynthia Epstein's entry into consultation. Ellie Gilfoyle strongly and consistently encouraged Evie to write a book to share with others my firm conviction that roles in primary prevention, health promotion, and consultation would be essential for occupational therapists in the future of health care. Ellie's inspiring views of occupational therapy and her interactions with both of us helped create the impetus for this book. It is only fitting that this book should start with some historical perspectives of consultation by Wilma West, our consultation role model and mentor, and end with the inspirational message of Elnora Gilfoyle about the future directions of consultation in occupational therapy.

Each of us has been influenced by many colleagues in the course of our professional growth. Of particular importance for Evie during her early professional development were three key individuals: Barbara Jewett, Elizabeth Boles, and Martha Moersch. Barbara Jewett's dedication to the profession instilled an understanding of the importance of occupational therapy in the health and care of individuals and provided Evie with some direction for future professional roles. Libby Boles, director of the occupational therapy program at the Neuropsychiatric Institute at the University of Michigan Medical Center, allowed Evie the freedom to explore some of her nontraditional ideas. These ideas included developing a community fieldwork program for occupational therapy students in the well-community, exploring primary prevention programming outside the medical institution, and studying and practicing principles and theory of consultation. Martha Moersch nurtured and reaffirmed Evie's professional ideas and firmly encouraged and prodded her involvement in professional organizational activities.

Mentors and colleagues who have played an important part in Cynthia's development include: Barbara Neuhaus, Ricki Cunninghis, Jerry Johnson, and Joan Rogers. Barbara Neuhaus' reflective counseling and support helped Cynthia expand vocationally oriented consultative skills, working within industrial and sheltered workshop settings. Ricki Cunninghis' collegial consultative relationship has spanned the years, providing Cynthia with objective encouragement along with extensive resources. Working with Jerry Johnson during the AOTA reorganization provided Cynthia with opportunities to refine her consultative skills while expanding knowledge of systems and organizational theory. A consultant's knowledge and skills are developed further through mentorship. Joan Rogers' mentorship to Cynthia has engendered continuous appreciation of the breadth and depth of consultation.

No project of this duration is possible without the understanding, patience, and encouragement of those closest to you. We owe many thanks to our husbands, Bob Jaffe and Alan Epstein, and to all our children for their steadfast love and support during this long-standing project.

Evelyn Jaffe and Cynthia Epstein

Foreword

Some two decades ago, a few occupational therapists assumed roles as consultants in public health programs. These roles required a duality of function that combined the previously more discrete role of therapist to individual patients with that of participant-adviser to systems. It also called for a changed setting of operations from the supportive environment of the self-contained hospital to the relatively unstructured teams of outreach personnel providing health surveillance and monitoring that typically led to case-finding in the medically indigent populations served. Contributions of therapists in these roles were principally evaluation of those at risk for developing physical and emotional problems—the initial therapist role—and participation, as integral members of the health care team, in referral and programming for treatment as indicated—the interdisciplinary consultant role. Although these roles were effective, thus supported in state services where they were modeled, and despite their description in the literature of the times, there was little real growth in the number of occupational therapists attracted or recruited to such positions.

Inevitably, however, as the health care system changed, similar and considerably greater needs for occupational therapy consultation in multiple other settings have become increasingly apparent in recent years. Visibility of these has been sharpened by major shifts in the employment settings of occupational therapists, which, in turn, have been occasioned by such trends as deinstitutionalization of the mentally ill, "mainstreaming" of handicapped children, establishment of a broad range of community-based treatment facilities, increase of day care programing for preschoolers and the elderly, and many other factors related to escalating costs of traditional medical care in hospitals. These trends have dramatically changed the locus of work for most categories of allied health personnel, including occupational therapists, and led to their entry into new arenas of practice. In these new arenas, traditional one-on-one treatment skills have been substantially supplemented by skills essential to intervention strategies and programs jointly planned and effected by a constellation of health care providers, many of whom have effectively combined treatment and consultation skills to extend the benefit of their services to patients. Public health physicians and nurses are prime examples of such practices.

The 1990 Member Data Survey conducted by the American Occupational Therapy Association contains figures that support the relevance and usefulness of this book to several groups of occupational therapy personnel. Most obvious among these are the 39.6 percent of OTRs and 26.3 percent of COTAs who list consultation as their primary or secondary work function. Somewhat less evident but implicit in the nature of function required is the need for communication and consultation skills by several other groups of occupational therapy personnel classified by employment setting or form of work. For example:

In the school system, which employs 18.6 percent of OTRs and 17.0 percent of COTAs, consultation to teachers, special educators, parents, and administrative personnel has become a function superceding direct treatment.

In rehabilitation hospitals/centers and rehabilitation units of general hospitals, which are the primary work setting of 16.7 percent of OTRs and 16.4 percent of COTAs, the multidisciplinary character of staff and the interdisciplinary nature of function require communication and consultation skills of an above average level.

Skilled nursing homes and intermediate care facilities, the primary workplace of 6.4 percent of OTRs and 20.1 percent of COTAs, characteristically utilize the consultation of a broad range of medical and allied health disciplines.

For the 7.7 percent of OTRs and 2.7 percent of COTAs in private practice, consultation to parents, caregivers, teachers, and other medical and allied health personnel is essential to effective therapeutic and related functions.

Finally, smaller, but in the aggregate, significant percentages of the occupational therapy workforce are employed in acute care, day care, and community mental health centers where collaborative and consultative skills are essential if the total needs of patients and clients are effectively served.

These data offer quantification of the need for consultation skills in the repertoire of significant numbers of today's occupational therapy practitioners. Over time, many other changes, both philosophical and real, have affected our concepts of optimal health care, and will inevitably have further impact on occupational therapy roles of future practitioners.

Among philosophical changes are the premises that health, like education, is a basic human right; that tomorrow's health care will be designed for the community as well as the individual; and that health care of the future will be as concerned with prevention as with rehabilitation. In the category of real changes, there may be listed shifts from institutional, clinical, and medical care models to broader community-based delivery systems designed to promote health and well being and prevent disease and disability.

The indicated need for occupational therapists to utilize consultation skills in public health and other community, out-of-hospital service settings was one motivation for undertaking this book. Another was the increasingly apparent need for the skills of consultation in programs addressing disability prevention and health promotion.

The already plausible case for occupational therapy's role in prevention of disability and promotion of health is given additional credence in this book by the authors' perceptive postulates that such a role is a natural extension of the profession's traditional role—that is, from improving function of the individual to helping improve function of the health care system. Agnostics of this goal raise the dilemma of proving the value of prevention efforts by asking how either the cost or the effect of prevention can be measured. Such doubts are reminiscent of questions raised about the cost and effectiveness of rehabilitation more than 50 years ago. The economic validity of rehabilitation that transformed the severely disabled from the role of tax burden to that of taxpayer has long since been demonstrated, and similarly creative logic and computations could do much to strengthen advocacy for prevention.

A third persuasion of the Jaffe-Epstein team to compile this book was their conviction of the need for a text for occupational therapy courses in both basic and graduate educational programs. To the extent that they convincingly document the need of current practitioners for knowledge of consultation theories, principles, and practices, they justify a corrective need in professional preparation for the future.

An important final feature of this book is Part II. To supplement their well-researched and clearly presented rationale for occupational therapy consultation, Jaffe and Epstein invited more than 30 contributing authors to describe models of occupational therapy consultation specific to their respective areas of expertise and practice. Thus, a considerable portion of the book is devoted to examples applied in the wide variety of settings indicated by titles in Part II, which concludes with technological, legal, and ethical issues in consultation. The total result is a comprehensive model for occupational therapy consultation practice.

No less should have been expected from these two respected colleagues. With 70 years of occupational therapy experience between them, the majority of which for both has been in consultation, they assuredly know whereof they write; and their separate and co-authored sections in both Parts I and II of this book display knowledge that highly qualifies them to discuss their subject in the depth that characterizes this publication. I concur with their premises, commend the results of their efforts, and believe this book will make a substantive and valuable contribution to the professional literature.

Wilma L. West, M.A., O.T.R., F.A.O.T.A.
Reston, Virginia

Preface

The concept for a textbook and practical guide to occupational therapy consultation evolved during the early 1970s. As our consultation activities expanded, we noted an increasing need for broader understanding of consultation theories and principles. While the importance of consultation was recognized in the occupational therapy literature, a substantive work on occupational therapy consultation was not available to guide us. The need for this information was reflected in comments from many of our colleagues. During the 1980s, the demand for occupational therapy consultation services continued to escalate and broaden. A comprehensive text addressing the multiple issues emerging in this field was needed. We were encouraged by colleagues and leaders in health care to develop a text that would draw on our consultation knowledge and experience as practitioners, lecturers, and authors.

This encouragement translated itself into *Occupational Therapy Consultation: Theory, Principles, and Practice,* a comprehensive book written for occupational therapy faculty, students, and practitioners. The text encompasses many of the theoretical concepts inherent in consultation, the dynamics of consultation, including basic process and procedures, and current models of occupational therapy consultation practice.

Today's health care delivery system has changed the role of the occupational therapist. It has expanded from practice in traditional clinical arenas to broader health care settings. As we move into new or nontraditional arenas, there is a growing need for increased communication skills, information, and expertise in the field of consultation.

Many therapists now are engaged in community health care services, while others are involved in political lobbying for health care legislation, consumer advocacy activities, and regulatory and reimbursement areas. Our rapid growth in private practice has led to an increased need for consultation skills. Occupational therapy managers in hospital facilities now collaborate closely with community and other health agencies. Additionally, the greatest number of occupational therapists who are considered "consultants" are currently working in the public school systems. With the enactment of Public Law 94–142, many therapists moved into the schools with little or no experience or training in consulting, a role required of them.

Academic occupational therapy programs do not uniformly include coursework on either the theory or practice of consultation. Therefore, graduates of many of these programs are not prepared with the theoretical background nor the technical skills needed to engage in consultation activities. *Occupational Therapy Consultation: Theory, Principles, and Practice* is directed to intermediate and advanced students, at both the undergraduate and graduate level, and will most likely be used in administration and/or management courses.

Occupational therapy administrators, directors, and therapists will find this book a useful resource as they develop or enhance the consultative aspects of their practice. The section Models of Occupational Therapy Practice, presented by experts in each of the settings described, will help the reader view the breadth of areas available to therapists choosing a consultation practice.

This book is organized to provide a comprehensive overview of consultation, including a historical perspective and basic theoretical concepts. It will provide an understanding of the background and skills required. Examples of occupational therapy consultation, provided by contributing authors in the Models of Practice section, follow a format allowing the reader to compare and contrast consultation practice settings. The appendix will provide additional resources, sample forms, and suggested readings.

The generic concepts presented provide the reader with background in the consultation process. The theory of occupational therapy consultation practice that we present is based on the philosophical principles and tenets that form the core of all occupational therapy practice. Our purpose is to offer a comprehensive context from which to develop a practice that is appropriate and current with trends in the health care system.

Evelyn G. Jaffe, M.P.H., O.T.R., F.A.O.T.A.
Cynthia F. Epstein, M.A., O.T.R., F.A.O.T.A.

Contents

PART I

Theory and Principles of Consultation

CHAPTER 1

The History of Professional Consultation: An Overview

Evelyn G. Jaffe, M.P.H., O.T.R., F.A.O.T.A.
Cynthia F. Epstein, M.A., O.T.R., F.A.O.T.A.

"The most general term for (the) helping process is consultation".
—*G. Lippitt and R. Lippitt*[39]

DEVELOPMENT OF CONSULTATION AS A PRACTICE

Historic Evolution

The art and practice of consultation, as a process of helping solve problems, can be traced throughout history and in practically all cultures. The health field in particular has had individuals known and revered for their sage advice and counsel, from primitive tribal medicine men, to healers and physicians in the Middle Ages, to contemporary health counselors. Most of the early individuals did not receive formal training in developing helping skills, but rather were charismatic leaders who developed followers, and, through role modeling and apprenticeships, passed these skills down from generation to generation.[19, 39]

The evolution of these helping roles can be linked directly to social needs. As the body of knowledge in a culture grows, and the numbers of the group increase, specialist roles emerge.[19] Societies developed around an agrarian culture had individuals knowledgeable about tools, shelters, and the properties of plants and herbal medicinal characteristics; those concerned with acquisition of territory created specialists in weapons and warfare; other societies, concerned with issues of life and death, had religious advisers, wise men, sorcerers, and high priests. The evolution of helping roles as a practice can be followed from these primitive beginnings to the highly refined roles now assigned to consultants as a result of the technology explosion in today's society. Modern consultation practice can be said to be derived from the prototype specialists in these early cultures: the healer, the technological adviser, and the sage.[19]

The *healer* is known in all cultures, from the most primitive to the most highly developed. The ancient healer's expertise came from both the study of medical techniques and the supernatural. Thus the medicine man or woman was both physician and sorcerer.[52] Today, people still attribute some supernatural qualities to physicians and lay a heavy dose of miracle curing on top of advances in medical technology. The modern medical consultant is often expected to assume the role of healer and to provide information that will lead to a complete amelioration of the patient's illness.[61]

All societies depend on the *technological adviser* and the skilled technician to help others learn new methods. In primitive societies, the technological adviser taught others how to hunt and how to construct tools, weapons, and shelters. They were not doers, but trainers, who transmitted their particular knowledge and skills to others.[61] In today's society, the technological adviser is particularly sought after to provide training and education in complex technical advances. The specialized scientific expertise and technical skills of these consultants have enabled our rapidly changing society to solve many problems, from social and human needs to the demanding and precise technical assistance required within our exploding world of technology.

The role of the *sage,* as the individual who proclaimed moral or political judgments about what was right or wrong in the society, helped ancient leaders make decisions. The modern-day use of this type of advice often creates dilemmas for today's consultant. When the consultant's views are requested about the moral or social consequences of certain policies or procedures, the consultant must be careful not to fall into the role of all-knowing, all-powerful sage. Political advisers are often vested with these powers. But the consultant must be sure that the information or opinions presented are based on objective fact-finding and the sage advice is a result of professional expertise and technical knowledge, not moral or political jdugments.[19, 61] (The pitfalls of consultation are discussed in detail in Chapter 6.)

The Industrial Revolution brought an increased need for the helping professions. Previously, the American ethic was based on self-reliance, precluding the need for professional specialists. The expansion of technology in the 1800s created many changes in medical care and increased the need for more health care professionals. These changes included a preponderance of home care in the beginning of the 19th century, the growing use of hospitals and clinics, and an increased understanding of hygienic techniques.

Clinical consultation evolved to address these changes. The centuries-old traditional medical practice of physicians consulting with one another in a collegial manner about the diagnosis and treatment of patients expanded to a hierarchical model of consultation, in which the physician also consulted with other independent practitioners. These individuals, usually "apothecaries," did not have formal medical training and needed the consultative services of the physician.[19, 34] Social reforms also created human service agencies and the development of a body of helping professionals who practiced both the collegial and hierarchical model of clinical consultation. This early use of the clinical consultant model is a forerunner of the collaborative style of consultation often used in health care and educational practice today. Then, as now, problems of competition emerged among colleagues, between the consultant and professional consultee, for the patient's favor. Additionally, hierarchical consultation could evolve to a superior/subordinate relationship in which the main focus of the relationship was not clinical consultation, but rather the supervisory role the consultant was required to perform.[48] (These problems are explored in Chapter 6.)

The Formalization of Consultation

The need for outside experts has grown steadily since the early 1900s. After World War I the demand for management help expanded and a body of helping practitioners was developed. By 1929 it was recognized that ethical and service standards for these practitioners were needed and the Association of Consulting Management Engineers (ACME) was formed.[56]

After World War II, the gradual shift from a production-oriented economy to a service-oriented economy had a major impact on the growth of the helping services. It was around this time that documentation of the role of occupational therapy consultants first appeared. In 1944, the Office of the Army Surgeon General established five occupational therapy consultant positions to maximize the services required for wounded personnel returning from the front lines.

Consultation in the 1950s was used mainly in the traditional fields of law, taxes and accounting, and collegial consultations among physicians. At this time, field consultant positions were established by the American Occupational Therapy Association (AOTA), in response to needs voiced by therapists practicing in rural areas or isolated from professional input. The consultant's activities included identification of resources, provision of support and advocacy, assistance in problem solving, and clarification of the role and function of occupational therapy for the therapists. Through this consultation process, other health professionals, physicians, and administrators also were apprised of the occupational therapist's role.[25]

With the tremendous surge in science and technology in the 1960s, consultation in technical industries came into its own.[35] At the same time, expanding health and human services programs, developed under the Johnson Great Society mandates, created increasing needs for occupational therapy consultants in nursing facilities, early intervention programs, school systems, vocational rehabilitation services, and other community models of care.[16] In the past 25 years, the practice of consultation has proliferated and become a recognized professional field in business, politics, labor, and economics, as well as in the legal, social, religious, educational, and health spheres.

Perhaps most well known as a general practice of consultation is organizational development (OD), which arose out of what Drucker[12] called "the mid-20th century phenomenon," the applied science of management. Management science, as taught in many business administration programs, focuses on quantitative analysis of business decisions and the tangible aspects of finance, marketing, and planning. Additionally, it emphasizes economics, administration, and organizational behavior and change. OD in the 1950s and 1960s was used extensively in large complex organizations, including private corporations, government, and nonprofit groups for long-term, large-scale progams and planning.

At the same time, both during and after World War II, the U.S. government employed consultants in the applied behavioral sciences of social psychology and sociology to study group behavior. This gave rise to the study of group dynamics as an academic discipline. The noted social scientist Kurt Lewin developed his force-field analysis theory and studied the process of participation in leadership styles, both autocratic and democratic.[38] The famous "T Group" study of group dynamics followed in the National Training Laboratories' (NTL Institute) Human Interaction Labs. In the 1950s and 1960s, the NTL emphasized psychological processes, personal growth, adult education, individual needs, feelings, and human relations.[38]

By the early 1970s, OD theory had expanded and integrated many of these concepts of the applied behavioral sciences. OD consultants often were asked to study the need for organizational change. Human problems in organizations were recognized as an important component of management. Personnel management became an academic field of study in business schools under the subject of organizational behavior. Organizations employed both external OD consultants and internal human resources consultants to deal with issues of personnel management. Personnel departments in many organizations are frequently referred to as the "human resources section." It has been estimated that 3% of personnel costs is spent on personnel management and human resource development, a growing area for consultation opportunities.[36]

Affirmative action initiatives further opened new challenges for organizational consultants. This trend continued in the 1970s and 1980s with the tremendous growth of high-technology industries and the rise of sociotechnical systems. Organizational consultation expanded from the social system of an individual organization to the broader technical system; from parts of the organization to the entire organizational structure; and to the external environment, including economic and social systems.[51]

Business and corporate management, although a major arena for consultants, as demonstrated by the Dun and Bradstreet listing of over 100 business management subspecialties, is only one area in which consultants are used today.[35] We need only to look in the telephone book of any metropolitan area to see the preponderance of consulting firms for any number of different sectors, from consumer services to education, data systems, conservation, health and human services, hospital administration, management, marketing, public relations, real estate, recreational events, safety, taxes, transportation, and weddings. There are consultants in almost every field, from large corporate industries to private homes where you can hire a consultant to help organize your home, provide suggestions to create a personal image, and recommend effective ways to run your garage sale!

The passage of health care and educational legislation in the 1970s and 1980s increased the demand for professional consultants. Collaborative consultation among professional colleagues, with its roots in the early model of clinical consul-

Diagnostic techniques may include interview and observation of key power individuals in the system and in the community or group requesting help with change. The consultant also may conduct a needs assessment or survey to obtain pertinent information from group members regarding the situation. This includes immediate and future client goals and the tasks and activities necessary to achieve them. Diagnostic techniques, including surveys and needs assessments, will reveal the ability of the community to organize and utilize a social action model of consultation. The methodology of data collection, analysis, and authoritative interpretation is usually the responsibility of the consultant.

The consultant has major responsibility for fostering communication within the client system to develop group cohesiveness through common cause. It is essential to acknowledge the unique contributions of individual members of the group and of various interests represented within the community. Understanding and agreement on the scope of expectations and goals require a collaborative approach, so that the client may assume an active role in the diagnosis and collection of information. The client, therefore, shares equally in the responsibility for development of strategies relevant to the community issues. The consultant may utilize a variety of methods and combinations of activities to provide the client with training in organization, strategy development, and self-determination to implement action plans that will accomplish the goals. Included in the helping techniques are assisting the client adapt to shifting political and economic circumstances and mobilizing the motivational forces of the community.

Evaluation is not usually in terms of formal measures but is related directly to the outcome of the social change, and, therefore, is assessed by the client. There may be continual evaluation and modification of strategies throughout the intervention. Termination of the consultation may take place when change has occurred and the desired goal reached. Consultation also may terminate when the client has attained a degree of efficiency and expertise in organizing the group and developing appropriate power strategies to accomplish the desired system changes.

This is not a traditional consultation model for most health professionals. But as health professionals, and occupational therapy consultants in particular, expand their practice to more global community settings, the social action model becomes an important tool. Occupational therapy consultants may use advocacy techniques to obtain greater services for children in school systems. They may be advocates for individuals who are physically, mentally, or emotionally challenged, helping groups organize to obtain more programs and job opportunities. Advocacy services also may be used to help develop health promotion and wellness programs and architectural barrier-free environments in communities and the workplace. As occupational therapists become more involved in the legislative and health policy arena, the concepts of social action consultation can be particularly valuable.

Assessment of the Model

The social action model is extremely useful for organization and mobilization of groups to help them develop systemwide social changes strategies. It values political action as a means of achieving social and economic changes. The emphasis is on a redistribution of power from the bottom up, which differs from the organizational model that values shared power from the top down. Often the focus is on community organization to gain community control through circumvention of the social structure. When this occurs, there is increased intergroup conflict and adversarial power struggles, which the consultant must acknowledge.

Constraints of this model include problems that may occur because participation is from a limited constituency. This model defines a particular group. It does not refer to the entire social system, thus it ignores participation and accountability to the larger system. The focus is on conflict between the structural system or societal organization and the needs of a specific group. There may be detractors in the system that lead to lack of support from the total system. A further limitation is that the model does not usually provide a framework for intergroup relationships. Conflict may be unresolved and may escalate, as seen in examples of community demonstrations and rioting. Additionally, because of the revolutionary nature of this model, the action or changes desired may not be integrated in the evolution of a social system.

Systems Model

The systems model, as we present it here, has an ecological perspective with roots in the scientific concepts that formed the basis for general system theory, described by von Bertalanffy in 1947. Research attempts to understand biological phenomena led to a systems approach that considered the interrelationship between all elements in living matter, from the study of a single cell to that of a society. This theory was refined and modified to the open system theory by von Bertalanffy in the 1960s, defined as "a system in exchange of matter with its environment."[58, p141] Open systems theory is discussed further in Chapter 3.

The systems model is based on the concept that there is a dynamic interaction between all components of a society. It is derived from basic concepts of ecology developed by the biological sciences and the adaptation of these theories to the social sciences. Therefore, the systems model includes both biological and sociological theories of ecology. The biological aspects of the systems model focus on relations between organisms and their environment. Sociological aspects of human ecology are concerned with the roles of people and institutions and their interdependency.[32]

The adaptation of these concepts to a systems model of consultation focuses attention on the relationship between community systems and the behavior of populations at risk. Although certain aspects of this model parallel the social action model, in that the consultation is concentrated on a community, the emphasis and definition of the community are different. In contrast to the view of a community as a specific constituency lacking power to effect change, in the systems model, a community is viewed as a unit in the relationship of the community to its environment.

Unlike the social action model of revolutionary change, this model considers the channeling of environmental resources to anticipate and deal with naturally occurring change as it affects the specific values and culture of a given system. The consultant must focus on all aspects of the environment and the interdependence of roles and behaviors in the system. The emphasis is on long-range changes in the social system.

Perceptions

In this model the consultant is perceived as a catalyst, planner, or interventionist. As in the social action model, professional skills in communication are essential. The consultant may be seen as the leader and organizer of plans to effect change in the system. The client may be part of a group or agency within the community. The consultant assumes a collegial role with the client, working collaboratively with community members.

Motivation, Entry, Goals

The client system (community or particular community group), is motivated to request consultation when there is a crisis within the community, initiated by maladaptation or a malfunction in the social system. The locus of the problem is the population at risk, which does not have the ability to be self-sustaining. The client lacks the knowledge, coping skills, and adaptive resources required to develop appropriate change strategies to address critical issues. The consultant is usually invited for an indefinite or long term that goes beyond the immediate presenting problem, in order to help adjust or adapt community processes to respond to changes in the system.

The primary consultation goal is to improve client skills to restructure the social system, thereby facilitating system adaptation to change. Goals are focused on maximizing the community potential by channeling the social resources and enhancing the positive aspects of human development. The target population is usually a subgroup of the system operating within the total environment. The target for consultation may be a group or agency having direct effect on segments of a disadvantaged or at-risk population. (For example, the target may be a particular school district in a community with a disadvantaged or at-risk student body.)

Strategies, Techniques, Responsibilities, Evaluation, Termination

As discussed in other models of consultation, the client presents the consultant with the problem, which the client and consultant jointly define in terms of a community intervention. In this model, after presentation of the precipitating problem or situation, the consultant works collaboratively with the client to identify the issues and analyze the system. Diagnostic techniques in this model may include interview, observation, participation, and interaction with individuals in the system at large and in the specific subsystem or community group requesting help with adaptation to change. The consultant may conduct a needs assessment or survey research to obtain pertinent information from group members regarding the situation and the cultural and social folkways of the community. Before recommendations or strategies for change are considered, knowledge of the current social structure is essential.[32] Immediate and long-range goals and the tasks and activities necessary to achieve these goals are discussed between consultant and client.

In the systems model, which embodies concepts of community enhancement, it is assumed that the client exists in a total environment. The consultation, therefore, should be a team effort, with participation by the professional consultants and nonprofessional community members. For example, in urban renewal projects that include both the physical environment and social system, urban and regional planners join with the helping professions and members of the community to modify the environment to meet the needs of the population.

The consultant has a major responsibility for fostering understanding of the total environment and helping all members of the community reach their full potential. It is essential to acknowledge the unique contributions of individual members of the group and various interests and resources represented within the community. There is a collaborative approach to the scope of expectations and goals and a sharing in the responsibility for the consultation intervention. The client assumes a very active role in the identification of issues, collection of information, and development of modification/adaptation strategies relevant to the community.

The consultant may utilize a variety of methods and combinations of activities to provide the client with training. Specific knowledge and skills relevant to planning and adaptation are presented. Most often, a collaborative, educational approach to strategy development is used to accomplish the goals. Important activities of the systems consultant include strengthening community resources through development of professional and research services, educational and/or staff training seminars, and new or modified community service programs. Additionally, the consultant may assume the role of a change agent, helping the client adapt behaviors to changes in the social environment. This requires an understanding of adaptive behavior theory and the relationships between individual behavior and social structures that affect various forms of adaptive behavior.[32]

Evaluation may involve formal research measures using pre- and postintervention methodology. Continuous analysis of community behavior is essential. This may be accomplished by informal, continual observation and assessment and by modifying of strategies throughout the intervention. Termination of the consultation occurs when the environmental modifications are in place and the client's skill in planning and adaptation forecasts positive enhancement of the community.

Health professionals, including occupational therapy consultants, often utilize systems concepts. Consultants to school systems; community programs for the physically, mentally, or emotionally disabled; or community programs for older individuals must consider the interrelationships of the specific program and the community as a whole. The ability to adapt and change is related both to needs and perceptions within the specific consultation site and to needs and perceptions within the community at large. General systems theory and principles are particularly important for occupational therapy consultants who are involved in the development of community prevention, health promotion, and wellness programs. Analysis of adaptive behaviors, community structures, and sociocultural influences is crucial to primary prevention activities, program development, and planning for change.[17]

Assessment of the Model

The systems model has considerable value as a consultation approach to improve and develop community resources. Because this model conceptualizes community processes as natural and evolutionary, it is not necessary to create forces, such as intergroup conflict and adversarial power, to achieve social and economic change. The intervention is designed to address locally defined problems with an emphasis on direct participation by the members of community organizations and social structures.

Another strength of this model is the awareness of the impact of change on the total system. Anticipation of change and the need for behavioral adaptation to social change are part of the continuing function of the consultative process. High value is placed on integrating the views of the individual and community through emphasis on the interrelatedness of behavior and social systems.

Table 2–1 compares the nine theoretical models of consultation described above.

EVOLUTION OF THE LEVELS OF CONSULTATION

In addition to using various models, consultation interventions may occur on several levels. The levels consider the *service target,* such as the individual client, health care agency team, entire agency or social system; the *intervention goal;* and the *approach required* to achieve needed change. Early work by Caplan in the field of mental health laid the foundation for this conceptual framework. Subsequently, other theorists, including Cooper, Rhodes, and Nagler expanded this work to include community and social systems.[19, 47]

Caplan[16] described four fundamental categories of consultation that influence the specific goals of the consultant and consultee:

- Client-centered case consultation
- Program-centered administrative consultation
- Consultee-centered case consultation
- Consultee-centered administrative consultation

In Caplan's typology, the client refers to the specific patient, and the consultee is another professional who is the direct recipient of the consultant's recommendations. The problem under consideration involves the treatment or management of the specific client(s)/patient(s), consultee, or program. (In this review of Caplan's typology, we use his terminology.)

Client-Centered Case Consultation

The focus of this consultation is the problem encountered by the consultee with a specific client/patient. The primary goal of the consultant is to help the consultee

TABLE 2–1
Comparative Theoretical Models

Model	Definition	Perceptions	Motivation of Client System	Entry Into System
Clinical or Treatment Model	"Patient" or case centered, client focused	Consultant viewed as expert, specialist, resource, client may be expert in own field	Anxiety, conflict, crisis	Invited, administrative sanction (usually short term)
Collegial or Professional Model	Case-specific, peer-centered collaborative, egalitarian mutual problem-solving	Consultant viewed as equal peer; consultant and client may be experts in own fields	Broaden base of knowledge to expand or modify programs; resolve problems	Invited, may have administrative sanction (short or long term)
Behavioral Model	Case-centered or problem-specific behavior change	Consultant viewed as expert or specialist, highly directive role	Anxiety, conflict, crisis as a result of negative behaviors	Invited, administrative sanction (usually short term)
Educational Model	Information-centered, instructional training, in-service staff development	Consultant viewed as teacher, expert, resource specialist, may also be peer.	Broaden base of knowledge to expand or modify programs to respond to environmental changes	Invited, administrative sanction (short term)
Organizational Development Model	Organization centered, management focused based on organizational structure	Consultant-viewed as expert, resource specialist, facilitator	Organizational change to respond to internal and/or external environmental changes	Invited, administrative sanction (short or long term
Process Management Model	Organization centered, focused on organizational process and dynamics	Consultant viewed as expert, resource specialist, facilitator, catalyst	Ineffective functioning of certain operational aspects, inability to respond to internal and/or external pressures	Invited, administrative sanction (time-limited short term)
Program Development Model	Focused on development or modification of service programs	Consultant viewed as expert, resource, or program specialist	Broaden or modify programs to respond to internal or external environmental and technical changes	Invited, administrative sanction (short term)
Social Action Model	Focused on social values and policies to effect change	Consultant viewed as advocate, activist, mediator, interventionist	Group conflict, community crisis, lack of power to implement social change	Invited or opportunistic, with or without sanction (indefinite term)
Systems Model	Focused on mission, goals, values and culture of the system	Consultant viewed as catalyst, planner, facilitator, interventionist	Community crisis from malfunction or maladaption in system	Invited for indefinite or long term

Goals	Diagnosis Responsibility	Diagnostic Techniques	Strategies/ Techniques	Evaluation	Termination
Clinical or Treatment Model 1. Improve understanding and skills 2. Generalize learning to future, similar problems	Consultant	Interview, observation, data analysis	Advising, teaching, skill development, modeling, discussion	Consultant perceptions, reports of client (no formal evaluation)	Resolution of crisis or problem
Collegial or Professional Model 1. Improve understanding and skills to generate creative solutions 2. Generalize learning to future, similar problems	Joint consultant/client	Interview, observation, joint data collection and analysis	Consultant fosters communication through brainstorming, joint development of options, skill development, discussion	Joint Consultant/client assessment	Mutual decision on goal achievement or resolution of problem
Behavioral Model 1. Improve consultee's skills in managing and changing understandable behaviors 2. Generalize learning to future, similar problems	Consultant	Interview and observation, data collection and analysis	Advising, teaching, skill development, modeling, designing behavioral change programs	Consultant-designed empirical studies (pre- and posttest measures)	Behavioral change, resolution of problem
Educational Model 1. Broaden knowledge base 2. Generalize learning to future issues	Consultant and/or consultant and client	Needs assessment and analysis	Instructional material, seminars, role play, lectures, discussion	Informal feedback, pre- and postinstruments, participant assessments	Completion of training, goal achievement
Organizational Development Model 1. Improve structure and function of organization 2. Reallocation of internal resources	Consultant and/or consultant and client	Interview, observation, survey, research data collection and analysis	Skill development in communication techniques, decision making, conflict resolution, power distribution, reward systems	Survey feedback, assessment	Achievement of organizational goals

(continued on next page)

TABLE 2–1 (continued)

Goals	Diagnosis Responsibility	Diagnostic Techniques	Strategies/ Techniques	Evaluation	Termination
Process Management Model 1. Enhance and improve understanding of organizational processes 2. Integrate interpersonal and group skills	Joint consultant and client	Interview, observation, survey research, data analysis	Skill development of groups through communication techniques, role playing, modeling, goal setting, group interaction	Continuous self-evaluation, group feedback, participant assessments and surveys	Achievement of process improvement goals
Program Development Model 1. Broaden or modify client system's programs 2. Improve general effectiveness of future program design	Consultant and client (unless consultant for highly technical program)	Needs assessment, program analysis	Program design, modification, and development	Formal outcome measures and test instruments	Completion of program design and evaluation methodology
Social Action Model 1. Improve skills to organize and develop systemwide social changes 2. Increase consciousness of common community concern	Consultant	Interview, observation, needs assessment and survey research	Skill development of groups and key power individuals with training in organization, strategy development, and self-determination	Informal, continuous self-evaluation of outcome of social change	Achievement of goals, client-attained expertise in organizing and developing power strategies
Systems Model 1. Improve skills to restructure system's ability to adapt to social changes 2. Maximize community resources	Consultant	Interview, observation, needs assessment, interaction with key individuals in system, survey research	Skill development of groups through educational seminars, strategy development and training to strengthen community resources	Formal research methodology, pre-and postintervention tests, continuous self-evaluation of outcome of system adaptations	Achievement of environmental modifications and client skills in adapting system to future changes

find the most appropriate and effective treatment for the client. Therefore, the consultant's activities are centered on the client through a specialized assessment and diagnosis of the client's problem and a judgment regarding the treatment to improve or ameliorate the client's condition.

Program-Centered Administrative Consultation

In this type of consultation, the consultant is requested to help with problems in the administration of programs. The primary focus of the consultant is an assessment of the current program or policy, followed by recommendations for a plan of action to resolve the difficulty. The consultant alone is responsible for the diagnosis of the problems, with little, if any, influence from the consultee.

Consultee-Centered Case Consultation

The precipitating problem in this category is again the specific client/patient case. However, in this instance, the consultant concentrates on the consultee's handling of these problems, rather than directly on the client. Therefore, the primary consultant focus is the consultee's difficulties in addressing the client issues. The goal is to improve the consultee's functions and ability to deal effectively with the client. Diagnosis of the problem is not through an assessment of the client, but rather by the consultee's actions and attitudes. Consultee difficulties may stem from a lack of understanding, skill, objectivity, or confidence and self-esteem.

Consultee-Centered Administrative Consultation

In this consultation category, the focus is again on the consultee, but in relation to consultee problems regarding administration of programs, rather than with specific client/patients. The consultant may work with an individual consultee or with a group of administrators. The primary goal is to help the consultee administrator(s) function more efficiently and effectively by enhancing knowledge, skills, and expertise in program development and administration.[17]

Caplan's impact on the growth and development of consultation in general, and mental health consultation in particular, led to expanded theoretical concepts that may be generalized to levels of consultation. The Caplan model was considered too narrow or conservative in its approach to consultation because it emphasized the sick, either in terms of the patient/client or the malfunctioning professional consultee.[47]

Further Conceptual Development

Cooper expanded Caplan's model to provide greater breadth to a consultative approach in clinical, community, and social systems. Using the theoretical framework of Caplan's typology model, Cooper conceptualized the following levels of consultation intervention focused on attempts at planned change:

- **Level I:** *Case-Centered Consultation,* where help is needed for the client and/or clientele. Derived from a clinical or treatment model.
- **Level II:** *Educational Consultation,* where help is needed by client or client system to enhance knowledge and thereby promote change.
- **Level III:** *Program and/or Administrative Consultation,* where help is needed by a client system to promote institutional/system wide change.

In this typology, Cooper considered three variables:

- The *target* of the attempted change
- The *goal* of the attempted change
- The *means* to achieve change, which depends on the locus of operation.

There also is a parallel between the levels of consultation intervention and the sequence followed in the three stages of prevention programs. Consultation, like prevention, may be considered *proactive.* It frequently takes place before the symptoms or incident develop into chronic illness or maladaptive functioning. Another similiarity between consultation and prevention is that both may empower people and encourage self-responsibility. Frequently, the consultant acts in a preventive capacity to promote the "health" of the client (the individual, an organization, or an entire system) rather than just remediating or ameliorating a situation. This function differs from that of the clinical therapist involved in treatment, which often is described as the *reactive* level. Treatment also places the individual in the role of the patient, which may tend to encourage passivity rather than active involvement in developing strategies to change the situation.

Therefore, in addition to the variables described by Cooper, we compare the consultation on the level of its potential for social and health preventive programming. We consider this to be the consultation's ***preventive potential.*** The potential is viewed from a tertiary, secondary, or primary perspective.

Tertiary prevention consists of rehabilitative programs that are aimed at reducing the after effects of the presenting problem or illness. It is more remedial in nature than primary or secondary prevention and is directed toward preventing further problems, loss, or disability through maintenance of function. Tertiary prevention is a component of all treatment and remediating activity.

Secondary prevention consists of early diagnosis, identification, and detection of populations at risk, and development of change strategies, with the intent of preventing the condition from becoming so serious that chronic dysfunction or permanent disability occurs. Secondary prevention programs should include proactive and educational elements that will build skills to prevent further problems.

Primary prevention refers to activities undertaken prior to the onset of the problem. The goal is to avoid the occurrence of malfunction or disability and to build resistance and coping strategies in a population *potentially* at risk. The intent of primary prevention programs is usually to provide long-term impact and major change through ongoing education, consultation, and collaboration. An awareness of the social, political, economic, and cultural influences that affect attitudes and functioning are basic to primary prevention. Onetime presentations or short-term activities are unlikely to be effective at the primary prevention level.[22, 27]

As the ultimate goal of all consultation is the prevention of future problems, the consultant must determine the appropriate level of consultation activities to achieve this purpose. Usually there is sequential movement from these various stages or levels through the different models of consultation. When the focus of the consultation begins to shift, the consultant must maintain awareness of the change and help the client understand when modification and adaptation is necessary.

In addition to the preventive potential of consultation, the consultant must consider the impact the activities will have on the system. Study and analysis of the specific client needs during initial and ongoing interactions will help determine desired outcomes of consultation. This *outcome or impact on the system* varies within the level of consultation. The three levels of consultation presented below are described in relation to the five variables we have just discussed. These are: target, goal, means, preventive potential, and outcome or impact on the system.

LEVELS OF CONSULTATION

Level I: Case-Centered Consultation

This level is targeted to a specific client and/or their clientele, with the focus being case-centered. The primary goal is to produce appropriate behavior or physical change, or psychological well-being in the individual. This level of consultation is derived from a traditional clinical or treatment model and the degree of change is limited to the single client. The strategies or techniques to achieve change usually involve clinical interview and case-centered consultation. The preventive potential is at the tertiary level of change and the impact on the system or outcome of the intervention is a modification of behavior.

Level II: Educational Consultation

This level is targeted on the client who may be a community caretaker, program director, or professional staff, therapist, teacher, manager, or an administrator. The focus is client-centered with the major goal of improving functioning, efficiency, and ability. The strategies or means to achieve the goal are through enhancement of knowledge, skills, and expertise, using an educational approach, which may consist of inservice training, community conferences and seminars. This level of consultation, derived from an educational model, has a secondary level of preventive potential and the outcome is a modification of behavior through skill development.

TABLE 2–2
Levels of Consultation

Level	Target	Goal	Means	Preventive Potential	Outcome or Impact on the System
Level I: case-centered consultation	Specific client or clientele	Behavior or physical change	Client/clientele focused, via clinical interview or case-centered consultation	Tertiary	Modification of behavior
Level II: educational consultation	Community caretaker, program director, or professional	Enhanced functional efficiency	Educational consultation through skill development	Secondary	Modification of behavior
Level III: program and/or administrative consultation	Overall system	Produce institutional change	Administrative and/or program consultation	Primary	Transformation and social system change

Adapted from Nagler and Cooper in Cooke, 1970.[47]

Level III: Program and/or Administrative Consultation

This level is targeted on the specific social system which may include the schools, churches, police, social agencies, corporations, or health facilities. The focus of the consultation is centered on that paticular system, with a major goal of promoting institutional change. This level of consultation is derived from several models, including systems, program development, and organizational development. The strategies or techniques at this level include program planning, enhancing management skills, and administrative consultation. The preventive potential is at the primary level of change and the outcome of the intervention is a transformation and change in the system.

Table 2–2 compares the levels of consultation described above. Consultation may progress through several levels, during which the model may also change. There is a direct relationship between the theoretical models and the levels of consultation. Figure 2–1 illustrates the different levels at which the various models may occur.

FIGURE 2–1

The interrelationship between models and levels.

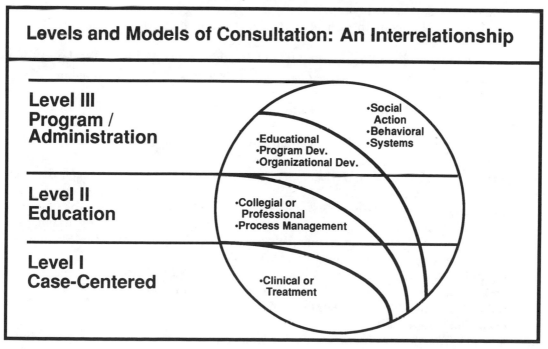

Levels and Models of Consultation: An Interrelationship

Level III
Program /
Administration

•Educational
•Program Dev.
•Organizational Dev.

•Social
Action
•Behavioral
•Systems

Level II
Education

•Collegial or
Professional
•Process Management

Level I
Case-Centered

•Clinical or
Treatment

SUMMARY

"Help is never really help unless it is perceived as "helpful" by the person on the receiving end . . ."—*Richard Beckhard*[8]

The theoretical constructs of consultation, as presented in this chapter, provide some of the basic information you need when considering a consultation practice. Study of various theoretical consultation models and levels will help you assess given situations and determine the appropriate approaches you need. As a consultant, it is essential to understand developmental shifts and stages of consultation and choose the model or combination of models most appropriate to the situation. Keys to successful consultation include the ability to diagnose situations accurately and to develop, organize, and help implement strategies for change. The structure suggested in this chapter provides a framework both for the potential consultant and client. Chapters 3 through 6 provide additional background information as precursors to the establishment of a consultation practice.

REFERENCES

1. Abramovitz AB: Methods and techniques of consultation. *Am J Orthopsychiatry* 1958; 28:126–133.
2. Alinsky S: *Reveille for Radicals*. New York, Vintage Books, 1969.
3. *American College Dictionary* New York, Harper, 1950.
4. Anderson SB, Ball S: *The Profession and Practice of Program Evaluation*. San Francisco, Jossey-Bass, 1978.
5. Argyris C: Explorations in Consulting-Client Relationships. *Hum Org* 1961; 20:121–133.
6. Argyris C: *Intervention Theory and Method*. Reading, Mass, Addison-Wesley, 1970.
7. Beckhard R: *Organization Development: Strategies and Models*. Reading, Mass, Addison-Wesley, 1969.
8. Beckhard R: *The Leader Looks at the Consultative Process*. Wash. DC, Leadership Resources, 1971.
9. Benne K: Some ethical problems in group and organizational consultation. *J Soc Issues* 1969; 15:60–68.
10. Bennis WG: *Organizational Development: Its Native Origins and Prospects*. Reading, Mass, Addison-Wesley, 1969.
11. Bennis WG: *Changing Organizations*. New York, McGraw-Hill, 1969.
12. Bennis W, Schein E: Principles and strategies in the use of laboratory training for improving social systems, in Bennis, W, Benne, W, Chin, R (eds): *The Planning of Change*. New York, Holt, Rinehart and Winston, 1969, pp 335–357.
13. Bergan JR: *Behavioral Consultation*. Columbus, Ohio, Merrill, 1977.
14. Block P: *Flawless Consulting*. Austin, Tex, Learning Concepts, 1981.
15. Bradford LP, Gibb JR, Benne KD (eds): *T-Group Theory and Laboratory Method*. New York, Wiley, 1964.
16. Caplan G: *The Theory and Practice of Mental Health Consultation*. New York, Basic Books, 1970.

17. Caplan G: Types of mental health consultation, in Cook PE (ed): *Community Psychology and Community Mental Health*. San Francisco, Holden-Day, 1970.
18. Chin R, Benne KD: General strategies for effecting change in human systems, in Bennis W, Benne W, Chin, R (eds): *The Planning of Change*. New York, Holt, Rinehart and Winston, 1969.
19. Cooper S, Rhodes W: Consultation course, Guest faculty, Ann Arbor, Mich, July 1972.
20. Coser L: *The Functions of Social Conflict*. New York, Free Press, 1956.
21. Dunn W: Models of occupational therapy service provision in the school system *Am J Occup Ther* 1988; 42:718.
22. Epstein CF: Consultation: Communicating and facilitating, in Bair, J, Gray, M (eds): *The Occupational Therapy Manager*. Rockville, Md, 1985.
23. Gagne RM, Briggs LJ: *Principles of Instructional Design*. New York, Holt, Rinehart and Winston, 1974.
24. Gallessich J: *The Profession and Practice of Consultation*. San Francisco, Jossey-Bass, 1982.
25. Heller K, Monahan J: *Psychology and Community Change*. Homewood, Ill, Dorsey Press, 1977.
26. Idol L, Paolucci-Whitcomb P, Nevin A: *Collaborative Consultation*. Austin, Tex, Pro-Ed, 1986.
27. Jaffe E: The role of the occupational therapist as a community consultant: Primary prevention in mental health programming. *Occup Ther Ment Health* 1980; 1:47–62.
28. Jaffe E: The occupational therapist as a consultant: A model of community consultation, in Cromwell FS, Broiller C (eds): *The Occupational Therapy Manager's Survival Handbook*. New York, Haworth Press, 1988.
29. Jonas MR: Asking for advice *US Air*, XI:18, 1989.
30. Katz D, Kahn RL: *The Social Psychology of Organizations*. New York, Wiley, 1978.
31. Keller HR: Behavioral consultation, in Conoley JC (ed): *Consultation in Schools: Theory, Research, Procedures*. New York, Academic Press, 1981.
32. Kelly JG: Ecological constraints on mental health services, in Cook PE (ed): *Community Psychology and Community Mental Health*. San Francisco, Holden-Day, 1970.
33. Lawrence PR, Lorsch JW: *Developing Organizations: Diagnosis and Action*. Reading, MA, Addison-Wesley, 1969.
34. Lawrence PR, Lorsch JW: *Organization and Environment*. Homewood, Ill, Irwin, 1967.
35. Leopold RL: Consultant and consultee: An extraordinary human relationship, some thoughts for the occupation therapist. *Am J Occup Ther* 1968;22:72.
36. Lewin K: *Field Theory in Social Science*. New York, Harper & Row, 1951.
37. Likert K: *The Human Organization: Its Management and Value*. New York, McGraw-Hill, 1967.
38. Lippitt G, Lippitt R: *The Consulting Process in Action* 2nd ed. San Diego, Univ Assoc, 1986.
39. Lippitt R: Dimensions of a consultant's job. *J Soc Issues* 1959; 15:5–12.
40. Lippitt R, Watson J, Westley B: *The Dynamics of Planned Change*. New York: Harcourt Brace and World, 1958.
41. McGehee W, Thayer PW: *Training in Business and Industry*. New York, Wiley, 1961.
42. Mann FC: Changing superior-subordinate relationships. *J Soc Issues* 1951; 7:56–63.
43. Mann FC: Studying and creating change: A means to understanding social organization. *Res Ind Hum Rel* 1957; 17:146–167.

44. Mann P: *Community Psychology: Concepts and Applications*. New York, Free Press, 1978.
45. Matuzek P: Program evalution as consultation, in Conoley JC (ed): *Consultation in Schools: Theory, Research, Procedures*. New York, Academic Press, 1981.
46. Nadler DA: *Feedback and Organization Development: Using Data-Based Methods*. Reading, Mass, Addison-Wesley, 1977.
47. Nagler S, Cooper S: Influencing social change in community mental health, in Cook PE (ed): *Community Psychology and Community Mental Health*. San Francisco, Holden-Day, 1970.
48. Perloff R, Perloff E, Sussna E: Program evaluation. *Annu Rev Psychol* 1976; 27:569–594.
49. Rhodes W: Conceptual overview of behavioral consultation. Consultation course, Guest faculty, Ann Arbor, Mich, August 1971.
50. Rogawski AS: New directions for mental health services: Mental health consultations in community settings, no 3. San Francisco, Jossey-Bass, 1978.
51. Russell ML: Behav Consultation, Personnel and Guidance 1978; 56:346–350.
52. Schein EH: *Process Consultation: Its Role in Organization Development*. Reading, Mass, Addison-Wesley, 1969.
53. Sherwood JJ: Essential differences between traditional approaches to consulting and a collaborative approach, in Lee RJ, Freedman AM (eds): *Consultation Skills, Reading*. Arlington, VA, NTL Institute, 1984.
54. Steinberg D: *Interprofessional Consultation*. Chicago, Mosby Year Book Medical Publishers, 1989.
55. Tharp RG, Wetzel, RJ: *Behavior Modification in the Natural Environment*. New York, Academic Press, 1969.
56. Thorndike F: Animal intelligence, in Gallessich, J (ed): *The Profession and Practice of Consultation*. San Francisco: Jossey-Bass, 1982.
57. Townsend R: *Up the Organization*. New York, Alfred A. Knopf, 1970.
58. von Bertalanffy L: *General System Theory*. New York, Braziller, 1968.
59. Vogel G, Johny A: Consulting focus: Process management. *Nurs Admin Q* 1986; 10:69–76.
60. Walton RE: Two strategies of social change and their dilemmas. *J Appl Behav Sci* 1965; 1:167–179.
61. Walton RE: *Interpersonal Peacemaking: Confrontations and Third Party Consultation*. Reading, Mass, Addison-Wesley, 1969.
62. *Webster's Ninth Collegiate Dictionary:* Cambridge, MA, Merriam-Webster Publishers, 1983.

CHAPTER 3

Related Theories: Challenges of the 1990s

Evelyn G. Jaffe, M.P.H., O.T.R., F.A.O.T.A.

Those who cannot remember the past are condemned to repeat it;
Those who do not study the future are condemned to be unprepared for
it.—*(source unknown)*

As we discussed in Chapter 2, a study of the theoretical constructs and models of consultation are essential to the development of the knowledge and skills necessary for successful consultation. Additionally, there are associated concepts that have a direct bearing on the process and practice of consultation. This chapter presents several theories related to basic concepts of consultation that provide additional background information for the potential consultant.

Included in this chapter is a discussion of the process of change, systems theory and the open system approach, environmental and system analysis, the importance of the study of trends, and the significance of forecasting and strategic planning to address the influences and impact of environmental changes and trends. Although described in separate sections in this chapter for the purpose of clarity, all of these concepts are interrelated. We discuss these concepts in relation to their impact on organizational systems and the community.

An *organization* is used to describe any of the social systems having a somewhat defined and specialized function that comprise a community. The organization is made up of a group of people with a relatively systematic relationship and coordinated by an administrative or leadership structure. There are inherent internal interactions among the subparts or various departments of an organization, as well as external relationships of the organizational system with its environment. The *community,* whether a specific community or a larger structure such as state government, is considered a dynamic social system, composed of many subparts or subsystems within which there is continuous interaction. The various systems of a community may include hospital facilities, social agencies, educational institutions, government bureaus, community service agencies, consumer organizations, and business organizations. The internal processes of all organizations are affected by external forces that challenge the system to change its structure.[57]

We should think of change itself as a *process* that has a direct bearing on the general system (*the community*) and the subsystem (the *organizations* within the community). The external driving or causal forces of change in the environment are multifaceted, having greater or lesser impact at different moments in society. A study of these factors helps determine an organization's ability to forecast and plan for the changes occurring in the social system. Additionally, all these forces have a direct influence on the development of an organization's strategic vision, the first phase in the consideration of strategic planning.[5, 6, 13, 14]

As consultants develop their practice, which may include many of the models described in Chapter 2, it is important to be cognizant of these multifaceted forces of change in the environment and their effects on systems that are open to all these influences. Particularly in consultations involving educational components, organizational and program development, advocacy, and a systems approach, the consultant should be able to help the consultee identify environmental influences and manage the related issues for effective implementation of new or modified programs and/or organizational restructuring.[14, 32]

CHANGE PROCESS

The pace of events is so fast that unless we can find some way to keep our sights on tomorrow we cannot expect to be in touch with today.—
Dean Rusk

Change and the process and rapidity of change in this century have been the focus of study by many social scientists and humanists.[8, 51, 55, 58] Since the 1950s, there has been a proliferation of scientific and popular writings on this subject. Several theoretical constructs of change have been expounded. Some of the popular proponents of change theory were Bennis, Benne, Chin, Hoffler, and Lippitt in the 1950s and 1960s; Argyris and Toffler in the 1970s; and Drucker, Naisbitt, Peters and Waterman, and Ferguson in the 1980s.* Regardless of the author, it is obvious that the imperative to adapt in this era of rapid acceleration has occupied considerable thinking in recent years.

Change in one's personal life and in society often is cause for feelings of discomfort and even foreboding. Most people do not like experiencing something new and different. Dostoyevsky wrote, "Taking a new step, uttering a new work is what people fear most."[31] Hoffler describes feelings of great uneasiness when people experience drastic changes. These stirrings of emotion often erupt into "an orgy of action." A population that undergoes drastic change must find opportuni-

---

* References 2, 4, 5, 6, 13, 16, 19, 31, 57, 63, 65, and 73.

ties for individual action and self-advancement. When these opportunities are not available, or denied, people may resort to unbalanced and perhaps explosive forms of behavior, or may reach out to fanaticism and defiant actions. Hoffler feels that drastic change sets the stage for revolution, generated by the difficulties and frustrations inherent in the attempt to address radical changes.[31]

Reactions to Change

Scientists have described the relationship of changes in the environment to physical and emotional health. Studies by many social scientists reveal that the health of individuals is intimately bound up with the adaptive demands placed on them by the environment and rate of life changes.[73] Hinkle termed this theory *human ecology* and wrote extensively about the importance of environmental factors in medicine.[30]

Adaptation

Adaptation is considered the organized process of modification, accommodation, and integration of new information. The adaptive reaction, also referred to as stress, can be triggered by shifts and changes in the psychological and/or physical climate and even by anticipation of change. Selyle has stated that no one can live without experiencing some degree of stress.[70] This stress occurs when our environment is altered in some way. When the environment is altered, the routine repetitive patterns of signals that are normally transmitted through the sensory channels to the nervous system are interrupted and responses are modified. This change in stimuli triggers what has been termed an *orientation response,* or OR and involves complex bodily responses.[73] This OR is humans' key adaptive mechanism and occurs when new information or a novel event has not yet been processed, filed, or reconciled by the body. The OR provides the quick spurt of energy to ready the body for action. When the body is in a situation in which the pressure is sustained, requiring a complex set of physical and psychological reactions, the *adaptive reaction* is activated. These two processes form the basis for humans' adaptability and functioning in a changed environment.

Levi demonstrated that even small changes in the emotional climate or interpersonal relationships can produce marked changes in body chemistry.[54] Dubos found that stimulation of the entire endocrine system can be effected by such circumstances as competition or functioning in a crowded environment.[18] Overstimulation, as a result of rapid and irregular changes in the environment, can interfere with humans' rational behavioral responses and produce maladaptive behavior and even dysfunction. This overstimulation occurs on three levels: *sensory, cognitive,* and *decisional.*[73]

- Disorganized, patternless, or chaotic stimuli can cause sensory overload.
- Cognitive distortions or interference with the ability to think can occur when there is too much new or distressing information to process.

- Decision stress may occur when the newness of the circumstances requires changes in the nature of decisions to be made and crises demand rapid responses.

The sudden injection of change into the environment can upset the delicate balance of programmed (routine) and nonprogrammed (creative) decisions. The individual's balance, which allows and fosters creative pursuits, has been upset. Therefore, individuals may react with maladaptive behavior, gravitate toward fusion with a group for united action or collective undertakings that provide identification and a measure of security, pull inward and resist the change by refusing to acknowledge the need to adapt, or respond with rational, internal adjustments and the learning of new strategies to cope with changes. Rational behavior includes an intricate combination or routinization and creativity. It is essential to program behavior with routine activities to free creative energies for dealing with new and baffling problems appropriately.[26] "Change is not merely necessary to life; it is life." . . . and "by the same token, life is adaptation."[70]

The Process of Change in Society

Change is the process of responding to a variety of forces in the environment. No society in history has experienced such tumultuous effects wrought by the rapidity of social change as in the 20th century. The rapid rate of change and the nature of the forces involved have brought a new society into being. The influences of social change, particularly those of the last 20 years, have resulted in new class alignments, new ethnic, sexual, and generational struggles, new media power, new values, new technologies and economic climates, and, of specific interest to health professionals, new policies in the health arena.

Change is also the process by which the future can invade our lives.[73] Until the 20th century, the pace of change allowed people the opportunity to incorporate change while feeling a sense of stability. But during this century, the scope, the scale, and, above all, the current rate of change have been accelerated to keep up with the rapidity of the directions in which our society is changing. Social change before the 1900s was so slow that it almost could pass unnoticed in a person's lifetime. It was possible for the individual and society to make the transition to change gradually. New ideas and methods could replace formerly held concepts and practices within the slow process of evolution.[20, 38, 39, 71]

Today, the demand to act is often presented to us before we have had sufficient time to understand and assimilate the meaning and significance behind the demanded actions. We are presented with a need and the pressure to respond to that need without the necessary time to reflect on the knowledge and skills required to respond effectively. Reality is continually outdistancing the preparation essential to respond to it. Societal change has developed a visibility and an imperative that former generations did not have to address. Man has a limited biological capacity for change. "When this capacity is overwhelmed, the capacity is in future shock."[p. 342 in 73] Toffler's warning over a decade ago has even greater significance today. He stated that it is no longer possible to ignore the "roaring current of change, a current so powerful that it overturns institutions, shifts our values, and shrivels our roots."[38, 39, 73 (p. 1)]

The responsibility, challenge, and need for individuals and organizations to make changes in the focus and direction of their activities has been discussed extensively in recent years by many social scientists.[32] Ferguson dramatically describes the current "Aquarian conspiracy," the leaderless, loose network of innovators: individuals committed to examining old assumptions, articulating new options, and postulating new paradigms. These individuals provide the direction for new challenges, a chance for renewal, and the vision for the future.[19] Although these conspirators may create stress by their revolutionary thoughts, this type of stress is thought to allow transformations in society that can "thrust us into a new, higher order." Prigogine feels, as does Hoffler, that crises create a natural response of evolution, perhaps even revolution, innovation, and transformation.[19, 66]

However, new paradigms are not embraced easily. History has ample examples of how new concepts are viewed with skepticism at best, but most often with hostility or rejection, and invariably resisted (e.g., Copernicus, Galileo, Darwin, and Semmilweiss). The tried and familiar views are more comfortable than new perspectives or paradigm shifts.[19, 50] As changes in society accelerate, we can either fall prey to the upheaval from collapsing institutions and former methods of doing things, or attempt to understand the forces of change. "The current disequilibrium (personal and social) foreshadows a new kind of society. Roles, relationships, institutions, and old ideas are being reexamined, reformulated, redesigned."[p 27, 19] It is possible that this turmoil in society can lead to an expanded consciousness, providing opportunities and new frontiers. For this positive transformation to occur, personal and institutional fear and denial must be considered and overcome. Toffler states that the prevention of future shock demands transitional models, or "change-regulators" to act as buffers and balance wheels by which societal acceleration can be harnessed or channeled.[73] Organizations in general, and health systems in particular, therefore, must be cognizant of the effects and prepare their members for the transformations that will occur. By reexamining priorities, reconceptualizing roles in the health care system, developing new techniques for managing health services, and certainly addressing biotechnical advances, it will be possible to make the necessary transformations.

Barriers to Change

> Let man proclaim a new principle. Public sentiment will surely be on the other side.—*Thomas Reed*

Regardless of the situation, change is apt to create resistance that causes individuals and organizations to set up barriers. The thought of making changes, no matter how positive or rational, often evokes feelings of fear, uncertainty, and even resistance.[38] In the early 1970s we were warned that change processes at best are not pleasant, but in times of a rapidly accelerating society, change can produce shattering stress and disorientation.[73] Robert F. Kennedy often propounded the need for progress in our social institutions. However, he also was aware of its pitfalls. He stated, "Progress is a nice word, but change is its motivator and change has its enemies."[64] This enemy may bring about feelings of loss of control, pain, and helplessness. The anxiety created by the threat of change is most acute before the change actually occurs, when it is still a threat.[43]

Kotter and Schlesinger[49] suggest that the four most common reasons people resist change are the following:

1. A desire to prevent losing something deemed of value
2. A misunderstanding of the meaning of the change and its implications
3. A belief that the change is not appropriate
4. A personal frustration with and low tolerance for any changes

A perceived change in values is often the most upsetting reason why people resist change. This strikes at the fundamental core of one's feelings and raison d'être. When values are threatened by the possibility or reality of change, people may react negatively out of what they feel is a violation of the basic principles on which their actions are founded. In the health professions, models of practice have changed considerably during the last decade from the traditional medical approach to treatment to a broader scope of services, not part of former educational theory or practical experiences. A more wholistic approach to health care has created new roles of health promotion and wellness that pose not only a threat, but are regarded by some as foreign to their concept of their profession and therefore to be rejected. These changes in practice have engendered feelings of fear by some professionals that a new or different system of health care delivery could create completely different patterns of services and that basic values of health care have been threatened.[32, 38, 39, 41, 42]

Misunderstanding the implications of new models of services also can create barriers to acceptance. A communication gap between the individuals who act as change agents and those affected by the change is the most frequent cause of misunderstandings. For example, when health professionals are not aware of current changes in practice as a result of new technologies, or have not read recent studies that might lead to new directions and theories of practice, resistance can occur.

A belief that the change will not provide any advantage or might actually cost more than would be gained is another major obstacle to acceptance of change. For example, recent legislation to address issues of employment for disabled individuals or educational opportunities for all children has increased possibilities of liability, greater capital investment for advanced technological equipment, and more staff. Required changes in worksites or school systems have caused some employers to resist conforming out of their belief that the changes are not cost effective.

A lack of tolerance for the process of change may create fear of a lack of skills and anxiety over the ability to cope with these new demands. Even though there may be an intellectual understanding of the need to change modes of operation, some people are unable emotionally to make the transition.[38, 39, 49]

In addition, there are other conditions that create resistance and provide a barrier to accepting change which include the following:[69]

- *Lack of clarity about the nature of change:* When the change agent, consultant, or other individuals proposing the change do not present the new concepts or modification of programs clearly and logically, in a way that those who will be affected can understand, resistance to the ideas often occurs.
- *Not knowing who will be affected by the change:* Frequently, changes are proposed by top management and staff hears rumors before actually receiving formal notification or opportunities to participate in the decision making. When this occurs, those not involved in the change decisions have concerns (both legitimate and perhaps unfounded) about how and if the changes will affect them directly.
- *Assigning different meanings to the change:* Some people regard change as an indication that they are doing a good job; others fear that their job will be abolished. Without complete understanding of the nature of the change, many misconceptions and conflicting ideas can occur.
- *Being caught between two strong forces:* Again, lack of clarity or understanding the rationale for the change provides the climate for rumors and manipulation. Administrative changes present a strong force from the top; peer resistance or banding together against management allows a pull from another, equally and sometimes more powerful force.
- *Feeling forced to make the change:* When authoritative pronouncements are made, again without an opportunity to participate in the change decisions, staff or lower level management may feel coerced into making changes they do not understand or do not want, and resist just because they feel the ideas are dictates being forced on them.
- *Perceiving that the change was made on personal grounds rather than on impersonal requirements:* Misunderstanding the rationale for change may cause others to personalize the change, thinking they either caused the changes to occur because of something they did or did not do, or because their manager has a personal vendetta against them.
- *Introducing a change that ignores established institutions:* When changes are proposed or implemented that do not take into account the organizational values, attitudes, and procedures that have evolved over the years and have long been regarded as sacred rituals (the "corporate culture"), there is apt to be great anxiety and resistance. This is a particular problem for a new executive officer or external consultant.[15] Individuals, or groups, may react to change by exhibiting certain types of behavior. Resistance may take the form of hostile or aggressive behavior, often directed against the change itself or the person deemed the change agent. Some individuals may exhibit a more passive-aggressive stance with obsequious, fawning submissiveness, or even

by performing poorly through sloppy efforts. Some may actually become apathetic, discouraged, or depressed to the point that their personal and professional aspirations are lowered and they operate inefficiently. Certain individuals may need the support of others and band together with equally unhappy people, forming demoralized cliques.[69]

Coping with Resistance to Change

One of the most common problems of consultation is handling resistance to new ideas and proposed organizational or procedural changes. At times, resistance will occur even when these proposed changes are presented with clarity, logic, and a full rationale for the need for change. As discussed earlier, most people react to change with anxiety, discomfort, and even active resistance. The consultant, whether an individual hired from within an organization (an internal consultant) or a consultant outside of the system (an external consultant), frequently has to develop methods to deal with resistance to these changes. Management leaders also must handle employee resistance to changes that definitely will be, or already have been, implemented. Often, the consultant can help suggest the most appropriate technique to address resistance. The following methods have been used to cope with resistance, many of which will be useful for consultants to consider[7, 28, 49, 63, 73]:

- Identification and awareness
- Education and communication
- Participation and involvement
- Facilitation and support
- Negotiation and agreement
- Manipulation and cooption
- Explicit and implicit coercion

Identification and awareness of negative reactions to change are crucial factors in coping with and managing change. It is important for the consultant to understand and to help management leaders realize that resistance is a natural reaction when someone is faced with new concepts that challenge or change formerly held ideas and procedures. The consultant also should anticipate an occasional rebuff and not take it as a personal attack or a reflection of incompetency.

Education and increased communication will clarify the need for changes and help prevent gaps and misunderstandings. Clearly communicating the objectives that the anticipated change will accomplish and the specific changes necessary are particularly important for people who resist change because of inadequate or inaccurate information. Education regarding the specific forces of change and how the change will occur should ideally take place before the change takes place. "The most reliable way to anticipate the future is by understanding the present."[63, p2] When there is a perceived need for change from within the organization, education and communication efforts are most effective to prevent staff resistance.

Resistance to new ideas is considerably lessened when people are part of the decision-making process. This involvement is what Naisbitt calls "participatory democracy."[63] Requesting support for the new ideas through active participation and involvement frequently leads to prior commitment, thereby increasing accountability and the feeling of shared responsibility and credit.

Supportive techniques may be necessary to deal with the fear and anxiety that usually accompany change and cause resistance to change. These techniques may include emotional support as well as specific skill building. As mentioned earlier, these are the change-regulators Toffler described.[73] Innovative programs may fail because individuals get caught up in the accelerative thrust of change without careful consideration of the need to move slowly with transitional activities that act as buffers to channel the effects of change. Consultants can help decrease the obstacles to change by lending continued support, allowing the client to express the resistance directly, and providing understanding of the impact of the new ideas and policies.[39]

Negotiation is another effective way to deal with resistance when one party stands to lose something as a result of a change in procedure or policy. By presenting alternatives and focusing on options or substitutes for previous policies, the individuals affected may be willing to agree to the changes.

The least desired techniques for a consultant are the last two on the list. When manipulation techniques and cooption are employed, there may be an increase in resistance, often accompanied by overt negative behavior. Obviously, explicit and implicit coercion are the most direct and, perhaps, powerful means of addressing resistance to change. However, in some cases, these two methods have been used successfully by organizations for immediate effect. Certainly, in authoritarian or totalitarian societies, these methods are used most often. However, in democratic societies, it would appear that use of these techniques for long-term effectiveness is doubtful.

The preceding techniques to cope with resistance should be assessed for their appropriateness to the situation, the speed of the effort required, the amount of preplanning, and the cost-benefit ratio. It is essential for the consultant to plan ahead and prepare for all contingencies as much as possible.

Strategies for Implementing Change

As a result of the many changes occurring in our society, organizations will certainly have to alter their process, procedures, and even their overall objectives. As we have seen, change creates stress, often resistance, and even hostility. To implement changes that will create a more efficient operation, produce effective outcomes, and reduce resistance, organizations must develop strategies that are internally consistent with the situation. Frequently, organizations will request objective consultative help to assess the situation and develop a process to implement changes.

The use of a problem-solving approach should improve the chance of success in organizational change efforts. Some strategies for implementing change include the following steps[40, 41, 42, 43, 49, 69]

- An organizational analysis should be conducted to identify the current situation, the real problems, and the forces and issues causing the problems. Included in this analysis should be identification of the need for change and the kind of changes appropriate to the situation.
- Further analysis should be conducted regarding the factors relevant to producing the desired change. Questions such as who might resist the change, who has information that can be used to design the change, and whose cooperation is essential to enlist to implement the change should be included in this fact-finding analysis.
- Selection of change tactics should be based on the analyses just described. The effort must be internally consistent with the situation. A clear plan should be developed with a list of sequential steps that include the amount of preplanning required, the degree of involvement of others, the time frame required to institute the change, identification of targeted groups or individuals, and selection of specific tactics.
- Presentation of the proposed changes to the targeted population follows. When the targeted group has been an active contributor to the development of the plan, change may be viewed by them as an exciting opportunity for innovative approaches to new services and programs.
- Careful monitoring of the implementation process, evaluation of the effectiveness of the strategies, and revisions when necessary are, finally, the key to any successful change effort.

As we have seen, these concepts are very similar to the strategies and techniques of the consultation models we discussed in Chapter 2.

OPEN SYSTEM THEORY

Man shapes himself through decisions that shape his environment.—
René Dubos

The profound changes that have occurred in this century have had a significant impact on all systems, both human and natural. Our environment and social structure have been shaped by all these forces as they interact with systems. The notion that none of these forces can be studied or understood in isolation, nor considered as single causal factors but rather as part of many variables that influence the system, formed the basis for von Bertalanffy's general system theory and open system approach.[75] As described briefly in Chapter 2, open system theory had its roots in the scientific attempts to understand biological phenomena and the interrelationship between all elements in living matter. Von Bertalanffy, in 1947, proposed a model that would embrace all levels of science, from the study of a single cell to that of a society. He referred to this model as "general system theory."[75]

In his early student years in the 1920s, von Bertalanffy was concerned with the life sciences and the systems of biological organisms. He formulated basic concepts on the laws of biological systems. Complex biological phenomena were explained, not only in terms of their components or the sum of their properties, but also in regard to the entire set of relations between the components.

From the initial application of his theories to "organismic biology," later studies of social organizations led to his consideration of general systems theory for interdisciplinary applications. During the 1960s, von Bertalanffy postulated that the general system approach was founded in the openness of all systems to environmental influences and had applicability to all organizations. All of nature, including human behavior, is interconnected. Therefore, according to this theory, nothing can be understood in isolation, but must be viewed as a part of a system. Each variable in any system interacts with the other variables, so that cause and effect cannot be separated.[75]

Social psychologists, economists, sociologists, and others concerned with the problems of social organizations and social structure embraced these concepts. A growing movement among social and behavioral scientists developed, referred to as the "systems movement," "systems approach," or "systems research." Laszlo, a disciple of Von Bertalanffy, called this a "new paradigm of contemporary scientific thought,"[52] thereby broadening the concept from a theory to something far wider in nature and scope, a paradigm, as described by Kuhn.[50]

General systems theory led the way for increased interdisciplinary research and the application of humanistic approaches to systems concepts. During the late 1960s and early 1970s, a growing consensus among systems theorists developed to address social problems, the solutions of which were considered to be based on models of humans, nature, and society.[44, 56, 57, 68] Contemporary systems research was translated into the practical application of operational programs to address concrete societal problems.[52]

General systems theory was refined and modified further by the open-system theory, defined as "a system in exchange of matter with its environment."[75] As social scientists studied human behavior in organizations and institutions, there was greater awareness of the need to deal with social-structural problems. The traditional approaches of social psychologists to consider individual cognitive processes (such as attitude change, cognitive dissonance, and causal attribution), personality development and socialization, and interpersonal and intragroup processes expanded to acknowledge the importance of social structure. The late 1960s saw an upsurge of studies in many disciplines, including sociology, psychology, economics, ecology, health care, and industrial psychology, addressing the impact of environmental forces, relationships with other systems, and the effects of organizations on individuals and members of society. Research, which started by studying behavior of individuals in organizational settings, expanded to include the effects of the organization or system in shaping that behavior.[44]

Open system theory is a comprehensive approach to the study of every facet of organizational life and the interactions of the system with its environment. It emphasizes the *character* of a system, including the dynamic events and predictable cycles that occur in organizations (e.g., budgeting, hiring, evaluation, termination), and its *openness* to environmental influences.[23, 44] Specific constructs of this theory, as identified by Katz and Kahn,[44] include the following:

- *The close relationship between a structure and its supporting environment:* Most social systems rely on human effort and motivation to sustain and maintain the system. The concept of *entropy,* or the measure of the capacity of a system to undergo spontaneous change, must be considered as the sources of the maintenance of the system are studied.

- *The ability to survive interruptions in the sources of support and maintenance:* Many organizations go into bankruptcy or out of existence because they have not been able to replenish or store their basic resources, or "sources of energy." The open system approach emphasizes the need for social organizations to improve their survival capabilities by acquiring a margin of reserves.

- *The cycle of input, throughput, and output:* Another consideration is the identification of environmental influences, or *input,* on the activities of the organization; the subsequent processing of these influences, or *throughput,* and the final product or services, considered *output,* of the system.

- *The critical nature of negative feedback:* Information inputs, or feedback, provide signals to the system, both in regard to the character of the external environments and to the functioning of the system in relation to the environment. The system then processes, or codes the information. Not all information can be coded or processed. The system makes selective choices about what information is accepted, rejected, or processed depending on the specific nature of the functions of that system. Often, negative feedback provides the greatest information by which a system can correct problems or malfunctioning to put the system back on course. Miller states that a system's negative feedback is crucial to its existence. If this feedback is discontinued, the steady state of the system may vanish and its boundaries may disappear, thus causing the system to terminate.[61]

- *The interaction of the organization with the field of forces in the environment:* Continual study and monitoring of the many divergent forces in the external environment are an inherent part of open system theory. The nature of that environment, its stability, turbulence, degree of change, or structure must be investigated.

- *The characterization of open systems that survive by the condition known as a steady state:* Although the system is exposed to a continual influx of information and influences from the environment, it is able to maintain a *dynamic homeostasis,* or balance of functions, in relation to these impacts. The maintenance of equilibrium, while responding to internal or external factors that might threaten to disrupt the system, is considered the steady state of a system.[9] The system learns to anticipate disturbances, mobilizing strategies to forestall or counteract the effects, thereby restoring or maintaining the system to its basic state. This state is not static, but must be considered in terms of dynamic homeostasis, which is the result of the response to the external stimulation causing a more complex and comprehensive equilibrium.

• *The characteristic of systems to exhibit growth and expansion to survive:* To preserve their basic character, systems often react to changes in the environment through a series of organizational growth. By adapting to or coping with external forces, the system may attempt to control the environment through expansion or incorporation of external resources. The open system regards change as a continual reorganization of the system as a result of the system's responses and actions to the environment. Therefore, the organization may deem it necessary and expedient to grow in size to address changing societal and/or economic needs or to forestall or deal with competition (e.g., corporate takeovers, hospital and health care agencies consolidation, or small business growth as a result of increased demands).

• *The interconnection and interrelationships of subgroups in the system:* The hierarchical relationships of organizations, from top management to the line staff, affect behavior patterns in the systems. Additionally, the interactions within and between subgroups often have a profound effect on the behavior and outcome of the work groups. Therefore, internal analysis of the autonomy and the interdependence of the system parts and levels are an important consideration in understanding the system as a whole.

• *The characterization of open systems by the principle of equifinality:* Von Bertalanffy proposed this principle in 1940 to explain the ability of systems to reach their goals or "final state" from different conditions and a variety of paths.[44] Therefore, systems do not have to maintain the exact same method of operation to achieve their goals. Alternative methods may be employed dependent on the differing conditions.

The open system approach developed during the rapid rate of societal changes that occurred during the middle of the 20th century. These rapid changes required organizations to be cognizant of the effects and impact of the changes on their system. Adaptation resulted in changes in the organizations and formations of new or different relationships to other systems. Openness to the environment, however, must be qualified. Complete openness to all influences could mean the destruction of the inherent properties of the organization. This approach encourages organizations to be selective in the incorporation of external inputs. Analysis of the effects and benefits of elements in the environment could mean the difference between growth and survival and extinction. Increased organizational effectiveness will lead to greater support of environmental change and the ability to incorporate internal system change and develop appropriate programs.

An example of general system theory and the open system approach in occupational therapy may be seen in the work of Kielhofner, Burke, and Igi.[45-48] In the 1980s, Kielhofner and Burke described a conceptual model of human occupation based on general systems theory.[45] This model was proposed to provide the field of occupational therapy with a conceptual foundation on which to develop theory and guide research and practice. Human behavior is considered "occupation," and a basic assumption is made that occupation is a central aspect of the human experience. Within the framework of an open system approach, the human system is represented by "man," and the dynamic interaction of this system with the environment is considered "human occupation." Humans' occupational behavior, including the mental, physical, and social aspects of occupation, is conceptualized as the output of that open system. "Within the model of human occupation, the environment is conceptualized as external objects, people, and events that influence the system's actions" and the "physical, social, and cultural setting in which the system operates."[p 573, 45]

Kielhofner further describes the process of change, or ontogenesis, in the open system according to the model of human occupation. The steps and process of change as the system responds to internal tendencies and the demands of the environment are outlined. Human occupation evolves during the life span from changes that occur in patterns of work and play throughout the developmental stages of life, as a result of the system's occupational choice.[46]

Using the open system approach as the basis for this model, Kielhofner, Burke, and Igi continue discussion of the model of human occupation to develop explanations for adaptive and maladaptive changes in behavior and to illustrate application of this model for the clinical practice of occupational therapy assessment, treatment, and intervention.[47, 48]

The open system approach as just illustrated may be used by practitioners as the framework for developing a professional model that explains changes in human behavior and by organizations to address societal changes. The open system concept provides the potential to investigate the dynamic forces that affect systems and to develop specific, yet flexible, programs or interventions that foster appropriate growth and mechanisms to cope with environmental influences.

ENVIRONMENT AND SYSTEMS ANALYSIS

The most reliable way to anticipate the future is by understanding the present.—*Naisbitt*

The challenge for the future for health professions, and occupational therapy in particular, is to monitor the trends in this tumultuous era of change; anticipate and predict the implications of change in the larger societal context; and to identify, through a systems approach, the significance of these changes for the health professions. We have an obligation to know and understand the circumstances we face in today's environment to develop strategies for the coming days, years, and even decades. Understanding the driving forces that are shaping today's environment and that of tomorrow will help the process of managing change. Key social, economic, political, and technological forces should be analyzed to provide a framework for a systems approach to program planning and interventions.[10, 39]

Our present environment is in a state of continual change and transition. In recent years, in all phases of society, there have been considerable shifts in demographics, economics, geopolitics, ideologies, lifestyles, institutions, markets, and management.[10] During the 1960s and 1970s the world was swirling with changes that had a direct effect on all organizations, institutions, and social systems. These changes altered many traditionally held concepts, including the view of women in the workplace, the hierarchical structure of large organizations, and an autonomous management style,[63] all of which made their way into the health care arena. During this decade and into the 21st century, shifts in demographics, technology, the health care industry, and the new health paradigm, often a result of the many changes that were taking place 20 years ago, will continue to have an impact on present and future health programs.

Demographic Shifts

In the United States, significant demographic shifts have occurred over the past few decades. Of all external changes, demographics are the clearest and most unambiguous. Although demographic shifts may be unpredictable in this era of rapid change, there is usually some lag or lead time before impact. Therefore, they are good predictors of future forces, have the most predictable consequences, and are usually the first environmental factors to be analyzed.[16] Recent demographic shifts include the following:

The Aging of the Postwar Baby Boomers

The baby boom generation, born after World War II, provided a considerable working force during the 1970s. However, American birthrates have been steadily declining since 1965. These baby boomers will soon reach the upper limits of available human resources, and, as we enter the year 2000, we can anticipate a shrinking labor force of under-25-year-old workers.[10] This gap will have a direct effect on the availability of professional health workers.

Another factor of the baby boom generation is that many of the women are better educated than their parents, may go into professions traditionally dominated by men (such as law, surgery, engineering, and corporate management), and have become a vital part of the American working force. These women have fewer children than the previous generation, may delay childbearing until their mid-30s to early 40s, and often return to work quickly.[10] This trend has economic, service, and health implications. The increased proportion of working mothers has intensified the need for day-care services, with a resulting increase in the amount of their salary spent for child care. To offset potential loss of work days due to the need to be at home with children, many large corporations now include child-care services as an employee benefit, often having the child-care facility on site. However, this is a relatively new concept for American businesses. The United States is far behind other industrial nations, including the Scandinavian countries and Japan, which have had both corporation and government child day-care services for many years.

Children of the baby boomers, called the "baby boom echo," are being born to women at a high-risk maternal age. A serious implication of this shift is the increase of babies born to older women and to teenagers, often resulting in low birth weight infants at risk, needing more extensive and expensive health care. Another high-risk factor is the increase in adolescent pregnancy. America has the highest teenage pregnancy rate of these five other industrialized nations: Sweden, France, England, Canada, and the Netherlands.[12] The issue of abortion is mentioned frequently when teen pregnancy is discussed. A recent study by the Alan Guttmacher Institute indicated that black urban unmarried teenagers who had (professionally performed) abortions suffered less stress, were more apt to stay in school, and had greater economic opportunities than peers who became young mothers.[27] However, the indication is that more unwed teenage mothers are keeping their babies. This trend will have a significant impact on immediate use of health care resources, teenage unemployment, and school dropout rates. The long-range impact of increased single parenthood, potential for child abuse, greater economic deprivation, dependence on the welfare system, continued need for expensive health services, potentially higher divorce rates, and possible serial marriages will have a direct effect on social agencies and the health care delivery system.[10, 34, 35–37]

Increases in the Influx of Immigration

The vast flow of immigrants in the growth decades following World War II has had a profound effect on our economic, social, and political systems. More people have emigrated to this country, (over 1.5 million) in recent years than in the peak immigration years of 1906 and 1914.[10] The recent wave of Southeast Asian and Hispanic immigrants have had a significant impact on population shifts. The 1990 U.S. census shows a profound change in the racial makeup of the American population, with a dramatic shift toward minorities in the past decade. Nearly one in every four Americans had African, Asian, Hispanic, or American Indian ancestry. The rate of increase in the minority population was almost twice as fast in the 1980s as in the 1970s, creating a greater population shift than at any time in the 20th century.[3]

This change in population must be considered in studying allocations of resources, resource use (particularly health care), and the potential for the labor force. Minority groups struggling to adapt to a new culture, especially the recent immigrants from Asia and Central America, are under considerable stress. They often take any job they can get, including those that do not require English language skills, and may assume menial jobs other Americans do not want.

However, many cannot find any work, and unemployment, poverty, and chronic illness (both mental and physical) are prevalent among all the minorities. These factors increase the need for adequate health services for this population particularly geared to their cultural or ethnic issues and concerns. Cultural differences should be considered in both the patient population and the worker pool. Employment of minorities in the health care field is an effective use of cultural diversity in health professional workers, who could provide important services to unassimilated, monolingual clients and patients.

The Graying of America

Older people in the United States are healthier, better educated, and more productive than ever before. There has been an unprecedented return of previously retired employees to the work force. Individuals over age 55 represent over 20% of the U.S. population and comprise about one fifth of part-time labor. As health care, scientific advances, and special programs focus on the older population, people are living longer and with a higher quality of life. Consideration of the older population as potential for the human resource pool should not be overlooked.[10]

However, it must also be recognized that as the population of older individuals in our society increases, their accompanying illnesses and injuries will require greater health services and health care workers. When older people are no longer in the work force, their decreased incomes will cause increases in the number of the elderly living below the poverty line, without adequate housing or access to services. The social and economic realities of the graying of America have serious implications for service provision. Private companies are beginning to look at the long-term care benefits that corporations in some other industrialized countries already provide, again including Japan and the Scandinavian countries. Indicators show that there is an increase in U.S. insurance company policies that include long-term care options for corporate employees. Many corporations now offer policies that cover nursing home and home health care for employees and their families. Retirement packages are broader and often are recruitment incentives.[22]

Increased Mobility

Americans are considered the most mobile people in the world because of their frequent changes in residences and work sites. There is still a dominant movement to suburban areas, causing increased commuting and the inherent problems of traffic, time, and stress. However, many cities are involved in urbanization and gentrification projects to boost the urban economies. Corporate workers, choosing to live in the gentrified city projects, displace the lower income population who previously lived in these communities. This trend compounds the problems of the urban poor. Also, there are shifts in populations from east to west and a rapid growth in the south Atlantic and mountain states, in large part linked to changes in economic conditions and opportunities for employment.[10]

These geographic shifts have a direct effect on the number of available health workers in a given area. Rural populations now may have difficulty obtaining adequate health services because of their geographic isolation, the lack or inadequacy of public transportation, and the paucity of services. Trends toward greater population growth in mountain and rural areas increase the possibility of a change of locus for health professional services and the need for more consultative services.

Technology

Advances in technology, particularly in biotechnology, information and communications technology, and use of new materials have caused an unprecedented explosion of radical changes in the past few decades. Never before have new inventions or discoveries changed our lives so quickly and drastically. Technological progress may account for the greatest changes in society by the year 2000, having a greater impact on life in the United States than almost any other factor.[10, 24] This technological revolution is continuing at such a rapid pace that it is difficult, if not impossible, to keep up with the latest advances. The changes occurring in the computer industry, artificial intelligence programs using robots, fiber optics and telecommunication systems, development of new materials to augment or replace natural sources, and the tremendous biotechnical advances that have allowed scientific endeavors envisioned only in science fiction are all mind-boggling. Technological advances are awesome in their power, creating profound changes, with a "promise for tomorrow—(of) even greater change."[10, p 53]

We have seen this awesome power in the weapons of war in the Persian Gulf War, with both the fear of nuclear and chemical warfare, the damage and success of Scud and Patriot missiles, and the speed and accuracy of computer-controlled air and ground weaponry. This power is also demonstrated in the genetic engineering that has allowed scientific altering of plants to be more disease and drought resistant, or the development of monoclonal antibodies to aid in the understanding and treatment of diseased cells, especially in the war on cancer and AIDS. Biotechnology has had a profound impact on the medical and ethical issues of reproduction, including genetic surgery in embryos, in vitro and in vivo fertilization, and prenatal testing for birth defects (amniocentesis, ultrasound). Exciting developments in technologically assisted devices for people with disabilities have provided access to the mainstream of life for many individuals who were previously excluded from the work force or participation in social commerce.[10]

The impact of these technologies on the health care industry is vast. The extraordinary advances in the biomedical sciences, in both basic scientific research and knowledge and in technical equipment have a direct effect on treatment interventions. Not only will there be an increased demand for more efficient, quality health care, but consumer demand for high-tech medical information, techniques, and treatment will increase the cost of health care at a time when there are greater cuts in health dollar program support.

However, these new technologies are expanding the health care job market. For example, individuals with expertise are needed to perform computer analysis for screening and diagnosis, for highly skilled microsurgery, and for specialized research using advanced technology. The implications, especially for the occupational therapy consultant, may be seen in the need for greater expertise in the field of assistive devices for the physically and mentally challenged, ergonomics in industry and the community, and communication assistance for the blind, hearing impaired, and others with communication deficits. The occupational therapy health consultant may provide help and information to other professional colleagues, patients, and families. Consultation expertise in the uses of advanced technological assistive devices and new communication technologies are described in Chapter 15.

Health Care Industry

In the early 1990s, the United States was concerned with the ailing economy. In almost all sectors of the economical world, businesses were in severe trouble: banks were failing; the automobile and airline industries had considerable problems; manufacturing and construction industries laid off more than half a million workers; wholesale and retail sales were down and many businesses filed for bankruptcy.

Yet, in the same period, the health care industry saw remarkable growth. It is clear that health care is big business. It is the third largest industry in the United States, with the cost of medical care rising faster than any other consumer service. As an example, in 1972 national health care costs were $100 billion, in 1984 they rose to almost $400 billion, in 1990 to $600 billion, and estimates are that if this upward spiral continues, by the year 2000 health care will cost over $3 trillion. In 1990 the health care industry made up almost 12% of the Gross National Product (GNP); by the year 2000 it is estimated that it will reach 15% of the nation's GNP.

The demand for professional health workers is unprecedented. The need for health professionals has far outstripped the available supply. It appears that the health care industry will continue to grow in the future. The Bureau of Labor Statistics projects that medicine (health professions) will account for seven of the ten fastest growing occupations through the year 2000. Other predictions estimate that health care employment will grow twice or three times as fast as the population through 1995. Employment of nurses, technicians, home health aides, medical assistants, and physical and occupational therapy personnel will grow between 48% to 81%, as compared to a 32% increase in all other occupations. By the end of this decade, the Department of Labor predicts that at least 12 million Americans will work in health services, even though the general population growth is slowing.[21, 60]

Specifically for occupational therapy personnel, the U.S. Bureau of Labor Statistics predicts a 49% projected job increase during the period from 1988 to 2000.[11] Although new occupational therapy programs have shown an increase every year from 1985, the output of new students will not be enough to keep up with projected demands.

The current shortages of skilled health personnel will become more critical as our aging population lives longer and requires more health care; as the health crisis as a result of AIDS and substance abuse in all stages of population development, from infancy through old age, increases; as technological advances become more and more complex requiring more highly trained specialists; and as the demand by consumers for faster and better quality care expands.

A positive effect of these trends will be that the rising demand and limited supply of health personnel should result in an increase in wages for services that have been traditionally at the lower end of the salary scale. The salary growth of therapists (including physical, occupational, speech, and inhalation therapists) was over 25% higher than the increase of consumer prices between 1985 to 1989.[21] In this decade we may see a trend of career changes or new students choosing the health care professions over the business and computer fields that were so popular in the 1970s and 1980s.

The New Health Paradigm

In the 1970s and 1980s a self-help movement blossomed in all spheres of society, from neighborhood crime watch groups; groups that provided food for the homeless and the elderly; support groups for all kinds of problems, diseases, and substance or human abuse (including child molestation, wife and husband battering); growing parental involvement in school system policies; to organizations that provided home building and small business assistance; and legal aid. One of the most prominent of the self-help activities was in the area of medicine.[63]

The idea that we should be involved in the promotion of a healthy society has gained momentum and increased recognition in the last 15 years. Americans have not always realized that they can exert influence on their own health and that of the nation. In the past decade there has been a greater interest in issues of health than ever before. Three important changes in thinking about health and well-being have occurred:

- The assumption of personal responsibility for our health destinies. A movement away from total reliance on medical institutions to greater awareness of the individual's ability to effect positive changes in personal health.
- The need to make good health available and accessible to all citizens regardless of their socioeconomic status. "Good health must be an equal opportunity, available to all Americans."[72]
- The importance of the concepts of health promotion and disease prevention to cut health care costs and to prevent the premature onset of disease and disability.[29]

The self-help movement has fostered this shift from institutional treatment, where the authority lies with the professional, to the consumer of health services. Naisbitt described three trends in this new health paradigm of personal responsibility to achieve healthier, more productive lives.[63]

- *New habits to achieve personal health.* More Americans are aware of the need for fitness through exercise, good nutritional habits, cessation of smoking, and reduction of job and personal stress than ever before.

- *Self-care for health issues not requiring the use of traditional medical services.* Individuals (laypeople) are making decisions about their own care. Home health care has resulted in a shift from using medical facilities for some simple screening procedures (such as pregnancy tests, blood pressure monitoring, and simple urinalysis) to at-home medical kits.

- *Promotion of health and wellness activities.* The concept of improved quality of life through a wholistic approach to health has gained increased recognition from health professionals and the general public. The notion that the body, mind, and spirit (or emotions) contribute to the existence of a positive state of wellness are basic to this new paradigm. Participation by the individual in the prevention and treatment of disease and disability through healthier lifestyles has become a major force in the last decade. This concept has created tremendous growth in private for-profit and nonprofit organizations including fitness centers, weight control organizations, hospice support services, alternative birth centers, smoking cessation programs, and 12-step recovery groups for every thing from drug and substance abuse to gambling and over-spending.[63]

Treatment approaches must adapt to this new paradigm and to the consumer's demand for involvement in health care decisions. Consumer advocacy and involvement has become an influential force affecting service providers and patterns of intervention. The increase in health education in schools, the media, community programs, and corporate health programs has brought a new awareness to the consumer of a personal role in health decision making.

Forces of Change

It is important to monitor these shifts and trends and analyze their impact on our society in general and on the delivery of health services in particular. A comprehension of the forces of change in the health care arena, using a systems approach to analysis, may permit us to anticipate the future. We then can adapt to these changes, modify traditional approaches to health care, and develop expanded consultant services. The development of specific strategies and techniques will assure a dynamic role for the consultant in the health care system that leads to effective, efficient, and systematic health programs.

Six interrelated forces of change specific to health care have been identified that will have direct implications for health consultation in the design and delivery of health services:

1. The extraordinary advances in biomedical science.
2. A heightened public expectation of improved health care services as a result of the awareness of the advances in modern technology.
3. An increased demand for a more efficient and extensive system for delivery of health services.
4. The changing nature and size of the demand for a variety of health personnel and the gap in the availability of the needed professional skills.
5. The many demographic, social, and economic variables that may create obstacles to obtaining optimal health services.
6. The paradigm shift to increased participation by the health consumer in self health care, health care decisions, and demand for wholistic approaches to prevention of disease and promotion of health, wellness, and quality of life.

Awareness of the forces of change in health care and analysis of relevant societal changes should be followed by active participation in shaping the environment to meet the needs and demands of the public. Reevaluation of professional theoretical assumptions, technical services, and consultative approaches will be necessary to develop effective health care programs. The need for health professional consultants will be greater than ever in the following decade as health personnel are in greater demand. Help will be needed to train colleagues, clients, and families in the use of new technologies; to develop new or modified health programs in hospitals, home health, and industry; and to assist other professionals in school systems, community agencies, and community programs to address the demographic and population trends we have described. This climate of change provides the health professional consultant an opportunity to assume a more frequent and contributory role in the planning of health services.[38, 39, 40, 41]

TRENDS ANALYSIS: FORECASTING/RESTRUCTURING/ ADAPTATION/STRATEGIC PLANNING

Our plans miscarry because they have no aim. When a man does not know what harbor he is making for, no wind is the right wind.—*Seneca* (4 B.C.–A.D. 65)

All organizations and systems need a clear vision of where they are headed. To achieve their mission and goals, they must develop strategies to strengthen their structures and programs if they are to be successful in the context of societal change. As we have described, the current upheaval in the health care system is significant. There is an essential need for individuals, organizations, agencies, facilities, and communities to develop specific approaches and strategic plans to assure continuity of care. A health care delivery system or organization must be able to reevaluate its structure or focus and reconceptualize basic ideas in response to changes in the environment. This may require the development of several different organizational characteristics and behavioral patterns, responsive to differing external conditions.[38] Many organizational leaders have a gut feeling about where they are headed, but cannot articulate this clearly enough to translate into plans. Additionally, differing opinions among the system's key individuals may create conflicting visions of the future.[74] Help with the process of reconceptualization, restructuring, and formulating a cohesive view often can be provided by either internal or external consultants who are able see the broader picture, help distill discussion into a common language, and provide focus for the development of the strategic plans.

However, strategic planning, in and by itself in this changing world, is useless unless preceded by a clear image of what is hoped to be achieved. This image is considered strategic vision, and provides the framework for the direction and organization of activities to achieve the goals. Naisbitt cogently uses the example of NASA's successful strategic vision to "Put a man on the moon by the end of the decade." This very specific goal was the strategic vision that provided the organizing focus and direction for the entire space program.[63, p94] This same specificity of where we are heading must be applied to health care goals.

Tregoe et al. have defined five key elements that must be considered and discussed before proceeding with strategic planning, to provide a clear and focused direction for all organizational planning. These "dimensions of strategic vision" include the following[74]:

1. The thrust or focus of the organization's future development
2. The scope of products, services, or markets to be considered
3. The future emphasis or priority of the products, services, or markets within that scope
4. The key capabilities required for successful implementation
5. The implications of this vision or strategic direction on the future return or outcome.

To develop this strategic vision, every organization must have a basic foundation or governing principle that provides the building blocks on which to construct the strategic plans. From this concept evolves the mission of the organization, or as Tregoe calls it, "the driving force" that integrates the dimensions of strategic vision.[74] Organizational and program development consultants frequently are called in to help an organization review their major ideology, reconceptualize their mission and goals, and design the planning process.

The purpose of an organization's mission statement is to express the basic philosophy or identity of the organization. Determination of this mission statement or driving force must include:

- the fundamental purpose and boundaries of the organization's activities (what business they are in, and what business they should be in as a guide to action);
- current verses future appropriateness of these activities;

- the scope of the organization's activities and the impact on present and future actions;
- identification of the organization's strengths and weaknesses; and
- development of broad goals to address the mission statement.[40, 59]

The mission and goals of the organization form the foundation and backbone of all the organization's planning. Strategic planning is the systematic process to determine the preferred future state of an organization by which the overall mission and goals of the organization can be implemented, providing the basic direction and focus to achieve the goals. It is not financial planning, budgeting, or marketing, but the future planning for the organization as a whole.[59] The strategic plan may be considered the long-term *destiny* of an organization.[1] The formulation of a strategic plan provides a flexible mechanism through which the organization can respond to issues and coordinate the overall planning process.

A system of strategic planning for health organizations should include a study of the environmental impact of the social, political, economic, and technological forces influencing the health care delivery system in general and the particular organization.[33, 37, 40] The strategic plan should be used to:

- *Forecast* emerging issues affecting the health care system and the specific facility or organizational system in question;
- *Accommodate* to changes and respond rapidly;
- *Integrate* the responses and concerns of members of the organization;
- *Identify* and *analyze* these issues to form the framework for the development of policies and recommendations; and
- Provide the *planning objectives* for implementation and management.[33, 37]

Basic Steps in the Development of a Strategic Plan

1. *Environment or situation analysis.* As we have seen in our discussion of environmental and system analysis, it is essential to identify the external, social, economic, political, and technological forces that have an impact on the organization. Environmental scanning and assessment, or situation analysis, enables the organization to review the trends and patterns that will influence future activities. This situation analysis also must look at the internal as well as external environmental patterns affecting the organization. The internal factors include the organization's services or products, the financial and labor resources, its facilities, and management strengths and weaknesses. The purpose of this study of the environment is to be able to anticipate change and thus prevent being caught unaware.[40]

2. *Decision making.* The next step in the development of a strategic plan is to link all aspects of the environment to the decision-making process. Consideration of the relationship of the macro, or external environment, to the institutional, or internal environment, the competitive market environment, and the specific organizational environment is important. If management is not able to articulate the signals from these environments, a consultant may be called in to help identify these trends as they relate to the organization's direction. The consultant may also be asked to help develop a process for the creation of a new, more appropriate vision. An essential part of the planning process is to involve the people within the institution or organization who will be affected by the planning and development of a new vision. In our discussion of strategies to resist change we described the need to provide the feeling of shared ownership in the decisions. "People whose lives are affected by a decision must be part of the process of arriving at that decision," without which any plan is doomed to fail."[63, p129]

3. *Identification of strategic issues.* Once the trends from all these environments have been identified and linked to the planning process, the next step is to determine how an internal or external development could impact the organization's activities and which are the key factors. The organization must then conclude if it can respond to these key elements and if it can exert some influence over these issues. The final step in this phase is to prioritize the issues in order of current importance.

4. *Development of general objectives.* The purpose toward which activities are directed form the basic goals of the organization. A clear understanding of these goals will diminish confusion about what is expected as the planning process progresses. Consideration of several general planning objectives that elaborate on the basic goals will serve as the foundation for developing more specific objectives and will help determine the overall course of action. Following the designation of general objectives, they should be ranked, placing the most important first, to address the key strategic issues.

5. *Development of specific program objectives.* Specific, concrete objectives necessary to accomplish each of the general planning objectives should be formulated. These should state measurable criteria that consider the significant impact of the planning objective, if it is achievable and cost effective, and a time period over which it can be accomplished. A specific listing of the action steps necessary to achieve the program objectives will guide the activities to follow.

6. *Formulation of the strategic plan.* The strategic plan will provide the broad direction to achieve the objectives. It is the road map or chart to head us toward the desired harbor. Without this plan, an organization will surely flounder, regardless of the prevailing wind. The strategic plan also provides a general time frame for achieving the mission and goals, and is usually developed for a 2- to 5-year span.

Existing and proposed programs should be reviewed and evaluated in light of the specific objectives. There is no one way to ensure success of a plan. Organizations may hire consultants to facilitate the entire process or this specific aspect of planning. However, the process includes a determination of the most appropriate program mix: a continuation, modification, or deletion of existing programs, or the initiation of new programs. The next step is to prioritize the overall strategic issues and planning objectives, considering the advantages and disadvantages of going ahead with specific objectives. The risks and opportunities, the negative or positive consequences, must be included in this evaluation.[37]

7. *Formulation of an operational plan.* This is the next phase in translating the organizational focus and strategy into a blueprint for action. Operational or tactical plans are very specific, detailed, highly structured, and short term. They include a determination of what can be accomplished realistically during a given time period, the specific target group, who will implement certain activities, and the allocation of financial and human resources. Frequently, separate operational plans are developed for the various components of the system.[59]

8. *Development of an evaluation, monitoring, and tracking system.* The last phase of the planning process is the development of an evaluation system to assure that the plan is still current and the specific tactics are being followed and achieving their purposes. This system should provide a mechanism for an ongoing review of the plan, methods to monitor the results, and data gathering and comparison and control mechanisms to assess the progress and success of the plan.

Equally important are mechanisms to provide continual monitoring and tracking of environmental trends. Study of trends and environmental influences should be an ongoing process by which issues and objectives are reviewed and revised, based on internal organizational information and the impact of external trends.

Some issues and planning objectives may shift in rank order within a given year, others remain fairly constant for a length of time, and new issues and objectives may emerge. The strategic plan is a process and should be flexible enough to accommodate change. The issues identified should reflect the evolution of the environmental assumptions and their implications and provide the focus for determining the major activities of the organization.

The strategic plan should accomplish these four things:

- Establish strategies to allocate resources effectively and efficiently in the future.
- Focus on results.
- Highlight tradeoffs and alternatives.
- Equip the organization to deal with contingencies and future opportunities.

Assessment of the impact of the strategic plans is essential if the organization is to survive.[40]

Signals of change must be recognized so that as society changes, organizational ideas can be reconceptualized. However, by appropriate forecasting and restructuring, the driving force(s) or mission of the organization will provide the framework to take advantage of future environmental opportunities, internal beliefs and strengths, and offset environmental threats.[74] Strategic planning can then adapt to these changes and make the transition from formulation to action.

SUMMARY

> Our age of anxieties is, in great part, the result of trying to do today's
> job with yesterday's tools—with yesterday's concepts.—*Marshall
> McLuhan*

We have discussed the accelerations of social change in the 20th century that have been intense and pervasive, causing not only values changes but a "values revolution."[53] Awareness of external changes and their concomitant impact on our lives may allow us to analyze these new values and develop methods of balancing the stress of environmental change within the human ability to synthesize, respond, and adapt to this social and values revolution.

Individuals must learn to adapt to the fast pace of change in today's rapidly accelerating society. We are in a changing era and there is no turning back. Regardless of resistance, changes in the environment have occurred and will continue to occur. The years ahead promise to bring an equally fast, if not faster, rate of change. However, rarely does the future "sneak up from behind and overwhelm us."[67] There is usually ample warning of the changes that might occur; but it is when we do not recognize the signals of change, misinterpret them, or choose to ignore them that problems arise. Complacency or the demand for consistency and adherence to old methods or precedents may mean that we will be as ignorant today as a year ago.[38, 39] In the health care arena, professionals and health systems must reexamine priorities and develop new techniques for managing health services.

Resistance to change can be overcome. If innovation and change are viewed not as a force to be feared or subdued, but as an opportunity for advancement, transformation, and renewal, the natural stress that occurs during crises can be positive and foster healthy changes in society.[19]

The importance of studying trends and forecasting, restructuring, and adapting to changes in the environment are basic to the functions of a consultant. As changes continue to occur in the external environment at an accelerating rate, the importance of these concepts for the professional consultant become increasingly cogent. An organization and its members must be able to change structure or focus in response to changes in the environment. Organizations or systems that continue to maintain a bureaucracy or formal organizational structure to deal only with the routine, day-to-day business, or to maintain ideas simply because they worked in the past, will surely fall by the wayside and soon be out of business.[25, 65] Gardner spoke of "organizational rot" when he described the usual organizational structure that is designed to solve problems which no longer exist. If methods are not examined and the necessary changes made, someone else will make them.[25, 38] There is a need for "organizational fluidity," a concept that addresses new issues and allows organizations and agencies to use communication strategies, problem solving, and decision-making techniques that address our rapidly changing society.[38]

This fluidity may require the development of several different modification and behavioral patterns responsive to differing external conditions. As rapid changes occur in a society, with the eruption of new discoveries, new technologies, and new social arrangements, a new level of adaptability is required.[38] In the discussion of environmental trends, we have seen there is no one single dominating causal force determining the changes that have or will occur. Rather, it is important to consider the many factors, variables, and interrelationships of mutually interactive open systems as we analyze the environment, study the trends, and plan for the future. The need for professional help, especially in the health care arena, to assist organizations adapt their systems, adjust programs, and reorganize their structure will become more acute with the projected growth of the health industry and the diminishing availability of health personnel.

We have seen that the concepts discussed in this chapter are directly related to one another and cannot be considered in isolation, but rather as a series in a process of complex interactions. They have a direct effect on a system or organization's ability to survive and thrive. These basic concepts are especially important to the health professional consultant. We have discussed the tremendous changes in the health care delivery system and how specific forces of change have mandated that caregivers address these issues. The health consultant can assess the impact of these changes, review the structure of the system, and help the organization address the key determinants for a strategic vision, thereby helping provide the organization with a clear definition and a focus for strategic planning, linking vision to action.[38, 39, 40, 74]

> The rapid rate of change in values and technologies have left some of us overwhelmed. We intend to catch up, but we become left behind when we stop to rest, and we end up just standing still. (source unknown)

Preparation for the future involves awareness and understanding of the meaning of the forces of change; adaptation through modification, accommodation, and development of new approaches; assumption of expanded roles; and training "in a new mold rather than a recasting of the prototypes of an earlier time."[76] Preparation for the future also provides opportunities for the health consultant to help organizations or agencies identify the issues and study and manage change, utilizing an open system approach through analysis of environments and systems, to develop strategies and a plan of action to assure a dynamic role in the health care system.

REFERENCES

1. Argenti J: Corporate Planning: Getting to Grips With Your Company's Destiny. *Director,* April 1979, p 61.
2. Argyris C: *Intervention Theory and Method.* Reading, Mass, Addison-Wesley, 1970.
3. Barringer F: *NY Times,* Mar 11, 1991, p A1, A12.
4. Bennis W, Benne W, Chin R (eds): *The Planning of Change.* New York, Holt, Rinehart and Winston, 1969.

5. Bennis WG: *Changing Organizations*. New York, McGraw-Hill, 1969.
6. Bennis WG: *Organization Development: Its Native Origins and Prospects*. Reading, Mass, Addison-Wesley, 1969.
7. Block P: *Flawless Consulting*. Austin, Tex, Learning Concepts, 1981.
8. Boulding K: *The Meaning of the 20th Century*. New York, Harper & Row, 1964.
9. Bradley DF, Calvin M: Behavior: Imbalance in a network of chemical transformations. General Systems. *Yearbook of the Society for the Advancement of General Systems Theory* 1969; 1:56–65.
10. Brown A, Weiner E: *Supermanaging, How to Change for Personal and Organizational Success*. New York, McGraw-Hill, 1984.
11. Bureau of Labor Statistics: 1990–91 Job outlook in brief. *Occup Outlook Q*, Washington, DC, U.S. Dept. of Labor, Spring 1990.
12. Children's Defense Fund report, Washington, DC, 1990.
13. Chin R, Benne KD: General strategies for effecting change in human systems, in Bennis W, Benne W, Chin R. (eds): *The Planning of Change*. New York, Holt, Rinehart and Winston, 1969.
14. Cooper S, Rhodes W: Consultation course, Guest faculty, Ann Arbor, Mich, July 1972.
15. Deal TE, Kennedy AA: *Corporate Cultures*. Reading, Mass, Addison-Wesley, 1982.
16. Drucker PF: *Innovation and Entrepreneurship*. New York, Harper & Row, 1985.
17. Dostoyevsky, in Hoffler E: *The Ordeal of Change*. New York, Harper & Row, 1952.
18. Dubos R: *Man Adapting*. New Haven, Yale Univ Press, 1965.
19. Ferguson M: *The Aquarian Conspiracy*. Los Angeles, JP Tarcher, 1980.
20. Finn GL: The occupational therapist in prevention programs. *Am J Occup Ther* 1972; 26:59–66.
21. Freudenheim M: Business and Health, *NY Times*, Mar 5, 1990, p C1.
22. Freudenheim M: Business and Health, *NY Times*, Feb 5, 1991, p C2.
23. Gallessich J: *The Profession and Practice of Consultation*. San Francisco, Jossey Bass, 1982.
24. Gallup G Jr: *Forecast 2000*, New York, Morrow, 1984.
25. Gardner J: *Self-Renewal: The Individual and the Innovative Society*. New York, Harper & Row, 1964.
26. Gross BM: The state of the nation: Social systems accounting, in Bauer RA (ed): *Social Indicators*. Cambridge, MIT Press, 1966, p 250.
27. Guttmacher A: *Study Jan 1990*. New York, Alan Guttmacher Institute, 1990.
28. Harlock S: Managing change, in Bair J, Gray M (eds): *The Occupational Therapy Manager*. Rockville, Md, AOTA, 1985.
29. *Healthy People 2000:* Washington, DC, U.S. Dept. Health & Human Services, Public Health Service, 91-50213, 1990.
30. Hinkle LE: The doctor, his patient, and the environment. *Am J Public Health* 1964.
31. Hoffler E: *The Ordeal of Change*. New York, Harper & Row, 1952.
32. Jaffe EG: Expanding the role of the occupational therapist. I: The mandate, challenge and barriers to change. Address to Michigan Occupational Therapy Association, 1973.
33. Jaffe EG: AOTA Vice President's Responsibilities. Rockville, Md, AOTA, 1983.
34. Jaffe EG: Historical Perspectives of Family Life and Sex Education in the Public Schools, Research Highlights, vol 1, no 5. San Francisco Institute for Health Policy Studies, University of California, San Francisco, October 1983.
35. Jaffe EG: Policy Implications and the Practice of Family Life and Sex Education, Research Highlights, vol 1, no 6. San Francisco, Institute for Health Policy Studies, University of California, San Francisco, December 1983.

36. Jaffe EG: Family Life and Sex Education in the Public Schools: An Overview of Current Practice and Policy. San Francisco, Monograph, Institute for Health Policy Studies, University of California, San Francisco, January 1984.
37. Jaffe EG: AOTA Vice President's Annual Report. Rockville, Md, AOTA, 1984.
38. Jaffe EG: Transition in health care: Critical planning for the 1990s, Part One. *Am J Occup Ther* 1985; 39:431–435.
39. Jaffe EG: Transition in health care: Critical planning for the 1990s, Part Two. *Am J Occup Ther* 1985; 39:499–503.
40. Jaffe EG: Long range and strategic planning. Presentation for Dept. of Occupational Therapy, San Jose State University, 1985.
41. Jaffe EG: The change process: Forces of change, barriers to change, strategies for survival, in Robertson SC (ed): *SCOPE*. Rockville, Md, AOTA, 1986.
42. Jaffe EG: The occupational therapist as a change agent: A model of preventive mental health, in Robertson SC (ed): *SCOPE*. Rockville, Md, AOTA, 1986.
43. Kanter RM: *The Change Masters*. New York, Simon & Schuster, 1983.
44. Katz D, Kahn RL: *The social psychology of organizations,* ed 2. New York, Wiley, 1978.
45. Kielhofner G: Burke JP: A Model of Human Occupation, Part One. *Am J Occup Ther* 1980; 34:572–581.
46. Kielhofner G: A Model of Human Occupation, Part Two. *Am J Occup Ther* 1980; 34:657–663.
47. Kielhofner G: A Model of Human Occupation, Part Three. *Am J Occup Ther* 1980; 34:731–737.
48. Kielhofner G, Burke JP, Igi CH: A Model of Human Occupation, Part Four. *Am J Occup Ther* 1980; 34:777–788.
49. Kotter JP, Schlesinger LA: Choosing strategies for change. *Harvard Bus Rev* March-April, 1979; pp 107–114.
50. Kuhn TS: *The Structure of Scientific Revolutions,* ed 2. Chicago, Univ of Chicago Press, 1970.
51. Lawrence PR, Lorsch JW: *Organization and Environment*. Homewood, Ill, Irwin, 1969.
52. Laszlo E (ed): *The Relevance of General Systems Theory*. New York, Braziller, 1972, p 3–11.
53. Lerner M: Values and education. *JC Penney Forum* May 1984; pp 30–31.
54. Levi L: *Stress*. New York, Liveright, 1967.
55. Lewin K: *Field Theory in Social Science*. New York, Harper & Row, 1951.
56. Likert K: *The Human Organization: Its Management and Value*. New York, McGraw-Hill, 1967.
57. Lippitt R, Watson J, Westley B: *The Dynamics of Planned Change*. New York, Harcourt Brace and World, 1958.
58. Mann FC: Studying and creating change: A means to understanding social organization, *Res Ind Human Rel* 1957; 17:146–167.
59. Marrus SK: *Building the Strategic Plan*. New York, Wiley, 1984.
60. Marshall J: *SF Chronicle,* March 7, 1991, p A1, A16.
61. Miller JG: Towards a general theory for the behavioral sciences, *Am Psychol* 1955; 10:513–531.
62. Nagler S, Cooper S: Influencing social change in community mental health, in Cook PE (ed): *Community Psychology and Community Mental Health*. San Francisco, Holden-Day, 1970.

63. Naisbitt J: *Megatrends, Ten New Directions Transforming Our Lives*. New York, Warner, 1982.

64. Peter LJ: *Peter's Quotations: Ideas for Our Time*. New York, Morrow, Inc, 1977.

65. Peters TJ, Waterman RH: *In Search of Excellence, Lessons from America's Best-Run Companies*. New York: Warner, 1982.

66. Prigogine I: in Ferguson M (ed): *The Aquarian Conspiracy*. Los Angeles, JP Tarcher, 1980, p 25.

67. Renfro WL: The future. *Association Management* Nov 1983; pp 140–143.

68. Rhodes W: Conceptual overview of behavioral consultation. Consultation course, Guest faculty, Ann Arbor, Mich, August 1971.

69. Robertson SC (ed): SCOPE: Strategies, Concepts, and Opportunities for Program Development and Evaluation. Rockville, Md, AOTA, 1986.

70. Selye H: *The Stress of Life*. New York: McGraw-Hill, 1956.

71. Snow CP: *The Two Cultures and The Scientific Revolution*. New York, Cambridge Univ Press, 1959.

72. Sullivan LW: Foreword, *Healthy People 2000*. Washington, DC, U.S. Dept. Health & Human Services, Public Health Service, 91-50213, 1990.

73. Toffler A: *Future Shock*. New York: Random House, 1970.

74. Tregoe BA, Zimmerman JW, Smith RA, Tobia PM: *Vision in Action: Putting a Winning Strategy to Work*. New York, Simon & Schuster, 1989.

75. von Bertalanffy L: *General System Theory*. New York, Braziller, 1968.

76. West WL: Professional responsibility in times of change. *Am J Occup Ther* 1968; 22:9–15.

CHAPTER 4

Approaches to Consultation

Evelyn G. Jaffe, M.P.H., O.T.R., F.A.O.T.A.

The next best thing to knowing something is knowing where to find it.—
Samuel Johnson[18]

Chapter 2 and 3 dealt with the theoretical concepts that form the basic body of knowledge of the consultant practitioner. In this chapter we present an overview of when consultation is needed, with a discussion of the specific indicators for a consultative approach to problem solving, the possible focus of consultation, and the characteristics of a consultant. As we stated in Chapter 2, we define the *consultant* as the professional who provides an indirect service in a helping role.* The terms *client* or *consultee* may be used interchangeably to describe the person or group with whom the consultant works, but usually the client refers to a system or organization and the consultee to an individual recipient of the consultative service. Additionally, the client/consultee may be involved with other people. The term *clientele* is used to describe those receiving the services of the consultee or client organization including other agencies, patients, families, and students.**

This chapter also addresses a key factor of consultation: the diversity and multiplicity of the consultant's roles. There are many similarities in the process and function of the consultant, as we see when we discuss the basic steps common to all consultations in Chapter 6. However, a major weakness of consultation practice, especially with the inexperienced consultant, is the lack of awareness of the variety and alternatives possible in the consultative approach.[5]

An understanding of this diversity can give the consultant considerable leeway to choose the role most appropriate to the situation. In Chapter 2, we reviewed the

---

* For the remainder of the text, we call the consultant "she." This is not to slight our male consultant colleagues, but to help the public become aware that more and more women are entering the consultation arena.
** See Appendix—Glossary

various theoretical models of a consultation practice. In each of these models, a specific approach may be required. There may be a need to choose one role initially and then shift roles as the consultation progresses. In addition to our discussion in this chapter of the multiple roles of the consultant and role choice, we address the issue of the internal and external consultant, with a description of the differences and similarities between these approaches.

INDICATORS FOR CONSULTATION

When is consultation needed? As we discussed in Chapter 3, today's rapid technological changes; decreased availability of health care resources, both financial and human, and, therefore, the continued emphasis on cost containment; an increased older population; a better informed and more demanding health consumer; and shifts in geographic and population demographics will all require health systems to make changes in organizational structure and provision of services. Change, as we noted, creates uncertainty and anxiety. People look for advice to address the issues resulting from these changes and for help to predict their future impact. Using consultant services to identify issues, trends, resources, and opportunities can provide organizations and individuals with invaluable help to manage change.

Consultation may be indicated when the following conditions exist:

- An organization has a policy or operating problem it cannot handle;
- An organization cannot identify issues causing the problem;
- A new proposal or program requires planning and development for which the organization has neither time nor adequate staff;
- Organizational objectives are not being achieved;
- An organization cannot determine why it has failed to achieve its objectives or it needs strategies to address internal or external issues affecting its efficiency or productivity;
- There is an inappropriate or unbalanced distribution of power within the organizational system of a specific department;
- There is a lack of communication between the subparts or departments of the organization;
- The expertise of the consultee needs redirection, refocusing, or change in the manner of application of the consultee's abilities; or
- The organization or consultee lacks specialized expertise in a given area;
- The consultee or members of an organization need stimulation or training in new methods or techniques;
- There is not consensus within an organization about exploring an alternative method of handling an issue or problem;
- There is a lack of clarity or commitment about taking action to achieve goals;
- The organization or consultee needs an objectve evaluation of performance, plans, decisions, and program objectives.[6, 8, 12, 17, 25]

DETERMINING THE FOCUS OF THE CONSULTATION

The consultant must determine the appropriate focus and duration of the consultation depending on the needs of the client system and the type of activities chosen for the situation. The consultation may concentrate on many different levels of work problems and may be informal or formally delineated. It may occur in various settings and over different periods of time. It also may focus on a single client, group of clients or potential clients, or an entire agency or system. Thus the consultation may have differing areas of focus, time, or emphasis.

For example, consultation may vary in one of the following ways:

- a single contact consultation in a time-limited, one-to-one relationship, or a one-day workshop, seminar, or in-service training session possibly for an urgent situation;
- a single consultation that may not be of an urgent nature, which includes a sequence of follow-up contacts;
- a series of planned contacts of predetermined length, which may include several sessions or phases of training;
- an ongoing relationship of undetermined length, which will be mutually terminated when the project, problem, or task is completed. [11, 23]

Additionally, the emphasis of the consultation may be on a particular target population:

- *The total system, such as an entire agency or organizational structure:* The consultation may focus on the overall long-range plans of a system. It may require an analysis on internal and external trends that affect the organizational system's implementation of program goals and objectives. It may involve planning for agency objectives such as developing a program for children with special needs in a school system; organizing a consortium of health facilities; planning community health programs; or reviewing the overall family structure to develop future home and community plans for an individual with special needs.
- *The structure of a section or department of the organization or system:* The focus may be the organizational structure of the subpart of a system and a review or reconceptualizing of the procedures of this division. For example, the focus may be on the mental health division of a multiservice hospital occupational therapy department, the occupational therapy department in a rehabilitation center, or the graduate program of an allied health college.
- *Relationships between two parties such as staff relationships (collegial, interdepartmental, interagency) or relationships between the client and their clientele:* Here the focus of the consultative work is on relationships involving team treatment concerns and/or staff conflicts; consultation between professional colleagues; interdisciplinary programming; or interagency coordination and/or liaison between directors from two different community agencies.

It also may involve the people with whom the client works: their patients and families, students and other teachers, and other clientele.

- *A single case related to a specific problem or issue:* This focus may follow the more traditional clinical model of case consultation. The consultant helps a specific client, referred to as the consultee to diagnose the problem or identify the issues related to a specific case (patient, student, staff member, other agency professional—the clientele of the consultee) and provides expert recommendations. Additionally, the focus may be the consultee, related to a specific issue that the individual needs help resolving. The consultant in this situation may provice support and guidance to help develop the consultee's ability to deal with stress-related problems.

  The consultation may focus on an urgent issue or a specifically planned project, such as consultation regarding a particular patient problem; conflicts in management style that have created an individual crisis; clarification of values for a staff member demoralized by abrupt or overwhelming changes; and identification of communication problems impeding programs. This focus may be most familiar to the occupational therapy consultant.[5, 6, 11, 23]

The consultant may provide a variety of services to help with those issues identified in an organizational system, agency, specific department, or individual as indicators for consultation. In addition to the length of time and target population, the focus of the consultation is on the type of activities or work in which the consultant is involved.

Problem Identification and Definition

A consultant may provide one of the most important services basic to solving any problem in an organization or with a specific client/consultee. Sometimes the organization or client has vague concerns about operating efficiency or is troubled by problems that cannot be solved without help. By facilitating the identification of the issues, the consultant helps the client system in the first step to problem resolution.

Joint exploration (collaboration) with the client for problem diagnosis, clarification, and eventual problem resolution is the most desired method of problem or issue identification. It requires informed consent on the part of the client, so that they know that entering into a consultative relationship will involve joint identification and clarification activities. The consultant can help clients examine their own motivations in requesting help and also help the client become aware of the interrelationship of both internal and external issues to the possible problem. Also, in a collaborative approach to identification of issues, if the "organization" is treated as the client and members are involved in the generation of information, they are more apt to share concerns about perceived or actual problems.[13, 22]

Specialized Expertise

At times, the specific skills of an outside expert are required. In the health care industry, particularly, the changes in service technology and biomedical approaches have required most health care providers to update their knowledge and skills and to adapt their programs to accommodate these advances. Specialized expertise in particular programs for targeted populations or in technical aspects of projects can be provided by a consultant who is trained and experienced in a specific body of knowledge. With this focus, the consultant may need to involve the client in a new process, procedure, or technique and help develop new or advanced skills.

Impartial Situation Analysis

Acute internal problems, either as a result of leadership conflict or organizational stress due to external pressures, can precipitate the call for help. A consultant, outside of the hierarchical structure of an organization, may be hired to review a management/staff problem, conflict between administration and management, or an overwhelmed or polarized staff. An impartial, objective analysis of the situation can give the organization a fresh view with an unbiased opinion that can make a valuable contribution to appropriate identification of issues, problem solving, decision making, and evaluation.

Training

The focus of training is to provide additional information so that the client will be more effective in dealing with the issues. This consultation may involve formal educational seminars and workshops or informal in-service staff training. For example, the consultant may provide informal staff training for specific programming problems or new methodologies, lead departmental workshops to develop more effective and/or new policies or procedures, or present formal organizational or community conferences or seminars to explain environmental influences and the need for new programs and overall system changes.

Innovation and Idea Generation

Consultation may be the most effective way to infuse the organization with creative thinking. Often the client and staff have the necessary basic skills to institute change in a program or department, but prefer to stick with the old way because it is secure or they cannot come up with anything different because they are too close to the situation. A consultant may be hired to develop new ideas and a fresh approach to organizational procedures and services. The consultant acts as the catalyst for facilitating innovation and change skills in the client system.

Planning and Design

Another focus of a consultant's tasks may be to design and plan new programs and methods or modifications in existing programs for organizations, agencies, or individuals. The health care consultant may focus activities on new programs for a given target population such as a church or community program for the elderly; corporate health programs for retiree health education to improve understanding of the health system or worksite wellness programs for employees; or school programs for children with special problems. The activities related to planning and design may also focus on the community or organization. For example, the consultant's tasks may be devoted to planning new organizational procedures or modifying environmental barriers in the home, workplace, school, or community.

Strategy Formulation

Another focus of a consultant's activities may be strategic planning. As we discussed in Chapter 3, it is essential for organizations to develop strategies to strengthen their structures and programs if they are to be successful in this rapidly changing society. In the health care system especially, an organization must be able to change its focus in response to changes in the environment. Many organizations enlist the help of consultants to analyze environmental trends and to review, and perhaps restructure, major goals and objectives through the development of strategic plans. Help in the formulation of specific strategies to address the issues may be a prime task of the consultant. However, the consultant must be aware that for strategic planning and strategy formulation to be effective, the client organization must understand the process. Therefore, a major activity of the strategic planning consultant is to provide the necessary training and information about the planning process so the plan can be implemented effectively.

Evaluation

Hiring an outside consultant to evaluate a program or organization's effectiveness has become increasingly popular in business. As health care funds diminish, demonstrating the cost-benefit of programs and services has become essential. Evaluation consultation is becoming an increasingly specialized field in the health care arena, requiring specialists with skills in survey research design, data collection measures, and statistical analysis.[5, 6, 9, 12, 23]

CHARACTERISTICS OF THE CONSULTANT

The most important basic characteristics of the consultant are the ability to identify issues, analyze data, transmit ideas, understand the frame of reference and values of the client system and the functions and responsibilities of the specific client, and utilize the interpersonal relationship to maximize the participation of the consultee in the problem-solving process.

As we discussed in Chapter 2, there are a variety of approaches and models of consultation from which a consultant may choose, depending on the consultant's own style and the given situation. But regardless of the method, there are certain characteristics common to all consultants. We view the consultant as:

- A *professional* with a background in the theory and process of consultation and with a body of knowledge in the health care system. The consultant may have additional specialized expertise in a specific area of health care, such as occupational therapy rehabilitation, technologically assisted devices, health education, school and community systems and agencies, health promotion and wellness, or a targeted population (such as children, adolescents, adult workers, the elderly, or minorities).

- A *peer* with the client. The relationship between consultant and client is unique. The consultation process is dependent on the give-and-take relationship between both parties in an atmosphere of mutual trust and respect. Each has different areas of expertise and responsibility. The client is usually the expert in a specific field, but has encountered a problem. The consultant does not focus on personal concerns of the client unless directly related to the situation. The consultant helps the client develop the necessary skills to address and resolve the problem effectively. The client determines the areas of immediate concern and the consultant helps facilitate the identification of issues by encouraging the client to share facts, impressions, and opinions, and to be amenable to new ideas and suggestions.

- An *outsider* to the consultative issue. The consultant may be either an internal consultant, contracted from within the organizational structure, or an external consultant, contracted as an independent agent from outside the organization. In either case, the consultant should consider the relationship with the client as independent. Even though an internal consultant may hold a position in the organization and be called in to review a particular department problem or issue, when wearing the consultant hat she becomes an outsider to the system. As a consultant she is outside the hierarchical structure for the duration of the consultation and should not have an integral role within the client system.

  As such, the consultant lacks direct authority for decision making and is also outside the power system of the client. The final decisions and actions are the domain of the client. The consultant, therefore, has no direct responsibility for operational intervention to the target population served by the system. The leverage of the consultant is indirect and is based on knowing the system and understanding the spheres of influence and the significant person-to-person relationships. If the consultant is especially skilled, she can organize latent forces and power blocs within the system or related to the system.

- An *indirect service provider*. The consultant works as a helper, which may include identification of issues, organizational restructuring, assessment of the condition or situation, design and development of programs, modification of existing programs, and training staff in new approaches to address issues. The consultant herself does not implement the changes. At times, the consultant is asked to manage a program or provide specific services as an expert in the area. In this case, she moves outside the consultation role and becomes a direct service provider.
- An "*idea person*." The consultant remains the facilitator or catalyst for the generation of ideas, but the client is the key operator. The client may accept or reject the ideas generated during the consultation process. It must be emphasized that the client has the ultimate responsibility for decision making, implementation of the program development ideas, and carrying out the day-to-day program operation.[5, 6, 11, 13, 19]

The consultant also may be

- An individual with recognized knowledge and expertise in problem solving in a given area or field, but not necessarily an expert in the particular profession. Many expert professionals never become consultants.
- An independent contractor who offers specialized technical services or skill to clients for a fee.
- A counselor or adviser either internal or external to the organization, employed for his or her special experience and judgment to infuse new information, perspectives, and values in an organization.
- An individual or group that is usually project or task oriented and devotes full attention to the specific issue.
- An individual who resolved a similiar problem successfully in the past and subsequently is asked to provide help to someone else.[9]

ROLES OF THE CONSULTANT

The health care delivery system has always been a people-intensive industry, noted for its interdisciplinary team approach to service. However, the increasing emphasis on technological expertise has sometimes meant hiring individuals with excellent technical skills at the expense of good interpersonal skills. The efficiency of the labor intensive and interdependent health care system will be determined by the abilities of its members to work well with one another. Inherent in all the roles of a consultant are good communication skills and the goal of increasing client effectiveness.[25]

Just as we have seen that consultation may have different foci and be based on differing theoretical models depending on the situation and what help is required, there are many dimensions to the actual role of the consultant. Within a given situation, the role of the consultant may evolve over time as changes occur in the cycle of the consulting relationship and in the client system itself. The consultant may begin the relationship in a nondirective role as she analyzes the environment, identifies the need for changes within the organization, and helps the client system understand and clarify its goals in relation to the changes needed.

As the consultant works with the client system, there may be a shift in this role to a more directive position of educating and/or training the clients to learn the appropriate skills to attain their new goals and adapt to the changing environment. Consultants who work with organizations or groups often have a greater challenge in determining role shifts than those who maintain their consultative relationship with an individual client.[13] However, there are certainly shifts in the role of the consultant, even with an individual client, as the relationship develops and new information is presented.

These are natural role shifts that occur in any consultation experience as the consultant facilities change. It is important for the consultant to be cognizant of when these changes are occurring and to adjust her role accordingly. Change efforts will be effective only if the consultant is aware of these shifts and is experienced and proficient in the roles required in the situation.

Lippitt and Lippitt discuss these roles as dynamic components of the consultant's work at the various stages of the consultative relationship. They have developed a descriptive model which presents the multiple roles of the consultant that may occur along a nondirective and directive continuum, as presented in Figure 4-1.[12]

A *nondirective role* is defined as one in which the consultant provides data as a guide for the "client's self-initiated problem solving."[12, p58-59] A *directive role* is assumed when the consultant provides active leadership in directing the activities of the client group or teaching specific skills and procedures to achieve the client goals.

Nondirective Roles

Nondirective roles may include the objective observer/reflector, the process counselor, the fact finder, or the alternative identifier/linker.

Objective Observer/Reflector

This is the most nondirective consulting approach. In this role the consultant asks reflective questions to help the client clarify the problem and gain insights on the appropriate directions for change and to stimulate the client to make decisions himself. The reflector role assumes a philosophical stance while providing an empathetic ear. However, the client assumes all responsibility for decision making.

FIGURE 4–1

Nondirective and Directive Roles

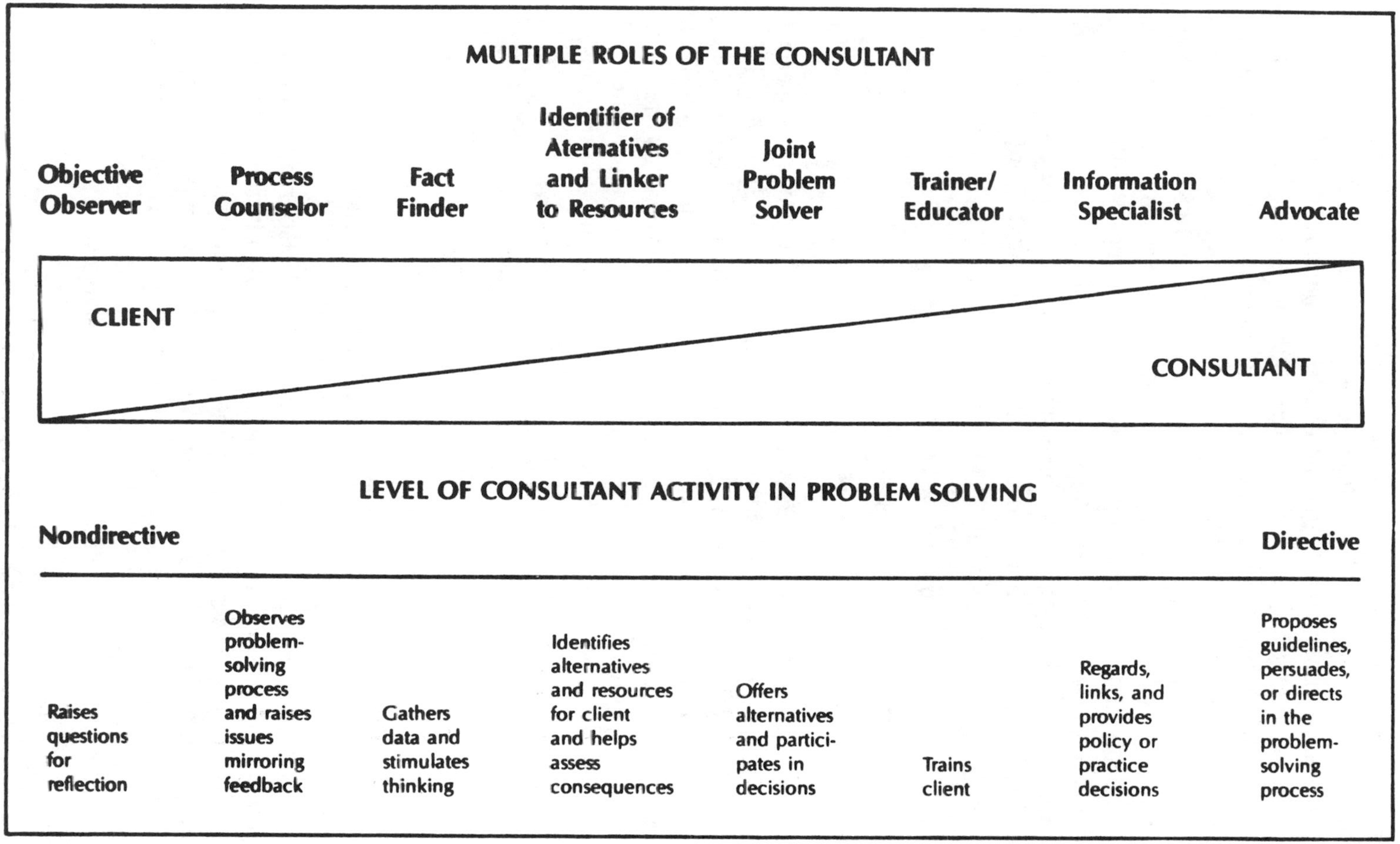

MULTIPLE ROLES OF THE CONSULTANT

Objective Observer	Process Counselor	Fact Finder	Identifier of Alternatives and Linker to Resources	Joint Problem Solver	Trainer/ Educator	Information Specialist	Advocate

CLIENT — CONSULTANT

LEVEL OF CONSULTANT ACTIVITY IN PROBLEM SOLVING

Nondirective ———————————————————————————— Directive

Raises questions for reflection	Observes problem-solving process and raises issues mirroring feedback	Gathers data and stimulates thinking	Identifies alternatives and resources for client and helps assess consequences	Offers alternatives and partici- pates in decisions	Trains client	Regards, links, and provides policy or practice decisions	Proposes guidelines, persuades, or directs in the problem- solving process

From G. Lippitt & R. Lippitt, in *The Consulting Process in Action*, 2nd ed., 1986, p. 61. Reprinted with permission of the publisher; University Associates, Inc., San Diego, CA.

Process Counselor

Process consultation has been defined by Schein as "a set of activities on the part of the consultant which help the client to better perceive, understand, and act upon process events which occur in the client's environment."[20, p9] The major focus of process consultation is the development of joint client-consultant diagnostic skills. The emphasis is on how things are done, the process, rather than only on the specific problem. The process consultant uses observational skills to identify and diagnose organizational problems. Additionally, the consultant in this role provides feedback to the client and helps the client integrate interpersonal and group skills to improve organizational relationships and processes, thereby hoping to develop in the client the necessary skills to address future problems. Organizational efficiency and improved productivity of individual departments and members are the goals of the process counselor.

Fact Finder

Fact-finding, or identifying the issues, is basic to all approaches in consultation and should be considered one of the most integral parts of the process. It is the essence of developing a database and is crucial to diagnosis and problem solving. The fact finder may simply listen or may actually develop highly sophisticated survey research techniques. Depending on the client environment, the consultant must develop a method for fact-finding and data collection appropriate to the situation and learn how and when to use specific techniques to gain the most information from the client system.

Alternative Identifier/Linker

The selection of an appropriate solution to a problem usually involves the identification and proposal of several alternative suggestions. In this role, the consultant acts as the *identifier* of both internal and external resources and alternatives, and the *linker* of the client to them in order to provide a broader range of options for organizational intervention.[11] The consultant develops criteria for assessing the alternatives and presents them to the client, but does not participate in the decision making or selection of the options. This role also may be considered as networking, in which the consultant helps the client develop the necessary links or networks with others who have similar problems or possible solutions.[25]

Directive Roles

A shift in the continuum from these nondirective roles may begin to occur when the consultant becomes a collaborator with the client in the "action-taking process" of solving the problem. Directive roles may include the joint problem solver, the trainer/educator, the information specialist, and the advocate.

Joint Problem Solver

In this role, the consultant works with the consultee in a collegial manner, with both parties collaborating to define the problem, weigh the alternatives, and determine the course of action. The consultant may help clarify the issues from an objective perspective, confront sensitive interpersonal conflicts in the role of a third-party mediator, encourage team building, reinforce the client's skills and resources, and provide the catalyst for action. Throughout this role there is an emphasis on joint decision making and collaboration. "The consultant and consultee have a co-equal relationship, where each respects the other's expertise."[23, Foreword] This role is used extensively in an occupational therapy model of consultation, either as an internal or external consultant (see Chapters 8 through 16).

Trainer/Educator

The role of educator and trainer is frequently chosen in occupational therapy consultation. This role requires development of strong interpersonal and communication skills and demonstration of competency as an educator. In this role, the consultant may plan and design educational events, such as conferences and seminars for a large audience, or develop experiential workshops as in-service training for staff and/or administrators. The consultant may develop learning experiences related to organizational restructuring; strategic planning; budget and/or management information systems; group process and interpersonal conflict resolution; enhancement of job performance; and problem identification, problem solving, and decision making. The occupational therapy consultant also may use this role in working with a direct service therapist to provide additional information and learning experiences for the patient or patient's family regarding coping with the disability or illness, environmental barriers, technical equipment, community resources, and other help related to the specific needs of the patient. The trainer/educator role is considered a primary one for all consultants, internal or external, and a major role of occupational therapists in particular.

Information Specialist

This role often is considered the traditional role of a consultant by the client, that of giving expert information in a specific area. However, as Steele points out, this can be the most seductive role of the consultant. It has the potential for ego satisfaction and personal excitement and gratification for the consultant, but also the danger of increasing the dependency of the client on the "wise and all knowing expert."[11] The client may demand or expect an expert to provide all the solutions to present and future problems, thereby never developing problem-solving skills in the client system. (This concept is discussed in greater depth in Chapter 6.) As discussed earlier in this chapter, the consultant is not a technical specialist, but may provide information or suggestions on specific methodology. Schein feels that the role of process specialist is appropriate for the consultant and distinguishes between the expert that *helps* an organization or client learn and cope with the problem and the expert that *solves* the problems.[20]

Advocate

The role of the advocate is the most directive role of the consultant and is viewed frequently as a role of strength and influence. Lippitt and Lippitt discuss two advocate-consultant behaviors: the content advocate and the process advocate.

The *content* advocate attempts to influence the client's choice of goals, values, or actions. The consultant in this role may be perceived as a persuader, provocateur, and defender of certain ideas specific to the client's needs. For example, the occupational therapy consultant to a school system may assume an advocate role for the school therapist and child's family by presenting the case before the review board for specific program planning, using persuasive behaviors in defense of the client to exert pressure on the system.

The *process* advocate influences the client to use certain methods of problem solving, types of strategy, and general approaches to the process of problem resolution. Again, as an example, the occupational therapy consultant to a school system may suggest the process or approach by which the school therapist and child's family exert pressure on the system, rather than the consultant promoting the specific program.

> Both these views of the advocate involve the values of the consultant. Both assume that the consultant will intervene in some way that exerts pressure on the system. However, the scope of the goals or values is quite different. The goals of the content advocate are rather specific, but those of the process advocate are broad and more flexible.[11, p32]

In all helping relationships, the consultant uses some aspects of process advocacy, whether as a conscious choice of roles or as a part of other consultant roles. The choice of advocate behavior is directly related to the consultant's own values and beliefs about what is the appropriate approach and/or content of the intervention.

ROLE CHOICE

As we saw in the preceding discussion, there are numerous roles of the consultant, which may change as the consultation progresses. The choice of intervention strategies for a given situation is based on the personal values and sensitivities of the consultant and the specific needs of the client. At times there is a blurring of roles, which should not be construed as a problem or viewed negatively. It is a false economy and also a waste of energy to attempt to peg a consultant into one role throughout a consultation experience. Usually, the consultant cannot consciously pinpoint when she has assumed a specific role. The individual trained in the full range of consultative role possibilities can react to a given situation by responding appropriately to the needs of the moment. Thus the consultant, often unconsciously, assumes one or more of the roles described. However, it should be emphasized that the overriding consideration in role selection is the choice of the most effective role at any given moment for a specific client's needs.[25] It is more important for the consultant to recognize why these role shifts occur, which role is predominant at a given time, and which role is most effective to achieve the goal, than to dwell on the choice of the role.[11]

Lippitt and Lippitt describe the following criteria as the most common factors in role selection.

The Nature of the Contract

The contract, whether a formal written document or oral agreement, is the initial mutual understanding between consultant and client and sets the stage for the hierarchy of consultant roles. (Negotiation of the contract is discussed in Chapter 6.) The terms of the contract may change as the consultation develops, which will determine subsequent roles of the consultant.

Goals

It is essential to understand the ultimate goals of the client system and the outcomes expected by the consultation. In addition, the consultant must determine goals for herself that are feasible and constructive. The goals and priorities for achieving them for both consultant and client may change within the development of the consultation. Therefore, the identification of mutual goals must be considered in the choice of the consultant's role.

Norms and Standard of the Client System and the Consultant

Lippitt and Lippitt define norms and standards as the "full spectrum of values from etiquette to morals and lifestyle."[11, p72] In terms of the client, we also would include the corporate culture of the client system as a major determinant of role choice. Values and standards basic to the organization resist change and occur slowly, if at all. The how and why of the client system must be considered as the consultant chooses the appropriate role.[11]

Personal Limitations and Inclinations of the Consultant

Determinants to role choice are based on the consultant's personal style, natural predilections and competencies, and the role in which she feels most comfortable. If the consultant chooses the role most personally suited to her in a given situation, the consultation is apt to be more effective and successful. Therefore, the greater the training, versatility, and repertoire of consultation roles, the broader the choice the consultant will have to be effective in a variety of settings.[11] The need for a wide perspective is especially crucial when the consultant must work with varied clients and adapt to different settings within changing contexts.

What Worked Before

Previous experience can be both a help and a trap. Although tried and true methods may create a strong comfort level in the consultant and boost her feeling of confidence to proceed with the consultation, it is important not to fall into the trap of complacency. Recognition of the need for a repertoire that includes a variety of roles is crucial if the consultant is to adapt to the changing needs of different clients.

Events

Personal life events affecting the consultant and/or client (weddings, births, deaths); external social happenings (earthquakes, hurricanes, war, racial tensions, stock market fluctuations); or internal organizational changes (change in leadership, layoffs, bankruptcy) will have profound effects on both the consultant and client system and the role choice of the consultant.

Internal and External

Additionally, role choice is related directly to whether the consultant is an integral part of the client system.[11] As we discussed earlier, the internal consultant is an individual who functions within an organization, as a member of the client system, but has been asked to serve as a consultant to another department or program within the same organization. Whereas the external consultant is hired by the organization from the outside, as a private contractor or a member of a consulting firm, with no or minimal organizational or political relationship with the client system.[24]

Role expectations, therefore, are usually different for the internal and external consultant, as each behaves quite differently even when working in the same situation. Consulting behavior must be adapted to the particular situation and can be adjusted appropriately if the consultant is aware of the major differences between the internal and external consultant. The consultant's effectiveness depends on her awareness of the situational differences. For example, the external consultant, who is an independent agent, is less constrained and can be more aggressive than the internal consultant, who must be more cautious because she "lives with the client." Her role and functions may be specified and limited. The option of which role to select is based on the client needs at the time.[24, 25]

There is often confusion about when to hire a consultant from outside an organization and when an individual who is part of the organization can perform consultative activities. An organization may not recognize the advantages or disadvantages of the internal versus the external consultant. Ulschak and SnowAntle describe four primary internal consulting roles: the *director*, the *counselor*, the *facilitator*, and the *delegator*.[25] However, these roles are not limited to the internal consultant. The external consultant often performs the same roles. Then, what is the difference and does it matter which an organization hires? Because there has been considerable misunderstanding about these terms and the choice of one over the other, we devote some additional attention to this particular role choice. A comparison of the two will be helpful in the discussion of approaches to consultation.

INTERNAL VERSUS EXTERNAL CONSULTANT

The difference between the internal and the external consultant is an important consideration, not only for role choice, but for the general consultation process. The way the consultant perceives the client system depends to a large extent on whether she is on the outside looking in, or the inside looking out. As a member of an organization, a consultant has certain loyalties, responsibilities, hopes, and fears that color her perceptions of the organization. The frame of reference of the internal consultant is significantly different from that of the external consultant.[11] Each has certain assets and strengths, advantages and disadvantages. Depending on the needs of the organization, one type may work better than another. The following discussion outlines the similarities and differences and the advantages and disadvantages of the internal and external consultant.

Internal Consultant Advantages and Strengths

The internal consultant is a member of the organization and knows the organizational culture and, perhaps, the strengths and weaknesses of the organization. As an insider, the internal consultant will know what will work and what does not work within her organization. She knows more about the internal concerns, operational problems, and existence of potential difficulties. She also has firsthand knowledge of what policies, procedures, and rituals are held dear that would create untold resistance if an attempt is made to change them.

The internal consultant may be regarded as a "member of the family," understanding the power and politics of the organization. Knowledge of the key individuals in the organization is one of the greatest advantages of the internal consultant. Understanding the subtleties of corporate power within the organization usually is not determined initially by someone who doesn't "live in the house." Knowing the corporate language, the norms and political realities, the background of the problem, and who has the power to sanction changes or implement them once instituted is very important. For example, knowledge that the top administrator may not be the key power person, or that access to a secretary or even the maintenance man is more important for a particular program gives the consultant an inside edge.

The internal consultant is "here to stay," committed to the organization as an integral part of the system. She has a primary allegiance to the organization and is committed to the success of its programs. She has an opportunity to see the recommendations from a successful consultation implemented, providing a measure of personal satisfaction.

Entry into the client system is not an issue. Usually, the internal consultant is asked to perform consultative activities by someone in the organization who knows of her particular abilities for a given project. As she is already part of the system, she does not have to present or prove her qualifications for the task. In addition, referral for consultation within the organization may be more acceptable because of convenience and most likely will be less expensive.

As a member of the organization, the internal consultant has a history in the system because she is known to other members. If she has functioned well within the organization and is respected by her peers, she is more apt to be accepted easily and well received in the role of a consultant, as she is a known quantity.

The internal consultant usually is more sensitive to potential impediments in the establishment of consultative relationships. Understanding the personalities and style of individuals within the organization can give the internal consultant insight into possible approaches for collaboration and to changes that might occur during relationships.

The internal consultant may have knowledge of the existing resources within the system. She may know of needed but unused resources. Awareness of pertinent diagnostic information and appropriate targets for data collection can save the consultant considerable time and effort. She also may be able to obtain feedback at strategic points in the consultation process because of greater knowledge of the linkages with other parts of the system.

The internal consultant has access to information about the value of key individuals in the consultation process. Knowledge of the potential human resource pool in the organization can help the consultant identify issues and solve problems more easily.

The internal consultant has greater opportunities for continuous observation of activities. Although the actual consultation may not be long term, the internal consultant has had the prior advantage of being able to assess the skill level of staff who will implement changes and the need for further skill development. She also has the opportunity to continue to observe the actions of staff related to the consultative recommendations and determine when additional support is needed to maintain the new procedures or structure.[*]

Internal Consultant Disadvantages and Weaknesses

As a "member of the family," the internal consultant may be too close to the organization. Because of her loyalty to the organization, she may overlook pertinent information or not be able to look at issues objectively. She may be too tied to old traditions herself, lack the perspective to see the broader issues, and not see the possibilities for new methods or procedures.

---

[*] References 6, 7, 11, 14, 24, and 25.

The internal consultant may be involved, knowingly or not, in the middle of internal power plays. As an integral member of the organization, the consultant may inadvertently take sides in an issue and may favor particular staff because of previous work relationships. She also may have a vested interest in some aspect of the internal issues. Individuals involved in a staff conflict could put the consultant in the middle of their problem, providing damaging information and using the consultant to play one against the other. In either case, involvement in internal politics could weaken the role and render the consultant ineffectual.

As an insider, the consultant may not devote sufficient fact-finding time. Because the consultant feels she has previous knowledge of issues or situations, she may not develop data gathering methodology or take the time to interview key individuals thoroughly or survey staff knowledge and attitudes.

The internal consultant may take the consultative work for granted. Since entry into the system was probably a given, either too easily accepted by the organization or considered a job responsibility by the consultant, there is the danger that an internal consultant will be too casual about the consultant functions. She may assume an informal stance in demeanor and when contracting for service, thereby appearing less polished and professional in her approach. She also may not identify the role and functions of the consultant appropriately.

The work history of the internal consultant may have a negative consequence. If the consultant has had previous difficulties and her work in the organization has been viewed negatively, her capabilities, credibility, and trustworthiness may be in question. This previous history could render the current consultant role ineffective.

The organization may have limited role expectations. The internal consultant may not be considered an independent agent (although technically she should be). As part of the organization, her role and function may be limited, with lesser expectations in terms of competency, professionalism, and scope of activities. She may not have a diverse background or independence of movement within the organization.

The internal consultant may encounter staff resentment. Other organizational members may become defensive and resist the efforts of the consultant if they perceive that "a member of the family" is attempting to tamper with traditions and interfere with the system by interviewing and collecting information about her own culture. The concept that familiarity breeds contempt may lead to role constraints in the consultant's sphere of operation.

The internal consultant may encounter stereotyped preconceptions of her responses. Familiarity also may lead the client to anticipate, often incorrectly, what the consultant will ask and suggest. Preconceived ideas developed out of prior experience in a working relationship can color both the consultant's ability to accept the client's responses at face value and, equally, the client's ability to develop an objective consultative relationship.

The internal consultant may have more difficulty in requesting participation of high-powered figures in the client system. Although the consultant may have greater knowledge of the key individuals, she may not have an adequate power base or be viewed as having much influence. By the very fact that she is an employee of the organization, she may not have access to the power players or be able to enlist their participation. It may be difficult for these high-powered individuals to admit the need for help from an employee of their organization or to accept her suggestions.

Internal consultation fees may be charged to the general organizational budget. When the fee for consultation services is absorbed as part of the general overhead, rather than directly to the specific subpart of the client system involved in the consultation, the client may feel that the consultation is not directed specifically toward him or his department. This reaction can cause the client to be less committed to accepting the consultant's recommendations, thereby rendering the consultative activities less effective.

The internal consultant may encounter difficulties in determining timing or criteria for evaluation. Due to the ongoing nature of internal relationships, the consultant may find it difficult to develop evaluation criteria and may have a problem determining the appropriate time for terminating the consultation contract.[*]

External Consultant Advantages and Strengths

The external consultant brings an objective view of the organization. Because the consultant is not blinded by internal traditions and rituals, she may view the issues with a different perspective to the situation, have a fresh new approach, and present an unbiased opinion.

The external consultant brings a variety of skills from previous experiences. The external consultant has a more diverse background and may have developed an extensive repertoire of roles and approaches from working with other organizations that provide her with greater options. Additionally, she may have encountered a variety of responses that have added to her own knowledge and skills.

The external consultant usually presents a professional manner. Since the external consultant must prove herself to the organization, her approach to contract negotiation, presentation of audiovisual materials, and interpersonal relations creates a general feeling of professionalism. The organization may assume a greater expertness or competency because of the initial impression.

The external consultant usually will devote more time to the fact-finding process. As the consultant may not be as aware of the concerns or issues in the organization, she may spend considerable time gathering information and identifying the issues. She may then be more selective about what can be accomplished in the consulting process.

The external consultant may be able to determine the readiness of a potential client. By viewing the situation objectively, the consultant may have a better feel

---

[*] References 6, 7, 11, 14, 24, and 25.

for when the client system is ready to become involved in a consultation experience and participate in the initial information gathering process.

The external consultant may have a wider perspective. Because the consultant is not limited by the narrow view of an insider, she may see a broader picture of the entire organization and be able to determine more possible goals, alternative courses, and needed changes in the system.

Greater acceptance of unfamiliar means of data collection is possible by the external consultant. The use of different or new methodology in fact-finding efforts often are expected and more readily accepted by members of the organization when presented by an outsider.

As an outsider to the organization, the external consultant is less likely to be caught up in internal politics. The external consultant is independent of the power structure. Usually the consultant has not had a close working relationship with the members of the organization; therefore, she will be able to develop a consultative relationship that is not biased by previous experiences. Staff members will not attempt to involve her directly in their internal conflicts. The consultant may propose a test period to determine the mutual compatibility of a consultative relationship.

The external consultant can usually address more sensitive problems. As the external consultant is not considered a "member of the family" and, therefore, would not be betraying the "family trust," she may be able to tackle thorny internal issues without creating fear or defensiveness.

The problem-solving process is usually faster. Since employees are apt to be less reluctant to discuss issues with an outsider, they have less need to provide politically correct answers. Their particular job or potential career in the organization usually is not a concern; therefore, they may be willing to provide more usable information to determine the key issues.

The external consultant may have greater access to top administrators. Because the consultant is not a peer or employee of the organization, she often will have greater leverage in involving the key power individuals in the client system.

There is usually less resistance to utilization of data and outside resources. The external consultant, viewed objectively in the organization, can combat resistance to the analysis of the information gathered in the fact-finding process. Suggestions to use outside resources and the data findings are accepted more readily from the external consultant.

The external consultant can provide an objective second opinion. The recommendations of an outsider to test, market, or reinforce new programs may provide the organization's decision makers with the support they need to implement organizational change.

Clients usually experience greater ease in accepting recommendations. The external consultant can introduce new skill development activities, propose periodic reviews, and suggest changes in procedures to create effective action more readily.

Both client and consultant find it easier to evaluate and terminate the consultation. Evaluation procedures proposed by the external consultant are usually accepted because they reflect an objective view. There often is greater commitment by the client to participate in the process of evaluation to determine the point of termination of the contract.[*6, 7, 11, 14, 24, 25]

External Consultant Disadvantages and Weaknesses

Entry into the system may create challenges for the external consultant. If there has not been a direct invitation for consultation, the consultant may have to prove the need for the intervention. The external consultant, not well known in the organization, also has to demonstrate credibility and her qualifications for the job.

The external consultant lacks history within the organization. When the consultant is hired by leaders to work with staff, the consultant is an unknown quantity and viewed as a stranger to the system. Staff may be wary of this new person, and acceptance into the system may be more difficult.

As an outsider to the system, the external consultant may not understand the corporate culture. By virtue of being a stranger to the traditions of the organization, some of the procedures proposed or the consultation approach may be inappropriate.

Previous experiences with many organizations may create a pattern of behaviors. The external consultant may develop a set repertoire and present activities that have been used in all other consultations without examining the particular situation and the needs and style of the client system.

The external consultant may develop strategies outside the organizational structure. Because of experiences outside the current client system, the consultant may be aware of external resources. This can be a disadvantage if the consultant does not study the specific situation. Rather than involving the employees in the identification of issues, decision making, and problem solving, the consultant may develop tactics that are external or foreign to the operations of the organization.

The external consultant does not remain with the organization. Most external consultations are time limited and shorter than internal consultations. Once the consultation has terminated and the consultant is gone, the commitment to her recommendations may not be as strong and the organization may revert to old behaviors.[*]

Reviewing the internal versus the external consultant in chart form may help you compare the advantages and disadvantages of each role. Table 4–1 illustrates this comparison.

In some situations, a combination of consultative approaches may be desirable. Internal and external consultants may work collaboratively within the organization as a team, creating a very effective working relationship. Organizational as-

---

[*] References 6, 7, 11, 14, 24, and 25.

T A B L E 4–1
Comparison of the Internal versus External Consultant

Advantages	
Internal Consultant:	*External Consultant:*
• Part of the system (knowledge of culture)	• Objective, fresh view of the organization
• Insider and "member of the family"	• Variety of skills and experiences
• Committed to the organization	• Professional approach
• Entry not an issue (already part of the client system)	• More time identifying issues
• History in the system (known to other members)	• Test client readiness
• Insight into approaches for collaboration	• Broader perspective to goals and changes
• Aware of pertinent diagnostic data	• Fact finding more readily accepted
• Access to information and resources	• Not involved in internal politics
• Opportunities for continuous observation	• Not betraying the "family trust"
	• Problem solving faster (less reluctance to discuss issues with an outsider)
	• Access and leverage with power people
	• Combat blockages more readily
	• Less resistance to use of outside resources
	• Provide objective, "second opinion"
	• Better acceptance of evaluation process
	• Better acceptance of recommendations
	• Easier to terminate consultation

Disadvantages	
Internal Consultant:	*External Consultant:*
• Too close to organization	• Entry difficult if lack of direct invitation
• Possible involvement in internal power plays	• Lacks history in organization (stranger to the system)
• Insufficient fact finding time	• Lack understanding of corporate culture
• Informal demeanor, less professional	• "pattern" of consultation activities (may lead to routine behaviors)
• Negative history can render consultant ineffectual	• Develop strategies outside of the organizational structure
• Limited role expectations	• Comittment may not be as strong
• Resentment for perceived interference ("familiarity breeds contempt")	
• Stereotyped preconceptions possible	
• Difficulty in obtaining participation of power players	
• Budget ties may render recommendations less effective	
• More difficulties in terminating consultation	

sessments, especially, can be extremely effective when there is a team approach by an internal consultant who understands the corporate culture and an external consultant who can provide an unbiased view. This team provides the unique opportunity to build on the strengths of each consultative role and thus minimizes the weaknesses or disadvantages just described.[19] It is critical for the team to be aware of their individual similarities and differences so they can complement each other's strengths and limitations.[24] The internal consultant can provide basic knowledge and information regarding the dynamics and culture of the organization, the power politics and key individuals in the system, and the internal resources available. The external consultant can eliminate the problems many internal consultants have of inside invisibility and blindness to issues by being too close to the family structure.

DEFINITIONS AND COMPARISONS OF OTHER HELPING ROLES: DIFFERENCES AND SIMILARITIES

Some similarities exist in other communication and interpersonal relationships found in the roles of health professionals and the occupational therapist in particular. There are major differences and some parallels in responsibility and function between the consultant and other organizational roles. Often both the consultant and the client confuse these functions, leading to disappointing outcomes. To understand the role of the consultant, and the overlap and applicability of some traditional skills of the health care professional, and the occupational therapist in particular, we outline the differences and similarities, contrasts and parallels of the following helping roles: consultation, administration, advocacy, management, collaboration, supervision and therapy. Table 4–2, on pages 114 and 115, presents a matrix of various helping roles to compare and contrast their similarities and differences.

Consultation

Purpose.—To enable the client to work through a particular problem.

Goal.—To help clients broaden and improve their knowledge, skills, and attitudes, thereby making the appropriate changes to solve the problem and achieve their goals.

Style.—Consultation uses an interactive style in which both consultant and the client develop a relationship of mutual respect. Therefore the consultant must establish rapport with the client before the consultation can proceed. Consultation is offered in a manner adapted to the needs of the client.[16, 26]

Authority.—The consultant has influence over an individual, a group, or an organization, but has no direct power to make changes, implement programs, or insist on compliance. The consultant is an outsider to the system and has neither the authority nor responsibility to direct the actions of the client. The client has the freedom to initiate, refuse, interrupt, modify, or terminate the process. However, the consultant may withhold consultation.[2, 26]

Qualifications.—The consultant must possess technical knowledge and communication skills that are valued by the client. The client must also possess skill and technical competence which may be equal or superior to that of the consultant. It requires self-confidence to give and receive consultation. The consultant must have insight into her own feelings about the consultation and be sensitive to those of the client.[26]

Duration.—Consultation is usually time limited: may be a one-time, one-day session with the client, a series of sessions, or in some cases can be ongoing.

Role and Function.—The consultant, in an indirect role, facilitates logical decision making by helping define the problem through the gathering of pertinent facts and analyzing the situation, the people involved, the time, location, and the cause of the problem.[1] The consultant acts as a catalyst by providing alternative solutions through fresh ideas, recommendations, and suggestions. The consultant may provide support to the client by strengthening the client's coping skills. Additionally, the consultant may motivate the client by inspiring, encouraging, and impelling him or her to take required action to solve the problem and improve their effectiveness.

Administration

Purpose.—To define the philosophy or mission and corporate culture (or values and beliefs) of the institution or organization and identify the goals and objectives to accomplish this mission.

Goal.—To determine the long-range plan and structure of the institution or organization and help management develop strategic plans to implement the policies that will facilitate the mission of the organization.

Style.—Administrative styles vary from the unapproachable, authoritative president of a company to the informal administrator with an open-door style. The administrator may be a myth or hero depending on the style of the person and the culture adopted for the company.[4]

Authority.—The administrator makes final decisions, establishes policy, and has direct influence over the organization to make changes or implement programs.[2]

Qualifications.—The administrator must possess knowledge of the entire structure of the organization and have the communication and organizational skills to convey the corporate philosophy to management. The administrator must have broad insight into both external and internal influences (environmental, social, political, economic) that will affect direction of the organization and future policy.

Duration.—Administration is ongoing.

Role and Function.—Administrators define the philosophy and structure of the organization and provide leadership for the overall goals and objectives.

Advocacy

Purpose.—To espouse the cause of the organization.

Goal.—To facilitate and assure the success of the mission and goals of clients (either individuals, groups, or organizations) and serve their needs by exerting pressure on the system or power source.

Style.—Advocacy is an action-oriented role that usually utilizes an adversarial style of demands, confrontation, and pressure to achieve its ends. The advocate may use direct force, active demonstration, or political or judicial influence.

Authority.—The advocate is responsible directly to the client or client system. Usually the advocate is an outsider to the system and therefore may take more risks in exerting influence. The advocate does not usually make final programming decisions or establish policy, but advises the client on the most effective strategies to make changes or implement programs. However, the advocate usually makes a conscious effort to influence the choice of methods and the means to achieve the client's goals.[5, 6, 11]

Qualifications.—The advocate must possess knowledge of the entire structure of the organization, understand its missions and goals, and have strong communication skills to convey these goals to appropriate power sources. The advocate must have broad insight into the external influences (environmental, social, political, economic) that will affect the direction of the organization.

Duration.—Advocacy is usually time limited: may be a one-time, one-day session, a series of sessions, or in some cases can be ongoing.

Role and Function.—Advocates develop and actively pursue strategies that apply appropriate pressure to accomplish the mission, goals, and objectives of their clients. The external advocate's responsibility usually includes exerting strong pressure to bring about organizational, political, or social change.

Management

Purpose.—The purpose of the manager is to clarify and implement the mission and goals of the organization by providing a sense of common direction for employees.

Goal.—Effective and efficient organizational functioning is the major goal of the manager.

Style.—Management involves the "persuade style" to get the audience (staff) to act.[16] The manager may adopt any number of styles in order to carry out the goals of the organization, depending on the general corporate culture of the particular organization. The appropriate choice of management style is crucial to the effectiveness of the manager and may include an authoritative manner, collaborative style, or egalitarian style with shared decision making.

Authority.—The manager has direct control over actions or procedures and has the responsibility to coordinate decisions and guidelines for the day-to-day behavior of his or her staff.[1, 2]

Qualifications.—The manager must possess technical knowledge and evaluation and communication skills specific to the organization. The manager must have insight into his or her own feelings about the situation and be sensitive to those of the staff. Additionally, the manager must be able to recruit, select, orient, and develop personnel to accomplish the goals of the organization.[14, 15]

Duration.—Management is an ongoing process.

Role and Function.—The manager plans, organizes, staffs, directs, and implements policy, programs, schedules, procedures, and budgets.[14, 15] The manager is responsible for developing job descriptions and performance standards, evaluating and measuring performance, and controlling operations.

Collaboration

Purpose.—To achieve resolution of a problem through shared responsibility between professionals.

Goal.—To help an agency, organization (corporation, health facility, department, school, etc.), or family improve their ability to make the appropriate changes to improve a situation or solve a problem through the joint effort of the professionals.

Style.—Collaboration is considered a "join style," or egalitarian relationship in which both parties join in action. There must be a mutual exchange and respect for the expertise of both parties.[2, 16]

Authority.—Collaboration implies that there is shared responsibility for data collection, analysis, decision making, planning, and implementing change. There may be prior negotiation and agreement regarding the scope of mutual expectations and responsibilities.

Qualifications.—Both the professional colleagues (health professionals, teachers, managers, administrators, etc.) must possess technical knowledge, interpersonal, and communication skills necessary for the specific situation. They must have insight into their own feelings about the situation and be sensitive to those of the other colleagues.

Duration.—The collaboration may be time limited: may be a onetime relationship to work on a problem or issue; may be a series of sessions; or in some cases can be ongoing.

Role and Function.—The functions of a collaborative relationship include joint enquiry and exploration and mutual program planning, development of techniques, modalities, and policies and procedures.

Supervision

Purpose.—To direct staff to perform effectively.[26]

Goal.—To facilitate program effectiveness by overseeing and evaluating staff performance.

Style.—Supervision uses an "inform style," or one that requires the staff to learn. It involves a directing and instructional style and therefore is hierarchical in nature. Although supervision is given, the supervisor must establish rapport with the supervisee.[16, 23, 26]

Authority.—The supervisor has direct responsibility for and influence over an individual or group, and acts in a somewhat judgmental role that may involve a superior/subordinate relationship. The supervisee does not have the freedom to refuse, interrupt, or terminate the process as long as the relationship exists. However, the supervisee may make suggestions for modifications in the relationship. Supervision may not be withheld. Supervision is geared to the demands of the job. The extent to which it is adapted to the needs of the supervisee is limited by the specifics of the job and the capabilities of those involved.[26]

Qualifications.—The supervisor must possess technical knowledge and communication skills that are necessary to the job. The supervisee does not necessarily possess technical competence in order to utilize the supervision. It requires self-confidence to give and receive supervision. The supervisor must have insight into his or her own feelings about the supervision and be sensitive to those of the supervisee.[26]

Duration.—Supervision is an ongoing process on a regular basis.

Role and Function.—The supervisor oversees policy and is responsible for evaluating and correcting performance.[16] The supervisor also may motivate the supervisee by inspiring, encouraging, and impelling people to take required action to perform effectively.

Therapy

Purpose.—To correct or ameliorate a diagnosed health problem.

Goal.—To help people (the patient or client) improve their endurance, knowledge, skills, and attitudes, thereby making the appropriate progress and changes to remediate the problem.

Style.—Therapy uses an interactive style in which both the therapist and the patient should work together to deal with the problem. Therefore the establishment of rapport with the patient is an important aspect of successful therapy. Therapy generally involves a learning process through direct intervention. Treatment is usually *given* by the therapist, though in some cases the therapy style may be *offered*.[26]

Authority.—The therapist has influence over an individual or a group to make changes in the direction of the therapy and to implement programs. Therapy is adapted to the needs of the patient. The patient has the freedom to accept, refuse, or interrupt the treatment process. However, the therapist also may withhold treatment.[26]

Qualifications.—The therapist must possess technical knowledge and communication skills that are valued by the patient and effective in the modification of the problem. The patient does not have to possess technical competence to benefit from the treatment process. It requires self-confidence to give treatment and willingness to receive it. The therapist must have insight into his or her own feelings about the treatment and be sensitive to those of the patient.[26]

Duration.—Treatment is usually time limited: may be a onetime, one-day session with the patient for evaluation, a series of sessions, or in some chronic cases can be ongoing.

Role and Function.—Therapy is a direct service that may involve program planning and the development of specific techniques and modalities to deal with a

T A B L E 4–2
Comparative Table of Helping Roles

	Consultation	Administration	Advocacy	Management	Collaboration	Supervision	Therapy
Purpose	enable client to attain problem resolution	define mission and corporate culture, identify goals and objectives to accomplish the mission	espouse cause of the organization	clarify and implement mission and goals of organization	shared professional responsibility for problem resolution	monitor and direct staff to perform effectively	correct, remediate, or ameliorate a diagnosed health problem
Goal	broaden and improve client knowledge, skills, attitudes	determine long range plan, policies, and structure of organization; develop strategic plans	facilitate mission and goals by exerting pressure on system or power source	effective and efficient organizational functioning	improve a situation or solve a problem through joint professional efforts	facilitate program effectiveness	improve function: endurance, knowledge, skills, and attitudes
Style	interactive style of mutual respect	vary from authoritative to informal, may be myth or hero	direct action-oriented, adversarial style of demands, confrontation, and pressure	"persuade style" in authoritative manner; or collaborative, egalitarian style	"join style" or egalitarian relationship, mutual exchange and respect	"inform style," hierarchical directing and instructional style	interactive style between therapist and patient
Authority	influence but no direct power	direct influence, makes final decisions and establishes policy	strong influence but no final policy or decision-making authority	direct control over actions or procedures	shared responsibility for decision-making, planning, and implementing change	direct responsibility and influence, superior-subordinate relationship	direct influence and intervention

Qualifications	technical knowledge and communication/consultation skills	knowledge of entire structure of organization, broad insight into external and internal environmental influences, communication and organizational skills	knowledge of entire organizational structure, strong communication skills, broad insight into external environmental influences	technical knowledge, evaluation and communication skills specific to organization	technical knowledge, interpersonal, and communication skills	technical knowledge and communication skills necessary to the job	technical knowledge and communication skills
Duration	usually time-limited	on-going	usually time-limited	on-going	time-limited or on-going	on-going	usually time-limited, or in chronic cases can be on-going
Role and Function	indirect role as facilitator, analyst, catalyst, educator, motivator; provides recommendations, encouragement, support to strengthen coping skills and improve effectiveness	define philosophy and structure of organization, provide leadership for overall goals and objectives	direct responsibility to client system to exert strong pressure to effect change, develop and pursue strategies to accomplish mission, goals, and objectives	plans, organizes, recruits staff, directs and implements policy, programs, schedules, procedures, budgets; develops job descriptions and performance standards, monitors and evaluates performance	joint exploration, data collection and analysis, mutual program planning, development of techniques, policies, and procedures	oversees policy, evaluates and corrects performance, motivates and encourages supervisee	define treatment plan, development of specific treatment techniques and modalities, direct program planning and implementation

problem. The therapist is involved in logical decision making when defining a treatment plan through the gathering of pertinent facts and analyzing the situation, the people involved, and the cause of the problem. The therapist may act as a catalyst by providing alternative solutions through ideas, recommendations, and suggestions. The therapist also may motivate the patient by inspiring and encouraging the individual to take the required action to remediate the problem. In the provision of direct service, the therapist implements the plans designed and treatment is given to the patient to ameliorate the problem.[6, 15, 16, 23, 26]

Our discussion of the various consultation approaches paves the way for the actual consultation. In the next two chapters, we examine in greater detail the preparation desired for the potential consultant and the process of consultation.

SUMMARY

When a man comes to me for advice, I find out the kind of advice he wants, and I give it to him.—*Josh Billings*[18]

Discussion of the various approaches, foci, and roles of the consultant has described the diversity in the practice of consultation. Understanding the wide choice available to the potential consultant should help guide your decisions on role and style and help you determine your approach to intervention.

Regardless of which approach is used or which consultant role is chosen, the process is similar—that of an interactive relationship between the "helper" (the consultant) and the "helpee" (the client/consultee). The goal and purpose of any consultation is to assist the client system or consultee in decision making, problem resolution, and strategies to prevent future problems.[11, 25] The expected outcome of the consultation is a greater level of awareness of the situation and an increased ability on the part of the client to cope with the present problem and resolve future similar problems within the framework of the client system. The ultimate goal of the consultation process is the delivery of more effective service to the client system's population (the clientele), who remain the responsibility of the client.

REFERENCES

1. Allen L: *Professional Management: New Concepts and Proven Practices*. New York, McGraw-Hill, 1973.
2. Block P: *Flawless Consulting*. Austin, Tx, Learning Concepts, 1981.
3. Cooper S, Rhodes W: Consultation course, Guest faculty, Ann Arbor, Mich, July 1972.
4. Deal TE, Kennedy AA: *Corporate Cultures*. Reading, Mass, Addison-Wesley, 1982.
5. Gallessich J: *The Profession and Practice of Consultation*. San Francisco, Jossey Bass, 1982.

6. Jaffe EG: *Consultation: Theory and Practice*. Faculty, consultation course, Department of Continuing Education, San Jose State University, 1977–1978.

7. Jonas MR: Asking for advice. *US Air,* XI:18, 1989.

8. Kelley RE: *Consulting: The Complete Guide to a Profitable Career*. New York, Scribner's, 1981.

9. Lant J: *The Consultant's Kit*. Cambridge, JLA, 1986.

10. Lee RJ, Freedman AM (eds): *Consultation Skills Reading*. Arlington, VA, NTL Institute, 1984.

11. Lippitt G, Lippitt R: *The Consulting Process in Action*. San Diego, Univ Assoc. 1978.

12. Lippitt G, Lippitt R: *The Consulting Process in Action, 2nd Ed*. San Diego, CA, Univ. Assoc., 1986.

13. Lippitt R: Dimensions of the Consultant's Job. *J Soc Issues* 1959; 15:1–12.

14. Marriner-Tomey A: *Guide to Nursing Management*, ed 3. St Louis, CV Mosby, 1988.

15. Miner JB: *The Management Process: Theory, Research, and Practice*, ed 2. Macmillan New York, 1978.

16. Munter M: *Guide to Managerial Communication*. Englewood Cliffs, NJ, Prentice-Hall, 1982.

17. Nackel JG, Jacoby TJ, Shellenbarger MT: *Working With Health Care Consultants*. Hospital Management Systems Society, American Hospital Association, 1986.

18. Peter LJ: *Peter's Quotations: Ideas for Our Time*. New York, Morrow, 1977.

19. Rhodes W: *Conceptual Overview of Behavioral Consultation*. Consultation course, Guest faculty, Ann Arbor, Mich, August 1971.

20. Schein EH: *Process Consultation: Its Role in Organization Development*. Reading, Mass, Addison-Wesley, 1969.

21. Sherwood JJ: Essential differences between traditional approaches to consulting and a collaborative approach, in Lee RJ, Freedman AM (eds): *Consultation Skills, Reading*. Arlington, VA, NTL Institute, 1984.

22. Steinberg D: *Interprofessional Consultation*. Chicago, Mosby Year Book Medical Publishers, 1989.

23. Swartz DH: Similarities and Differences of Internal and External Consultants. *J European Industrial Training,* 1975; 4:5.

24. Ulschak FL, SnowAntle SM: *Consultation Skills for Health Care Professionals*. San Francisco, Jossey-Bass, 1990.

25. Uris A: *101 of the Greatest Ideas in Management*. New York: Wiley, 1986.

26. West W: The principles and process of Consultation, in Llorens LL (ed): *Consultation in the Community: Occupational Therapy in Child Health*, Dubuque, Iowa, Kendall Hunt, 1973.

CHAPTER 5

Preparation for Consultation

Evelyn G. Jaffe, M.P.H., O.T.R., F.A.O.T.A.
Cynthia F. Epstein, M.A., O.T.R., F.A.O.T.A.

It is the function of creative men to perceive the relations between
thoughts, or things, or forms of expression that may be utterly different,
and to be able to combine them into some new forms—the power to
connect the seemingly unconnected.—*William Plomer* [13]

Consultation is not always considered a profession in and of itself, but rather a set
of additional skills that enhance and further expand one's original field. The health
care professional desiring further enhancement of knowledge and skills may turn to
consultation activities for this growth. It is a demanding activity and the requirements for success also are demanding.[9] Additional training in the theoretical
concepts of consultation are necessary so that one's own field of expertise is
elaborated, but does not interfere with or detract from the consultation process. In
this chapter, we discuss what it takes to be a consultant, the inherent attitudes and
skills and the type of training and experience that are helpful for the potential
consultant.

PRECURSORS TO CONSULTATION

Why does an individual choose to become a consultant? Most potential consultants
feel they have good problem-solving skills and a particular background and expertise that could be utilized in a more productive manner outside a traditional
institutional job. Individuals who choose consultation as an area of practice desire
a vehicle for channeling these skills.

Other people want the freedom of a flexible working schedule. Still others feel
that consultation is an easy way out of the typical hierarchical job description
found in most institutions or organizations. This latter group will come to realize
that consultation is no easy job. However, it can be very rewarding, and, when

developed as a private practice, consultation does provide the opportunity to "be your own boss."[3] The establishment of a private consultation practice is discussed in Chapter 17.

When making a conscious choice to move from a traditional or direct service position to that of a consultant, all of these motivating factors come into play. Other incentives that may entice the uninitiated are, in fact, myths. Schiffman describes three of these.[14]

- *Myth 1:* Once you embark on a career as a consultant, you need never worry about working for a difficult boss. "You're your own boss." You are accountable only to yourself.

  Fact: Most consultants have many bosses. Consultants are usually hired for specific tasks, for time-limited periods, and must, therefore, answer to a number of clients, who, in reality, are the bosses. Additionally, the consultant is directly accountable to the client or person who hired her for the consultation. The consultant is also accountable for her consultation skills and the ability to focus on the client's concerns.

- *Myth 2:* Consultants are highly respected members of the professional community, like doctors and lawyers, and as such need only announce the opening of their practice to ensure steady business.

  Fact: Marketing is an essential aspect of consultation. Consultants who are not knowledgeable or ignore marketing strategies are "marked for failure." Some agencies or organizations feel that anyone can provide consultative services, and may choose someone inside the organization just to save costs. Others only choose external, well-established firms. Whether you provide services as an internal or external consultant, it is essential to develop a reputation for competency and respect, which may require selling yourself and demonstrating your skills and abilities.

- *Myth 3:* Being a consultant is, by the very nature of the job, less stress-oriented and time-sensitive than most other fields. When you're a consultant, you can establish your own hours and work as little or as much as you want and still be successful.

  Fact: The key to myth 3 is success. You *can* have flexible work hours and determine the amount of work for which you are willing to contract. But to be successful, you must adhere to deadlines, which are usually set by the client. The consultant's work time, in general, is usually determined by the best schedule for the client not for the consultant.

We would like to add the following myths:

- *Myth 4:* As a consultant, you have complete authority to control the outcome of your work. You are able to identify a problem, demonstrate your expertise, provide recommendations and solutions, and assure that they will be appropriately implemented.

  Fact: Nothing could be further from the truth. This assumption is a primary cause for failure in consultation. The consultant may offer suggestions, provide alternative solutions, and influence client decisions, but in reality has no direct power to make changes or implement programs. "The moment you take direct control, you are acting as a manager."[1] Taking responsibility for implementation of recommendations is a major obstacle to effective consultation.

- *Myth 5:* Consultants earn big bucks for a few hours of work. You don't have to work many hours to earn lots of money.

   Fact: Consultants may spend days, weeks, and sometimes months without a paid client. The "feast" time, when you do have a client, must help pay for the "famine" time, as well as all the ongoing business overhead costs. The realities of taxes, sick time, vacations, rent, phone, and much more must be factored in to costs.

- *Myth 6:* Only big consulting companies make money and become very successful. The solo consultant or small partnership groups cannot make it in a highly competitive marketplace.

   Fact: Smaller firms sometimes have a distinct advantage over larger ones when it comes to the ability to act quickly. For example, let us suppose a new state regulation goes into effect mandating specific changes in the garment industry. The regulation is aimed at helping more disabled individuals obtain jobs. Your town has a big manufacturer in the industry. The big consulting company, tied up with many projects, has no time to research the implications of the new regulation for potential area clientele. The little company, more responsive, quickly assesses the situation, prepares a proposal for the leading firm in the area, and sets out to obtain the contract.[15]

Attitudes and Attributes

There is no mold to determine who can become a successful consultant. Each person brings their own internal resources to the job. However, regardless of the motivation for choosing to practice consultation, certain character or personality traits and inherent attitudes and attributes are suggested as basic to the successful consultant.*

These basic personality traits, attitudes, and attributes are illustrated in Table 5–1.

Professionalism

The consultant's manner indicates that she has the appropriate skills and knowledge to assume consultant responsibilities. She demonstrates integrity and competence in her relationships with others and in helping others identify and address certain problems or issues. She expresses herself clearly and with convic-

---

* References 3, 5, 9, 10, 11, 16, and 17.

TABLE 5–1
Attitudes and Attributes

Professionalism
Maturity
Credibility
Personableness
Honesty and sincerity
Flexibility
Creativity
Objectivity
Intelligence and sound judgment
Humanism and insight
Self-Motivation

tion. An attitude of confidentiality is maintained in her work activities and in her relationships.

Maturity

A professional consultant conveys an attitude of self-confidence, reliability, and assurance of her convictions. She demonstrates emotional stability in her behavior and actions. The mature consultant is able to accept rejection and knows that often the client system will react with suspicion and perhaps hostility. She can understand and cope with resistance and rejection. She is self-motivated, has a profound respect for self and others, and handles herself with poise and confidence. This is especially important when entering a new situation or in a new system.

Credibility

Establishing a solid reputation built on sound judgment, character, and high performance levels will help the consultant convey credibility. Presenting credentials (academic standing, educational courses, and references) that demonstrate competence, experience, and knowledge also help establish client trust.

Personableness

First impressions are very important, especially for the consultant who is a stranger to the system. A favorable appearance and personal impression help create a positive atmosphere for the start of a consultative relationship. Professional etiquette and courtesy also are important attributes.

Honesty and Sincerity

The professional consultant has high principles and maintains an attitude of interest in and willingness to listen to others. Her demeanor conveys the attitude of a very trustworthy, ethical professional who has a commitment to the client. Accepting the client and maintaining the confidentiality of the situation are hallmarks of this commitment. One of the consultant's most valuable assets is a good reputation. Following a personal or professional code of ethics that precludes conflicts of interest and assures monitoring of the consultant's performance will contribute to a standard of excellence.

Flexibility

Remaining open to new ideas and situations is essential for the professional consultant. She is able to adapt easily and quickly to unfamiliar and perhaps ambiguous circumstances. By accommodating her time to that of the client, she is not rigid about schedules or procedures. By moving with the client in this manner, she continues to build a strong relationship.

Creativity

Maintaining an open-minded attitude allows the consultant to be innovative in her approach. She seeks new ways to view situations and learn and comprehend issues. She develops viable alternatives for client consideration. Clients appreciate her ability to generate new ideas and the optimistic approaches she uses to develop diverse problem-solving strategies.

Objectivity

It is imperative that the consultant maintain an objective point of view. Personal values, prejudices, or attitudes must not interfere with her ability to maintain an open mind. This is more difficult for the internal consultant who is part of the value system of the organization. However, objectivity is a key to accurate diagnosis and problem identification.

Intelligence and Sound Judgment

By portraying a comprehensive grasp of the situation and the ability to understand the issues, the consultant conveys intellectual competence and acute, clear thinking in problem identification. Consultation skills combined with specialized expertise help the consultant demonstrate her competence and ability to make rational and considered judgments.

Humanism and Insight

The possession of a personal belief system that values the importance of the individual and a trust in people is essential for the successful consultant. She possesses a sensitivity, insight, and perception that will create an atmosphere of trust and demonstrate a sincere interest in helping the client. Her own value system must be considered in the association or disassociation with that of the client. When the consultant is clear about her own values, she is able to come to grips with her own internal constraints, attitudes, and aspirations. This allows her to negotiate the many complexities encountered during consultation.

Self-Motivation

Successful consultants possess the internal drive and tenacity to take advantage of new opportunities and challenges. They derive satisfaction from their work and do not need to be told what to do by others. They are usually leaders, rather than followers, and demonstrate their leadership capabilities in their interpersonal competence, their achievements, and their zest for learning. These self-starting abilities usually are coupled with a conscientious nature and personal ambitions.

Knowledge and Skills

The development of competency must be viewed from the basic premise of the consultative process: the relationship between the people trying to solve a problem. The skills of the consultant depend on her ability to influence the relationship with the client or client system. Lippitt and Lippitt describe this influence in four ways:

1. The behavioral competence of the consultant
2. Communication of appropriate concepts and ideas
3. The degree of acceptance by the client for these ideas and of the consultant
4. The client's "legitimization" of the consultant's role

The consultant must be accepted by the client and viewed as having a legitimate role in the problem identification and problem-solving process. Without this, no amount of skill and competence will compensate for a client's total resistance to the consultant.[11]

An important cornerstone of consulting is the interaction between consultant and client, where the ability to provide help to a client is based on the skills and expertise of the consultant. Interpersonal skills are essential to the success of any consultation. The ability to listen, establish rapport, and form a good relationship with the client is the forerunner to identifying problems, providing support, and proposing solutions. The prospective consultant must have a thorough grounding in basic technical and interpersonal skills before considering the field. The techniques of consultation may be acquired, but they also must be built on a level of expertise in a particular specialty area.

Consultation is based on three major areas of skill:[1]

- Interpersonal skills
- Technical skills
- Consulting skills

Interpersonal Skills

The consultant seeks to create a climate of comfort for the consultation relationship. During the consultation process, the consultant helps the client work through many issues. Developing a positive relationship, communicating effectively, understanding group behavior, and reflective counseling are necessary interpersonal skills.

Development of Relationships.—The ability to develop rapport and form relationships with others built on trust and respect is foremost and often determines the potential success of the consultation. These human relations skills include a sensitivity to others' interests, feelings, needs, preferences, and hopes. Consultants often work with clients from diverse personal, professional, and educational backgrounds. They must convey an attitude of openness, caring, and willingness to help and be able to form relationships with a great variety of people. The successful consultant must inspire confidence, cooperation, and trust. However, the consultant cannot rely solely on her ability to form good relationships; she cannot "substitute a relationship for having something to offer."[17]

Communication.—Seventy percent of consultation time is spent communicating with others.[9] Therefore, the consultant must possess the basic communication skills of listening, observing, identifying, and reporting and be able to use these skills with a variety of client systems. The ability to listen with a third ear often is considered the most basic communication skill. Additionally, the ability to communicate ideas, articulating the issues clearly and accurately, is important in verbal and written presentations. The consultant also must consider the client's communication style and preferences. Knowledge of the client system may determine the type of communication most appropriate for the specific situation.

Group Dynamics.—The ability to analyze the sociometrics within groups and the phases of group development is essential. Understanding the roles of individuals in a group, the leaders or key power people, the decision makers, the resistant forces or ring leaders, and the helping agents in the client system is crucial to the consultant's ability to effect change. An effective consultant assesses and diagnoses group functions and dysfunctions, analyzes the effect of group norms, standards, and peer pressure on group members' behavior, and assists the goal-setting and decision-making processes in groups.

Counseling.—As a good listener, the consultant must hear the real concerns of her client and exhibit good judgment. About 45% of total communication time is spent listening to the client.[9] Sorting through a number of the clients' voiced issues, the consultant must be able to counsel clients or lead them in an appropriate direction to identify the key problems.

Technical Skills
The consultant's special expertise must be used in conjunction with other important technical skills. Through the use of comprehensive data collection, the consultant develops a picture of client problems. Planning and intervention strategies help the client review and implement an effective organizational plan.

This step should be followed by an educational process to help the client integrate new information.

Specialized Training.—The consultant must have something specific to offer the client. Consultation usually is requested because of a consultant's expertise, training, and experience in a particular area. The consultant may be a specialist or a generalist, but in either case she brings her background and expertise to the client system to provide help on particular issues, strategies, modalities, or organizational problems. The *specialist* has in-depth, state-of-the-art knowledge of a particular field, function, or technique and is usually brought in after the problem has been identified. The *generalist* has knowledge and experience in a variety of fields and can transfer her consulting skills from one type of situation to another. Generalists usually apply diagnostic skills over a broader view of the client system and often are consulted when the client is aware of an issue but has not identified the real problem.[9, 10]

Data Collection Skills.—Most consultants gather information about the client system and the presenting issues immediately after their entry into the system when they conduct their "dilemma analysis," or diagnosis. Therefore, it is important that the consultant be versed in a variety of data collection methodologies, including the use of surveys, questionnaires, interviewing, and pre- and posttest instruments. The consultant may collaborate with research analysts and statisticians who have very specific technical knowledge regarding the design of data collection instruments and the methodology of data analysis. However, the consultant must provide the research analyst with an overview of the client system and information regarding the specific needs of her client so that the data collection methodology is appropriate for the client system. The consultant, then, must have the knowledge and skill to understand and use these instruments appropriately.

Planning Strategies.—Consultants often are asked to help review an organization's overall mission and goals and conduct strategic planning sessions. Basic knowledge of the planning process and skills in organizational structure, idea gathering and idea generation in relation to the organization's objectives, goal setting, and prioritizing, and the development of measurable, time-bound objectives are essential for the consultant planner. The consultant must be skilled in presenting the process, which includes the development of an evaluation, monitoring, and tracking system.

Intervention Strategies.—Intervention strategies are the heart of consultation. All consultants must be versed in their development. The actual work of the consultant implies that she will perform certain activities to address the issues and problems for which consultation has been requested. She must be able to design, plan, and present specific strategies that will intervene in the progression of the problem. Intervention strategies may be presented directly to the individual client; conducted in educational and training sessions for staff, community groups, or families; or proposed to the client organizational system. A comprehensive knowledge of the client system is essential. Expertise in the specific area in question, creativity in designing innovative approaches, skill in presenting new methodology, and knowledge of building evaluation and monitoring measures are important components. The consultant must have these skills in order to develop effective intervention strategies.

Teaching.—The ability to design learning experiences and impart new ideas is another essential skill. It is especially needed in an educational model of consultation when workshops, in-service training, and other educational activities must be developed. Teaching skills include the ability to design programs based on the appropriate timing, sequencing, and pacing of the information presented. In addition to knowledge of educational methodologies for the preparation and design of training materials, the educational consultant should develop skills in the actual delivery of educational programs, integrating training goals with learning needs. Skillful involvement of the participants in the learning process is essential.

Consulting Skills

A broad range of consulting skills are needed to enter the consultation marketplace. The ability to examine and clearly diagnose the client's situation effectively is paramount. Through advance preparation and effective diagnosis, the consultant sets the stage. Important component skills include problem solving, facilitation of groups and teams, working as a change agent, and administrative abilities. The successful blending of these skills allows the consultant to move effectively within the client system.

Preparation.—The consultant, armed with her own technical knowledge and skills in her specific area of expertise, also must enter consultation activities with some prior knowledge of the client system. She should study the nature of the organization and its structure, the request or stated need for consultation, the individuals she most likely will contact initially, and her own reasons for accepting the consultation request. Her overview of the organizational system and initial perception of the organization's readiness to address the issues and make appropriate changes also must be considered and be subject to modification as she becomes involved in the consultation.

Diagnosis.—An examination of the client system and the presenting issues is the first step in consultation. Diagnostic skills are essential to any consultation and should include the ability to perceive the relationships between the various subsystems of an organization, the interdependent nature of individuals and groups, and both the internal and external environmental influences that have an inpact on the system. Lippitt and Lippitt call these diagnostic skills the ability to make a "dilemma analysis." As the consultation was no doubt requested because the client needs help with a problem, the consultant must recognize that a dilemma exists. "The consultant's role is to discover the nature of the dilemma (whether real or not) and to help determine what really is causing it.''[11] The consultant must possess insight, perception, and intuition to make this dilemma analysis. She must develop inductive reasoning skills that enable her to penetrate complex issues; locate sources of help, power, and influence; and isolate the situational variables to make an accurate diagnosis of the situation. These diagnostic skills will enable the consultant to help the client with problem identification and determine the client's readiness for change.

Problem-Solving Skills.—Facilitation of problem-solving skills is a major activity of many consultants. The consultant usually does not solve the problem herself but rather helps in the problem-solving process. Therefore, she must understand the process thoroughly and have skill in using problem-solving techniques and in helping improve client skills. She also must have the deductive reasoning skills to analyze the situation and the creativity to develop a variety of alternatives for problem resolution.

Group Team Facilitation.—Skill as a group facilitator or team builder is especially important for the individual who assumes the role of a process consultant. Basic to group facilitation is knowledge of group dynamics. The group facilitator must be thoroughly grounded in the process of group development, be able to assess typical group issues, and have a conceptual grasp of what works in groups and what does not. Similarly, to help individuals work together as a team requires designing a sequence of steps and activities for effective team building. The consultant's team-building skills will help these clients develop a clear picture of how they function. The facilitator must develop a repertoire of group intervention strategies to encourage feedback and help the group/team function effectively.

Change Agent Skills.—We have already discussed the need for consultants to be cognizant of change theory and process. Many consultation activities require the consultant to assume the role of a change agent. Knowledge of how to recognize and anticipate change is a basic skill of the change agent. Additionally, the consultant must understand her own attitudes toward change and how they affect her credibility and effectiveness as a change agent. The consultant must develop techniques to reduce both natural and, sometimes, inappropriate resistance to change efforts, to manage transitional states prior to the implementation of the proposed changes, and to guide the change efforts. Developing strategies specific to the client system to help ensure the success of the change effort must be considered.

Administration.—Administrative skills are important for all consultants. A considerable amount of the behind the scenes consultant work involves coordinating the consultative project or program and integrating the activities and recommendations with people involved in the client system. The consultant, as owner or manager of a consulting practice, needs administrative skills to operate a business. Managing resources of time, people, and money are administrative functions, as are skills in marketing, documenting, and financial planning. The business and marketing aspects of consultation are discussed in detail in Chapters 17 and 18.

Table 5–2 summarizes the components of interpersonal, technical, and consulting skills.

TABLE 5–2
Consultation Skills

Interpersonal Skills	Technical Skills	Consulting Skills
Development of relationships	Specialized training	Preparation
Communication	Data collection	Diagnosis
Group dynamics	Planning strategies	Problem solving
Counseling	Intervention strategies	Group/Team facilitation
	Teaching	Change agent
		Administration

These attitudes, abilities, and skills are applicable to all types of consultation, and are inherent in any field and with any client system. Basic to the development of consultant attributes and skills is the fundamental knowledge of oneself. Additionally, knowledge of the behavioral science, social systems, and the process of consultation is essential.

Self-Knowledge.—A consultant must understand her own motivations, values, and biases and have insight into her strengths and weaknesses. The old adage "know thyself" is especially important if the consultant is to be successful in analyzing others. A major responsibility of the consultant is to foster this insight in her client, thus enabling the client to pursue problem resolution. This personal self-knowledge is essential so the consultant can proceed with appropriate, unbiased, and objective suggestions.

Knowledge of Behavioral Sciences.—Basic knowledge of the social and behavioral sciences provides the foundation on which consultants build their skills in interpersonal relationships, the essential ingredient in all consultation. An understanding of human nature, attitude formation, and capacity for change is essential: why people react the way they do; how internal and external stresses can motivate, deter, or derail individuals' attainment of their goals; the impact of the environment and sociocultural influences on the human system; the development of a value system; and how people react and cope with these stresses and influences. These are vital aspects of a consultant's knowledge, as all determine the character of the consultant relationship.

Knowledge of Social Systems.—An understanding of organizational systems, including administrative philosophy and corporate culture, and the establishment of policies, procedures and practices is essential for all consultants, whether working with large client systems or an individual in an organization. As we discussed earlier, it is important for the consultant to have an overview of the organizational system in which she will work and its interrelationship with subparts of that system and other external systems or agencies or the community at large. Therefore, it is important for the consultant to understand how social systems function and have knowledge regarding the stages in the growth and development in individuals, groups, organizations, and communities.

Knowledge of the Basic Phases of Consultation.—Prior to assuming the role of a consultant, it is essential for the potential consultant to understand the process and procedures that are basic to all consultation: the sequence of consulting, or "what to do, when to do it, and why it is done in that way." The process of consultation is discussed in detail in Chapter 6.

The development of this knowledge and the major qualities of the consultant provide the background and the support for the consultative relationship. With this foundation, individuals have a much greater chance to implement the helping process successfully.*

EDUCATION AND TRAINING

How do you become a consultant? The preceding discussion referred to the precursors to consultation: the personality traits, attributes, and attitudes and the skills and knowledge required to be successful. Can a person with these abilities just hang out a shingle and establish herself as a consultant? Although the successful consultant is always learning new strategies and methods and buidling a repertoire of techniques from her varied experiences, consultation is too demanding an activity to enter into the field without adequate preparation and training. Lippitt and Lippitt aptly state, "the process of consultation is challenging, awesome, rewarding, and humbling."[11] It takes considerable knowledge and skill to be a professional consultant. There are two major training avenues for entry into the world of consultation: formal education and on-the-job training.

Formal Education

In our historic overview in Chapter 1, we pointed out that the art and practice of consultation was passed on in certain societies and cultures to individuals who had some of the inherent charismatic qualities, personality traits, and skills we have just described. In previous centuries, there was no formal education in the practice of consulting. Training and development were learned from observation, appren-

---

* References 1, 5, 9, 10, 11, and 17.

ticeship, and experience. When consultation became recognized as a growing field, there was an attempt to define it and to formalize the training process. These early attempts were haphazard at best.

Resistance to the establishment of a new specialty area, occurring as a natural phenomenon to change, was evident in the slowness of universities and professions to recognize the need for consultation training. Although the rapid changes in society created the need for outside help in many organizations and institutions, established departments in universities and professional organizations often ignored the impetus to make the necessary changes in their educational programs.[4, 5, 7, 8, 11]

Professional School Coursework

Over the past 40 years, a greater awareness and understanding of the breadth of consultation has developed. The growing demand for consultants in many fields (professional, technical, governmental, and personal) highlighted the need for special training. It was recognized that specific skills were needed.

Now, many professional schools have specific course work in consultation. Schools of business have highly developed formal courses in organizational development and management consultation. Other professional schools, including law, engineering, education, and the biological sciences, have course work and training in consultation. Consulting is usually viewed as a subspecialty or area of practice of a profession.[4]

In the health care field, schools of public health and departments of psychiatry developed educational course work in consultation. Formal training for postdoctoral mental health professionals was offered at the Harvard School of Public Health in 1955.[2] Mental health consultation, as discussed in Chapter 2, had a specific model and guidelines for practice, which were modified and refined as consultation became more important during the community mental health movement in the 1960s. Many of the early mental health concepts of consultation were adapted by other health fields.

A number of health professional educational programs are beginning to include aspects of consultation in their curriculum, particularly in administration courses. In these university-based programs, consultation often is considered as a subspecialty at an advanced level of practice and is studied in graduate degree courses. Frequently, however, mention is made of consultation as a potential area of practice without providing the detailed training in the specific skills required for a successful consultant. It is our hope that more health professional schools will acknowledge consultation as a vital and growing area for the practice of their profession and include the basic concepts, process, and procedures in the curriculum.

In addition to specific formal training in consultation theory and process, a broad general background is essential. At the undergraduate level, a strong liberal arts background paves the way for the basic information helpful for all potential consultants. A thorough grounding in a wide range of subjects provides the foundation on which to build a diverse consultant practice. Advance training or course work that addresses general systems theory and analysis; the impact of social, political, and economic influences on society; and the psychology of human behavior provide information that increases the breadth and scope of the potential consultant's knowledge. Study in these and other areas, including administration, management, and business principles, is invaluable. However, in-depth knowledge in certain specialty areas may be required to develop the expertise necessary to provide clients with the specific help they need. This broad-based background, coupled with specific expertise, will provide the diversity required for a broader practice and greater opportunities for the consultant.

Continuing Education and Postdegree Seminars

In response to the demands of practicing professionals, consultation training has developed outside traditional educational institutions.[4] Considerable information and skill building is available to the potential consultant through continuing education. Workshops and experiential seminars are now becoming increasingly available throughout the country. These workshops are sponsored by university-affiliated continuing education programs or by professional member organizations as continuing education courses.

Other independent, for-profit educational companies offer workshops in a variety of subjects pertaining to consultation and human relations. These training workshops, usually most easily accessible and often the most appropriate, are presented by consulting practitioners in the professional discipline of choice. The content of these consultant workshops can be designed to meet specific needs of the participants.

Informal and On-the-Job Training

Many opportunities exist for the potential consultant to acquire consultation experience through on-the-job-training and as a part of volunteer or professional organizations. Work environments offer innumerable consultation opportunities. Local and state organizations that are related to one's profession, the health care consumer, and other health care and political organizations offer valuable experience. Volunteer organizations such as environmental, health-related, and social service groups also offer opportunities to expand consultation skills informally.

On-the-Job

On-the-job, the potential consultant may "take a page" from the approach to consultation that we have discussed and begin by assessing her work setting (system) to identify possible consultation experiences.

For example, one quickly realizes that the very nature of occupational therapy service delivery provides opportunities to explore various aspects of consultation. Take the case of a potential occupational therapy consultant working with geriatric clients in a long-term care facility. Here the goal is to return the client to the community. The therapist must not only develop a specific treatment plan for the client, but also must address environmental issues involving caregivers in the facility, at home, and possibly in the community. She must be involved with the team(s) who will support the established goal, and in many cases, will be the facilitator or change agent to help everyone involved problem-solve issues that may stand in the way of discharge.

While the therapist is performing the important role of treatment, aspects of her work may require consultation skills. Analyzing these demands and understanding the differences in approach and methodology is a beginning point for the therapist to gain consultation experience.

Therapists who are fortunate to work in settings with experienced clinicians and mentors have multiple on-the-job training opportunities. Internal and external consultation opportunities are usually available in these large departments. Today's concern with access for all disabled, for example, has led administrators and community organizations to seek occupational therapy expertise in such areas as job descriptions and architectural barriers. When these consulting opportunities arise, the novice consultant may accompany or participate with a mentor to address the particular issue at hand.

Within the workplace, in-service education programs, weekly papers, monthly journals, texts, and visiting clinicians or educators provide additional sources of information. Student programs may offer opportunities for the potential consultant to develop special programs that could not otherwise be offered. One such experience described a community mental health program that was developed with the assistance of students participating in their mental health fieldwork placement.[6]

Other opportunities arise when the potential consultant seeks outside job experiences, perhaps with consultants who are in an established practice. This may be an after-hours or part-time endeavor. Here there may be additional opportunities for a mini-apprenticeship or mentorship program. Working with recognized experts, the novice consultant has an opportunity to assume responsibility for some aspects of the consultation while the major role is assumed by the mentor.

In order to utilize on-the-job experiences effectively, you must arrange time for performance evaluations. The potential consultant's self-evaluation is an important tool. Equally vital is an evaluation provided by a mentor or experienced consultant. This feedback will help structure the learning path for future on-the-job experiences.

Informal and Volunteer Experience

As we noted, professionalism is a key consultant trait. Participation in professional and community organizations helps build this skill. Volunteer organizations provide multiple opportunities for expanding consultation abilities. For example, we have both been active participants in our local, state, and national professional organizations. The experiences provided through many years of volunteer service have broadened our knowledge base and expanded our visibility within the health care community. Participation in other community and health-related organizations provided additional specialized information and networking in our own particular specialty areas. These are some of the natural resources that you may easily access through professional and community environments.[3]

Another important aspect of informal training is your daily paper and various news weeklies. Consultation needs are frequently driven by legislative mandates. For example, innumerable occupational therapy consultation opportunities have developed as a result of the Education for All Handicapped Children Act, Technology Act, Americans With Disabilities Act, and Omnibus Reconciliation Act of 1987, to name just a few. In each case, the information regarding the act was detailed in an edition of the daily paper.

Keeping abreast of important legislative and professional trends helps the potential consultant to see the macro picture, which often has important implications for specific consultations. Once developed, this awareness should become an integral part of your consultation skills.

SUMMARY

Consultation is a professional skill that can expand and enhance your role in health care. The professional with specialized expertise who contemplates a consultation role must consider the important attitudes, attributes, skills, and knowledge required for success.

The successful consultant is a self-directed, highly motivated person whose value system is clearly defined. Using intelligence and sound judgment, she establishes a solid reputation as a credible, mature professional. Her demeanor and personableness help establish a positive client relationship. These and other attributes assure an open and mutually respectful relationship.

To establish an effective relationship, the consultant must merge attitudes and attributes with critical interpersonal, technical, and consulting skills. Interpersonal skills help create a "climate of comfort"; technical skills incorporate the consultant's expertise and are integrated with a broad range of necessary consulting skills.

The potential consultant must possess self-knowledge if she is to provide appropriate, unbiased, and objective recommendations. This knowledge, coupled with knowledge of behavioral sciences, social systems, and the basic phases of consultation, forms a strong foundation for successful implementation of the consultative process. Formal education, continuing education, on-the-job training, and informal learning opportunities are also available. The potential consultant should take advantage of these many learning options to develop a broad knowledge base.

The considerable knowledge and skill needed for the practice of consultation is usually acquired over a period of years. Learning does not stop when you enter the field. Rather it is a continuous growth process that includes ongoing study and training.

REFERENCES

1. Block P: *Flawless Consulting*. Austin, Tex, Learning Concepts, 1981.
2. Caplan G: *The Theory and Practice of Mental Health Consultation*. New York, Basic Books, 1970.
3. Epstein, CF: Consultation communicating and facilitating, in Bair J, Gray M (eds): *The Occupational Therapy Manager*. Rockville, Md, AOTA, 1985.
4. Gallessich J: *The Profession and Practice of Consultation*. San Francisco, Jossey Bass, 1982.
5. Jaffe EG: *Consultation: Theory and Practice*. Faculty, consultation course, Department of Continuing Education, San Jose State University, 1977–1978.
6. Jaffe EG: The role of the occupational therapist in community consultation: Primary prevention in mental health programming. *Occup Ther Ment Health* 1980; 1:47–62.
7. Jaffe EG: Transition in Health Care: Critical Planning for the 1900's, Part One. *Am J Occup Ther* 1985; 39:431–435.
8. Jaffe EG: Transition in Health Care: Critical Planning for the 1990's, Part Two. *Am J Occup Ther* 1985; 39:499–503.
9. Kelley RE: *Consulting: The Complete Guide to a Profitable Career*. New York, Scribner's, 1981.
10. Kishel G, Kishel P: *Cashing In on the Consulting Boom*. New York, Wiley, 1985.
11. Lippitt G, Lippitt R: *The Consulting Process in Action*. San Diego: Univ Associates, 1978.
12. Naismith D: Educational opportunities and consulting skills, in Lippitt G, Lippitt R (eds): *The Consulting Process in Action*. San Diego: Univ Assoc, 1978.
13. Peter LJ: *Peter's Quotations: Ideas for Our Time*. New York, Morrow, 1977.
14. Schiffman S: *The Consultant's Handbook: How to Start & Develop Your Own Practice*. Boston, Bob Adams, 1988.
15. Shenson H: *Complete Guide to Consulting Success*. Wilmington, Del, Enterprise, 1987.
16. University Associates: *Consulting and Training Services:* San Diego, Univ Assoc, 1991.
17. West WL: The principles and process of consultation, in Llorens LA (ed): *Consultation in the Community: Occupational Therapy in Child Health*. Dubuque, Iowa, Kent/Hunt, 1973.

CHAPTER 6

The Process of Consultation

Evelyn G. Jaffe, M.P.H., O.T.R., F.A.O.T.A.
Cynthia F. Epstein, M.A., O.T.R., F.A.O.T.A.

It isn't that they can't see the solution. It is that they can't see the
problem.—*G. K. Chesterton*[2]

Previous chapters presented an overview of the history of consultation and the
theoretical foundations and multivariate roles possible in consultation. Also discussed were when consultation is needed, what the focus may be, and the preparation necessary to become a consultant. Now, how do you begin? First, consultation must be considered a *process,* in which help is given to address certain
problems, issues, and concerns. It is usually requested when an individual, group,
or organization cannot solve a problem alone.

Often a major difficulty is the inability of the person(s) requesting help to see the
real problem. Therefore, consultation as a process includes working with the
client to identify the basic issues. This requires give-and-take between the consultant and the client. Thus the major thrust of the practice of consultation is the
process of interaction, which includes several phases, whether the procedures are
formally delineated as a contracted professional service or informal arrangements
are made between two parties.

In this text, we consider the practice of consultation in its professional sense,
especially as it relates to the health care arena. The basic process and phases of
consultation are the same, regardless of the setting or model. The differences in
procedures and the number and type of interventions and activities that are chosen
are a result of the roles required of the consultant and the specific needs of the
client system. The consultant may work as either an internal or external consultant, assume singular or multiple roles as the consultation progresses, and provide
a variety of services as indicated by the needs and setting of the client.

The theoretical models of consultation discussed in Chapter 2, considered
together with the empirical model describing the procedures and basic steps of
consultation, form the conceptual framework for an analysis and systematic description of the consultation process. In this chapter, we discuss the basic steps in

the process of consultation and what we refer to as the four Ps of consultation: power, politics, problems, and pitfalls and their relationship to regulatory, legal, and ethical issues.

BASIC STEPS OF CONSULTATION

The cycle of the consultation process includes the following basic steps:

- Entry into system
- Negotiation of contract
- Diagnostic analysis leading to problem identification
- Goal setting and planning through establishment of trust
- Maintenance phase of intervention and feedback
- Evaluation
- Termination
- Possible renegotiation[9, 10, 14, 16]

These steps are also illustrated in consultation case studies presented in the models of consultation section of the text (Chapters 8 through 15).

Entry into System

The first step in the consultation process is entry into the prospective system or organization. This entry is usually based on exploration of the possibilities and an initial contact with the potential client. A potential consulting relationship may develop in several ways. We consider four ways to enter a system (see Table 6–1).

TABLE 6–1
Ways to Enter a System

Type of Entry	Definition
Planned entry	The individual develops a strategy and presents a proposal.
Opportunistic entry	The situation arises spontaneously and the individual seizes the moment.
Uninvited entry	The individual perceives a need and attempts to enter the system.
Invited entry	The individual is invited because of specific skills.

Planned Entry

In a planned entry, the consultant explores a specifically targeted system or organization for the express purpose of entering the system for a consultation. The individual (or consulting firm) develops a deliberate, systematic strategy chosen for a particular possible client system that appears to have the potential to be influenced by consultative methods. The consultant may be motivated by a search for new clients, by the knowledge that this system is not functioning effectively and might benefit by consultation, or by the consultant's experience and skills in helping other systems with similar issues and concerns. In planned entry, the consultant develops specific tactics for entry that include phased or sequential steps before presenting a proposal to the prospective client system.[10, 14, 16]

Opportunistic Entry

Another way to enter a system may be through hearsay, media announcements, or articles about an organization in trouble or needing specific assistance. This initial involvement in a system is considered opportunistic. Knowledge of a potential client may occur spontaneously because of a crisis situation or when circumstances within the system suddenly open the possibility of entry. Opportunistic entry usually occurs without prior planning or preparation of the system for a consultation. It is pursued by the consultant on her own initiative, based on interest in the issues or programs of the system. Due to the spontaneous nature and lack of preparedness by the client for consultation, opportunistic entry initially requires more accommodation to the system.

Uninvited Entry

Uninvited entry, as with opportunistic entry, involves consultant initiative to establish a consulting relationship with a particular client system. In this case, the consultant may be referred through a third party who perceives that a particular system has a need for help and suggests that the consultant contact key people in the system. Often in uninvited entry it is helpful to contact someone in the organization who has access to these key individuals within the potential client system. This may involve having the third party set up an informal meeting with the appropriate person(s) through whom entry may be arranged.

Uninvited entry also requires some preplanning. The consultant should determine entry level, initial approaches, potential gains for consultant and client, and, of particular importance, what the consultant has to offer the system.

Other questions to be considered include the history, if any, of a relationship between the client system and potential consultant, common interests, or possible collaborative efforts. The current role of the consultant in regard to the system is important. If the individual is an insider, who therefore would be serving as an internal consultant, intimate knowledge of the problems may create difficulties for both consultant and potential client. The potential client may find it difficult to admit to a need for help that has not been requested, especially when suggested by a peer in the system. Referral by a third party may make the initial contacts more acceptable.

An external consultant, unknown to the system, may also have difficulties approaching a potential client. In this situation, credibility must be developed by the consultant. However, referral by a third party in this case could establish a link between the consultant and the potential client system. The client system may find it easier to share problems with an impartial outsider. A review of the advantages and strengths and disadvantages and weaknesses of the internal versus the external consultant will help the potential consultant determine the appropriate approach for an uninvited entry (see Chapter 4).

Invited Entry

Obviously, the easiest way to enter a system is through invitation. It also is the most preferable form of entry because diagnosis of the system and problem identification may proceed more quickly.

When a potential client is aware of the need for help to improve the functioning of the system as a whole or a subsystem in the organization, he may request the services of a consultant, either internal or external. An existing crisis or normal changes in the environment may demand review and revision of current procedures, or staff may need additional training. Consultant services may be a routine part of an organization's operating procedures when strategic planning is necessary or new programs are to be instituted. Usually an individual consultant or consultant firm is contacted because of the client's prior knowledge of the consultant's reputation, expertise, or skills in a particular area.[14]

Planned, opportunistic, and uninvited methods will fail if the individual ultimately is not invited by the client to enter the system. During the phase of entry, after the potential consultant has made the initial contact with the potential client, there are other factors that should be considered, which are outlined here.

Potential for a Mutual Relationship

The consultant and client must explore the potential for developing a working relationship. This tentative relationship usually is based on the consultant's skills, interests, and values and the client's attitude and openness toward inquiry and the conducting of a needs assessment. The client, at first, may not have the ability to explain the situation clearly, truly understand the basis of the problem, or be up front about the issues. This situation requires sensitivity on the part of the consultant to perceive the client's motivation for consultation and for both to determine if there is enough mutual respect and trust to establish a relationship. Successful consultants actively involve the clients in the process and provide a common frame of reference. A technique to ensure this success is to foster mutual goal setting and clarification in initial interactions.[3, 6]

Initial Assessment of Needs

The consultant should have a discussion with the client regarding the reasons and need for help. This stage may require preliminary fact-finding and a tentative diagnosis of the system. The consultant should assess the client's willingness to comply with requests to interview groups and key individuals and to visit and observe various parts of the system.

Involvement of the client in data gathering and analysis will help lead to a successful consultation outcome.[3] The readiness of the system to accept a stranger, if the consultant is an outsider, or a peer, if the consultant is a part of the organization, should be considered. Having had a good working relationship with the client prior to a consultant relationship contributes to greater success. Knowledge of the client's interests, problems, and personality from a former interaction eliminates much of the consultant's background work, allowing the relationship to proceed at a faster rate with greater success. It is a time to get acquainted or reacquainted and to explore needs and issues that may possibly be creating problems within the system.

Readiness for Change

Exploration of the system's initial openness, its ability to tolerate intrusion, and its readiness for intervention in the specific area of need should be addressed. The consultant must assess the system's ability to accept change. Potential interactions within the organizational structure, the flexibility or inflexibility of the system, and the degree of openness in communication should be studied. The system's readiness to devote the necessary time, effort, and commitment to problem identification and the change process is important at this phase.

The success of the consultation also depends on the openness of the client in working with the consultant. When the client has no personal investment in the situation, he or she may be more open to the alternatives suggested by the consultant, without becoming threatened by new suggestions. Contributing to a feeling of openness may be the extent of the client's knowledge about the situation. Clients who do not possess prior knowledge may be less concerned, lack a vested interest, and, therefore, be more open to recommendations.

These initial contacts also provide the client with an opportunity to assess the consultant's competence, credibility, and trustworthiness. This is the time for both parties to test the potential for and explore the possible nature of the consultation activities. Some consultants and/or clients advocate a trial period to determine if there is mutual compatibility before entering into a formal contract.

Negotiation of Contract

Consideration of the important factors during entry just described help prepare consultant and client to reach considered judgments regarding a formal agreement. Development of a contract is a standard part of the consultation process. This formal agreement may be a written contract executed by both parties, a letter of agreement prepared by one party and accepted by the other, or a more casual verbal agreement.

The written contract, which we focus on here, should be a specific and detailed document that serves as a preamble describing the reason for the consultation and delineating the scope of services to be provided, method and amount of compensation, accountability provisions to protect both parties, and options for renegotiation.[19] The consultant should also keep in mind the important role the contract can play in marketing her services.

The information gathered during the entry phase regarding attitudes, skills, preliminary objectives, and working conditions will provide both parties with a realistic determination of the value of further consultation. The contract preamble will then draw from this to introduce the consultation purpose.

Preamble

After the client and consultant have been identified formally in the contract, a preamble sets the stage by presenting background information and a rationale for the consultation. Here the identified concerns and overall goals can be stated, thus assuring clarification for both consultant and client. A consultant engaged by a nursing facility to provide program development that would address specific requirements for improving resident quality of life, would, for instance, be sure the preamble included a reference to the regulations mandating change and the identified program goals. Given the nature of such consultation, the consultant also would want to provide an opening that would allow her to extend her services to other program needs should the opportunity arise.

The next section on scope of services details more specifically the nuts and bolts of the agreement. In this part of the contract, both parties should be able to define clearly the envisioned scope and extent of services.

Scope of Services

The role of the consultant and the expectations of the system or client should be mutually understood. Both parties should know the degree of time and energy each will put into the change effort and their respective responsibilities. For example, staff management and decision making are not consultant responsibilities, but staff training may be. Additionally, there should be clarification of internal and external resources and identification of the consultation target recipient.

Using information gained in preliminary discussions regarding described outcomes, goals, and objectives, the parties then are able to identify and agree on responsibilities and services. This statement may include the type of consultation to be provided, such as case, program, or educational consultation, as well as the provision of feasibility studies, needs assessments, and staff training. Each setting and client will determine the specific content of this section.

Compensation

Determining the method and amount of compensation is a key factor in negotiating a contract successfully. The consultant must determine whether she will be paid by the hour, day, or job. Will the fee include travel, telephone, secretarial costs, copying costs, and so on, or are these expenses an additional client cost?

Payment may be made on a performance basis. When this is the case, the performance criteria must be identified carefully. For instance, a consultant contracts to provide case consultation. She is to be paid per case and will evaluate patients and provide a written assessment, using a collegial consultation to the treating therapist or other specialist, who will provide ongoing services. Who decides whether the consultation service has been satisfactory? How is it measured? Performance criteria should be realistic, understandable to both parties, and measurable.

Payment for services should be spelled out clearly so that there are no misunderstandings. In some cases, a specific payment schedule is established. The consultant also may submit monthly statements or may agree to payment upon completion of particular portions of the consultation.[21]

Accountability

A good contract provides protection for client and consultant. Time frames, liability, termination, confidentiality, and the individual to whom the consultant is accountable are among the important issues.

Both parties must agree to time periods for each aspect of the consultation including expected times for completion of various phases of the work, reporting dates, and the nature of such reports. Since problems and constraints do arise, there must be specific requirements for the client as well. The consultant will require information from the client in order to move forward with the consultation.

Liability is of major concern to everyone in today's litigious society. Both parties must provide adequate insurance coverage related to the consultant's activities and interactions within the client's environment.

Options for termination also should be included. Either party may find that the other is not living up to the agreement. When considering this issue in the formation of the contract, provisions should be made for reasonable payment of consultation fees.

The contract must identify an individual within the system to whom the consultant reports. The confidential nature of this relationship must be stated clearly. This is particularly critical when the consultant's task involves work with this individual's subordinates. Information given to the consultant by subordinates may have a negative effect on the relationship with this party or may jeopardize the subordinate's job. In such cases, the consultant must be able to provide assurances of confidentiality.

Renegotiation

Contracts should be reviewed periodically and reaffirmed or renegotiated depending on the progression of the consultation. Renegotiation should be considered as the consultant moves from one role, level, or model to another. For example, a school consultant initially may be requested to provide a level I (case) consultation about a particular student, using a collaborative model with the teacher, for a specific time period. Contact with other teachers may result in involvement in the special education division of the school, leading to level II (educational) consultation. Staff in-service training may be required using an educational model. Further, the consultant's skills may be sought to help assess overall programs within the school system, leading to a level III (administrative) consultation. The consultant's role and approach will change to a program development model if she is requested, for instance, to examine the organization and structure of programs for students with special needs. If the contract is not renegotiated as the consultation progresses, there is opportunity for misunderstanding and the consultant may be perceived as having overstepped her bounds as her role expands.

In some consultation experiences, an addition or change in consultants or specific client may necessitate revising or renegotiating the contract.

Marketing

Contracts also serve as a tool in the marketing process (see Chapter 18). The methods used to establish and negotiate a contract indicate the consultant's operational policies, ethics, concerns, and perspective. The client's satisfaction and appreciation of the consultant's methodology lays the groundwork for the work at hand and for future relationships. It also acts as a networking tool. Satisfied clients share their experiences with other potential referrals, thus widening the consultant's referral base.

The contract is a key aspect of the consultation relationship and must be carefully planned and skillfully executed. As you enter the substantive phases of the consultation process, this tool acts as a guide. Sample contracts and structured formats are helpful as you begin (see Appendix D).

Diagnostic Analysis Leading to Problem Identification

The preliminary diagnostic work done in the entry phase helps to delineate the interactive structure of the system. Once the contract negotiation has been completed, a more intensive diagnosis of the system is crucial to success. During this phase there is an intensive study of the organizational structure. The internal and external trends and resources that influence the system's functioning and the corporate culture, mission, and goals of the organization are examined in detail. Chapters 2 and 3 emphasized the importance of this environmental and systems analysis.

Lippitt and Lippitt, among many others, have discussed the force-field method of diagnosis developed by Lewin in 1951, based on general system theory.[12, 14, 20] This model, shown in Figure 6-1, identifies those forces that impede movement toward current or future goals and those that facilitate progress. It is a useful tool for the consultant in the data collection and information gathering process because it can help identify the forces preventing the system or individual client from offering open access to fact-finding. Because this process may be viewed as intrusive, it is essential to assure the client and other individuals providing the information that all sources will be protected and confidences respected.

The ability of the consultant to diagnose the problem accurately within the context of the situation contributes greatly to the success of the consultation. Assessment skills should include an objective and open mind prior to diagnosis, validation of the assessment, and validation of the client's definitions of terms and roles.

FIGURE 6-1

The Force-Field Analysis Model

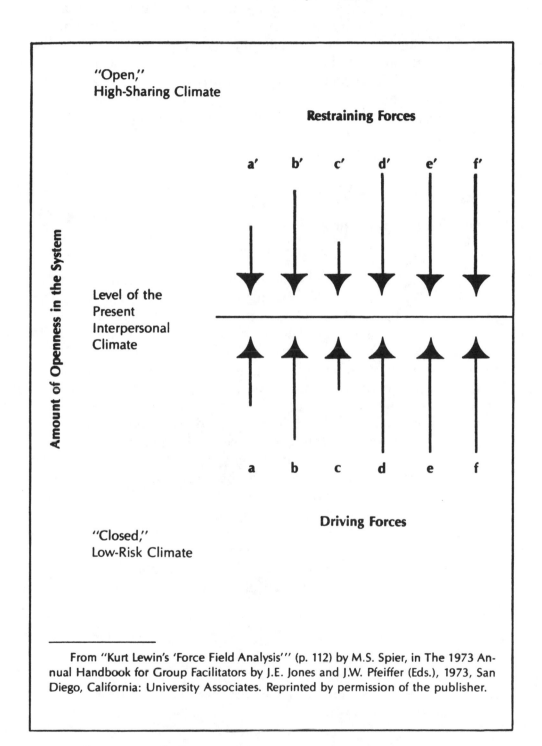

From "Kurt Lewin's 'Force Field Analysis'" (p. 112) by M.S. Spier, in The 1973 Annual Handbook for Group Facilitators by J.E. Jones and J.W. Pfeiffer (Eds.), 1973, San Diego, California: University Associates. Reprinted by permission of the publisher.

Source: Lippitt G, Lippitt R: *The Consulting Process in Action.* San Diego, University Associates, Inc, 1978, p 19. By permission of the publisher.

The diagnostic process may include a number of data gathering methodologies, including observation, interviews, records, surveys, needs assessments, questionnaires, and specially designed protocols or test instruments. In some situations, the consultant may develop the methodology and proceed independently; in others, data collection is done in teams or collaboratively with the client. The choice of data collection methods must be considered in terms of a number of variables, including the *needs* of the specific client, the *nature* of the client system, the *time* available to gather information, and the *cost* of the fact-finding methodology.[14] Usually, the consultant is responsible for the synthesis and analysis of the information, using inductive as well as deductive reasoning, to help the client system identify the basis for the problem and interpret the implications for change. Figure 6–2 details this process.

Goal Setting and Planning Through Establishment of Trust

The diagnostic process identifies the needs and problems in the system. It also helps provide the framework for the next step in the consultation process. The goal setting and planning phase of consultation requires a broad understanding of the system in which the consultation will take place. The establishment of mutual respect is a key to a successful consultation. The consultant achieves this through in-depth knowledge of the formal and informal lines of communication, awareness of the politics of the situation, identification of key power figures, and an understanding of the decision-making process that occurs in the system.

The internal consultant usually has prior knowledge of these factors and has the advantage of beginning the goal setting phase earlier than the external consultant, who must get to know the system before planning strategies. However, as we saw in our discussion of the internal and external consultant, it is important not to prejudge or skip over the data gathering phase because of inside information.

Sharing the diagnostic analysis and working in collaboration with the client to identify problems and desired outcomes helps establish the trust necessary to set meaningful goals. The consultant works with the client to determine the feasibility of attaining these goals. During these contacts, the bond of mutual trust and respect is built. The consultant should keep the following key strategies in mind when establishing trust:

- Knowledge of lines of communication
- Awareness of system politics
- Identification of key power individuals
- Understanding of the decision-making process
- Collaboration on diagnostic analysis
- Mutual identification of problems and goals

It is important that the consultant be aware of the mission and goals of the overall system. This assures that specific consultation activities do not conflict, but

FIGURE 6–2

The Diagnostic Process

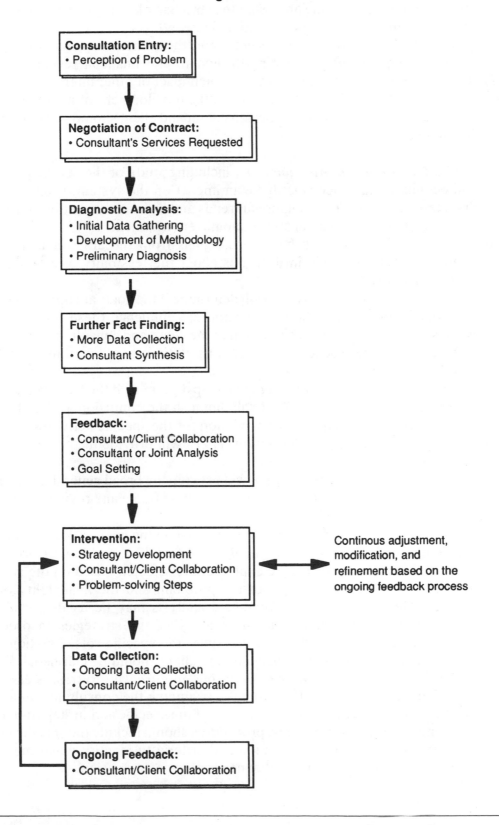

rather enhance the thrust of the organization's future development. Although the consultation focus may not be exclusively for strategic planning, all consultants can benefit from understanding and using the strategic planning process described in Chapter 2 when reaching the goal setting phase.

The projection of future goals helps determine the immediate plans. These must be considered sequentially, depending on human and financial resources; staff availability, interest, and commitment; and the impact of other internal and external influences. A brief review of the steps in the development of a strategic plan highlights the factors and sequence the consultant and client should consider in the planning and goal setting phase.

- *Environment and situation analysis,* including study of the social, political, and economic influences that have an impact on the system, is an essential first step. Local, state, and national trends and legislation must be addressed as well as the local political and economic environment.
- *Decision-making* that will link these signals from the environment to the planning process will aid in decisions about the feasibility of attaining the proposed goals.
- *Identification of strategic issues* will determine if the goals are appropriate for the organization and if the organization can influence these issues by the proposed activities. It is at this point that the client and consultant may decide if the goals can be reached and if the consultation should continue or terminate here.
- *Development of general objectives* will help determine if the basic goals of the organization are addressed. This will diminish the confusion as the planning process progresses and lay the foundation for the specific activities.
- *Development of specific program objectives* will provide the concrete, measurable steps to guide the activities.
- *Formulation of the (strategic) plan* will provide the broad general direction to the planning objectives, including a general time frame and review of existing and projected programs.
- *Formulation of an operational plan* will translate the goal setting into action, providing the detailed steps of who does what, when, and how. During this step, intervention strategies are explored and selected based on the specific needs of the client, the nature of the problem, and the availability of resources. Here also, Lewin's force-field analysis may be used to rank the issues or forces and determine the priority of the strategies in order of importance and achievability. At this time, the specific role, function, and responsibilities of both the consultant and client should be clarified.[7, 11, 14]
- *Development of an evaluation, monitoring, and tracking system* is essential at the time of planning so that from the beginning the consultant can assure that the plan is functioning effectively and if the specific action steps or tactics are achieving their purpose. The procedures should include the specific methodology and schedule of evaluation and criteria to identify when the steps have been achieved and if the plan needs change or revision.

Maintenance Phase of Intervention and Feedback

The ongoing aspect, or the actual implementation of the consultation, is considered the maintenance phase, during which a communication network should be developed. Linkages both within and without the system are essential to assure that the information received is accurate and that the consultant's perceptions are on target. During this stage the consultant uses her information to assess the hierarchical power base of the system, build and increase power blocks to facilitate the consultation activities, review internal and external alliances and resources, and gain a perspective of the supporters or detractors of the project. The consultant may need to confront resistive forces, develop alternative strategies, and provide educational activities and training for staff. This is the phase when the consultation progresses and the consultant can assume a variety of roles at different levels. In addition to educational roles, in which the consultant may provide specific training to staff or introduce broader concepts and new ideas to the client system, the consultant also may act as a mediator between subparts of the system or an advocate for the system to external agencies. Throughout the maintenance phase, the consultant must be cognizant of the internal and external environmental factors that affect the system.

Inherent in the communication network is a feedback system. The consultant, having been trained in communication skills, should develop a cognitive map, or that part of the feedback system facilitating a review of observations, perceptions, and progress. The feedback system is like an insurance policy, in that the consultant can check out her perceptions with others in the network to clarify impressions and assure that her views are shared by others in the system and that the activities are coordinated and running smoothly.[10]

The feedback system may consist of periodic reports by the consultant and staff and/or by planned feedback sessions. Eliciting feedback is an essential part of the consultant's role in the implementation phase.[14] The communication/feedback network is of ultimate importance to the success of the consultation. By listening to all cues in formal reports, feedback sessions, and casual conversation, it is possible for the consultant to ascertain concerns of the staff and the progress of the consultation activities. The consultant may become a sounding board for staff concerns, be able to assess the consequences or implications of the activities, and use this process to reexamine goals and revise strategies. The information provided to the client by the consultant must be nonjudgmental and relevant to the goals of the consultation. Figure 6–3 illustrates the continual gathering and feedback process essential to a successful consultation. The model also shows the possibility of reviewing the same problem in the various stages of the feedback process and progressing to identification of new problems that require different action.[14]

Evaluation

The ongoing feedback provides the background for the evaluation of the consultation. Monitoring and evaluation of consultant actions and outcomes of the intervention should be continuous. The evaluation process is an integral part of plan-

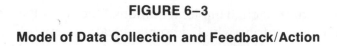

FIGURE 6–3

Model of Data Collection and Feedback/Action

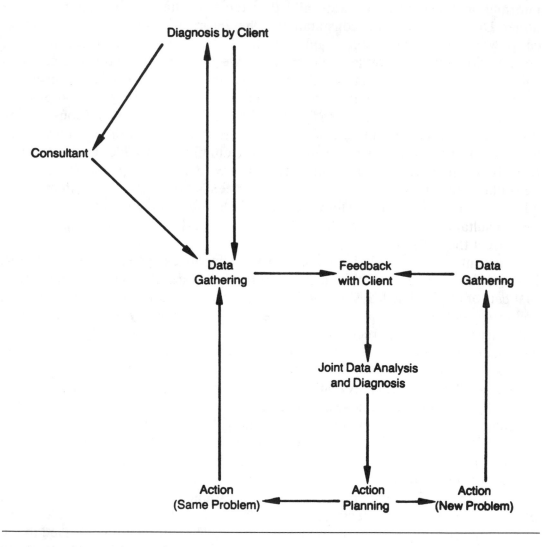

(Adapted from Lippitt G, Lippitt R: *The Consulting Process in Action.* San Diego, University Associates, Inc, 1978, p 88. By permission of the publisher.)

ning and implementation. It provides data to clarify goals, refine or revise intervention strategies, and develop future plans. Its purpose is to provide information for decision making and, to be effective, must be flexible in accommodating to changing needs.[7] Evaluation involves both *formal* and *informal* methods of assessment.

Informally, periodic observations and feedback from the staff and client system enhance the consultant's formal review. The client also may be involved in assessing activities and changes. This informal evaluation may be done independently by the consultant and client, or in collaboration with one another, or accomplished by a mix of the two methods. Periodic renegotiations or revisions of the consultant/client contract also are part of the informal consultation evaluation.

Formal evaluation may be conducted by the individual consultant, a consultant team, by the client or client system, a combination of consultant and client, or by an outside research evaluation analyst. The initial (or revised) contract should delineate evaluation responsibilities, methodology, and the schedule for evaluation. Selection of outcome measures, as discussed in the initial fact-finding techniques, is dependent on several variables: the particular *model* of consultation, the most *appropriate methodology* for the client system, *time,* and *cost* considerations. The client, who often can provide important information regarding the criteria for measuring outcomes in his system, should be involved in the initial discussion of choice of measures and the schedule for conducting the evaluation. Formal evaluation consists of data collection and analysis based on the specific outcome objectives desired from the consultation.

Information Desired
Gallessich describes several types of information useful to the evaluation process.*

- The degree to which the desired goals were reached
- The factors that contributed to both positive and negative outcomes
- Interim feedback about how an intervention is progressing
- The cost-benefit ratio of interventions
- The consultant's overall effectiveness and effectiveness in the various stages and processes of consultation

Sources of Data
Data for evaluation purposes may be collected from several places, including external as well as internal sources.

- The consultant should provide ongoing information regarding the consultation intervention strategies and activities.
- The individual client also should provide an assessment of the effectiveness of the techniques and the impact of the activities.
- Staff in the organization subparts who have been directly or indirectly affected by the consultation activities can provide both formal and informal feedback on their perceptions of the consultation activities.
- The client system as a whole, particularly administrative leadership, should assess the overall effectiveness of the consultation in terms of enhancement

---

* Gallessich J: *The Profession and Practice of Consultation.* San Francisco, Jossey-Bass Inc, 1982, p 338. By permission of the publisher.

or furtherance of the organization's missions and goals and cost-benefit to the system.

- Administrators or advisory boards of community agencies, external programs, social and other health care systems, and government officials, including legislators who may be influenced by the changes resulting from the consultation, are all very good sources of information.

Data Collection Methodology

As mentioned earlier in the diagnostic phase, information may be obtained in many ways.

Observation.—Informal, unstructured evaluation of the consultation is made through periodic observation throughout the intervention activities. More formal, objective observational instruments may be devised through flow charts and specific formats for recording observations so as to obtain baseline data and a comparison as the consultation progresses. Staff performance, individual and group behavior, and system functioning, as a result of the interventions, can be observed and recorded. The evaluator must ensure that structured observations are systematic and reliable. A disadvantage of this method is that observation of performance and behavior can be viewed as intrusive. Resentment and reaction, including the altering of behavior by the individuals being observed, may skew the results. Therefore, the consultant must be cognizant of these factors and skilled in using observation techniques.[7, 14]

Documented Organizational Reports and Records.—Review of the consultant's written reports provide information regarding progress of the activities, including barriers to overcome and changes in the system as a result of the interventions. The organization's current and archival records also may reveal considerable information about the impact of the interventions on employee status. For example, personnel demographic baseline data and changes, health benefit usage, employee absenteeism, employee accident and injury records, workers' compensation, and staff changes all provide valuable evaluation data.

Interviews.—Individual or group interviews, via telephone or in person, are useful means of assessing perceptions, attitudes, and feelings about the impact of the interventions. Additionally, because interviews are flexible tools, they may generate or elicit new ideas about problem-solving techniques. Interviewing also may be considered intrusive. Therefore, it is important to develop structured interview forms to provide quantitative data and prevent subjective distortions on the part of both interviewer and interviewee.[7, 14]

Questionnaires/Surveys/Protocols.—A most frequently used evaluation tool is a set of questions designed to elicit specific information and measure a number of variables. These may be standardized questionnaires or protocols to determine attitudes, perceptions, behavior, opinions, past history, present or projected activities, performance, and knowledge. Other questionnaires or surveys may provide demographic information, reveal trends, and be used as pre- and postinstruments for baseline and comparison data. These instruments may be standardized, providing a higher rate of reliability and validity than some other measures.

Test Instruments.—Certain specific tools may be devised for the particular consultation model and situation that provide pre- and postinformation for evaluation. These may be used to assess behavior and functional performance and also may be useful to facilitate discussion and feedback.

Termination

Actual termination preparation should begin at entry, during the development of the initial contract.[16] The preliminary goals and time frame of the consultation should be established prior to the onset of the consultation experience, preferably during the systems analysis and problem identification. If possible, these can be delineated earlier, when the consultant and client discuss the contract. Some contracts have a renegotiation clause at the end of the consultation time period built into the contract; others are of an indefinite nature and do not specify the termination point. However, the possibility of terminating the contract at any time during the consultation should always be an option for both client and consultant.

Early or Premature Termination
There are many reasons why a contract could be terminated prematurely. Most obvious is dissatisfaction with the consultation on the part of either the client or consultant or both. The consultant may be able to anticipate a rupture in the consultant/client relationship early on if there is a lack of openness in the client system that precludes access to crucial information. Additionally, the relationship may be unproductive because of a lack of mutual trust or an unwillingness to accept the necessary responsibilities to make the consultation activities work. Termination of the contract actually may help the client system redefine values and goals and encourage the consultant to be more astute in the initial entry, contract negotiation, and diagnostic analysis phases.[7, 10]

Obstacles to Termination
A long-term relationship between consultant and client may develop into mutual dependency. The consultant may prolong the consultation when in reality the work is over, and the client may fear letting go of the support and assistance provided by the consultant. The client and consultant may have formed such a strong, meaningful relationship, with considerable sharing of mutual problems and successes, that an emotional bond of personal closeness may have developed. The consultant may be ambivalent about leaving and find new problems or generate new ideas to help the client system.[7, 13]

Other obstacles to termination include the income needs of the consultant, the degree of comfort with and stability of the current work, and the desire to continue with the present client so the consultant does not have to look for other consultation contracts. The client, on the other hand, may not wish to assume the responsibilities of ultimate decision making and implementation of the consultant's suggestions.

Easing Termination

Some of the obstacles mentioned can be avoided if the consultant builds in some guidelines for herself and the client, initially and throughout the consultation. From the beginning there should be a clear understanding of the objectives of the consultation, with the intention that the client will take over when the intervention strategies are completed. Also, the client must comprehend the limits of the consultation in terms of time and function, with the client assuming the ultimate responsibility for decision making and implementation.

If the consultant progresses with activities in stages, she can transfer responsibilities to the client system and staff gradually at appropriate periods, allowing for a period of disengagement and eliminating abrupt termination. During this trial period the consultant can assess if the intervention strategies have provided enough training, modeling, and skill development to sustain changes after she has left the system. She then may be able to withdraw or reduce involvement in her activities so that the client system will gradually take over.[1, 7, 10, 16]

When the consultant and client are both comfortable ending the consultation activities, social rituals help all concerned resolve the emotional impact of termination. Final staff meetings, conferences, and social gatherings allow both consultant and members of the client system to say goodbye.[7]

Possible Renegotiation

As we mentioned, some contracts initially consider the possibility of renegotiation. Most renegotiation occurs at the conclusion of the consultation period, pending the outcome of the experience. However, sometimes there are changes in the client system that warrant renegotiation before conclusion of the consultant work, including a change in client or consultant or a change in levels of consultation, as discussed previously. Also, as a result of the consultant's findings and the evaluation of the consultation activities, it may be determined that the goals of the consultation have expanded and the contract should be renegotiated.

The basic steps or phases of consultation just described provide the foundation for all consultative activities. An understanding of these stages in the consultation process will help clarify the roles and functions of the consultant and serve as guidelines for developing the sequential steps necessary for problem identification and strategy intervention. In addition, they can assist the potential or practicing consultant in avoiding some of the pitfalls of consultation that may preclude success.

THE FOUR Ps OF CONSULTATION: POWER, POLITICS, PROBLEMS, AND PITFALLS

Power and politics are closely allied areas that influence the consultation process. In the health care arena, we think of the administrator and/or physician as keys to power, along with the director of nursing. The political infrastructure that supports and extends this network may have a far-reaching effect on the consultation.

Similarly, problems and pitfalls that have a direct impact on the client, consultant, and system will contribute significantly to the consultation's success or failure. Frequently, the precipitating consultation problem is not the issue. The underlying problem may be a sensitive and threatening area for the client. A pitfall for successful consultation will occur if the consultant is unable to discern the real issues from the stated problem or create a climate where the client can view and discuss the issues so that the consultation can proceed on target.

Keeping these four Ps in mind, the consultant can move more confidently through the process. Power, a strong and visible issue, is usually considered early in the consultation.

Power

When considering power, the consultant must recognize not only the visible players, but those beneath the surface. For instance, when consulting in a nursing facility, the gender of most key players is female. The administrator, on the other hand, is most likely a male. So it is very possible that male department heads may hold more power than their female counterparts. As the consultant reviews the organizational structure, she should keep this possibility in mind. The formal organizational lines may show all department heads at an equal level. When male gender is a factor, the informal structure may have elevated a male department head to a stronger power position.

If, for instance, the occupational therapy consultation is focusing on developing a restraint-free environment, the maintenance department, usually composed of men, must play a major role in program implementation. Should they feel negatively regarding the program, they can influence the administrator against the project. A knowledgeable consultant will recognize this important source of power and assure integration of these key persons into the planning and implementation phases.

Important power sources also may exist in less visible areas of the system, such as the volunteer arm of the organization. They usually are key members on advisory boards of organizations. Highly motivated, vocal, unpredictable, and potentially capable of quick access to regulatory and/or financial sources, volunteers can play a crucial role within the system and therefore within the consultation process.

Recognizing the many variations possible in regard to power, the successful consultant will move with care, using her diagnostic skills. Concurrently, the consultant will develop a clear understanding and awareness of the political under-currents in the setting.

Politics

Each organization has its own unique political situation, intimately related to formal and informal power sources. To analyze the political undercurrents suc-cessfully, which may have bearing on the consultation process, the consultant must develop a sensitive third eye and ear. Observing the nuances in client and system response, both to the consultant and each other, is essential. Avoidance behaviors, body language, conflicting or lack of critical information, and sudden changes in communication flow are but a few of the signs and symptoms.

If, for instance, the consultant has been engaged to help design a program that will meet new regulatory mandates and her work is viewed as a threat by the political infrastructure, this issue must be addressed first. Formal and informal opportunities must be used to help defuse and educate those involved. Similarly, a consultant may enter a system to provide case consultation for a highly motivated colleague, but the system may be very defensive. The consultant must be ready to utilize skills at consultation levels II and III (educational and administrative) on an informal basis to help achieve the goals identified for the sanctioned consultation at level I.

Building a supportive and mutually respected relationship with key power persons helps establish a strong foundation for the consultation process. Knowl-edge of the political climate and development of a smooth working relationship that is in concert with both the politics of the situation and the consultation goals should be an integral consultation strategy. Additionally, the consultant must maintain ongoing awareness of client problems and common consultation pitfalls that may have an impact on the situation.

Client Problems

Innumerable factors contribute to consultation success or failure. The client comes to the consultation process with his "baggage" and that of his "family," or system. Since the consultation may be a lengthy trip, it is important for the consultant to view the baggage closely in order to pull or smooth out problems that can interfere.

While the consultant hopes that the preliminary planning stages have clarified roles, responsibilities, and/or goals, it is possible that the client has not integrated this information successfully and during the maintenance phase has become con-fused and disruptive. When the client is not clear about his responsibilities versus those of the consultant or is uncertain about what is hoped to be gained from the consultation, the process can be halted abruptly.

Hidden Agendas

The client with a hidden agenda also poses a problem. For example, the consultant may be asked to address a specific problem in the negotiating phase and to identify possible solutions. In reality, the client has already chosen a solution. The client needs administrative support for this action and brings in the consultant to provide an objective viewpoint. In this case, the client will attempt to manipulate the consultant to assure favor for his strategy.

Unrealistic Expectations

Consultants often help resolve highly complex and difficult problems. Their reputations for "magically" solving problems precede them. New clients may expect magical solutions that do not require a heavy investment of their time and energy. The consultant must reinforce continuously the mutual involvement of all concerned when seeking resolution to the problem. The "magic" is what is created by this mutual relationship.

Resistance

Change is usually a part of the consultation process. Clients with a vested interest in maintaining the status quo may perceive the consultant as a threat and become defensive. New ideas and/or creative alternatives may be met with resistance and also may result from a lack of motivation and/or commitment. The client may be unprepared for meetings or fact-finding sessions scheduled as part of the consultation. There may be "cognitive dissonance"[3] within the client group if they perceive the consultation as a no-win situation.

Distrust

Entry into the consultation may be sabotaged unintentionally if the person or persons receiving the consultation are viewed negatively by members of the client group. This situation may be difficult to detect, requiring heightened awareness on the part of the consultant. Similarly, if the consultant was engaged specifically to implement mandated change or organizational change, the client group may display significant distrust.

These and many other client problems must be viewed and reviewed by the consultant as the process evolves. Client problems reflect one side of the coin; consultant pitfalls are seen on the other. The consultant must review the common pitfalls judiciously as she progresses through each phase of the consultation.

Consultant Pitfalls

The road to success can be detoured permanently if the consultant does not maintain awareness of potential pitfalls. Allowing personal needs and desires to override a professional manner and stance can create a negative environment. Relinquishing the objective consultation role and becoming enmeshed in the client system or misreading the system will have an adverse affect on the consultation. Most importantly, lack of consultation experience and expertise at both the task and process levels will be the final deterrent to success.[18]

Lack of Expertise and Experience

Consultation expertise has been cited as the single most important factor contributing to the success of a consultation.[3] This expertise includes knowledge of process in the particular consultation environment, expertise in specific task or technical skills related to the content of the consultation, knowledge of resources, and the ability to present a wide range of alternative solutions.

The dynamic, interactive consultation environment requires careful negotiation to avoid many obstacles. A lack of preparation, process, or content knowledge, inability to meet previously stated goals, and difficulty in communication are only a few of the common pitfalls. The consultant may view herself as the expert, when in fact her expertise is limited to the technical or task skills required for the consultation. Without the necessary process skills, she will be unable to help the client move toward a successful outcome.

For example, a consultant therapist is called in to a school for multiply handicapped children to help the related services team develop a lunchtime program emphasizing student independent eating skills. The related services team members are new to the district and have had limited experience working in schools.

Initially, the consultant uses her technical expertise to help focus the team's attention to seating and positioning issues, which are keys to functional eating skills. Concurrently, she provides resources and information regarding adaptive eating equipment. Assured by the team that they are well focused, comfortable with the technical information provided, and aware of available resources, the consultant concludes her intervention. She holds an exit meeting with the team to reinforce the information provided and allow time for any loose ends to surface.

As the clients attempt implementation, they are confronted by innumerable system blocks that neither they nor the consultant considered. A major process concern that should have been addressed was funding for the equipment and devices. The school administration considered these items to be medically, not educationally related. This important information was not communicated to the related services team until administration was asked and refused to allocate the necessary monies. Had the consultant carefully analyzed the environment and system influences, established a relationship with administration as well as the team, and clearly detailed her recommendations to the administrator, this major stumbling block would have been avoided.

Similarly, the consultant neglected to consider the role of cafeteria personnel in a lunchtime program. Issues of space reconfiguration or adaptation and the care and maintenance of special adaptive equipment required a knowledgeable and committed cafeteria staff. Lacking the commitment and understanding of this staff, the related services team again experienced failure when attempting to implement suggested strategies.

The consultant with a limited knowledge base will find herself easily frustrated, seeking cookbook solutions in situations that require creativity and flexibility. Lacking an understanding of the various models and possible roles that can be utilized in given situations, this consultant is unable to develop alternative strategies and possible solutions for her client. Misunderstanding the role of the client, misinterpretation of the expected outcomes of the consultation, a nonexistent or incomplete contract, poor follow-up, and ineffective listening and communication skills are other common pitfalls.

Listening and communication skills are central to the consultation role. When the consultant is not well prepared in this area, many pitfalls can occur. The consultant and client must define their respective roles. If the consultant lacks listening and communication skills, she may misinterpret the client role, inappropriately expecting the client to assume consultation responsibilities, or she may not respect the client's right of autonomy. She also may be afraid of rocking the boat when required to give negative feedback to the client. This fear will limit her ability to take the consultation process to its next stage, since a critical dynamic of communication is missing.

Accepting a consultation without a written contract is another major pitfall. Important communication between client and consultant may exist verbally, but both parties are at risk of misinterpreting the goals, expected outcomes, and key responsibilities if there is no formal definition.

The novice consultant can avoid many of these pitfalls through study and mentorship. Experiencing some of these pitfalls may heighten the consultant's awareness and motivate her to prepare more carefully for the next consultation experience. Other pitfalls, such as allowing personal issues to color the consultation process, can occur whether one is a novice or experienced consultant.

Allowing Personal Issues to Enter

A family crisis, physical problem, financial loss, personal relationship with client staff, or other stress can cause the consultant to deviate unconsciously from her appropriate role. While individuals each have their own method for dealing with stress, often the ability to handle routine but strategic aspects of a job are affected. The consultant must be wary of allowing these stress situations to lead to pitfalls such as not adhering to schedules or time lines, making judgments based on personal relationships rather than factual data, expanding the consultation to reap greater financial rewards, or seeking the limelight as an ego support.

In some instances, these pitfalls have ethical components. The consultant must draw on internal strengths to step back from these personal issues and look at the consultation process in an objective light. Often it is helpful to use a colleague or mentor at this juncture to guide consultant actions or act as a sounding board.

At times, the consultant may be drawn into the client system in a more personal way, so that her role as an objective facilitator is compromised. Becoming enmeshed in the client system not only reduces the consultant's effectiveness, it can bias perspective, leading to a misreading of the consultation findings.

Incorporation into the Client System

The temptation to be drawn into the client system beyond the boundaries of the consultation process may be great. Both client and consultant strive to find the "just right" relationship that allows them to maximize the consultation process. It is the consultant, however, who must monitor this status and withdraw from situations that will draw her in beyond appropriate limits. Should this pitfall occur, the consultant may find herself entering into the corporate culture in a manner that skews her relationships, findings, and effectiveness.

Once enmeshed, the consultant may become involved in the power politics of the system, unable to extricate herself to resume a more objective stance. At such a juncture, it may be necessary to bring in a consultant colleague who can help to reestablish appropriate boundaries for client and consultant.

Pitfalls are an important concern both for novice and experienced consultants. By developing an awareness of these issues, the consultant is constantly on guard, internally monitoring the status of each consultation experience. Closely related to the four Ps of consultation are regulatory, legal, and ethical issues. These areas of concern play a strategic role in the overall process of consultation.

REGULATORY, LEGAL, AND ETHICAL ISSUES

The very nature of the consultation process creates situations and interactions with regulatory, legal, and ethical implications. Legislation and public policy governing health care service delivery, as we have seen, are significant factors that drive the health care marketplace. As the consultant extends her practice into various environments, she must be knowledgeable about current regulations that affect her target markets, utilize risk management strategies to help avoid liability, and maintain an ethical stance in her consultation relationships. Chapters 38 and 39 provide an in-depth picture of these complex issues. This section focuses on some of the major concerns that affect the process of consultation.

Regulatory Issues

Health and social welfare legislation has opened multiple doors for occupational therapy service delivery and consultation in particular. As we move across the developmental spectrum, we note that growth in occupational therapy consultation services is closely linked to enabling health care legislation (the most recent example of this is the Americans With Disabilities Act [4]). Conversely, health care legislation can also be viewed as constraining. Nursing home reforms mandated by the Omnibus Reconciliation Act of 1987 were challenged by the state of California as being too costly and unwieldy to implement. Federal reviewers then restructured their interpretive guidelines to accommodate the constraints identified.[15] This continuously changing legislative scene requires that the consultant closely monitor regulatory issues in order to keep her practice current. The federal and state registers, the *Wall Street Journal* and other national papers, and topical newsletters specializing in particular aspects of health care legislation are examples of resources that can help maintain an up-to-date information base.

Regulation is multifaceted. It extends beyond federal mandates to state, local, public, and private perspectives. The consultant must be aware of regulations that emanate from third-party intermediaries, managed care groups, accreditation groups, and licensing boards.

Insurers carefully scrutinize reimbursement claims. The consultant providing case consultation may be required to complete a report for the insured party. The consultant must provide the appropriate credentials and generate a report that meets standards set by the insurer in order for the client to be paid. This is true for managed care groups also, such as health maintenance organizations (HMOs) and others.

Accreditation bodies, such as the Joint Commission on Accreditation of Health Care Organizations (JCAHO), have various professional advisory boards that help them develop standards to measure a facility's performance. Consultants providing services to such facilities must be aware of these standards and guidelines and their relation to the specific consultation problem under study.

Occupational therapy licensing boards and other state licensing mandates affecting occupational therapy practice should be part of the consultant's concern when negotiating a contract and implementing service. Should the consultant cross over to another state, she must know the law governing occupational therapy consultation practice there.

These special interest factions can play an important role in both the assessment and implementation phases of the consultation. In some cases, the regulatory bodies themselves require the expertise of an occupational therapy consultant (see examples in Chapters 31–33).

The consultation process is generally thought of as a specific, time-limited intervention. In occupational therapy, consultants often find the need for a more continuous relationship with clients because of regulatory requirements, for example in school settings and long-term care.

In these environments, the consultant's contract may call for her to perform therapist and supervisor roles. In such cases it is imperative that the contract clearly delineate the differences between these roles. This complex situation requires that the consultant understand the contrasts and parallels between consultation, supervision, and treatment.[5] She must help the client system to understand these differences, and may find it advantageous to assume some aspects of her consultation role in the stance of an internal rather than external consultant.

Legal Issues

Our litigious society has made everyone more aware of the need for careful planning and the development of practice strategies. The consultant must consider innumerable issues that may have legal implications. Therefore, she should utilize legal counsel, strategic planning, and risk management approaches to minimize and control risks.

Risk management represents the formal treatment of risk and its consequences, especially in relation to business practices and professional service delivery. The consultant must assume a proactive stance by reviewing critically all potential risks and then analyzing those that have the greatest chance for extensive loss. Such a loss would place the consultant in financial crisis, whereas manageable loss could be a factor in the implementation of a new project where risk taking is expected. Additionally, other risks related to regulatory issues such as licensure, professional standards of care, and federal, state, and local requirements must be considered.[8] Here, the consultant's technical expertise and understanding of complex regulatory issues pertaining to her practice will be of value as she considers risk factors.

From a bottom line business perspective, the consultant must manage her business operations carefully. Risks she must consider include business location and the related costs of rent, furnishings, equipment, telephones, and postage. Since the consultant's primary income is drawn from the contracts she negotiates, these also must be carefully scrutinized. Contracts should address specific risk factors, such as liability responsibilities, fee payment schedules, and penalties for late payment or default.

Liability issues are an ongoing concern. Professional liability is defined as negligent conduct on the part of a professional acting in his or her professional capacity.[17] Consumer protection, standards of care, negligence through omission or commission, and irreparable harm are trigger words commonly associated with malpractice issues. While the consultant therapist may be less likely to confront litigation, the possibility exists and should be considered a risk. Common examples can be found at all consultation levels and in various models.

Consultants frequently use their technical expertise for case consultation, for example, assessing a client's patient, designing a program for the patient in conjunction with the client, and/or training the client in specific treatment strategies. Suppose the patient suddenly experiences a seizure and falls and breaks an arm while the client is performing the program designed by the consultant? The patient had no prior history of seizures. Did the program cause the seizure? Is the consultant liable?

In educational consultation, the consultant may face other potential liabilities. For example, a consultant is called in to provide a back injury prevention training program for staff in the shipping department of a nearby firm. Upon completion of the program, all employees involved are given a written and performance test by the consultant to assure their understanding and application of the principles taught. The consultant leaves written guidelines and visual posters for the shipping room staff. A few weeks later, three employees are injured severely while lifting an oversized container designed to hold new equipment just brought on line at the company. The consultant had not addressed the specifics of lifting this container. Is she responsible for the injuries?

At times, the consultant may face regulatory issues that have liability components. For example, many states mandated reporting the abuse of a child or an institutionalized individual. If a consultant in the course of consultation has reason to believe such abuse occurred and neglects to report it, she may be held liable and could risk loss of her professional license.

In addition, the consultant may need to consider protection of specific materials, such as teaching and diagnostic tools she has created. In the course of a consultation, she may share these with the client. To protect her exclusive use of these materials, she advises the client that they are to be used only during the course of the consultation. She has not, however, copyrighted her materials. Months after the close of the consultation, the consultant finds out that the client has shared these documents with a nearby firm. Can the consultant sue?

Given these varied examples, it is obvious that the consultant needs to have legal guidance available and should obtain liability insurance. She must understand regulatory issues pertaining to her practice and maintain the professional standards of practice that govern her interventions. The policies and procedures governing her business practice must be well documented and provide specific details in regard to any and all issues with legal implications. Further discussion is found in chapters 38, 40, and 41 that deal with legal and business concerns in depth.

Ethical Issues

As the consultant moves through the process of consultation, various ethical issues will arise. Most are also closely related to legal and regulatory issues. Ethical practices are of concern to the consultant, the client, and those with whom the consultant interacts on a daily basis. Hansen, in her chapter on ethics, provides a detailed discussion. She points out that the occupational therapy code of ethics (see Appendix C) includes the role of consultant.

Multiple ethical issues can arise during the process of providing consultation. Ethical quandaries encountered by the consultant may vary to some extent in each specific setting, but the underlying ethical considerations remain the same. Our discussion focuses on four areas frequently considered as ethical concerns in a consultation practice: professional competence, confidentiality, professional relationships, and business concerns.

Professional Competence

Consultants are viewed as having expertise far beyond that of entry-level personnel. While the level of expertise will vary between individuals, the consumer/client expects the consultant to have acquired requisite knowledge and skills and to have maintained this competence through ongoing study. This requires self-discipline and allocation of monies for continuing education. The consultant may face an ethical quandary when considering the financial and personal effort required to fulfill this requirement. The constraining factors should be outweighed by the professional need for maintaining competence. The consultant must realize that her role choice demands a high level of proficiency and broader expertise.

Another quandary may arise when the consultant receives a referral in an area where she has limited competence. This may be particularly tempting for someone just beginning a practice. The client may expect all occupational therapy consultants to have the needed expertise for their particular problem, not realizing that occupational therapy consultants also have areas of specialization. If the consultant refuses the contract because she lacks the requisite expertise, she may not receive future referrals from this source. The consultant must carefully consider the ethical constraints and the consequences of refusal versus acceptance. A useful strategy may be a referral to a colleague who is more experienced and skilled in the specific area. In so doing, she has provided the referring source with the expert needed, opened a professional interchange and possible shared referral base with a colleague, and demonstrated her professional ethics to the marketplace.

Signifying professional competence and level of expertise to potential clientele may pose particular problems and ethical concerns. A master's degree in a specialty area of occupational therapy or allied field and/or recognition by professional organizations at local, state, and national levels both serve as affirmation of expertise. Awards, appointment to professional committees and task forces, and election to office provide a tangible record of the consultant's dedication and professional commitment. These experiences also infer a broader base that includes an understanding of systems and other theoretical constructs pertaining to consultation. This breadth of background contributes to the consultant's process skills.

Specialty certification, for example in pediatrics, hands, or sensory integration, offers credentials that signal higher levels of competence. Consultants who do not have these professional credits and hold themselves out as experts should be able to demonstrate significant experience in a particular area of practice and should obtain letters of recommendation from former clients.

Confidentiality

The consultant's awareness of the need for confidentiality is critical to the establishment of trust in the consultation process. This issue pervades many levels of interaction, involves professional and business considerations, and has both legal and ethical components.

During the course of a consultation the consultant may be entrusted with proprietary and confidential information regarding the client's business affairs. At times, this may include personal information. Ethically, the consultant is bound to maintain these confidences, using the information in a manner that will facilitate the consultation process without jeopardizing the trusting relationship.

Ethical quandaries may arise for the consultant if she is asked to provide consultation for a competitor. Will she bias her process with this new client, given her knowledge? If the client knows about her prior consultation, will he request that she divulge confidential information which would benefit his company? Should the consultant even consider accepting the second consultation?

Inevitably, the consultant who specializes in particular markets will find herself facing these issues. She must develop considered judgments regarding these ethical quandaries, taking into consideration the trust levels established with each client, her ability to separate and contain information from one consultation to another, and the potential for liability that must exist in each circumstance. She must set her standard of professional ethics and abide by it.

Issues of confidentiality are not limited to the client's business and personal information. A consultant may learn of strategic plans being set by her client that can benefit her personally. A merger of her client's corporation with a national health care conglomerate may create an insider position for a consultant in regard to purchase of the conglomerate's stock or the company stock. The temptation to make a quick buck may be exceedingly attractive!

Confidentiality may arise as an issue through less formal circumstances. A consultant may meet a prospective client at a dinner party. In the course of conversation, the client indicates an interest in hiring the consultant and proceeds to share some confidential information. After several subsequent contacts, made by the consultant to the prospective client, it becomes obvious that the client is not interested. Should the consultant be bound to hold the shared information as confidential? If she provides consultation to a competitor, should she use this knowledge to her contracted client's benefit?

Contracts between the consultant and client can be structured to help clarify issues of confidentiality. The contract can spell out the responsibilities of both parties regarding confidential information that arises during the course of the consultation. This may be of benefit when personnel issues are part of the consultation process. In such cases, the consultant may be reporting to the executive officer of the corporation while dealing with substantive personnel issues at a lower level that reflect negatively on the overall management style. Here, given assurances of confidentiality, subordinate personnel will feel free to share important perspectives with the consultant. This information then can be used by the consultant in a positive, nonthreatening, and ethical manner to develop change strategies that do not jeopardize the confidences given her.

Professional Relationships

Inevitably, consultation experiences require the establishment of intra- and interprofessional relationships. In some instances the consultant may be required to work along with other consultants or colleagues within her discipline to achieve the goal set by the client. In others, the consultant works closely with many different professionals, particularly when a collegial consultation model is used. Ethical quandaries arise in these relationships as well.

As discussed earlier, when the consultant is asked to wear several hats including that of consultant, therapist, and supervisor, her role is complex and the relationship often confused. For example, a consultant is contracted to provide services to a nursing facility. She is asked to provide program consultation services to the activity director, evaluation and some treatment services for patients, and supervision for the full-time occupational therapy staff. As consultant, she helps design a maintenance exercise program to be carried out by the activities staff. As therapist and supervisor she discovers that the rehabilitation department is not developing appropriate maintenance care plans for patients who are to be discharged to the new program. The rehabilitation staff have not received adequate inservice training regarding the development of such plans, and the consultant/therapist proceeds to provide inservice to the occupational therapy staff. However, the physical therapy department is opposed to receiving any instruction from the consultant/therapist. Which role is the consultant to assume in order to help overcome this resistance? Since the physical therapists now are aware of their deficient documentation skills, does this mean that they are jeopardizing the facility's compliance with regulations? Ethically, is the consultant bound to bring this problem to the administrator? Whose ethics are in question?

Business Concerns

The first ethical quandary that arises in regard to the consultant's business usually concerns fees. When establishing fees, the consultant looks at many factors that contribute to her costs, and she includes a reasonable profit margin (see Chapter 40 on developing a consultation practice). Ethical issues arise when the consultant does not develop a precise accounting of her costs, and instead meets with two other consultants who practice in the area to establish mutual fee structures. Such price fixing certainly falls into the category of unethical behavior.

Similarly, a consultant may have a long-standing relationship with a client and remain on call for him through a retainer agreement. If the consultant is called in by the client's competitor, can she ethically accept the contract, since she is still involved with the initial client? As a prudent professional, the consultant would need to discuss this issue with her long-standing clients before making a final decision.

The selected examples of ethical quandaries presented here are a small sample of those that can arise as you become involved in consultation. The knowledgeable consultant integrates her professional code of ethics into her daily professional life. She maintains self-discipline and evaluates her performance in regard to these standards, thus assuring a standard of excellence for herself and her clientele.

Regulatory, legal, and ethical issues are intimately interwoven into the consultation process. As the consultant broadens her understanding and appreciation of these important and complex issues, she will move with greater assurance and professional skill. Applying this knowledge in the practice of consultation will help the consultant establish a firm footing with clients, colleagues, and referral sources.

SUMMARY

The process of consultation involves a structured interaction between consultant and client. The basic steps include entry, contract negotiation, diagnostic analysis, goal setting and planning, maintenance or intervention phase, evaluation, termination, and possible renegotiation. Within each step, the consultant considers various options to find the right approach or strategy for a given consultation experience. These basic steps provide the foundation for all consultative activities.

The consultant's understanding and awareness of the four Ps of consultation—power, politics, problems, and pitfalls—will help her move successfully through each phase in varying consultation environments. Key power persons, the organizational structure supporting them, and the political infrastructure in a given system will have significant impact on the consultation outcome. Client problems that may be real, imagined, verbalized, hidden, clear, or confused must be analyzed astutely by the consultant throughout the consultation process. The consultant also must maintain an awareness of potential pitfalls. Personal needs, lack of objectivity, lack of experience, and expertise at task and process levels can be deterrents to consultation success. The knowledgeable consultant structures each consultation experience so that these four Ps are part of her ongoing, internal monitoring system.

Regulatory, legal, and ethical issues are the important threads in the consultation process. Working in varied environments with complex systems and multiple relationships requires a knowledgeable consultant who utilizes her professional skills to weave carefully through each new consultation experience. In so doing, the fabric of her relationships with clients, colleagues, and referral sources will be firmly established.

Effective utilization of the consultation process is the linchpin of a successful practice. It demands skillful integration of theory, principles, and technical expertise, along with an understanding of business and health care issues. It mandates ongoing study and self-discipline for each practitioner. The professional consultant will value the process, appreciate its complexities, and enjoy its rewards.

REFERENCES

1. Bell CR, Nadler L (eds): *The Client-Consultant Handbook*. Houston, Gulf, 1979.
2. Chesterton GK, in Peter LJ: *Peter's Quotations: Ideas for Our Time*. New York, Morrow, 1977.
3. Clark MJ: Factors enhancing the success of consultation. *Nurs Adm Q* 1986; 10:4.
4. Ellek D: Health policy: The Americans With Disabilities Act of 1990. *Am J Occup Ther* 1991; 45: 177.
5. Epstein CF: Consultation: Communicating and facilitating, in Bair J, Gray M (eds): *The Occupational Therapy Manager*. Rockville, Md, AOTA, 1985.
6. Ford CH: Developing a successful client-consultant relationship, in Bell CR, Nadler L (eds): *Clients and Consultants: Meeting and Exceeding Expectations* ed 2. Houston, Gulf, 1985.
7. Gallessich, J: *The Profession and Practice and Consultation*. San Francisco, Jossey-Bass, 1982.
8. Hertfelder SD, Crispen C: *Private Practice, Strategies for Success*. Rockville, Md, AOTA, 1990.
9. Jaffe EG: Consultation theory and practice. Faculty, consultation course, Department of Continuing Education, San Jose State University, 1977–1978.

10. Jaffe EG: The occupational therapist as a consultant: A model of community consultation, in Cromwell FS, Brollier C (eds): *The Occupational Therapy Manager's Survival Handbook.* New York, Haworth Press, 1989.
11. Lee RJ, Freedman AM (eds): *Consultation Skills, Reading.* Arlington, VA. NTL Institute, 1984.
12. Levinson H: *Organizational Diagnosis.* Cambridge, Harvard Univ Press, 1972
13. Lewin K: *Field Theory in Social Science.* New York, Harper & Row, 1951.
14. Lippitt G, Lippitt R: *The Consulting Process in Action.* San Diego, Univ Assoc, 1978.
15. National Citizens' Coalition for Nursing Home Reform: HCFA capitulates to California. *Quality Care Advocate.* Mar 1991, pp 1,4,6.
16. Rhodes W: Conceptual overview of behavioral consultation. Consultation course, Guest faculty, Ann Arbor, Mich, Aug 1971.
17. Roady T, Andersen W: *Professional Negligence.* Nashville, Tenn, Vanderbilt Press, 1960.
18. Shenson HL: *Complete Guide to Consulting Success.* Wilmington, Del, Enterprise, 1987.
19. Shenson HL: *Contract and Fee Setting Guide for Consultants and Professionals.* New York, Wiley, 1990.
20. von Bertalanffy L: *General System Theory.* New York, Braziller, 1968.
21. Woody RH: *Business Success in Mental Health Practice.* San Francisco, Jossey-Bass, 1989.

CHAPTER 7

Occupational Therapy Consultation Practice: An Overview

Evelyn G. Jaffe, M.P.H., O.T.R., F.A.O.T.A.
Cynthia F. Epstein, M.A., O.T.R., F.A.O.T.A.

We must go forward, but we can not kill the past in doing so, for the past is part of our identity and without our identity we are nothing.— *Carlos Fuentes*[14]

INTRODUCTION

As occupational therapists continue to respond to new and varied challenges from the health care marketplace, opportunities abound for diverse consultant roles. Public acknowledgment of the rights of all disabled individuals to equal access and opportunity has created unlimited service demands in a variety of settings.[2] Occupational therapy personnel shortages continue as a constraint in direct service delivery while legislative mandates and the escalating cost of health care services demand a more cost-effective and environmentally appropriate continuum of services. To address multiple service demands and environmental constraints effectively, occupational therapists will utilize consultation concepts and approaches with increasing frequency as we enter the 21st century.

Drawing from our historical roots in consultation, we note that early advocates of a strong consultative approach, including West, Finn, Mazer, Llorens, and Wiemer recognized the need to move out of the direct service or medical model, into a community-based, health-oriented model of consultation.* They counseled that occupational therapy's holistic view of the individuals' performance of occu-

---

* References 12, 13, 31, 36, and 47–50.

pation in a world fraught with change could be applied in the context of health promotion and the prevention of disability.[8] This indirect community service model mandated shifting the point of entry of occupational therapy practice from that of the presenting illness or disability, within a treatment or rehabilitative framework in an institutional setting, to early detection, screening, and prevention programming in the community. Consultation was the process identified as most feasible to maximize "man and mind power."[31, pviii]

Our view of occupational therapy consultation practice integrates prevention concepts with the levels of consultation we have presented. The consultant must have a thorough grounding in the principles of prevention in order to move effectively and efficiently through the consultation process. Emphasis is placed on the proactive nature of consultation, where intervention is sought before maladaptive functioning takes over. Through consultation, the client is empowered and encouraged to assume responsibility for positive action. Preventive health care and consultation are carried out in the natural environment of the consumer and both utilize an indirect service focus. The concepts of primary, secondary, and tertiary prevention flow naturally into occupational therapy consultation levels: program or administrative (level III), educational (level II), and case centered (level I). This chapter provides an in-depth discussion of this important relationship and its use in consultation practice.

Interwoven in the consultation practice process are the multiple roles and functions of the occupational therapy consultant. Occupational therapists are utilized frequently as internal consultants. Entering the consultation environment as an internal versus external consultant requires a shift in strategies and approaches. In either position, the consultant assumes multiple roles that evolve along a continuum as the consultation progresses. The consultant also may be required to assume conflicting roles and functions. The client system often needs direct intervention and/or management services as well as consultation. To assume diverse and possibly conflicting roles requires consultant and client to understand these functions and the concurrent constraints that may occur. This chapter discusses some of the diverse settings available for the practice of occupational therapy consultation and the inherent issues of status, role, and function, as well as parallels and differences that must be considered.

UTILIZING PREVENTION CONCEPTS IN CONSULTATION

As we have noted, the occupational therapy consultation literature is replete with references and discussions regarding the importance of health promotion concepts.* Study of the concepts of prevention reveals that occupational therapists traditionally practice at the *tertiary level of prevention,* developing programs to reduce the effects of further disability.[17, 23, 26, 47] The role of the occupational

---

* References 8, 12, 13, 17, 26, 27, 31, 36, 37, 47, and 48.

therapy consultant emerged with the shift from a direct treatment approach to one of planning and evaluating with others who would implement the treatment program for the specific patient.[9] This indirect model, an extension of traditional emphasis on direct patient care, resulted in a natural evolution of consultative services at the case consultation, or level I of the consultative typology. Level I is targeted at the specific client or patient, is adapted most easily from a reinterpretation of the clinical skills of the occupational therapist, and has a tertiary preventive potential.

However, the proponents of consultation as an area of occupational therapy practice in the later 1960s and early 1970s emphasized a *secondary level of prevention*. They suggested an educational approach in which the consultative activities were conducted in community settings and consisted of outreach, early diagnosis and detection, and intervention and skill building. The intent is to prevent the condition from becoming so serious that chronicity sets in. The advent of Medicare and Medicaid in 1965 also provided increasing opportunities for occupational therapy consultation for the aged in extended care facilities and home-care programs. It was suggested that the occupational therapy consultant for this identified population become an educator, evaluator, and clarifier. In this area of preventive community programming, the occupational therapy consultant provides educational consultation, or level II of the consultative typology.[7, 23] Additionally, the call for involvement in community health through program development and "advice-giving in specific areas of expertise" was sounded.[30,pix] Terms such as *participatory consulting* [13] or *action consultancy*[15, 35] were used to describe models of occupational therapy consultation in which the occupational therapist consultant "would collaborate with the community to identify its strengths and resources, its needs, and its impending dangers."[15,p130] This *primary level of prevention* refers to activities directed toward helping the client avoid malfunctions. The consultant seeks to help the client build coping strategies so that disability will not occur. Consultation is directed toward well populations and those with a potential for risk. Using educational and collaborative approaches to develop community resources, the consultant practices at level III, providing program and administrative consultation, where the preventive potential is primary in nature. The activities consist of assessment of needs, identification of community resources, collaborative education and enhancement of coping skills, and community program planning. The goal of level III consultation is to modify the environment to avoid the occurrence of malfunction or disability and to strengthen the community's ability to adapt to changes.

Merging the concepts of prevention with occupational therapy consultation practice at the various levels is congruent with the expressed goal of our profession, "enabling a person (client/system) to achieve optimum functional and adaptive performance, prevent occupational impairment, and promote health and occupational maintenance."[40] Case-centered (level I) consultation, which addresses the needs of a particular client or patient, has been utilized most frequently by practitioners. It is closely related to the traditional treatment model, and reimbursement for services has been more easily obtained. This model has been demonstrated especially in school systems, long-term care facilities, programs for the developmentally disabled and older adult, and in the use of technological approaches to enable greater personal independence.*

Today's mandate for a more holistic approach to health care, which emphasizes prevention, calls on the occupational therapy consultant to focus her entry at levels II and III of the consultation typology. As we have noted, extensive support exists for this move in the occupational therapy literature.

Llorens, as illustrated in Table 7–1, depicted a prevention model of consultative service delivery. This included entry at level II and progression to level III for health maintenance in the community, and involved community institutions, architecture, and community planning for optimal growth and development.

The concepts in these levels of consultation, level II and level III, were discussed in the occupational therapy literature of the late 1960s and 1970s. They were considered the direction for future occupational therapy practice. Izutsu called for the development of leaders that have a broad spectrum of thinking in social planning, public health principles and procedures, and health team collaboration in community-oriented settings. [22] The mandate was very clear for occupational therapists to develop new approaches, assume broader roles, and prepare for living in a different world to maintain a professional visibility and viability in the rapidly changing health care system.[48]

However, consultation, at levels II and III, was slow in receiving acceptance in the health care delivery system. Many attempts to develop community health promotion and disease prevention programs were met with resistance from politicians at all levels of government, community agencies, including schools, community members, and even health professionals, who regarded such programs as

---

* References 3, 11, 16, 33, 39, 44, and 45.

TABLE 7–1
From a Medical to a Health Care Model

Proposed Entry	Previous Entry	Proposed Follow-Through
Early detection	Illness	Health maintenance
Screening	Treatment	Programming
Prevention programming	Rehabilitation	Consultation
Consultation (Level II)	Supervision (Level I)	(Level III)

Adapted with permission from Llorens LA (ed): *Consultation in the Community: Occupational Therapy in Child Health.* Dubuque, Iowa, Kendall/Hunt, 1973, p viii.

superfluous, inexpedient, ineffective, and a waste of money.[27] Additionally, this move in the delivery of health care services was seen as a change that was interpreted by some, even occupational therapists, as against all medical tradition.

Political and economic forces in the 1970s and 1980s caused a shift from the social and health focus of President Johnson's Great Society programs of the 1960s. Federal and state monies for these previously funded health and social programs were reordered. Major government funding priorities in the 1970s and 1980s were in the areas of technology, space exploration, and defense. Monies for health promotion and disease prevention programs were limited. Occupational therapy clinicians and consultants, as well as other health personnel, had to seek positions that were reimbursable in the current health market. Treatment measures and case consultation (level I) were more readily covered by third-party payors. These activities were considered more reimbursable than educational and administrative consultation (levels II and III) efforts because outcome studies could prove effectiveness more readily than studies of the long-term effects of prevention programs.

Advice or help to develop preventive health programs and projects certainly is not new, having occurred throughout the history of civilization. Traditional consultation in health care, as seen at level I, is focused on the treatment of individuals who are ill or disabled. It is understood that prevention activities will never eliminate the need for treatment. No matter how effective we are in preventing disease, disasters, or disability, all will occur due to circumstances beyond our control. However, by giving priority to preventive activities, we may be able to reduce the incidence and severity of disease, thus also reducing the cost of treatment.[27, 34] The recent epidemic of acquired immune deficiency syndrome (AIDS) gives evidence to this fact. Although the burden of illness is still heavy, a growing body of facts relative to disease prevention has helped society open its eyes to new methods to combat disease.[18]

Wiemer, as early as 1970, long before AIDS was identified, cautioned that "intervention to prohibit occurrence of disease or lessen incidence of disability is usually exerted only upon obvious or profound hazards."[47] The preventive efforts to stem the current tidal wave from AIDS and its debilitating effects have been described in professional journals, consumer newspapers, and radio and television programs. Major publicity and health education activities related to AIDS have brought an awareness of prevention measures to the public in other areas of health as well that is unparalleled in history.[27]

Recognizing the need to deal effectively with the deep social problems that destroy health, the U.S. Surgeon General stated that most improvement in the health status of society would come about as a result not of the treatment of disease, but of the prevention of disease. In his 1979 report, he emphasized that "prevention is an idea whose time has come."[21,p7] It took business and industry, legislators, many health professionals, and society in general many years to recognize that prevention can reduce significantly the costs of disease and disability. In the last decade of the 20th century, it appears that the concept of prevention has finally arrived.

As consultants, occupational therapists can utilize their background and skills to become more involved in prevention activities and the documentation of their effectiveness. A major strength of occupational therapists is their ability to analyze situations and tasks, utilize problem-solving techniques, and employ an interdisciplinary approach. Occupational therapists are trained in the dynamics of inter-

T A B L E 7–2
Consultation Levels and Preventive Outcomes

Function ←————————————————————————————→ Dysfunction

	Level III (Primary)	Level II (Secondary)	Level I (Tertiary)
Situation	Precursors of dysfunction may exist 1. Environmental hazard 2. Socioeconomic hazard 3. Organizational change 4. Systems and individuals potentially at risk	Symptoms not apparent but problems exist Groups and individuals at risk	Symptoms apparent Groups and individuals in crisis
Status	Dysfunction/disorder not apparent Dangers reversible	Dysfunction/disorder in early stages May be reversible	Disorder or disability disrupting functioning May be irreversible
Goals	1. Modify environment (organizational restructure) 2. Build resistance to identified hazards 3. Avoid onset of malfunction 4. Motivate system/individuals to develop positive activities	1. Prevent further dysfunction/disorder 2. Outreach 3. Early intervention	1. Prevent further dysfunction 2. Rehabilitate to highest level of functioning
Methods	1. Education 2. Skill building 3. Program development 4. Administrative consultation	1. Education 2. Skill building 3. Program planning 4. Collaborative/training consultation	1. Education 2. Skill building 3. Rehabilitation 4. Case consultation

personal relationships and use these skills in their consultative activities with clients and their families, the public, and with professional colleagues. Occupational therapists' understanding of the need for analysis in planning programs enhances their ability to become involved as consultants in interagency and interdepartmental strategies. Health promotion and disease prevention activities require considerable interdisciplinary efforts, a collaborative problem-solving approach to consultation, and outcome studies to support and substantiate the impact of prevention approaches.[5, 27] Table 7–2 illustrates the goals and methods of the three levels of consultation and preventive outcomes, applicable in institutional, community, and industrial consultation settings.

The AIDS crisis, increased public exposure of child abuse in private homes and day-care centers, and the growing population of older adults have all contributed to a greater awareness of the need to develop community resources in prevention and health promotion programs through a consultative approach. Interestingly enough, it is in the field of business and industry that the concepts of prevention are being addressed most aggressively. Even in business and industry, rising workers' compensation costs have led many employers to press for new systems and programs to control injuries, thereby reducing the expense of injured employee payment settlements.[5]

In this economically driven society, where the cost-benefit ratio appears to determine all programs, corporations are seeking ways to hold down their spiraling employee health costs. With employee health care consuming over 24% of corporate income, with health costs of approximately $3,000 for every employee, industry must reduce the costs of lost worker productivity. This loss is the result of absenting related to environmental health hazards, injury, accident, stress-related disorders, and poor lifestyle habits. By the year 2000 it is estimated that health costs will increase sevenfold, resulting in costs of $10,000 per employee (see Chapter 28).

Consultation to industry has opened an ever-expanding market for occupational therapists in analysis of job activities, injury and accident prevention, and health promotion, education, and wellness programs. Recent occupational therapy literature demonstrates that not only is there interest in this type of consultation, but, most importantly, it is now considered reimbursable.*

SOCIAL POLICY AND HEALTH LEGISLATION: AN OPPORTUNITY FOR OCCUPATIONAL THERAPY CONSULTATION

The Occupational Safety and Health Administration (OSHA), established to control industrial hazards, has issued regulations related to ergonomic factors in the work environment. These standards have provided occupational therapy consultants who are knowledgeable regarding regulatory standards, policies, and procedures and who possess grounding in ergonomic analysis with an opportunity to be on the cutting edge as health and ergonomic consultants in industry.[10]

---

* References 1, 5, 6, 24, 25, 28, 29, 32, 35, 38, and 41–43.

In 1990, the Americans With Disabilities Act (ADA), Public Law 101-336, was passed prohibiting discrimination against people with disabilities. This landmark legislation requires consultants with expertise in technical assessments of places of employment, public transportation and accommodations, and telecommunications for the hearing or speech impaired—all within the purview of occupational therapy expertise. In addition, occupational therapists can develop an advocacy and advisory role as members and consultants to committees developing guidelines for implementation of the ADA in both the public and private sector.[4] In the future, occupational therapists may provide increasing consultation to lawyers interpreting the legal implication of this act, as expert witnesses or technical specialists (see Samson, Chapter 22, Kornblau, Chapter 38). This legislation is yet another example of a proactive health policy that will provide occupational therapists with opportunities to expand and redirect their clinical skills to a consultative role as they become involved at the cutting edge of service delivery.

OCCUPATIONAL THERAPY CONSULTANT ROLES AND FUNCTIONS

The multiple roles and functions of occupational therapy consultants have expanded and diversified over past decades. As health advocate, planner, and facilitator, the occupational therapy consultant helps the community understand and appreciate the important relationship between health and occupations that challenge the use of hand and mind.[47] The consultant, as an enabler, collaborates with the client to meet specific needs and seeks to influence the community at large to address health needs proactively.

Within a given setting, the occupational therapy consultant may be required to perform a broad spectrum of roles and functions. Role choice and its function in each consultation context is determined by a combination of factors. These include status of the consultant, the consultation setting, focus and duration, and issues precipitating the consultation request. The occupational therapy consultant must consider these factors when identifying specific roles and functions for each consultation.

Consultant Status

Study of the multiple roles and functions that can be assumed during occupational therapy consultation must consider consultant status. The consultant may be an internal consultant, contracted from within the client system, or an external consultant, contracted as an independent agent from outside the system. While general consultation literature has emphasized the outsider status, occupational therapy literature has identified internal consultative functions as part of the therapist's role for many years.* However, adequate clarification has not been provided to help the

---

* References 7, 19, 20, 37, 40, and 48.

therapist assume internal consultant status in a manner that allows her to perform effectively as a change agent and objective facilitator. When performing as an internal consultant, control and decision making are deferred to the client, who, in some cases, may be another employee in the system with whom the consultant has a supervisory relationship. As we noted in Chapter 4, the internal consultant is an employee of the system and has been called in to review or help resolve a particular problem or issue. When wearing the "consultant hat" she becomes an outsider to the system, as would an outside consultant entering the system to address specific issues.

Status also must be considered when the occupational therapist performs as a regulatory consultant. (See Harlock, Chapter 31). In this situation, the often repeated principle regarding decision-making power as the client's domain becomes shaded. Today's health care services are driven by reimbursement and regulation. Accrediting organizations, state and federal health care agencies, and health care insurers all utilize consultants as a part of their organizational structure. These consultants can perform internal and external functions. It is in their external function, where they perform as surveyors and consultants, that power surfaces as a factor. The nature of this consultant relationship is therefore modified.

For example, an occupational therapy consultant, as a member of an accreditation survey team, helps determine a facility's ability to meet specific standards. Her observations contribute to approval or denial of accreditation. This is her function as surveyor. However, a consultation role also is expected as part of the site visit. The consultant then may assume such roles as adviser, trainer, or diagnostician. She will, when requested, consult with rehabilitation service personnel to help resolve issues of concern that they have identified.

In order to build a relationship of trust and confidence when providing regulatory consultation, the consultant and client must discuss openly the factors of authority, influence, and control. In so doing they will clarify the issues and set the stage for effective communication.[8]

While both internal and external consultants may be qualified to address the same issues for a given client, their status creates fundamental differences in how they approach the consultation situation. It is important, therefore, to consider some advantages and disadvantages inherent in assuming the status of an internal versus external consultant. Consult the comparative Table 4–1 in Chapter 4.

Internal Consultant

Employee status provides the internal occupational therapy consultant with immediate access to information regarding the system. She is aware of formal and informal lines of communication, key power people, their personalities and style of communication, resources to speed her data collection process, and, as a person known to the system, she may be able to establish trust more quickly. On the other hand, the internal consultant must observe her own behaviors and relationships carefully in her new and changed status. Because she is within the system, her familiarity with its traditions and methodology may color her views, lessen her objectivity, and block her ability to assume the diverse roles required. Most importantly, the internal occupational therapy consultant usually is still involved as an occupational therapist within the system. Therefore, she must establish very clear demarcation lines for her consultant status, so that those in the system who have worked with her as a therapist understand her new role and can respond appropriately.

For instance, the director of occupational therapy in a community hospital is asked to consult with the personnel department about modifying job descriptions in order to comply with new regulations. These regulations require that job descriptions indicate the potential for individuals with disabilities to perform given tasks. The occupational therapist, hospital administrator, and director of personnel meet and develop a specific memorandum (contract) spelling out the parameters of the consultation, including allocation of 40% of the therapist's time to her new task. All departments in the hospital are advised by the administrator that the occupational therapy director will be providing this consultation service. However, the administrator still expects the occupational therapy department to meet its productivity levels.

In order for this internal consultant to address the demands of her job as both director of occupational therapy and internal consultant, she must develop an action plan. It should include negotiation for more therapy staff, assurance of support and cooperation from her department staff, development of open communication lines and ongoing support from key power figures in the system, and design of strategies to help hospital staff recognize her different roles.

The strategies chosen may include designated times for daily meetings with the occupational therapy staff; structured memoranda to specific department indicating when, what, where, and why she will be meeting with them; allocation of specific days for consultation versus occupational therapy status; verbal reinforcement of her status as consultant by administration at department head meetings and other facility gatherings; and the consultant's external message, conveyed by her personal appearance and manner. In the occupational therapy clinic, she may wear a lab coat or more casual clothes. As consultant, she dresses more formally, thereby giving an immediate message to the client regarding her task for the day.

The internal occupational therapy consultant also needs to pay particular attention to organizational politics. Her status gives her quick entry to the facility's upper management. This may create problems with peer department heads, who are part of her consultation agenda. She must use her observation and communication skills to monitor their responses. Additionally, she must educate them and obtain their cooperation for the task at hand.

Obviously, there are many other issues and concerns that you need to consider when assuming an internal consultation. Some of the chapters in the models of practice section present examples of the occupational therapist as an internal consultant. Utilizing key consultation concepts when assuming a dual status in your organization will help you as the internal consultant negotiate successfully through what can, at times, be very muddy water!

Occupational therapy consultants employed in one system may also be required to provide both internal and external consultation. A hospital system, for example, may need internal consultation services such as those described in the preceding example. Additionally, a community-based early intervention program may request that the hospital system assign the same occupational therapy consultant to help them meet new regulations which require changes in their transdisciplinary approach. Moving into the status of external consultant requires a shift in focus and structure.

While outside consultants appear to have a clearer path at the outset, remember that most occupational therapy consultants gained some of their early consultation experience through internal consultation tasks. These earlier experiences help you proceed with a seasoned eye in outside consultation situations.

External Consultant

The external occupational therapy consultant, an unknown quantity within the client system, initially may need more time to establish trust, lines of communication, and methodology required to obtain baseline data. However, as an outsider, she is not biased by organizational politics and structure, can provide an objective perspective to problem solving, and usually can draw from a diversity of experience in various settings.

The occupational therapy consultant frequently is invited in as an outside expert to help resolve specific issues. This status allows her to move effectively within the system, interacting with individuals at different levels and in various disciplines. Often this is particularly advantageous when there is an occupational therapy department in the client system. The consultant can facilitate and advocate for the department from a different perspective, such as handling a sensitive issue that may be blocking the department's functional ability. Using her expert status, the consultant can recommend necessary outside resources, which the client will accept more readily. Additionally, knowing that the consultation is time limited, the client and system are more focused and motivated to resolve the issue at hand.

The Consultation Setting

There are infinite occupational therapy consultation environments. Schools, long-term care facilities, acute care, community health programs, and industry are among the most familiar settings. Occupational therapy consultants also provide services in higher education programs, regulatory agencies, and technology centers. These settings and the diverse roles and functions required in each are discussed by authors in Part II.

While each consultation setting presents unique variables, the consultant must prepare to enter consultation using a set schema. This helps identify key roles and functions she must assume in the specific consultation environment.

This schema may be created as a background information form and can then be utilized as a basic part of the client's file. The information gathered should include the following:

- Initial date of contact
- Referral source (if client made the contact)
- Initial contact person and his or her position
- Authorizing person who will sanction the contract
- Stated reason for requesting consultation
- Environmental factors precipitating need
- Descriptive information regarding client system
- Mutual acquaintances for networking resources
- General information regarding similar systems
- Management and financial background data
- Support available to consultant at client site
- Possible model(s) and level(s) of service needed
- Time frame requested
- Date of initial site visit

As the consultation relationship takes form, this information will provide a guide to effective communication and more formal documentation. It will be useful in developing the contract and consultation plan and will help both parties to delineate their specific responsibilities.

Today's emphasis on cultural diversity, social advocacy, environmental protection, and fiscal management requires the occupational therapy consultant to broaden her knowledge base and enhance her skills. Neglected environments, such as prisons, Native American reservations, hospices, shelters for the homeless, crisis centers, and juvenile detention centers will benefit from the occupational therapy consultant's expertise. Currently, few occupational therapy consultants can be found collaborating in these settings or with planners in architectural, industrial, and community environments. Each of these important settings would benefit from occupational therapy consultation. With increased visibility and good marketing strategies such relationships can be more common in the future.

Focus and Duration

The specific model(s) and level(s) required in a given consultation provide the frame of reference and direction for development of the consultant roles and function. Within each model, the consultant may assume specific roles. For example, the occupational therapy consultant may be a trainer for the client colleague who is working with a head-injured patient in a community reentry program or an adviser to help a school district expand its vocational readiness program for special education high school students.

The consultation duration often affects the number and types of roles and functions the occupational therapy consultant is required to assume. When the consultant working with the community reentry program is involved as a trainer at level I, case-centered consultation, her collegial relationship usually involves training the colleague to follow a specific plan that is developed mutually and agreed upon by all parties. This is a short-term intervention. However, if the consultant follows the case and expands her consultation to other patients in the program, a long-term relationship may evolve, requiring a variety of models and higher consultation levels. In this instance, the consultant might expand into program development and systems models at levels II and III. She will use change-agent skills to help revise the program structure or assume an advocate role in order to help the program develop supportive employment opportunities in the surrounding community.

Precipitating Issues

Requests for occupational therapy consultation may be precipitated in many ways, such as a system's inability to respond to its client/employee health care needs; reaction to cited deficiencies subsequent to a state survey; or when the health care system is considering service expansion in an area related to occupational performance. In most cases, the consultant finds that the precipitating factor is the tip of the iceberg. As the consultant evaluates and diagnoses the situation, she must clarify underlying issues.

Often, occupational therapy consultation is sought to address therapy-related issues within the system. While the initial request may be addressed through consultation, underlying problems, which are related to occupational therapy service delivery, may require a more direct treatment approach. In this case, consultant and client must recognize these as discrete functions and determine the feasibility and appropriateness of assigning them to one individual.

As the occupational therapy consultant assumes various roles and functions in each consultation setting, she must have a clear understanding of the similarities and differences required to function as a consultant, supervisor, and/or treating therapist. Table 7–3 compares similarities and differences in the process of consultation, supervision, and treatment. Given the multiple demands placed on occupational therapists functioning as consultants, it is important that the consultant understand and clearly delineate these similarities and differences.

Role and Function

We have referred to many occupational therapy consultant roles and functions as we considered status, setting, focus and duration, and precipitating issues. Recognizing the diversity of descriptors available, we now discuss those roles and functions most commonly associated with occupational therapy consultation. The *Dictionary of Occupational Titles* states, "There is a commonality in (the consultant's) functions which include the need to identify, analyze, or solve a problem and recommend a solution."[46, p138] Certainly we should add the helping function to this definition since an inherent part of the occupational therapy consultant's function is to help clients make an informed choice or decision.

TABLE 7–3
Consultation, Supervision, Treatment: Similarities and Differences

Consultation	Supervision	Treatment
1. The purpose of consultation is to enable the client to work through a problem that is of concern to the client.	1. The purpose of supervision is to direct staff to do a job effectively.	1. The purpose of treatment is to resolve a problem.
2. Consultation is offered.	2. Supervision is given.	2. Treatment is both offered and given.
3. Consultation is a mutual learning and problem-solving process.	3. Supervision is a directing and instructional process.	3. Treatment is a directing/instructional, assisting process.
4. The essential characteristic of consultation is catalytic and facilitative in decision making.	4. The essential characteristic of supervision is responsibility for decision making.	4. The essential characteristic of treatment is improving individual functioning.
5. The client has the freedom to initiate, refuse, interrupt, modify, or terminate the process.	5. The process starts when the work relationship is established. The supervisee does not have the freedom to refuse, interrupt, or terminate the process as long as the work relationship exists. However, he or she may make suggestions.	5. The patient has the freedom to accept, refuse, or interrupt the treatment process.
6. The consultant may withhold consultation.	6. The supervisor may not withhold supervision.	6. The therapist may withhold treatment.
7. To be effective, the consultant must possess technical knowledge and skills that are valued by the client.	7. To be effective, the supervisor must possess technical knowledge and skills that are seen as necessary to the job by the supervisee.	7. To be effective, the therapist must possess technical knowledge and skills that are effective in the alteration of a problem.

TABLE 7-3 (*Continued*)

Consultation	Supervision	Treatment
8. The consultant must establish rapport with the client. To do this, you must have insight into your own feelings about giving consultation and about the client and be sensitive to how the client feels.	8. The supervisor must establish rapport with the supervisee. To do this, you must have insight into your own feelings about giving supervision and about the supervisee and be sensitive to how the person feels.	8. The therapist must establish rapport with the patient. You must have insight into your feelings about giving treatment and be sensitive to the patient's feelings.
9. To utilize consultation, it is necessary that the client possess some degree of skill and technical competence. Competence may be equal, even superior, to that of the consultant.	9. It is not necessary for the supervisee to possess technical or professional competence in order to utilize supervision.	9. It is not necessary for the patient to have technical professional competence to benefit from the treatment process.
10. It requires some self-confidence to give and receive consultation.	10. It requires some self-confidence to give and receive supervision.	10. It requires some self-confidence to treat and some motivation to receive treatment.
11. Consultation is adapted to the needs of the client; the consultant deals with the client's agenda.	11. Supervision is geared to the demands of the job. The extent to which the needs of the supervisee may be met are limited by the demands of the job and capabilities of those involved.	11. Treatment is adapted to the needs of the patient/client. The extent to which these needs may be met is limited by abilities of the therapist and the motivation of the patient.

Adapted with permission from Epstein, CF: Consultation: Communicating and facilitating, in Bair J, Gray M (eds): *The Occupational Therapy Manager*. Rockville, Md, AOTA, 1985, p. 308-309.

As we noted in Chapter 4, consultant roles may be viewed along a nondirective and directive continuum. While occupational therapy consultants perform roles across this continuum, those assumed with greater frequency fall into the directive model. The occupational therapy consultant is commonly sought as an information specialist, joint problem solver, trainer, and leader. As the most usual entry is at level I, case-centered consultation, these directive roles are necessary to address tertiary prevention concerns. As the consultation progress, another directive role, that of advocate, may emerge.

As we have discussed, in many cases the consultation evolves toward a more proactive and primary prevention stance at levels II and III. The consultant's roles at these levels also become less directive. These nondirective roles include observer/reflector, process counselor, and fact-finder. The consultant seeks to stimulate client growth by helping the client gain perspective and understanding for resolution of a given problem and to apply this same process to other problems. The following hypothetical case illustrates the many roles the occupational therapy consultant may assume during the course of her consultative activities regarding a specific situation.

As an *information specialist,* the occupational therapy consultant brings special expertise to the consultation environment to help the client solve a problem. For example, an adult day-care center may request occupational therapy consultation regarding services to a woman in mid-life with multiple sclerosis. The consultant may be asked to help identify appropriate environmental adaptations for this patient so that she is more functional in daily living skills while at the center. The information provided to the staff and the woman will help them make considered judgments regarding adaptations or changes that will meet her specific needs. The consultant also may provide a more direct evaluation of the woman, if appropriate. In so doing, the consultant must remember that the ultimate consultation goal is to help the center staff and their clientele learn how to cope with this and similar problems.

The consultant may encourage the clients to participate in the formulation and clarification of the problem by assuming the role of *joint problem solver.* The occupational therapist will use her technical and consultative expertise to guide and reflect ideas generated by the group. She will help them weigh various alternatives, and in so doing, provide a path that should lead to an action plan. When conflicting opinions arise, she clarifies and mediates as required.

To aid the problem resolution, the consultant may step into a *trainer* role. The focus will be education for all concerned. In the particular situation just described, the clients required a broader understanding of the many factors contributing to fatigue and increasing tremor with a diagnosis of multiple sclerosis. The day-care staff also lacked awareness of the many sensory deficits that occur in this disease process. Experiential inservice training and the provision of specific resource materials concerning the disease could be key tools used in the consultant's trainer role.

Resource information and ongoing support needs were identified by the client as a significant need. Assuming a *linker* role, the occupational therapy consultant provides information regarding support groups, national, state, and local multiple sclerosis societies, and names of other health specialists who could provide additional training in their particular areas of expertise.

As a result of these interactions, a new and important problem emerges that will require the consultant to assume an *advocate* role. The center's clientele were primarily older adults. This mid-life woman desired increased contact with other disabled adults in her cohort. She also wanted socialization opportunities in the evening. The center was available for evening activities, but none existed. Using both content and process advocacy roles, the occupational therapy consultant helps the staff, clientele, and surrounding community to mobilize around this issue to develop the desired evening program.

The evening program at the day-care center was a first for the community. A successful experience such as this may lead to consultation requests from other agencies, such as the Community Board of Social Services, to help them identify other social and recreational sites for disabled young and mid-life adults. This broader and more proactive issue will require the consultant initially to assume an *observer/reflector* role, where she will be able to help the board clarify the problem and determine strategies for change. Concurrently, in the role of *process counselor,* where consultant and client join forces to diagnose the community needs, she will work with the board in a collegial manner. Using her skills in group process and team building, she helps board members appreciate and utilize the knowledge available within their group. For example, one board member was active in the local YMCA program and identified possible interaction between the Y and the community disabled. Another member, who was an avid golfer, discovered that the pro at the community golf course was very interested in developing a golf program for physically challenged individuals. Stepping into a *fact-finder* role, the consultant develops a structured format that board members may utilize as they gather data regarding these sites. The consultant may also arrange mutually convenient times to conduct site visits with the respective board members and identify specific tasks each person would perform.

During the course of this consultation, the consultant may have assumed many of the directive roles she had utilized when providing services to the day-care program. Her understanding of each role and the skill with which she performed them helped move the consultation to a successful conclusion. The board recommended that the County Recreation Commission establish a coordinator position dedicated to the development and implementation of programs for the disabled.

Role Choice

The consultation continuum described highlights a variety of consultant roles and functions that may be required. The consultant's role repertoire is not limited to those we have discussed, as they are determined by innumerable variables. These include the consultant's skill and knowledge, frame of reference, and specific area of expertise.

Most importantly, the occupational therapy consultant must be knowledgeable regarding the similarities and differences that exist when requested to assume functions outside her domain as a consultant. To respond appropriately, she and the client must delineate and understand these differences.

Shifting consultation environments, expected outcomes, and unexpected events all contribute to the complex picture of role choice. Role selection is a process within a process. The consultant and her client must understand this concept and be comfortable with its evolutionary and changing nature.

SUMMARY

As we enter the 21st century, occupational therapy consultation practice beckons the experienced therapist. Health policy and social and health legislation, as well as traditional economic and political influences, are the driving forces that increase opportunities for occupational therapy consultation. An infinite variety of settings require the consultant's expertise and perspective. Diverse consultant roles challenge her skill and knowledge. An understanding of consultation concepts will help occupational therapists move more comfortably between the conceptual framework of their clinical skills and team treatment approach to that of an indirect collaborative model of service. Knowledge of the various roles and theoretical models of consultation and the integration of these models with that of an occupational therapy based consultation model (see Chapter 42) will provide potential and practicing consultants with the foundation to develop and expand their service delivery, maintaining a visibility in the health care system.

Recognizing and integrating prevention concepts within the levels of consultation, the consultant works in the natural environment of the consumer. Emphasis is placed on the proactive nature of consultation, where intervention is sought before maladaptive functioning takes over.

While each consultation experience presents unique demands, common factors help determine consultant roles and functions. The consultants' status, as an internal or external agent, will determine key approaches and actions taken. Major concern for the internal occupational therapy consultant is balancing the objective and nondirective consultant role with a managerial/treatment-oriented therapist role. The external consultant, while unencumbered, initially must spend more time to establish trust, communication, and baseline data.

Consultation settings are another determinant. Occupational therapy consultation services will emphasize case consultation in such settings as schools and long-term care facilities; systems consultation will be emphasized in community health environments. The consultant should utilize a set schema to obtain background information regarding the setting and presenting issue(s).

The length of the consultation and precipitating issues also must be factored in for consideration. A very important concern for occupational therapy consultants is the common request for a shift in service roles. Performing consultation, supervision, and treatment functions can be confusing for the consultant, the client (organization or facility), and those patients requiring treatment. Therefore, it is important that both consultant and client understand the differences and similarities.

Multidimensional consultant roles are viewed on a continuum, from nondirective to directive. Within the more directive roles (which are more closely allied to treatment), the roles of information specialist, joint problem solver, trainer, linker, and advocate stand out. The more nondirective roles include process counselor, observer/reflector, and process counselor.

Each consultation experience will require modification and/or adaptation of the most commonly chosen roles and functions and interjection of other roles as the situation demands. The consultant must understand that role selection is a process within a process and proceed accordingly.

"Occupational therapy as a profession needs to encourage the therapist towards the role of the consultant." [44, p4] Therapists have the specialty expertise required in many roles of a consultant, but they need to increase their knowledge and skills in the consultation process and develop the demand for their expertise.[8, 9, 26, 44] Occupational therapists should be part of the current catalysts for a changed outlook on health care. For years, community settings, including schools, social agencies, day-care centers, and industry were considered outside the traditional domain and locus of practice for occupational therapists. Consultation was thought of as a nontraditional role. We propose that the profession move from thinking of these settings and the use of consultation as a nontraditional approach to a recognition that they are inherent in occupational therapy practice. As health professionals and consultants, occupational therapists can contribute their skills in activity analysis, program planning, and interpersonal collaboration to develop ongoing techniques and strategies that will enhance health, prevent disease, and improve the social climate which fosters and promotes a healthy society.

REFERENCES

1. Allen VR: Health promotion in the office. *Am J Occup Ther* 1986; 40:764–770.
2. Americans With Disabilities Act: U.S. Pub Law 101-336, July 26, 1990.
3. Dunn W: Models of occupational therapy service provision in the school system. *Am J Occup Ther* 1988; 42:718–731.
4. Ellek D: The Americans With Disabilities Act of 1990. *Am J Occup Ther* 45:177–179.
5. Ellexson M: Personal correspondence, June 1991.
6. Elias WS, Murphy RJ: The case for health promotion programs containing health care costs. *Am J Occup Ther* 1986; 40:759–763.
7. Epstein CF: Directions in long-term care. *Gerontology Special Interest Section Newsletter* 1979; 2:4.
8. Epstein CF: Consultation: Communicating and facilitating, in Bair J, Gray M (eds): *The Occupational Therapy Manager*. Rockville, Md, AOTA, 1985.
9. Ethridge DA: Issues and trends in mental health practice: An update. *Mental Health Special Interest Section Newsletter* 1986; 9:3.
10. Falkenburg SA: Occupational therapists at the cutting edge of ergonomics. *Work Program Special Interest Section Newsletter* 1989; 3:3.
11. Ferraric: Toward autonomy: Consulting in geriatrics. *World Federation of Occupational Therapists (WFOT) Bulletin* 1988; 18:5–7.
12. Finn GL: The occupational therapist in prevention programs. *Am J Occup Ther* 1972; 26:59–66.
13. Finn GL: The children's developmental workshop, in Llorens LA (ed): *Consultation in*

the Community: Occupational Therapy in Child Health. Dubuque, Iowa, Kendall/Hunt, 1973, p 103.

14. Fuentes C in Terkel S: *The Great Divide.* New York, Pantheon Books, 1988.
15. Gillette N: Occupational therapy belongs in the community, in Llorens LA (ed): *Consultation in the Community: Occupational Therapy in Child Health.* Dubuque, Iowa, Kendall/Hunt, 1973, p 130.
16. Goldenberg K: Toronto's home-based mental health aftercare program: An exciting new model. *Special Interest Section Newsletter* 1986; 9:2.
17. Grossman J: Preventive health care and community programming. *Am J Occup Ther* 1977; 31:351–354.
18. Hamburg DA: Disease prevention: The challenge of the future. *Am J Pub Health* 1979; 679:1026.
19. Harnish SK, Schmidt DK: Developing and implementing an interdisciplinary feeding training program within a large institution: The manager's planning responsibility. *Occup Ther Health Care* 1988; 5:153–174.
20. Hartsook R, Angus GD, Bloom R: Structured job descriptions for occupational therapy. *Am J Occup Ther* 1972; 26:424–433.
21. *Healthy People: The Surgeon General's Report on Health Promotion and Disease Prevention.* U.S. Dept. HEW Public Health Service, Washington, DC, 1979, p 7.
22. Izutsu S: The changing patterns of patient care (position paper), in *Proceedings from Research Conference in Occupational Therapy and Occupational Therapy.* New York, AOTA, 1967.
23. Jackson BN: The occupational therapist as consultant to the aged. *Am J Occup Ther* 1970; 24:572–575.
24. Jacobs K (ed): *Occupational Therapy: Work Related Programs and Assessments.* Boston, Little, Brown, 1985.
25. Jacobs K (ed): From the editor. *Work: A Journal of Assessment & Rehabilitation* 1990; 1:5.
26. Jaffe EG: The role of the occupational therapist as a community consultant: Primary prevention in mental health programming. *Occup Ther Ment Health* 1980; 1:47–62.
27. Jaffe EG: Prevention, "an idea whose time has come": The role of occupational therapy in disease prevention and health promotion. *Amer J Occup Ther* 1986; 40:749–752.
28. Jaffe EG: Medical consumer education: Health promotion in the workplace, in Johnson JA, Jaffe EG (eds): *Occupational Therapy: Program Development for Health Promotion and Preventive Services.* New York, Haworth Press, 1989.
29. Kaplan LH, Burch-Minakan L: Reach out: A corporation's approach to health promotion. *Am J Occup Ther* 1986; 40:777–780.
30. Kuhn TS: *The Structure of Scientific Revolution,* ed 2. Chicago, University of Chicago Press, 1970.
31. Llorens LA (ed): *Consultation in the Community: Occupational Therapy in Child Health.* Dubuque, Iowa, Kendall/Hunt, 1973.
32. McCracken N: Conceptualizing occupational therapy's role within vocational assessment. *Work: A Journal of Assessment & Rehabilitation* 1991; 1(3):77–83.
33. McFadden SM: Private practice in mental health settings: A therapist's experience. *Special Interest Section Newsletter* 1986; 9:2.
34. Maddox GL: Modifying the social environment, in Holland WW, et al (eds): *Oxford Textbook of Public Health,* vol 2. New York, Oxford University Press, 1985, pp 19–31.
35. Maynard M: Health promotion through employee assistance programs. *Am J Occup Ther* 1986; 40:771–776.

36. Mazer JL: The occupational therapist as consultant. *Am J Occup Ther* 1969; 23:417–421.
37. Moersch M: The occupational therapist as a consultant, as a consultant, as a consultant, in Jantzen A, Anderson R, Sieg K (eds): *The Occup Therapist as Consultant to Community Agencies: Conference Proceedings*. Gainesville, Univ of Florida, College of Health Related Professions, 1975, pp 15–29.
38. Mungai A: The occupational therapist's role in employee health promotion programs. *Occup Ther Health Care* 1985/1986; 2:67–77.
39. Post KM: Seating workers with physical disabilities. *Work: A Journal of Assessment and Rehabilitation* 1990; 1(3):11–18.
40. Reed KL, Sanderson SR: *Concepts of Occupational Therapy*. Baltimore, Williams & Wilkins, 1980.
41. Schwartz RK: Prevention, in Jacobs K (ed): *Occupational Therapy: Work Related Programs and Assessments*. Boston, Little, Brown, 1985.
42. Schwartz RK: Occupational therapy in industrial accident and injury prevention. *Work Programs Special Interest Section Newsletter* 1989; 3(1):2–7.
43. Schwartz RK: Preventing the incurable. *Work: A Journal of Assessment & Rehabilitation* 1990; 1(1):12–25.
44. Tolan S: Using vocational assessment to become a consultant to the legal profession. *World Federation of Occupational Therapists (WFOT) Bulletin* 1988; 18:3–4.
45. Tomioka N: Housing consulting for the physically handicapped. *World Federation of Occupational Therapists (WFOT) Bulletin* 1988; 18:8–12.
46. U.S. Dept. of Labor: *The Dictionary of Occupational Titles,* "Consultant (Profess. & Kin) 189.167.010," Washington, DC, Author, 1981, p 138.
47. Wiemer RB: Some concepts of prevention as an aspect of community health. *Am J Occup Ther* 1972; 26:1–9.
48. West WL: The occupational therapist's changing responsibility to the community. *Am J Occup Ther* 1967; 21:312–316.
49. West WL: Professional responsibility in times of change. *Am J Occup Ther* 1968; 22:9–15.
50. West WL: Principles and process of consultation, in Llorens LA (ed), *Consultation in the Community: Occupational Therapy in Child Health,* Dubuque, Iowa, Kendall/Hunt, 1973.

PART II

Models of Occupational Therapy Consultation Practice

Chapters 8 through 37 describe a variety of occupational therapy consultative activities as practiced in multiple settings, using varying theoretical models and conducted at differing levels of consultation. These examples have been selected to demonstrate the broad range of occupational therapy consultation practice. You may compare and contrast consultant roles and functions in different settings and levels and consider the variety of intervention methodologies presented in each chapter.

Experienced occupational therapy consultants have contributed descriptions of their experiences to Part II. Within various settings there may be two styles of presentation: a shorter format that considers consultation highlights in occupational therapy practice or a longer description that utilizes a case study approach.

In general, the shorter chapters include an overview, a description of the target population and potential market in the specific area, and some key points to consider in the development of a consultation practice in the particular setting. The longer case study chapters follow a common format adapted for this text.* This consistent structure facilitates the study of a variety of occupational therapy consultative roles. The same major headings and subheadings are used throughout the case study chapters in Part II to provide a basis for comparative study. This will help you follow the basic process of consultation, which remains constant regard-

---

* The authors wish to acknowledge the source of the format, which was adapted from Cromwell, FS and Brollier, C: *The Occupational Therapy Manager's Survival Handbook* The Haworth Press, Inc., NY (1988) and Johnson, JA and Jaffe, E: *Health Promotion and Prevention Programs* The Haworth Press, Inc., NY (1989).

less of setting and despite the considerable flexibility in choice of roles, models, and levels of consultation. The major headings are as follows.

OVERVIEW

The author provides an introduction to his or her personal consultation experiences, with a description of the settings in which these consultations took place. The overview includes a short summary of the author's consultative experiences and a brief glimpse at the character of the activities.

ENVIRONMENT AND SYSTEMS INFLUENCES

The author describes the climate that fostered or precipitated the consultation. An analysis of the environmental factors, including the social, economic, and political trends or issues that affected the system, help the consultant determine the frame of reference for consultative activities.

FRAME OF REFERENCE

The specific consultative approach chosen for the models of practice is based on occupational therapy principles and theory and/or specific theoretical concepts of consultation. The frame of reference provides the consultant with the conceptual underpinnings for the analysis and the particular consultative strategies and interventions. In each case study, the contributing author identifies a frame of reference based on the theoretical constructs pertinent to his or her specific system. In some cases, more than one frame of reference may provide the basis for formulating and developing techniques and strategies.

CONSULTATION DESCRIPTION

The consultation description provides a comprehensive view of the actual consultation experience presented in case study form. The description is divided into several subheadings.

Organization

An overview and background of the organizational structure of the consultation setting, which may include an occupational therapy department, a health care facility, professional educational program, public school system, community or governmental agency, or an industrial corporation.

Support

A discussion of the financial and personnel resources and support obtained for the consultation activities, including the method of reimbursement for the consultant's services.

Participants

A description of the key individuals, including those with the power and/or authority, the target population (client system or individual client), contributing staff or team members, administrative or management personnel, and influential people, colleagues, and associates.

Services Provided

A complete description of the actual consultation intervention, including the goals, specific consultative strategies, and the process of consultation.

Outcome

The results of the consultation intervention, including a description of the evaluation methodologies and the changes that occurred in the target population.

SUMMARY

Each model of practice closes with a discussion of the conclusions drawn from this type of consultation, including the choice of strategies, program design, intervention approach, and recommendations, if any, for change or replication.

READER ORIENTATION

As descriptions of occupational therapy consultation practice, the following chapters serve as practice models to help you analyze the different situations, determine the possible scope of consultative activities, and conceptualize the many options available in designing your own practice. Each chapter has a table that summarizes the *theoretical models, levels of consultation, loci of activity,* and *goals of the consultation* described.

SECTION A

Occupational Therapy Consultation in School Settings

Since the mid-1970s, occupational therapy consultation in public and private school settings has expanded significantly. As described in the following models, legislation was the driving force that not only provided the opportunity, but mandated consultation by related services, which included occupational therapy.

Rourk describes the different roles and levels of consultation required of a consultant in a state education agency to facilitate the provision of occupational therapy services for students with disabilities. The need to understand the regulations, guidelines, and legislative mandates for related services is crucial to successful school consultation. Rourk traces the history and provisions of two of the most influential federal school acts, PL 94-142 and PL 99-457.

Dunn emphasizes a collaborative approach to case consultation for school-age children with special needs in the two case studies she presents. The focus of the consultative activities is on enhancing service provision for children within age-appropriate natural life environments. The expertise of the occupational therapy consultant is discussed in advocating for a comprehensive integration of the development of adaptive skills to the child and family's specific environmental needs.

Weiss presents an educational model for consultation in preschool programs for handicapped youngsters. The emphasis is on the enhancement of teacher communication skills through in-service training and the development of specific teaching aids.

This section concludes with a systemwide consultation description by Spencer. Administrative consultative activities are discussed that aided the development of a planning process to provide individualized transition services to secondary students with disabilities, preparing them to move more easily from the school setting to adult community life.

The following table summarizes the approach and goals for each chapter in this section.

School Settings

AUTHOR	MODEL	LEVEL	LOCUS	GOAL
Rourk	Systems	Levels II and III: Educational and administrative	Public school system	Facilitate occupational therapy services for students with disabilities
Dunn	Collegial	Level I: Case centered	Family and classroom	Support development of adaptive skills in natural child environments
Weiss	Program Development	Level II: Educational	Preschool classroom	Assist program planning by in-service training and generation of instructional material
Spencer	Program Development and Systems	Level III: Administrative	Public school system	Develop transition services planning process in three districts for secondary level special education students

CHAPTER 8

The Occupational Therapist as a State Education Agency Consultant

Jane Davis Rourk, O.T.R./L., F.A.O.T.A.

OVERVIEW

Author's Consulting Experiences

Involvement in both volunteer and employment positions provided the opportunity for the author to acquire the skills needed to be a consultant in a state agency. The earliest clinical experience was as an occupational therapist in a private psychiatric hospital and a large medical center hospital. There the caseload consisted primarily of adults and a small number of children. At the time, consultation was not recognized as a role for the occupational therapist in everyday practice. However, expertise in a clinical area is an essential component of consultation, and this work experience provided a practice knowledge that would continue to be expanded and later used in consulting situations.

Extensive hours spent in volunteer activities and leadership positions in political, church, civic, and professional organizations provided many of the personal and technical skills needed to function as a consultant. Experience gained from participating on local and state levels of the League of Women Voters helped in understanding the importance of analyzing a problem or issue and formulating possible solutions for effecting planned change. These efforts often involved working in collaborative relationships and preparing and presenting statements at public hearings or committee meetings of local governing bodies and the state legislature.

The public school system in the local community and the efforts by individuals and groups to improve the quality of public education were of particular interest. During this period, the consultant was a regular observer at meetings of the school board for the League of Women Voters, meeting with the school superintendent and other staff members to communicate concerns and share the league's ideas for solving a problem. These tasks taught the communication and listening skills that are also essential components of the consultation process. Even though it was not a deliberate education plan for becoming a consultant, the combination of professional employment and volunteer experience was good preparation for this role.

In the late 1970s, a new area of clinical practice was developing in the public schools. Public Law (PL) 94-142 (Education for All Handicapped Children Act), passed by Congress in 1975, provided a practice challenge, since it offered the opportunity to merge interest and knowledge about occupational therapy, legislation, and the public education system.

After accepting a position as an occupational therapist in a local school system, it quickly became apparent that the service delivery provisions traditionally used in medical facilities would not meet the needs of students with disabilities and educational personnel in school systems. The school therapist's role required both a direct service and a consultation component, but the latter had to be greatly expanded from the traditional role. The consultation services needed included communicating and sharing information and techniques with teachers, parents, and administrators so that occupational therapy services could be integrated into the educational program of students with special needs. Few practice models existed to use as examples for meeting the needs for occupational therapy services in the education setting. Therefore, school therapists often created new approaches to service delivery for this rapidly expanding community-based practice area.

As the consultant for occupational therapy services in the Division of Exceptional Children's Services, North Carolina Department of Public Instruction since 1978, the author has continued to augment consultation knowledge through reading, continuing education, and on-the-job training. An important part of the state consultant's role has been to assist in the establishment of policies, procedures, and best practice guidelines (relating to occupational therapy) for the division. Recommendations related to developing, implementing, and expanding efficient and effective occupational therapy services in public school systems across the state also were provided. Occupational therapists and occupational therapy assistants working in local school systems receive consultation on specific problems, such as defining occupational therapy as a related service, using models of service provision appropriately, and mediating conflicts between parents and a school system prior to the initiation of due process procedures. The original commitment was to remain in the position at least three years, but the consultant has continued longer because it has been a constant challenge. Each new request for assistance brings a fresh problem to be solved.

Levels of Consultation

The majority of consultation situations at the Department of Public Instruction fall into three major categories: student focused, therapist focused, and administration focused. As described in Chapter 2, the consultant follows a frame of reference outlined in the consultation levels of case centered, educational, and program and/or administrative. The following case descriptions illustrate these levels of the consultant's practice.

CONSULTATION DESCRIPTIONS

Student-Focused Consultation

The student-focused model is the same as case-centered consultation. The problems dealt with in this type of consultation relate to a particular student or group of students. The primary object is to provide occupational therapy services that will meet the identified needs of the student. A secondary objective is to increase the therapist's knowledge and skill so that similar situations can be managed more effectively in the future.

The initial contact with the state agency consultant regarding a specific student often comes from a telephone conversation with a school occupational therapist, the director of exceptional children, or a parent. Thus the consultant must first understand the problem from information supplied by other people. But the problem, as it is first described, is not always the primary issue. Therefore, a series of probing questions follow that help clarify the underlying issues to the problem. A visit may be scheduled by the consultant to the school system to meet with the occupational therapist, other school personnel, or parents to continue working on possible solutions. This visit can include a review of the student's records and observations of the student in the school environment. As an example: a local school system previously has shown minimal interest in providing occupational therapy services. The director of exceptional children contacts the state consultant, urgently trying to locate a therapist to provide services. This usually means that angry parents are threatening to request a due process hearing because occupational therapy services are not being provided for their child. Without the right question, or without a visit, the actual consultation needs may not be apparent.

The following examples illustrate the student-focused consultation.

1. A community agency has evaluated a preschool child with mental and physical disabilities that result in feeding problems. The child has difficulty taking in adequate calories by mouth and is chronically malnourished. After several months of hospitalization involving gastric tube feeding and occupational therapy to enhance oral feeding skills, the child returns to his home and kindergarten program. The school system does not employ an occupational therapist because no professional lives within the geographic area and recruitment outside the area has been unsuccessful. The occupational therapist treating the child in the hospital has recommended that occupational therapy be provided by the school system to maintain necessary oral feeding skills. The state consultant is asked to assist in locating occupational therapy contract services for the student while at school.

2. The director of exceptional children in a local school system asks the occupational therapist working under a contractual agreement with the district to consult each week with the teacher of a class of 15 educable mentally handicapped students (EMH) to provide gross motor and fine motor activities. The current individualized education program (IEP) for these students includes gross motor and fine motor objectives, and the director has instructed the occupational therapist to add occupational therapy to the related services listed on the IEP. The therapist contacted the state consultant regarding the need for student evaluations prior to providing consultation and the need to contact parents before changing the IEP.

3. Parents of a 9-year-old learning disabled student requested that the school occupational therapist treat their child four times a week. An occupational therapist employed in another agency had evaluated the child during the summer and had made this recommendation to the parents. It was the school therapist's opinion that the child's needs could be met by providing treatment twice a week and by incorporating related movement activities into the adaptive physical education program. The parents threatened to initiate a due process hearing if the school did not comply with their request. The occupational therapist contacted the state consultant for assistance in mediating the issue with the parents.

Therapist-Focused Consultation

In therapist-focused consultation, which is the same as educational consultation, the goal is to minimize problems that interfere with serving students. The consultant works in a collaborative relationship with the therapist to explore the problem situation and to facilitate necessary change by the therapist. The following examples illustrate therapist-focused consultation.

1. A local school system employs an occupational therapist for the first time. The therapist worked previously in the pediatric section of a large hospital. The state consultant helps the therapist interpret federal and state laws and regulations related to providing occupational therapy as a related service in schools. The consultant explains the role of the occupational therapist and the assistant in this practice setting to appropriate school personnel.

2. Parents of a 10-year-old student with cerebral palsy involving severe physical handicaps made a request for a due process hearing because they disagreed with the school system on their child's educational placement. The parents wanted a residential placement for their daughter because they did not think the school was providing an appropriate education with adequate occupational therapy, physical therapy, and speech therapy. The school system's occupational therapist requested the state consultant's help in preparing for and participating in the due process hearing.

3. An occupational therapist is employed by a school district that has employed two physical therapists for two years. After several months, the occupational therapist requests the state consultant's help to define the role of occupational therapy in this system. Clarification was needed because physical therapists were managing areas usually referred to as occupational therapy, such as feeding, fine motor skills, and adapting wheelchairs.

Administration-Focused Consultation

The questions at issue in administration-focused consultation concern therapist interaction with the school system, its organization, and its functions. Problems in this area can result in school administrators having communication, morale, and retention difficulties with their occupational therapy staff. The following examples illustrate administration-focused consultation.

1. Four occupational therapists employed by a school district each have caseloads of 60 to 70. The therapists requested that three additional therapists be employed so that caseloads would be reduced to a reasonable number. The director of exceptional children encounters resistance from the superintendent regarding the needed increase in budget. The state consultant is asked to assist the therapists in structuring their existing caseloads and to work with the director to help document the need for additional staff.

2. A large school system has eight positions for occupational therapists and four positions for occupational therapy assistants. During the past two school years, the system has had continued recruitment and retention problems. These difficulties resulted, in part, from large caseloads, noncompetitive salaries, and refusal to advertise in state and national publications. Occupational therapy staff attempts to resolve these issues with the administration were unsuccessful. The state consultant is asked to assist with finding solutions for the salary and retention problems.

3. A new director of exceptional children has been hired by a local school district that has been receiving occupational therapy services two days a week through a contract agreement with a self-employed therapist. The director wants to employ a full-time occupational therapist. The state consultant is requested to assist with conducting a needs assessment for occupational therapy services, developing a plan for establishing a program, and recruiting an occupational therapist.

ENVIRONMENT AND SYSTEMS INFLUENCES

Mandates of PL 94-142

Education has traditionally been the responsibility of state and local governments. The educational needs of children with disabilities had not been met by the nation's public schools, and many of these children had been excluded from educational opportunities. The federal government's concern about the rights of children with disabilities to an education evolved slowly until a series of federal legislation, litigation, and societal influences came together to strengthen support in Congress for education of all children.

During the 1950s and 1960s, parents became active advocates for their children with special needs, and many national support groups such as the National Association for Retarded Citizens and the Association for Children With Learning Disabilities (ACLD) were formed. These groups composed of both parents and professionals lobbied Congress and government agencies for improved health care and educational services. National leaders such as John Kennedy, Hubert Humphrey, and Lyndon Johnson used their influence to encourage changes that would correct existing inequities for individuals with disabilities.

In 1975, Public Law 94-142, the Education of the Handicapped Act (EHA), was signed into law by President Gerald Ford. This federal law mandated that all children with disabilities, aged 3 to 21, be provided with a free appropriate public education that includes special education and related services. This mandate did not include children in the 3 to 5 and 18 to 21 age brackets if services were not provided for nonhandicapped children in these age groups. The act committed federal money to help state and local education agencies provide programs to meet the educational needs of students with disabilities. States received the funds under the provisions of PL 94-142 through their state education agency, which has the responsibility of conducting annual compliance reviews of local education agencies to ensure appropriate use.[4]

The act also required the following: (1) a comprehensive evaluation before a student is considered for placement in special education; (2) an individualized education program (IEP) to describe the educational program before placement by school personnel and the child's parents; (3) students with handicaps be educated in the least restrictive environment; (4) parents or guardians be allowed to examine their child's school records; and (5) due process procedures are available to ensure that concerns of parents are considered before decisions are made.

In PL 94-142, children with handicaps were legally defined as those who are mentally retarded, hard of hearing, deaf, orthopedically impaired, other health impaired, visually handicapped, seriously emotionally disturbed, or children with specific learning disabilities who, by reason thereof, require special education and related services.[7] Special education was defined as specially designed instruction, at no cost to parents or guardians, to meet the unique needs of a handicapped child, including classroom instruction, instruction in physical education, home instruction, and instruction in hospital and institutions.[7] The act defined related services as transportation and such corrective and other supportive services (including speech pathology and audiology, psychological services, physical and occupational therapy, recreation, and medical and counseling services (except that such medical services shall be for diagnostic and evaluation purposes only) as may be required to assist a handicapped child to benefit from special education.[7]

Individual states also have passed laws to ensure that children with disabilities receive appropriate educational services. State laws may expand the services provided beyond those included in the federal law, but they may not restrict them. Occupational therapy has been included as a related service in state laws. These state and federal legislative mandates have contributed to the rapidly expanding employment of occupational therapists and occupational therapy assistants by school systems.

Mandates of PL 99-457

Public Law 99-457 passed in 1986 by the Congress revises and expands PL 94-142. It was authorized for five years. The act extended the mandate of Part B of PL 94-142 for special education and related services to all preschool children, ages 3 to 5. An important distinction for the preschool age group is that states can provide for them without having to use categorical eligibility criteria. There are many positive reasons for not identifying children at this early age by handicapping condition such as orthopedically impaired or learning disabled. Many local communities currently have nonpublic preschool programs for this age group. State education agencies are encouraged to contract with them to continue providing services when appropriate. Occupational therapy remains a related service for the 3- to 5-year-olds, which means that they must qualify for special education before being eligible for occupational therapy services.

PL 99-457 also established a new Part H—Handicapped Infants and Toddlers Program—for handicapped and at-risk children from birth to their third birthday and their families. If a state chose to participate in this program, the governor had to designate a lead agency to develop and oversee the statewide program and to administer the necessary funds. The act committed federal funds to assist states with planning and implementing early intervention programs and for training qualified personnel.

A second requirement was that an interagency coordinating council, composed of parents, service providers, state legislators, state agency representatives, and others was to be appointed by the governor to assist the lead agency in developing policies, establishing timetables, and defining eligibility criteria.

Part H lists special education, occupational therapy, audiology, speech/language pathology, psychology, physical therapy, social work, nursing, nutrition, and medicine as core components of early intervention programs. Occupational therapy is considered a primary service for the birth to age 3 group and can be provided apart from special education.

PL 99-457 recognized the importance of considering the individual needs of children at this young age in the context of the family and the environment. Parents have an important role in the development of their child. Services that assist parents in acquiring the knowledge and skills necessary to fulfill this role are considered allowable services under this legislation.[6]

Each child receiving these early intervention services must have a multidisciplinary assessment and an individualized family service plan (IFSP) written by the multidisciplinary team and the child's parents. The IFSP must include among other items (1) a statement of the child's present level of development, (2) a statement of the family's strengths and needs related to enhancing the child's development, and (3) a statement of major outcomes expected.[5] It should be reviewed and updated at least every six months and more frequently if appropriate.

University and State Education Agency Collaboration

In 1971, the Developmental Disabilities Council of the North Carolina Department of Human Resources, whose membership included an occupational therapist and a physical therapist, began examining the role of health care professionals in educational settings. This study resulted in three occupational therapists and three physical therapists being employed by school systems in the mid-1970s. This was an early commitment by the state to meet the special needs of students with disabilities. However, these programs experienced minimum growth until the federal mandate was passed in 1975.

When the North Carolina legislature passed Chapter 927 of the 1977 Sessions Laws, it brought the state into compliance with the requirements of PL 94-142. The state education agency had begun to consider how it would identify and provide the occupational and physical therapy services required by these new federal and state laws.

At the same time, many occupational and physical therapists working in clinical settings and in the professional education programs were becoming aware of the vast implications these laws and regulations would have on the future practice of the two professions. There was concern that therapy programs in the public schools be developed properly so that students with disabilities would have their individual needs met. Additionally, there was concern that there would be sufficient qualified therapists to provide the services.

In 1977, a partnership was established between the Department of Medical Allied Health Professions, School of Medicine at the University of North Carolina at Chapel Hill, and the Division of Exceptional Children's Services, North Carolina Department of Public Instruction. This partnership continues as a productive and successful working relationship. An essential first step was communicating information concerning the professional education and standards of practice of occupational and physical therapists, since the agency staff had minimal knowledge and experience regarding health care professionals.

Faculty members from the divisions of occupational therapy and physical therapy at the university spent several months negotiating a contract with the director of the division of exceptional children's services for an occupational therapist and a physical therapist to work as consultants with the division's staff. Appendix D contains a sample of the contract. The state education agency was to provide the university with funds from PL 94-142 (EHA Title VI-B) allocations to recruit and employ one occupational therapist, one physical therapist, and one secretary. The university agreed to provide office space and equipment for the project, and the two therapists were given clinical faculty appointments in their respective divisions. Being employed by the university and having the office on campus permitted the consultants frequent access to the occupational and physical therapy faculties, students, and university resources. The consultants participated in university-related activities including teaching modules of established courses, presenting individual lectures, conducting seminars, supervising students in independent study projects and fieldwork, serving on committees, and participating in faculty meetings. These activities provided opportunities for communication with faculty and students regarding therapy services in school systems. The consultants discussed the emerging role of occupational and physical therapy as a related service in schools and the growing need for therapists with the occupational therapy and physical therapy faculties. Suggestions were made for modifications in course content and clinical fieldwork that would better prepare students for employment in public schools. However, effective communication between the consultants and other staff of the division of exceptional children's services was more difficult to maintain because the offices were not located in the same building.

The major responsibility of the consultants was assisting the division of exceptional children's services. Initial activities included studying state and federal laws and regulations that could effect provision of occupational and physical therapy services in schools, becoming familiar with the organizational structure and operation of the state education agency, conducting a statewide needs assessment of therapy services, and presenting recommendations for developing, implementing, managing, and expanding therapy services for students with special needs.

The consultants provided information to both state and local educational personnel, parents, and staff of referring health care programs regarding the role and function of occupational and physical therapists and assistants in schools. Information also was presented including the need for integration of related services into special education programs, recruitment of therapists, with appropriate salary and fringe benefits, and the licensure laws, standards of practice, and codes of ethics under which they must practice. The consultants worked closely with directors of exceptional children and superintendents in local school systems. These interactions resulted in valuable support of the state consultants and the use of therapy services.

FRAMES OF REFERENCE

The frame of reference for consultants in state education agencies may follow different models and levels of consultation and involve various roles depending on the specific services required by the consultee.

Generalist Model versus Specialist Model

The state education agency in each state has a number of options for providing information and other services to its local school systems. Two models frequently used by state education agencies are the generalist model of consultation and the specialist model. There are advantages and disadvantages associated with both models. A generalist consultant can be responsible for more areas overall, but cannot function in the role of expert or information provider as effectively as a specialist consultant. Additionally, the generalist primarily uses the consultation process to facilitate solving problems, rather than developing specialized knowledge and skill in the consultee.

If an agency selects the specialist model, employing consultants who have acknowledged expertise in a specific area, a larger staff may be required to have consultants in each of the areas that school systems identify as needing assistance. The disadvantage of this model is that a larger personnel budget may be required. Therefore, the generalist model is used by the majority of state education agencies.

Working in a state agency that uses consultants with expert knowledge in a special content area, the author has found that the consultation process is more effective when a consultant has the technical knowledge and experience in the specific area for which she is responsible. This is especially true in the fields of special education and related services specified in PL 94-142, such as occupational therapy, physical therapy, speech therapy, and audiology. These therapeutic services, which have been provided traditionally in medical facilities, are specialized clinical areas that require consultants who can recommend the necessary technical advice and information needed in school systems. For example, clinical expertise in occupational therapy enables a consultant to recognize undeveloped subskills such as balance reactions, in-hand manipulation, or size discrimination that may interfere with a student's ability to perform tasks in the educational setting. An educator/consultant does not have adequate knowledge of occupational therapy theory or practice to analyze the specific deficits in subskills and to offer constructive recommendations.

Internal and External Consultative Models

A consultant in a state education agency must function simultaneously in both the internal and external consultative models. As an internal consultant, the individual works closely with the other consultants in the division developing position papers, policies and procedures, and recommendations for the delivery of special education and related services for students with disabilities, and planning and conducting statewide continuing education programs. For example, if the division of exceptional children's services issues or changes procedures for providing driver education for students with handicaps, the consultant for occupational therapy services might recommend which areas should be included in the evaluation, thereby determining if a student can learn the necessary skills to be a safe driver. The consultant may also assist with developing courses and instructional methods for the students enrolled in driver education.

As an external consultant one may be invited by local school systems to help the local school occupational therapist or occupational therapy assistant, director of exceptional children, or other administrators with specific problems. These could include recruitment and retention of occupational therapy staff, the state performance appraisal process, or the development of criteria for students to receive occupational therapy. The consultees in the local system may become involved in the consultation process voluntarily. The state consultant functions in an advisory capacity and has no direct responsibility or authority for the acceptance and implementation of recommendations. However, a state consultant often is perceived to have administrative authority when the request for assistance comes from the school superintendent, director of exceptional children, or other administrator.[2] Because the state education agency conducts annual compliance monitoring of federal and state standards and the use of funds, the consultee in a local education agency does not always feel free to reject the consultant's advice about implementing procedures required in the agency's regulations. This often creates ambivalence on the part of the consultee that may interfere with the effectiveness of the consultation process.

Dimensions of the Consultant's Role

A consultant in a state education agency functions in a multiplicity of roles depending on the problems that have been identified. The consultant may function in one or more of these different roles while providing consultation.[3] The roles include clinical specialist, problem solver, resource person, and teacher. Brief descriptions of each of these roles follows.

Clinical Specialist

The state consultant, utilizing clinical expertise, assists school occupational therapists to problem-solve questions related to the occupational therapy needs of specific students. The goal is to increase the consultee's knowledge and experience for dealing with similar situations in the future while simultaneously finding a solution to the student's problem. In some situations, all that is needed is support and reassurance from the consultant that what is being done for a student is appropriate. This is particularly important to therapists who work in isolated settings. A clinical specialist must have current knowledge about research, education, environmental trends, and procedures related to the practice of occupational therapy.

Problem Solver

To define a problem clearly and develop alternative solutions, the consultant uses good interview skills and asks questions that will ferret out additional pertinent information. The consultant works in collaboration with the consultee to select and analyze possible solutions for the problem.

Resource Person

Locating information on a variety of subject matters needed by individuals or agencies is an important role. Requests include assessment tools for blind-deaf students, advertising sources for occupational therapist positions, and appropriate activities to improve handwriting skills for developmentally delayed students. The state consultant seeks new and improved resources so that a variety of choices can be recommended.

Teacher

Sharing information with occupational therapists, occupational therapy assistants, and other education personnel on a formal and informal basis helps expand their knowledge and skill. Examples include demonstrating assessment and intervention procedures while visiting a classroom and conducting a statewide workshop to teach IEP goal writing skills to occupational therapists.

CONSULTATION DESCRIPTION

Organization

Planning Effective Use of Consultation

Careful advanced preparation by both consultant and consultee make the consultation process more successful. As a state consultant, it is important to become acquainted with a local school system before starting to work with the superintendent or staff. Copies of correspondence and compliance monitoring reports on file with the state education agency are reviewed. Additional information is collected by talking with other state consultants who have worked with the system and staff at the regional education center which includes that system.

The individual(s) from the local school system, requesting the consultation services, should define the problem and manner in which it is thought that the state consultant can be helpful. Compiling a list of questions for clarification helps to focus the process on the primary concern.[2]

Case Study Example: Student-Focused Consultation

During an IEP meeting, the parents of an 8-year, 7-month-old female disagreed with the school's recommendations for the provision of occupational and physical therapy services for the following school year. The evaluation results showed that the student had a three-year delay in motor skills, major communication problems, and a mild to moderate delay in all cognitive areas. Gross and fine motor skills were functional. The occupational therapist had used the following evaluation methods: Peabody Developmental Motor Scales, Developmental Test of Visual Motor Integration, Test of Visual Motor Skills, and clinical observations. Occupational therapy intervention during the past school year had focused on improving visual motor skills, fine motor skills especially prewriting, and self-care skills. The recommendations included providing occupational therapy treatment for 45 minutes once a week and providing physical therapy through consultation with the occupational therapist and the teacher. The parents were demanding occupational and physical therapy for 30 minutes each once weekly. When agreement could not be reached, the director of exceptional children invited the occupational and physical therapy consultants from the division of exceptional children's services to review the student's records and provide recommendations.

Support

The state education agency provides the services of all the program consultants and other agency staff to local school systems at no cost. A local system contacts the individual consultant and arranges for the needed assistance.

Participants

The student's parents, the director of exceptional children for the local school district, the child's special education teacher, and the state occupational and physical therapy consultants all participated. The director of exceptional children was the primary consultee during the process and the state occupational therapy consultant served as the primary consultant. The majority of the communication was between these two individuals.

Services Provided

Following the IEP meeting, the director of exceptional children telephoned the state occupational therapy consultant to discuss the issues and arrange a meeting. Since these two individuals had previously established a good working relationship, there was a free exchange of information. It was apparent that the parents did not trust the local school system. They expressed satisfaction with the therapy services that their child had been receiving. However, they were annoyed that physical therapy services had been terminated 2 months earlier without using the proper procedures. They expressed their concern that the physical therapist had made the recommendation for consultation services the following year based on administrative reasons, rather than the special needs of the student based on evaluation results. The parents requested that neither of the state consultants talk with the school therapists involved prior to presenting their recommendations. The state occupational therapy consultant did not think that this was a reasonable request, since it was important to have information from the therapists who had evaluated and treated the student during the school year. After several telephone conversations, the parents agreed that the state consultants could talk with the school therapists, but requested that they not attend the meeting. There were several telephone conversations between the state consultants and the school therapists to clarify issues and recommendations for IEP goals and objectives.

On the appointed day, the state consultants met with the director of exceptional children and the child's special education teacher for several hours to discuss the problems and to review the student's educational records, including the IEP. Later in the day there was a meeting with the parents. The state consultants observed the student during play and viewed a videotape made by the parents when she was 2 and 3 years old.

The consultants told the parents that based on the information they had available to them, they supported the continuation of occupational therapy services on a weekly basis, with consultation from the physical therapist not less than once a grading period for the next school year. The consultation services needed to be more frequent at the beginning of school to ensure that the student was functioning as anticipated. The parents stated their concern that this plan would not be adequate, but, after more discussion, agreed to consider it. The group agreed to meet again in a month to reach agreement on the IEP.

At the second meeting, many of the same issues were discussed. The parents finally agreed to sign the IEP after several amendments were made clarifying the amount of intervention. It was decided that 3 months after the beginning of school the group would meet again to review the student's progress and evaluate the effectiveness of the program. The parents agreed to allow the school therapists to attend this next meeting.

Outcome

When the group met to review the student's therapy programs and progress, it was decided that the student's needs in the educational environment were being met appropriately. Some progress had been made in her self-help skills and pre-writing skills such as maturing hand grasp, cutting, and tracing. The parents were assured that the therapy programs could be modified again if the student's needs changed. The parents involved in the consultation process were intelligent, articulate individuals. They become stronger advocates for occupational therapy services and the school system because they were active participants in the development of solutions to meet their child's related service needs. The fact that the student's skills and ability to function in school improved while receiving the recommended services probably contributed to the parents' acceptance of the plan.

SUMMARY

The consultation component of the school therapist's role continues to be an important one. It requires an occupational therapist with clinical expertise in pediatrics, knowledge of the legislative mandates for related services such as occupational therapy, and good problem-solving and communication skills. This chapter discussed the different roles of a consultant in a state education agency.

A variety of situations are described in which an occupational therapist in a state consultant's position works with therapists and school administrators to facilitate the provision of occupational therapy services for students with disabilities. More occupational therapists should be employed in state and national agencies that establish policies and procedures influencing the practice of occupational therapy.

REFERENCES

1. American Occupational Therapy Association: *Guidelines for Occupational Therapy Services in School Systems,* ed 2. Rockville, Md, Author, 1989.
2. Kadushin A: *Consultation in Social Work.* New York, Columbia Univ Press, 1977.
3. Lange FC: *The Nurse as an Individual, Group, Community Consultant.* Norwalk, Appleton-Century Crofts, 1986.
4. Mopsik SI, Agard JA (eds): *An Education Handbook for Parents of Handicapped Children.* Cambridge, Brookline Books, 1985.
5. Smith BJ: *P.L. 99-457 The New Law.* Written handout for Chapel Hill Training Outreach Project, 1987.
6. Szanton ES: Perspective: A new day for infants and young children. *Infants and Young Children* 1988;1:5–8.
7. The Council for Exceptional Children: *Public Law 94-142 and Section 504. Understanding What They Are and Are Not.* Reston, Va, Author, 1977.

CHAPTER 9

Occupational Therapy Collaborative Consultation in Schools

Winnie Dunn, Ph.D., O.T.R., F.A.O.T.A.

OVERVIEW

Service provision in pediatrics broadened considerably in the last two decades. The enactment of Public Law 94-142 and more recently Public Law 99-457 introduced new service environments for pediatric occupational therapists. Prior to this time, children were more likely to be seen in hospitals, clinics, and residential facilities. Now it is more common for children to be served in their natural life environments—their homes, schools, and day-care centers.[2] As therapists have spent more time observing and intervening within these natural environments, different needs have become apparent. Therapeutic expertise must now be applied directly to many self-care, learning, work, and leisure situations. Direct services address only a portion of the needs of children, other professionals, and family members; therapists must consider a wider range of service provision options to meet this broader range of needs. The introduction of consultation as a viable service provision option enables therapists to create more effective living and learning environments on behalf of children.

Consultative services are designed to enable others to meet their expressed goals. Occupational therapists use their professional skills in early intervention and school programs to enable parents, teachers, other professionals, and extended family members to become more effective at dealing with their children's needs. Each of these persons has a unique focus within specific children's lives, a focus that the occupational therapist must be ready to address.

Prior Consultation Experiences

The author has served as an occupational therapist within a variety of school and community programs for children birth to 21 years and their families since 1973. Early experiences were within suburban and rural school programs, but also included provision of consultative services in urban school districts. The author has collaborated with program administrators, classroom and special education teachers, other occupational therapists, physical therapists, speech pathologists, parents, and extended family members. Additionally, she has consulted with persons at state departments of education in various states.

Philosophy

There are several underlying philosophical principles that guide the author's personal approach to consultation. First, although consultation is a very effective intervention strategy, it is only one service provision option. Service provision models are chosen because of their ability to meet a need effectively; there is no other reason to choose one.[3] Consultation takes as much time as direct services, so time shortages cannot be a reason for choosing consultation. Direct service is an effective choice for establishing new patterns of performance. Consultation is the more effective choice for situations that require generalization of skills to life demands, task or materials adaptation, or which will be enhanced from other adults being taught a procedure or technique.[4]

Children with special needs generally process information differently than other children. It is not useful to presume that they will generalize skills to new situations without support.[10] These children also need many opportunities to practice before behaviors become part of the performance repertoire. It is unlikely that they will have sufficient opportunities to practice in 60 minutes of direct services per week. Therefore, therapists must apply interventions that facilitate more practice opportunities within naturally occurring activities throughout the day. Consultation techniques can also effectively extend direct service and facilitate its generalization to natural life environments.

Collaborative consultation is the most preferred style of school consultation.[9] The shared responsibility and partnership is a mutually satisfying and growth experience. Occupational therapists have many areas of expertise that are useful to others; collaborative relationships provide a mechanism for applying these specialized skills to children's and families' needs. Dunn[3] conducted a study comparing direct service and consultation provided to preschoolers, and found that both groups of children attained the same number of overall IEP goals, but that teachers who collaborated with therapists in consultation reported that occupational therapists contributed to 24% more of the overall IEP goals. The contribution reported expanded beyond their original targets of gross motor, fine motor, and self-help skills to include socioemotional development, cognitive, and language skills.

Case Studies

Two case studies are presented in this chapter. The first case involved an infant and family who sought the help of a community-based early intervention program to obtain assistance with feeding and socialization strategies. The second case involved a school-aged child who received services through the special education system in his school district. Each case illustrates the core principles of collaborative consultation, but present unique considerations that need to be made in specific situations.

ENVIRONMENT AND SYSTEMS INFLUENCES

Public Policy

In 1975, Congress enacted Public Law 94-142, the Education of the Handicapped Act.[6] This law states that all children have the right to an education, and that school districts have the responsibility to provide a free, appropriate public education to everyone. Occupational therapy is designated as a related service in this law; this means that occupational therapy is provided for those children who need these services to profit from their educational experiences. All services within school-based programs must be educationally related. Therefore, therapists who work in these settings must understand the educational demands of the environment and construct interventions that are compatible with educational needs.

Public Law 99-457[7] is more recent legislation that affects pediatric practice. This law extends the school-aged services to preschoolers, and designates services for infants, toddlers (birth through 2 years), and their families. Occupational therapy can be provided as an individual service or along with other needed services for the infants and toddlers. Family-focused intervention necessitates addressing needs in relation to the family priorities. Therapists must therefore provide expertise that will improve the family's ability to deal with their child.

Historical Evolution

In the 1960s, professionals and parents focused their energy on deinstitutionalizing individuals who had special needs. They believed that persons would be more successful in smaller, community-based service programs, rather than in large, segregated institutions. Community-based services and programming are now the norm rather than the exception. Now professionals and families are seeking to establish services that fully integrate individuals with special needs with typical individuals in age-appropriate learning, work, living, and leisure situations.[1, 10] We now believe that it is essential to ensure access to natural life experiences if we expect individuals with special needs to function as independently as possible when they grow to adulthood. This priority challenges professionals to address specific needs in relation to natural expectations and outcomes and minimizes an artificial approach to intervention services.

With the expectation that pediatric services address an individual's ability to function within age-appropriate life tasks, parents, other professionals, and administrators have become more aware of the need for adult interactions. Without ongoing adult interactions and problem solving, services for children can become irrelevant and artificial.

FRAME OF REFERENCE

Service provision is a complex process; the therapist must create an intervention plan that addresses an individual's particular needs within appropriate life tasks. A wide range of service provision options are available to the occupational therapist to better match the needs and the services.[4] The referral concerns usually frame the performance areas that need to be addressed (activities of daily living, work, play/leisure). The occupational therapist identifies those performance components that are either enabling or interfering with functional outcomes.[5] The therapist also records contextual variables that may contribute to or block functional performance. After the therapist identifies the level of interference of each problem area,[4] she then has the following options:

1. Provide no services, because functional performance exists;
2. Make recommendations for other community services;
3. Adapt tasks, materials, equipment;
4. Adapt posture or movement demands;
5. Teach an adult to carry out a procedure or technique;
6. Supervise an adult who carries out a procedure or technique;
7. Provide direct intervention.

In the preceding list, 3 through 7 are considered intervention options. Options 3, 4, and 5 are considered consultation, option 6 is monitoring, and intervention 7 is direct service.[4]

The organizational psychology, school psychology, and special education literature contain extensive discussion about the theories, models, and features of consultation.[11] Collaborative consultation is advocated by many of the researchers and theorists who are trying to apply consultative constructs to school-based issues.

Idol, Paolucci-Whitcomb, and Nevin[9, p1] define collaborative consultation for special education in the following manner:

Collaborative consultation is an interactive process that enables teams of people with diverse expertise to generate creative solutions to mutually defined problems. The outcome is enhanced, altered and produces solutions that are different from those that the individual team member would produce independently. The major outcome of collaborative consultation is to provide comprehensive and effective programs for students with special needs within the most appropriate context, thereby enabling them to achieve maximum constructive interaction with their nonhandicapped peers.

There are several advantages to a collaborative model of consultation. Collaboration in schools focuses on ongoing communication among team members and joint problem solving within the team, acknowledging the unique contributions and shared responsibility of each discipline. It has the potential of being a mutual growth experience for the collaborators while addressing student needs. This model also focuses on needs and functional outcomes for students, which is the primary purpose of school programs.

Additional features of consultation also guide implementation. Collaborators make decisions based on data collected about the student's functional performance; reinforcement mechanisms are built into the plans that are designed; situational leadership is used to guide program implementation; conflict resolution occurs based on mutual commitment to a common goal; and effective communication strategies are applied by all members at all times.[8]

CONSULTATION DESCRIPTION

- *Case 1:* Marilyn*
- C.A.: 5 months
- Diagnosis: Down syndrome

Organization

Marilyn's parents initially contacted the community early intervention program because of a recommendation from other parents in their support group, which they had been attending since Marilyn's birth. Marilyn is their third child (Karla is 5 years; Vince is 3 years); they wanted to make sure that they did everything possible to facilitate Marilyn's development within their family structure. Extended family members lived within the same community and were also requesting information about interacting with Marilyn.

The community early intervention program is an extension of the county and state developmental disabilities programs. This program receives referrals directly from families, other professionals, or other programs within the county. The program's mission is to provide services for families whose children have already been identified as at risk for developmental delays or who have a problem that is

---

* Names of individuals in this chapter are fictitious.

already interfering with their development. (When persons contact this program to obtain a diagnostic evaluation, they are referred to either the developmental disabilities regional center for the county or to the community children's hospital diagnostic teams.) Program staff include an occupational therapist, physical therapist, speech/language pathologist, social worker, nutrition specialist, and developmental psychologist. Medical consultation is provided by the family's pediatrician and pediatric specialists (e.g., neurology, orthopedics) from the community children's hospital staff.

Support

Services of this community early intervention program are supported by state funds, some of which are available through federal initiatives. Developmental disabilities monies are available through the mental health/mental retardation state budgets, which are renegotiated each year. The Department of Health provides funds through the crippled children's services of the state. This program is also involved with the state Interagency Coordinating Council, which is planning for the full implementation of PL 99-457 activities for infants, toddlers, and their families. Families are eligible for the services based on state identification criteria; although a sliding payment scale is part of the financial structure of the program, many families with limited resources receive services at no charge.

Participants

The primary participants in Marilyn's case were the parents and the occupational therapist. Marilyn's sister and brother also participated in the activities, and occasionally extended family members, such as grandparents, participated as well. The occupational therapist consulted with the speech/language pathologist to maximize her knowledge about the communication issues that would impact this service provision situation.

Services Provided

After the parents made the initial contact, the social worker conducted an interview to obtain a pertinent history and more detailed information about their concerns. He then brought this information to the team to identify the best professionals to serve Marilyn and her family. Since the family's questions centered on eating and socialization, the team decided that the occupational therapist, the speech/language pathologist, and the parents would comprise the intervention team. The occupational therapist would serve as the case manager and would have the regular contacts with the family, with support provided through collaboration with the speech/language pathologist.

The occupational therapist set up a home visit with Marilyn's family. The parents felt that this would provide a more accurate picture of Marilyn's functional performance, and the therapist wanted an opportunity to become familiar with the home environment. She planned to arrive during a play time and stay through the next feeding. The therapist primarily used skilled observation and parent interview to record data; she also conducted an oral motor exam and evaluated postural and reflex development to determine if these factors would contribute to or block Marilyn's functional performance. Analysis of information suggested that family members very much wanted to include Marilyn in family activities. Marilyn was willing to interact with her siblings and parents, but tired easily. She would initially arouse to their voices or faces and smile, but then would collapse, not being able to hold her head in position to keep them in view. She was attempting to reach for objects, but also had difficulty maintaining those movements. Marilyn's sister and brother interpreted her behavior as lack of interest and would then discontinue their play attempts. Her father commented that she seemed to do better when they held her up in their arms. He used a lot of movement when he demonstrated holding her in this way. During mealtime, Marilyn sucked on her bottle, but took frequent breaks. Mom was introducing cereal, and she had to pour spoon contents into Marilyn's mouth because Marilyn had trouble closing her lips around the spoon. She continued to encourage Marilyn throughout mealtime.

The therapist discussed her observations with the parents during their visit. She then summarized her findings and data from the diagnostic team using the Functional Skills Assessment Grid[4] (see Figure 9–1.) Since the parents were concerned with the socialization and eating, evaluation findings were considered within these contexts. As can be seen, several performance components were influencing or interfering with Marilyn's functional performance in eating and socialization. The therapist then considered the intervention options that would match this pattern of needs and the family's style. Table 9–1 provides a format for considering the level of interference of a problem in relation to the type of intervention that would be appropriate to provide. In Marilyn's case, the therapist decided that it would be helpful to adapt posture and movement, teach the parents some specific techniques (consultation strategies), and supervise the parents in other, more complex techniques (monitoring strategy).

The occupational therapist met with the speech/language pathologist to identify specific activities and strategies that would facilitate the communicative aspects of the family's interactions with Marilyn. Then she met with the parents to formulate the intervention plan (see Figure 9–2). The intervention plan describes the focus of the intervention, its purpose, and the parameters for implementation and evaluation to determine effectiveness. The parents and therapist agreed to meet once a week for the first 3 months to establish their routine. They met in the family home after school hours so the siblings could be present; the parents made changes in their work schedules to accommodate this time.

The therapist and parents began with simple alterations in positioning and handling. The therapist also strongly reinforced the skills the parents had already

FIGURE 9-1

Functional Skills Assessment Grid for Occupational and Physical Therapy Services

Marilyn

Program Outcome	Performance Components	NA	0	1	2	3	Comments
Learning: Skill Acquisition and Academics*	1 Manipulation/hand use						
	2 Interpretation of body senses						
	3 Perceptual skills organization of space and time						
	interpretation of visual stimuli						
	4 Cognitive skills problem solving						
	generalization of learning						
	5 Attending skills						
	6 Use of assistive and adaptive devices						
	7 Mgmt of body positions during learning						
	8 Mgmt of body positions during transitions						
	9 Movement within learning environment						

(continued on next page)

FIGURE 9–1 (Continued)

Category	#	Item							Notes
Work*	1	Mgmt of body positions during work							
	2	Mgmt of body positions during transitions							
	3	Movement within work environment							
	4	Manipulation/hand use							
	5	Use of assistive and adaptive devices							
Play/Leisure*	1	Mgmt body position during play/leisure							
	2	Mgmt body position during transitions							
	3	Movement within play/leisure environment							
	4	Manipulation/hand use							
	5	Use of assistive and adaptive devices							
Communication*	1	Oral motor movements							Note: socialization and eating problems noted in play also affect communication as Marilyn grows.
	2	Communication access							
	3	Manipulation/hand use							
	4	Mgmt body position during communication							
	5	Movement w/in communication environment							
	6	Attending skills							
	7	Perceptual skills							
	8	Use of assistive and adaptive devices							Observe this area carefully.

Socialization*			NA	0	1	2	3	
	1	Self-esteem	X					
	2	Recognition and use of nonverbal cues		X				
	3	Mgmt body position during socialization		X				
	4	Movement within social environment			X			
	5	Attending skills			X			
	6	Perceptual skills	X					to be evaluated later
	7	Cognitive skills	X					to be evaluated later
Activities of Daily Living*	1	Oral motor movements			X			
	2	Mgmt of body position during ADL		X				
	3	Movement within daily living environment		X				
	4	Attending skills			X			
	5	Manipulation/hand use		X				

* When acquiring new skills, use the Learning: Skill Acquisition section of this grid.

NA—No problems are identified in therapy evaluation

0—Although a problem has been identified through evaluation, it is not presently interfering with program outcome(s). Needs may be met by self, parents, or professionals in other programs or agencies.

1—The problem *influences* successful program outcome(s); simple instructional or environmental changes are likely to result in functional performance.

2—The problem *interferes* with specific program outcome(s); specific strategies are necessary to enable functional performance.

3—The problem *prevents* successful program outcome(s); multifaceted strategies are necessary to reach functional performance.

Dunn & Campbell (1988)

Dunn W, Campbell P: Designing pediatric service provision. in Dunn W (ed): *Pediatric Occupational Therapy: Facilitating Effective Service Provision*. Thorofare, NJ, SLACK Inc, 1991. (Form used with permission; student information pertains to this text.)

TABLE 9–1
Severity of Problems to be Addressed by Occupational and Physical Therapists

Through interview and observation, the therapist will create a hypothesis about how the problem is interfering with learning and will determine an assessment plan to confirm this hypothesis.

In collaboration with the team, the therapist will determine which level of interference is created by the problem(s). If documented evidence is available that the individual's behavior is currently interfering with his or her ability to benefit from therapist, the team reconvenes to reestablish priorities and create a new plan.

Rating	Parameter Definition	No Interv.	Consultation				Monitor	Direct Service
			Make Recommendations	Adapt Task Matls. Environ.	Adapt Posture Mvmt.	Tch. Adult	Spvs. Adult	Use Therapist Admin. Strategies
NA	No problems are identified in therapy evaluation.	X						
0	Although the problem has been identified through evaluation, it is not presently interfering with the program outcome(s). Needs may be met by self, parents, or professionals in other programs or agencies.		X					

#						
1	The problem *influences* successful program outcome(s); simple instructional or environmental changes are likely to result in functional performance.		X	X	X	
2	The problem *interferes* with specific program outcome(s); specific strategies are necessary to enable functional performance.	X	X	X	X	**
3	The problem *prevents* successful program outcome(s); multifaceted strategies are necessary to reach functional performance.	X	X	X	X	**

** This level of service is
1. Only provided in conjunction with other levels of service (e.g., adaptation, supervision).
2. Only chosen if ONLY the therapist can provide the intervention safely.
3. Provided as part of the life environment unless the intervention interferes with age-appropriate tasks.

Dunn W, Campbell P: Designing pediatric service provision, in W. Dunn (ed): *Pediatric Occupational Therapy: Facilitating Effective Service Provision.* Thorofare, NJ, SLACK, Inc, 1991, used with permission.

acquired through their own experimentation, such as Dad's holding and bouncing technique to keep Marilyn engaged in an activity with a sibling. For example, she recommended more frequent use of supported sitting to make it easier for Marilyn to interact with others; she would expend less effort holding herself up, and would therefore be able to interact longer. They also discussed techniques to increase Marilyn's muscle tone in order to support eating and more active interaction with the environment. The therapist would guide the parents through the techniques with Marilyn and explain the purpose of the technique so the parents would understand the critical features of the task. They would then practice with the therapist present in order to receive feedback. The next week they would demonstrate their skills again and ask questions; the therapist would use these opportunities to increase the complexity of some activities and reinforce their skills on other activities. They also practiced sibling interactions, cuing the children about better strategies when playing with Marilyn.

Outcome

After the initial three-month period, the parents and therapist agreed that they would invite extended family members to every other visit. This broadened the family's options by enabling others to feel confident in their handling of Marilyn, and the extended family members felt more comfortable learning what to do from the therapist than from the parents. After Marilyn's first birthday, a bimonthly visit schedule was established, and the therapist and parents shifted their focus to include mobility in play and total communication. The speech/language pathologist became involved with the family to introduce both vocal and sign language.

After Marilyn turned 2 years of age, the parents expressed concern about her contact with peers. The therapists suggested a center-based early intervention and preschool program that served both children with disabilities and typical children. This program also provided family support in the form of educational groups and consultative services and had frequent family get-togethers at the school (such as potluck dinners, picnics, and visits from Santa and the Easter Bunny). The professionals from the early intervention program provided records for this program and met with the staff to help plan Marilyn's next developmental experiences.

FIGURE 9–2

Intervention Plan

Child's Name: <u>Marilyn</u>   Date: _____

                                 Birthdate: _____

Agency Name: _____   Chron. Age: __0__ yrs. __5__ mo.

Outcome Statement: <u>Marilyn will eat independently. Marilyn will</u>
<u>interact with family members in age-appropriate ways.</u>

Outcome Category: _____ Learning   _____ Work
                  _____ Play/Leisure   _____ Communication
                  __X__ Socialization   __X__ ADL (eating)

Performance Components:

    ENABLING COMPONENTS: CONCERNS:

    <u>self-esteem</u>   <u>postural control</u>

    <u>initiation of attention</u>   <u>muscle tone</u>

    _____   <u>activity tolerance/endurance</u>

    _____   _____

Service Provision Models:

_____ Direct*   __X__ Monitoring   __X__ Consultation
                     _____ supervise adult __X__ teach adult
                                             __X__ adapt posture/mvmt
                                             _____ adapt task/matls
                                             _____ adapt environ

* Provided in conjunction with one or more other service models

_____ DIRECT   __X__ n.a.

__X__ MONITORING   _____ n.a.

(continued on next page)

FIGURE 9–2 (Continued)

Target Objective: Marilyn will eat independently.

Intervention
Approach: _____ remed. _____ compens. ___X___ prevent-interv.

   Describe: provide opportunities and support

   so Marilyn can develop needed skills.

Location of Services: family home

Intervention Procedures: supervise parents in oral motor facilitation
and jaw control procedures for eating.

Implementor: _____ teacher ___X___ family _____ aide _____
other: _____

Training and Verification Strategies: parents will perform technique while
therapist observes; parents will demonstrate technique one week after
it has been initiated in Marilyn's program.

Proposed
Meeting Schedule: ___X___ weekly _____ bimonthly _____ monthly

Location of meeting: family home

Method for Documentation of Performance:

   behavior to be observed: eating cereal from a spoon

   natural environment for observation: family kitchen

measurement/data to be collected: <u>number of spoonfuls obtained</u>

criterion for successful performance: <u>Marilyn will use her upper</u>

<u>lip to scrape the cereal from the spoon at least five times during</u>

<u>a meal.</u>

<u> X </u> CONSULTATION <u>   </u> n.a.

Area of Concern: <u>a. Socialization; b. Activities of Daily Living –</u>

<u>eating</u>

Identified by: <u>Mr. and Mrs.   </u> role: <u>parents   </u>

Statement of Area to be Addressed: <u>a. Marilyn will interact with family</u>

<u>members; b. Marilyn will eat independently.</u>

Location of Services: <u>family home</u>

Strategies: <u>teach parents about oral motor control; adapt seat for</u>
<u>Marilyn and explain its importance for placing Marilyn in optimum</u>
<u>positions for eating and interacting; teach parents about the</u>
<u>importance of working on postural control and endurance separately</u>
<u>from working on eating and socializing. Assist them in establishing a</u>
<u>family routine which balances all components of Marilyn's needs and</u>
<u>their family style.</u>

Proposed
Meeting Schedule: <u> X </u> weekly <u>   </u> bimonthly <u>   </u> monthly

(continued on next page)

FIGURE 9–2 (*Continued*)

Location of meeting: family home

Method for Documentation of Performance: a. Socialization

behavior to be observed: Marilyn's interactions with others

natural environment for observation: family home

measurement/data to be collected: number of responses Marilyn
produces.

criterion for successful performance: Marilyn will respond to sibling
interactions with eye contact and either a smile, vocalization,
or reach at least 10 times in a 3–minute period of play.

Method for Documentation of Performance: b. eating

behavior to be observed: eating cereal from a spoon

natural environment for observation: family kitchen

measurement/data to be collected: number of spoonfuls obtained

criterion for successful performance: Marilyn will use her upper
lip to scrape the cereal from the spoon at least five times
during a meal.

Dunn W, Campbell P: Designing pediatric service provision, in Dunn W (ed): *Pediatric Occupational Therapy: Facilitating Effective Service Provision.* Thorofare, NJ, SLACK, Inc, 1991. Used with permission.

CONSULTATION DESCRIPTION

- *Case 2:* Benjamin
- C.A.: 10 years
- Diagnosis: learning disability

Organization

Ben was diagnosed as learning disabled when he was in the first grade. He was in the fourth grade at his neighborhood public school at the time of the consultation. During his primary school years, he spent most of his school day in a self-contained classroom for students with learning disabilities. He also received occupational therapy as a related service. The educational team decided Ben had made significant progress and that it would be appropriate for him to enter the fourth grade in a regular classroom. After completing the reevaluation, the team identified that Ben would continue to need support from the learning disabilities specialist and the occupational therapist in order to make this new placement successful. Ben produced written work at a slower rate than others his age, was somewhat clumsy in his movements, and sometimes had trouble maintaining attention for the length of time necessary to complete tasks at the fourth grade level. He had demonstrated the ability to comprehend and utilize information at this level when these other variables were controlled or adapted.

The school district provided occupational therapy services through a contract with the local hospital. The same pediatric occupational therapist had been providing services to this school district for 5 years, and therefore had served Ben since the beginning of his school career.

Support

The school district uses local education funds and federal special education monies to support the provision of occupational therapy services. The special education administrator of the school district met with the director of rehabilitation services at the hospital to create the contract. They discussed the school district's needs and the hospital's financial requirements. The school district estimated that they needed a therapist 1½ days per week, but acknowledged that it was difficult to determine the exact amount of professional time they needed without a therapist on the teams. Due to this lack of information, they wanted the option to increase the amount of services if necessary. The hospital asked for an hourly rate to cover the therapist's salary and benefits, and requested a mileage rate to cover the therapist's travel to various schools. They discussed whether the hourly rate applied only to services provided to children, or whether it included meetings and travel time.

Since both parties were committed to providing comprehensive services, the hourly rate would have to be higher if it were only applied to service time in order to ensure adequate compensation. They decided to use a smaller hourly rate and charge for actual time spent, and they negotiated that the school district would pay the therapist directly for her mileage, using the district's mileage rate. They agreed that the hospital administrator would meet with the occupational therapy department regarding this proposal and would have one of the therapists contact the school administrator to make further arrangements.

The occupational therapy staff and director of rehabilitation services discussed the need to shift their focus when they provided services within the school district. It would be important to remember that the role of the occupational therapist within the public schools was a related service. It was posible the therapist would identify needs during evaluations that were not related to the student's ability to perform in school. Therefore, the administrator and the occupational therapists made a commitment to inform families of their findings and provide them with options for addressing these needs outside the public school. When the therapist met with the special education director, she restated this commitment, and was supported by the special education director and the school district's philosophy and scope of service.

Participants

The actual consultation in Ben's case included the occupational therapist, the classroom teacher, the physical educator, and the learning disabilities specialist. As just described, the administrators of the two agencies supported the service provision process by providing the mechanism to allow the therapist to work in the school system. Additionally, the school principal provided support by ensuring that the teachers and therapists had a place to meet and arranging for class coverage when necessary to work on Ben's program.

Services Provided

As Ben was completing the third grade, the team met to determine his needs for the next school year. As stated previously, the team determined that occupational therapy and learning disabilities services would be needed to support Ben, but that he could succeed in the regular classroom for the fourth grade. During the first and second grades, the occupational therapist used direct service and consultation to meet Ben's needs in the self-contained learning disabilities classroom. In the third grade, services were provided using consultation to the special education personnel within the learning disabilities classroom. By this time the teacher and aide had adapted Ben's educational routine to meet his needs throughout the day, and there was no need for the occupational therapist to provide direct services. Now that Ben would be in a new educational environment, his needs within this context would have to be reevaluated.

Ben always had good relationships with his peers, so this was not a concern. The primary concern from the team continued to be learning and academic performance. Although the therapist had a lot of information about Ben, she decided to spend some time in Ben's future fourth grade classroom and with his future fourth grade teacher so she would understand the demands of this environment. The therapist summarized her impressions from test data, intervention outcomes, teacher interview, and classroom observations using the Functional Skills Assessment Grid[4] (see Figure 9-3). Then she discussed her intervention options with the present learning disabilities specialist, using Table 9-1 as a guide.

The therapist, classroom teacher, and learning disabilities specialist agreed that Ben's slowness to complete written work and difficulty maintaining attention for the duration of the task would be his most significant problems in the fourth grade classroom. His clumsiness would not greatly interfere with classroom activities, but might affect physical education and free play experiences. They also agreed that Ben was not likely to develop a high degree of skill and endurance in relation to writing, and so decided to look at possible task adaptations to enable his writing success. The parents were happy to consider adaptations.

Ben's parents were pleased that he had made such progress, but were also nervous, stating that Ben felt safe in the special education classroom. The professionals and parents agreed they would monitor his performance closely and would increase their intervention support if he seemed to be frustrated or failing. They concurred it would be beneficial for Ben to learn to type; the learning disabilities specialist agreed to teach Ben. The occupational therapist planned to consult with the classroom teacher weekly to learn about Ben's assignments and to collaborate with the teacher to adapt the tasks, minimizing the use of fine motor skills. The therapist also explained the importance of a good seating position to support Ben's postural control, and the school staff decided to make necessary adaptations in the fall. They all discussed strategies for improving Ben's ability to attend to learning tasks and agreed to meet every other week in the fall to review the success of their strategies and make new plans. The team also decided that either the learning disabilities specialist or the occupational therapist would complete a classroom observation once a week during the first quarter to determine the success of the strategies and to identify possible needed alterations.

The occupational therapist also agreed to meet with the physical educator to discuss ways to enhance Ben's coordination and postural control. The therapist and physical educator would review the fourth grade physical education curriculum to identify effective class strategies that would be beneficial to Ben. The parents asked whether they could assist in this area, and it was suggested that they consider swimming, karate, or gymnastics. They also decided to increase Ben's responsibilities around the house in an attempt to improve his attention to tasks.

FIGURE 9–3

Functional Skills Assessment Grid for Occupational and Physical Therapy Services

Benjamin

Program Outcome	Performance Components		NA	0	1	2	3	Comments
Learning: Skill Acquisition and Academics*	1	Manipulation/hand use				X		
	2	Interpretation of body senses	X					
	3	Perceptual skills						
		organization of space and time						
		interpretation of visual stimuli						
	4	Cognitive skills						
		problem solving						
		generalization of learning	X					
	5	Attending skills				X		
	6	Use of assistive and adaptive devices	X					
	7	Mgmt of body positions during learning			X			
	8	Mgmt of body positions during transitions			X			
	9	Movement within learning environment			X			

Work*

1 Mgmt of body positions during work
2 Mgmt of body positions during transitions
3 Movement within work environment
4 Manipulation/hand use
5 Use of assistive and adaptive devices

Play/Leisure*

1 Mgmt body position during play/leisure
2 Mgmt body position during transitions
3 Movement within play/leisure environment
4 Manipulation/hand use
5 Use of assistive and adaptive devices

Communication*

1 Oral motor movements
2 Communication access
3 Manipulation/hand use
4 Mgmt body position during communication
5 Movement w/in communication environment
6 Attending skills
7 Perceptual skills
8 Use of assistive and adaptive devices

(continued on next page)

FIGURE 9–3 (Continued)

Socialization*		
1	Self esteem	
2	Recognition and use of nonverbal cues	
3	Mgmt body position during socialization	
4	Movement within social environment	
5	Attending skills	
6	Perceptual skills	
7	Cognitive skills	

Activities of Daily Living*		
1	Oral motor movements	
2	Mgmt of body position during ADL	
3	Movement within daily living environment	
4	Attending skills	
5	Manipulation/hand use	

* When acquiring new skills, use the Learning: Skill Acquisition section of this grid.

NA—No problems are identified in therapy evaluation

0—Although a problem has been identified through evaluation, it is not presently interfering with program outcome(s). Needs may be met by self, parents, or professionals in other programs or agencies.

1—The problem *influences* successful program outcome(s); simple instructional or environmental changes are likely to result in functional performance.

2—The problem *interferes* with specific program outcome(s); specific strategies are necessary to enable functional performance.

3—The problem *prevents* successful program outcome(s); multifaceted strategies are necessary to reach functional performance.

Dunn & Campbell (1988)

Dunn W, Campbell P: Designing pediatric service provision. In Dunn W (ed): *Pediatric Occupational Therapy: Facilitating Effective Service Provision*. Thorofare, NJ, SLACK, Inc, in press. (Form used with permission; student information pertains to this text.)

FIGURE 9–4

Intervention Plan

Child's Name: Benjamin _____   Date: _____

Birthdate: _____

Agency Name: _____   Chron. Age: ___10___ yrs. _____ mo.

Outcome Statement: Ben will perform successfully in the fourth grade. _____

Outcome Category: ___X___ Learning   _____ Work
                        _____ Play/Leisure   _____ Communication
                        _____ Socialization   _____ ADL

Performance Components:

ENABLING COMPONENTS: CONCERNS:

perceptual skills _____   fine motor skills _____

cognitive skills _____   attending skills _____

_____   postural control _____

Service Provision Models:

_____ Direct*   _____ Monitoring   __X__ Consultation
                        _____ supervise adult   __X__ teach adult
                                                      __X__ adapt posture/mvmt
                                                      __X__ adapt task/matls
                                                      __X__ adapt environ

* Provided in conjunction with one or more other service models

_____ DIRECT   ___X___ n.a.

(continued on next page)

FIGURE 9–4 (*Continued*)

_____ MONITORING   X   n.a.

  X   CONSULTATION   _____ n.a.

Area of Concern: Learning in a regular classroom environment

Identified by: Special Education Team   role: Multiple

Statement of Area to be Addressed: Ben will meet the demands of a regular
fourth grade classroom successfully.

Location of Services: fourth grade classroom; gym

Strategies: adapt seating to optimal configuration for postural
control; identify ways to adapt tasks so Ben can complete them
successfully; observe classroom activities and Ben's performance.

Proposed
Meeting Schedule: X   weekly _____ bimonthly _____ monthly

Location of meeting: conference room

Method for Documentation of Performance:

   behavior to be observed: class work

   natural environment for observation: fourth grade room

   measurement/data to be collected: amount of work completed
   accurately

criterion for successful performance: Ben will complete at least 80% of written assignments each day with 80% or more correct on each assignment.

Dunn, W, Campbell P: Designing pediatric service provision, in Dunn W (ed): *Pediatric Occupational Therapy: Facilitating Effective Service Provision*. Thorofare, NJ, SLACK, Inc, 1991. Used with permission.

Outcome

In the fall, Ben entered the fourth grade. The team implemented the plans they had made in the spring. A sample portion of the occupational therapy intervention plan for Ben is provided in Figure 9–4. Initially, the therapist and special education teacher spent a lot of time with the classroom teacher to ensure her success with Ben in the classroom. The principal made arrangements for Ben to have access to a computer for 1 hour per day. Initially he learned how to type, and then later in the year he used the computer time to produce written work for his class assignments. Ben's parents purchased a computer for Christmas, so Ben could practice at home and develop a lifelong skill.

Ben continued to progress. The occupational therapist met with him in the fifth grade to help him become more aware of the successful adaptations they had identified in the regular classroom. It was important for Ben to begin taking responsibility for his own adaptations, knowing when and how to implement them and when he needed to seek help from others. By high school, Ben was taking all regular classes and had incorporated many of the strategies learned in grade school into his routines.

SUMMARY

The cases presented demonstrate the expertise of occupational therapists in creating an interface between a person's skills and needs and the demands of particular environments. In the best possible service situation for children, therapists would provide services within age-appropriate natural life environments.[2] Therapists can advocate comprehensive integration by taking advantage of natural opportunities to apply their expertise. The model of collaborative consultation provides clear mechanisms for applying occupational therapy expertise to children's and families' needs in a way that immediately infiltrates their lives. When this occurs, children have more opportunities to practice within regular routines, and they expend less effort to generalize their skills. The environment and its natural characteristics support the development of adaptive skills.

REFERENCES

1. Brown L, Ford A, Nisbet J, et al: Opportunities available when severely handicapped students attend chronological age appropriate regular schools. *The Association for Persons with Severe Handicaps* 1983;8:16–24.
2. Dunn W: Integrated related services, in Meyer L, Peck CA, Brown L (eds): *Critical Issues in the Lives of People with Severe Disabilities.* 1991.
3. Dunn W: A comparison of service provision models in school-based occupational therapy services. *Occup Ther J Res,* 1990.
4. Dunn W, Campbell P: The service provision process, in Dunn W (ed): *Pediatric Occupational Therapy: Facilitating Effective Service Provision.* Thorofare, NJ, SLACK, Inc, 1990.
5. Dunn W, McGourty L: Application of uniform terminology to practice. *Am J Occup Ther* 1989; 43: 817–831.
6. Education for All Handicapped Children Act of 1975 (Public Law 94-142), 20 U.S.C., 1401.
7. Education of the Handicapped Act Amendments of 1986 (Public Law 99-457), 20 U.S.C., 1401.
8. Idol L, Paolucci-Whitcomb P, Nevin A: *Collaborative Consultation.* Austin, Tex, Pro-Ed, 1986.
9. Idol L, West J: Consultation in special education. II: Training and practice. *J Learning Disabilities* 1987; 20: 474–494.
10. Rainforth B, York J, Macdonald C: *Collaborative Teams for Students with Severe Disabilities.* Baltimore, Brooks Publishing Co., 1992.
11. West J, Idol L: School consultation. I: An interdisciplinary perspective on theory, models, and research. *J Learning Disabilities* 1987; 20: 388–408.

CHAPTER 10

Program Development Consultation for the Classroom

Donna Weiss, M.A., O.T.R./L.

OVERVIEW

The development of a full-time school-based consultation practice that could meet the needs of preschool handicapped students in a suburban/rural setting evolved over the past 18 years. Six years of experience in a private school for learning disabled children provided the author's basic experience in an educational setting. The frequent contacts with public school child study teams that referred children helped to establish visibility and create a network of potential clients. Isolated requests for in-district evaluations and technical assistance quickly grew into long-term consultation contracts.

Legal mandates[1] for the establishment of preschool handicapped programs in public school districts increased the demand for occupational therapy services. The dearth of qualified personnel required the development of service delivery models that focused on consultation rather than direct service. The author developed a practical model of occupational therapy consultation that emphasizes the use of multiple communication strategies which facilitate the incorporation of therapeutic recommendations into the school and home setting. A product line of in-service presentations, caregiver guides, and weekly lesson plans was developed to reinforce the consultation recommendations. These tangible products, created in a generic format, are individualized and personalized for each student and classroom setting.[6] Assistance with individual gross and fine motor and self-care evaluations and generation of related IEP goals, objectives, and classroom strategies facilitated the individualization of the generic plans.

The consultation model presented utilizes monthly scheduled visits to each class setting. It assumes that the consultant will be able to educate and motivate classroom staff to carry over recommended procedures.[2] The parent is viewed as

237

an important team member, and home carryover activities are an integral part of the program. Children requiring direct treatment services are identified and referred for more intensive intervention when necessary.

The model requires the consultant to possess a broad knowledge base, encompassing appropriate frames of reference, assessment tools, treatment approaches, and preschool curriculum design. The ability to synthesize this information and create appropriate and practical strategies that will enhance children's ability to function in home and school environments is an essential component of the consultation.

Active listening skills[4] along with strong written and verbal skills are critical, as is computer literacy. Administrators, educators, parents, and students derive maximum benefit from materials designed for their environment that are generated and distributed during or soon after a consultation visit. This personalized product line of school-based occupational therapy consultation recommendations addresses needs[5] that are expressed and/or observed during the consultant's site visits.

Familiarity with educational curricula and schedules is important in order to determine when and if occupational therapy consultation will enhance the educational goals of children. The consultant must be able to differentiate the need for medically based occupational therapy versus school-based service and must be able to inform clients when other services are required or when occupational therapy consultation is no longer necessary.[1]

POTENTIAL MARKET

Many school districts and regions face critical shortages in related serviced personnel. Occupational therapists who have a strong background in pediatrics and school-based practice may wish to consider this model of service delivery. The occupational therapy consultant utilizing this model must be able to perform the following tasks:

- Ascertain the status of a large number of children in a short period of time;
- Understand the skill levels of primary caregivers;
- Determine the assets and limitations of each educational environment (physical plant, administrative support, availability of time, space, and equipment);
- Develop skill in the use of computer and audiovisual technology; and
- Adapt a generic product line of activities and strategies to meet the needs of specific children within individual classrooms or at home.

This type of monthly consultation service increases parents', teachers', and administrators' familiarity with the range of occupational therapy services and facilitates the timely recognition and referral of students requiring more direct/intensive intervention to a direct treatment source.

Administrators value this type of collegial consultation and often have referred the consultant to regional learning centers, professional associations, or consumer groups that require in-service education programs. These, in turn, provide more exposure and lead to more requests for services. There are multiple markets for this type of consultation model, such as school districts, educational consortiums, commissions, private and state schools, and federally or state-funded infant/parent programs.

Federal and state committment to early childhood programs[3] ensures that there is and will continue to be a broad market for occupational therapy consultation services. The boundaries are drawn by the individual consultant's interest and motivation.

KEY POINTS

Case Example

The following case example exemplifies the approach described and highlights the varied communication tools that are utilized to ensure carryover and consistency in the consultation plan.

After attending a county in-service program presented by the consultant, the director of an educational service commission requested a 1-day paid consultation visit. The commission administered four preschool handicapped programs located throughout a suburban/rural county. Each program had a morning and afternoon session with no more than eight children in each session. A full-time teacher, full-time aide, and part-time speech therapist were assigned to each setting. Each child had been referred to the program by his or her local child study team. The administrator and teachers were aware of the importance of sensory motor experiences for this age group. An occupational therapy consultation was requested to assure that sensory motor aspects of overall programming were being addressed and that children who required more intensive therapeutic intervention were identified and referred in a timely fashion.

On the initial visit, an informal needs assessment was conducted by the consultant through discussions with the administrator and teachers and observations at the program sites. The consultant then met with the consultees to share observations and recommendations. Using a consensus method, the consultant and consultees identified the following needs: (1) Broader understanding of the relationship between sensory motor development and the acquisition of early educational skills; (2) Establishment of referral criteria for children whose sensory motor deficits might require occupational therapy services; (3) Development of methods for the incorporation of sensory motor learning into the classroom routine; (4) Establishment of a program of home carryover activities; (5) Identification of equipment and supplies needed to provide sensory motor experiences within the classroom.

During the needs assessment phase, it became apparent that teachers wanted suggestions to complement their existing group-oriented program. They did not want to be burdened with voluminous activity sheets for individual children who did not require direct treatment services. However, they wanted to ensure that children who had individual treatment needs were identified and referred to their home district for direct therapy services.

At a follow-up meeting with the director, the consultant presented a consultation proposal that included an initial in-service presentation, monthly site visits, and weekly gross and fine motor lesson plans that would incorporate sensory motor experiences into the already existing lesson plans. Since consultations were scheduled monthly, a written instructional guide for school personnel was also proposed to facilitate classroom implementation of the plan.

The consultant referred children who demonstrated severe functional lags to the program administrator with a recommendation for direct occupational therapy services. The program administrator relayed this recommendation to the children's sending district. Arrangements for individual treatment were the responsibility of the home districts.

The suggested program strategy reduced the teacher's burden of activity generation, was easily assimilated into the existing program, facilitated educational goals, and the proposal and consultant gained quick acceptance into the program.

The cost-benefit analysis for monthly visits to four different sites, in-service training, lesson plans, and related travel, preparation, and record keeping was prepared and presented to the director. This information was factored into negotiations for remuneration. Sources of secretarial support and copying facilities were also established. Since the consultant had office facilities that included a computer, it was agreed that the equivalent of one paid office day per site or not more than four office days per year could be conducted at the consultant's office.

A firm working relationship was established by delineating the expectations and goals of consultant and consultee. For example, a brief description of the occupational therapy consultant's role was prepared and sent to teachers and parents along with a description of what would be done for the children in the program (e.g., generate lesson plans, create home activities, assist in sensory motor evaluations). The timely completion of these projects along with an open invitation to ask questions and voice concerns assisted in the consultees' acceptance of the consultant.

Consultation strategies were then developed to help parents and teaching staff accept the consultant's program recommendations. Utilizing a market research approach, the consultant focused on understanding and identifying issues that would impact these consumers. By defining present needs and prognosticating future needs, product development could take place. Active listening[3] and awareness of the needs of the students, teachers, and parents in preschool programs also facilitated the generation of consultation strategies.

The consultant understood that preschool teachers must incorporate a variety of curriculum requirements into a short period of time, and that most parents have hectic schedules. Short duration activities for small groups were designed for teachers. Home activities capitalized on the therapeutic potential of daily living activities (rather than games, exercises, or craft projects requiring parents to set aside specific blocks of time or to acquire special materials) so that the busy home schedule would not be taxed. Parents also requested holiday toy suggestions and summer activities. A holiday toy suggestion list was created highlighting the therapeutic aspects of various toys. A booklet of summer activities based on gross and fine motor goals was also prepared.

The preschool handicapped classes had a wealth of volunteers, student teachers, and aides. The consultant provided classroom activity guides or charts that could be used by support personnel. Simple goals were stated and therapeutic methods for presenting materials and for positioning students were explained or depicted. All suggestions were demonstrated by the consultant during on-site visits. These strategies assisted both the teacher and support staff by assuring more efficient utilization of personnel in the classroom.

After conducting a thorough review of the children's needs, general goals for the classes and individual student goals were established. Gross and fine motor lesson plans were designed and distributed at each site at the beginning of each month. Teachers had access to these when drawing up their own weekly lesson plans. In addition, an activity sheet reflecting the gross and fine motor goals of the classroom was provided for home use.

The consultant was able to address both the global classroom needs and those of individual students during each monthly consult. Following assessment of individual students, the consultant's suggestions for a specific student might include the following:

- Alternative methods of movement to and from various classroom activities
- Alternative methods of positioning to enhance attention and facilitate responsiveness
- Alternative methods of material presentation to enhance ability to manipulate classroom materials

On monthly site visits new activities or strategies were demonstrated, changes/ additions to lesson plans were made, and children who demonstrated consistent difficulty with activities were identified as needing more comprehensive evaluation. This was carried out by the consultant or a therapist employed by the home district. The results of these evaluations were written in a format that included

1. Current functional status (age levels for gross motor, fine motor, and self-care skills)
2. Strengths and weaknesses
3. The educational significance of these findings
4. Goals and objectives of proposed intervention
5. Suggested strategies (e.g., direct occupational therapy—individual/group and frequency)
6. Specialized materials
7. Methods of evaluation

This report was shared with the student's child study team. The team and parents would make the final decision regarding implementation of direct occupational therapy services. The home district was responsible for the provision of these services.

Lesson plans, activity guides, and other written communication were generated and saved on a computer. This allowed the consultant to maintain a comprehensive and readily accessible library of products that could be easily tailored for individual client needs.

As the consultation progressed, staff became comfortable incorporating recommended therapeutic approaches into the daily classroom schedule. There was an increased number of questions regarding sensory motor aspects of children's performance. Staff, administration, and parents noted progress in children's sensory motor skills. These positive indicators resulted in increased requests for services and the product line developed through the consultation.

The prepared lesson plans, customized for the individual setting, and other programs were tangible results—products—of the consultation. Networking by teachers and other therapists created a demand for these products. School administrators expressed interest and a market for these services and a customized product line was developed. As interest in this type of service delivery grew, requests were made to present the concept to the state department of education and pupil personnel administrators. This resulted in a consultation role, targeted to school districts. Program planning and in-service training presentations regarding consultation strategies were then developed. These presentations were designed to help districts understand that direct service is not the only service delivery option for occupational therapy in the schools. They helped special service personnel utilize occupational therapy services more efficiently and created a better working relationship between school personnel and the occupational therapy consultant.

SUMMARY

The expanding market for occupational therapists in educational settings requires the development of skill in a variety of service delivery models. Employment of direct services alone will not fulfill the needs of children and staff in special education classes. Through appropriate consultation services, the potential for classroom caregivers and the classroom environment to carry over therapeutic recommendations can be developed. One therapist cannot personally provide daily opportunities for practice, follow-through, and carryover of specially designed activities. Time constraints make it impossible for one person to interact consistently with each child who may require a special intervention focus. One experienced and knowledgeable consultant can impart a great deal of information to concerned classroom staff who, in turn, can utilize that information to enrich the educational programs of many children.

There will always be children who require intensive, direct therapy in order to achieve educational goals. In most cases, however, a less restrictive consultation model, such as the one highlighted, can best meet the challenge of precarious educational budgets and chronic personnel shortages. The key to this type of practice is continuous communication and the utilization of individualized tangible products that are meaningful to and applicable within the consultee's environment. This creative and exciting approach to school-based consultation practice provides continual challenges and unlimited opportunity for professional growth.

REFERENCES

1. American Occupational Therapy Association: *Guidelines for Occupational Therapy Services in School Systems*. Rockville, Md, Author, 1987, pp 1–45.
2. Clark P, Allen A: *Occupational Therapy for Children*. St Louis, CV Mosby, 1985, pp 482–483.
3. Dunn W et al: *Guidelines for Occupational Therapy Services in Early Intervention and Preschool Services*. Rockville, Md, AOTA, 1989, pp 3–16.
4. Michelson DJ, Davis JL: A consultation model for the school counselor. *The School Counselor* 1977; 25:98–105.
5. Olsen T, Urban C: Marketing, in Bair J, Gray M (eds): *The Occupational Therapy Manager*. Rockville, Md, AOTA, 1985, pp 123–135.
6. Weiss D: *Goal-Oriented Gross and Fine Motor Lesson Plans for Early Childhood Classes*. Palo Alto, CA, VORT Corp., 1990.

CHAPTER 11

Transition Program Planning in the Public Education System

Karen C. Spencer, M.A., O.T.R.

OVERVIEW

As a result of extensive federal legislation, students with disabilities are now an integral part of the public education system.[4] There is widespread recognition that individuals with disabilities can and do benefit from individualized public education and related services that prepare them ultimately for adult life. Members of the educational team, including occupational therapists, share responsibility for enabling students with disabilities to achieve meaningful educational outcomes in the form of employment, community living, and recreation. The process of helping students move smoothly from public education to the vast array of adult opportunities and services is being widely termed *transition*.[1, 2, 5, 6, 7, 8, 10] Individualized *transition planning* refers to a team effort that includes the student and parents in designing a positive future for the student with a disability.

This chapter presents a consultation targeted at designing and implementing individualized *transition planning processes* for students with disabilities in three school districts. This effort was led by an occupational therapist who worked collaboratively with parents, teachers, related service personnel, school administrators, and representatives from the adult service system (e.g., State Division of Rehabilitation, State Division for Developmental Disabilities). A collegial consultation approach was used that involved active problem solving, planning, and action.

CASE DISCUSSION

The occupational therapist consultant identified the need for comprehensive transition-related services for secondary level students with disabilities. This need was demonstrated by three local school districts that included both urban and rural communities. These districts reported that most of their secondary level special education students lacked the necessary skills, experiences, and supports to allow them to move smoothly into integrated employment or community living options after graduation. On a statewide basis, it had been demonstrated that most special education graduates with significant disabilities were experiencing high rates of unemployment, underemployment, and dependency.[3] The problem, therefore, was of both local and statewide significance.

As the need for effective transition-related services was being explored and discussed, the occupational therapy consultant was serving as the director of a supported employment project based at Colorado State University. This project provided highly individualized functional assessment, job development, community job placement, on-the-job training, and ongoing support services for adults with significant disabilities. The overall goal of supported employment was to assist individuals in obtaining and maintaining meaningful, paid employment in integrated community settings. These services evolved as an alternative to unemployment and more restrictive or segregated employment options including sheltered workshops. The people being served at the time had a wide range of abilities, interests, and needs. Their disabilities typically resulted from one or more of the following diagnoses: mental retardation, seizure disorder, cerebral palsy, traumatic brain injury, chronic mental illness, blindness, or other neurological conditions.

Through the successful experience of developing and implementing supported employment services and integrating people with disabilities into a variety of typical community environments, the occupational therapist director felt that she and her staff had acquired the necessary skills and credibility to propose some interventions on behalf of younger individuals who were still in school. It was felt that intervention at the junior high and high school levels would help prevent the current pattern of unemployment, underemployment, and restricted living options that were so prevalent among adults with disabilities.

Having established a track record for providing innovative community-integrated services, the occupational therapist then assumed a consultant role and approached the special education directors of the three surrounding school districts. A series of meetings were scheduled to determine the school's perception of transition-related needs among their secondary level students. The consensus was that extensive needs were not being effectively addressed. It was believed that students were clearly in need of integrated employment, living, and recreation opportunities that would extend beyond high school. The special education directors stated further that in order to meet student needs, extensive training and support would be required by special education staff: teachers, aides, and related service personnel. Discussion also revealed that involvement of parents in all future transition-related planning activities would be critical. Parents were already beginning to approach the directors to voice dissatisfaction with current educational programming for their teenage sons and daughters who were rapidly approaching the difficult transition to life after school.

The consultant then offered to seek funding in cooperation with the participating school districts to conduct needed transition-related activities and to prepare a proposal to the U.S. Department of Education, Office of Special Education and Rehabilitative Services.[9] The proposal sought funding to pay for school-based consultation and training that would be provided by the consultant and her staff who would comprise the consultant team. The decision to seek external funding (U.S. Department of Education grant) to address local transition issues alleviated the following concerns that had been expressed by the districts:

1. Current lack of resources on the part of the districts (money and personnel) to institute a systems change project of this magnitude.
2. Current lack of administrative and district expertise in the areas of transition, community-based services, and establishment of linkages with the adult service system, all of which would be needed to train staff to meet the identified transition-related needs of students.
3. Current need for seed money to initiate comprehensive transition-related activities. Each district felt strongly that following an initial investment by the U.S. Department of Education, they would be able to continue transition-related activities with available resources. A 3-year project, therefore, was viewed as an appropriate short-term intervention that would be carried out on a long-term basis by the districts, without external financial support.

The proposal written by the consultant and her staff incorporated the ideas and concerns generated from several lengthy brainstorm/problem-solving sessions with the special education directors. The consultant felt it was imperative that the district directors, who would be ultimately responsible for overseeing transition planning activities, participate at this early stage in order to feel ownership of the overall plan. Had the consultant independently designed a consultation and training package for each district, it is very unlikely that it would have been accepted or implemented.

As discussions moved toward projecting the costs of such a project, the consultant asked that each district identify their contribution in terms of personnel and funds. Although the districts did not have the resources to fully support a multiple-year effort, they did have limited resources to contribute. The consultant felt that a school district contribution of personnel time, as a minimum, was imperative if the project was to succeed. Total district reliance on a federal grant to pay for a complete package of consultation and training might ultimately detract from each district's sense of ownership and long-term commitment to change.

Collaboration and joint decision making involving the district administrators and the consultant at this early stage allowed for the establishment of effective communication and trust among the participating parties. All of the preceding activity occurred before funding was actually obtained and may be regarded as a marketing strategy on the part of the consultant. The joint identification of needs and potential solutions was followed by active fund-raising to secure the needed resources to make solutions possible.

A proposal for a 3-year project was subsequently submitted and funded for $308,000—the resources needed to implement major system change in three districts that would ultimately benefit youth with disabilities, their families, and education and related service staff who would be the actual change agents.

The overall purpose of the project was to develop a transition planning process that could be implemented district wide for students with disabilities. This planning process was to be *student-centered,* promote active decision making on the part of the student and family, and address all the critical life areas for each student: employment, living, recreation, and community utilization. It was further agreed that the process should strongly promote community-integrated work, living, and recreation alternatives for students in lieu of more traditional segregated and restrictive options. The planning process was to culminate in a specific action plan for each student that identified goals, objectives, services to be provided, provider agencies (including both the school and adult service agencies), and time lines for completion. The transition planning process was to be integrated into the existing IEP planning process to avoid duplication of meetings and efforts. The quality of the transition planning effort would be evaluated based on four overarching criteria:

1. Student acquisition of a paid job prior to school exit with the necessary supports in place to assure continued employment beyond graduation
2. Student and team decision making regarding postschool living arrangements accompanied by needed supports
3. Student participation in a variety of community-integrated recreational activities based on individual interests and preferences
4. Active and timely referral of the student to appropriate adult services prior to graduation to prevent students and families from suddenly finding themselves in a service void

The specific roles assumed by the consultant team over the 3-year project period varied with each district depending on the local needs and capabilities. Overall, four major consultant roles were assumed:

1. Facilitation of communication among and between school personnel and related adult service agencies (e.g., State Rehabilitation, State Division for Mental Health, State Division for Mental Retardation) to allow for effective, long-range student-centered planning. This led to the development of formalized interagency agreements to serve youth with disabilities who were exiting the public schools.
2. Training of parents, school personnel, and adult agency staff in specific

transition-related activities including functional assessment, community job development, community-based instruction, and referral and funding patterns to assure that transition-related services are in place.

3. Training of school personnel and parents to conduct and facilitate effective IEP meetings with integrated transition components: planning related to future employment, living, recreation, and community utilization.

4. Preparation of school personnel to train others in the district to implement transition planning processes. This training would assure district-wide dissemination and continuation of transition activities beyond the federally funded project period.

As the project got underway, a core transition team was formed in each participating district comprised of parents, school personnel, representatives from adult service agencies, and the consultant team, who served as the leaders/facilitators. Each team had responsibility for designing and testing a transition planning process that would meet the needs of their students. Once a process was identified and tested, members of the core team, with consultant support, would train additional school teams. The overall goal by the end of the three-year grant period was for the transition planning process to be disseminated throughout each district by the core teams.

During the development of a transition planning process, the consultant team found that they had to play a very major role in generating and proposing ideas and alternatives that would address the transition-related issues identified by the schools. Core team members initially needed substantial guidance and support before they were able to assume an active problem-solving role. The consultants, therefore, presented options but did not impose solutions. The core team was then able to consider each option and adapt, accept, or reject as needed. The role of the consultants at this stage was to present information and facilitate active decision making on the part of the core teams. The consultants also shared their past and current experiences with functional community-based services that provided team members with ideas and a sense that effective transition planning was, indeed, possible. Additionally, core team members needed extensive reinforcement for their proactive stand on the issues and for the time and energy they were expending. They were involved in a major system change project which, to many, was very threatening and often perceived by other school personnel as a project to make their already busy jobs only busier. For this reason the consultants proposed a rule that when decisions were made to *add* new processes or services to the already busy schedules of school personnel, other more obsolete or ineffective processes or services would be dropped. The consultants relied on the special education directors to reinforce this rule so that the core team members would not fear reprisals for changing well-entrenched protocols.

When the core team met during the summers or after regular school hours, the grant was able to pay the members of the core team for their time. This arrangement greatly enhanced the district's ability to commit personnel, particularly during the time-consuming start-up phases of the project. It also alleviated time pressures on the part of team members who, in many cases, were addressing the transition issues in addition to their other job responsibilities during the project's initial stages. As the project continued, the need for the grant to pay for release time decreased as project activities were incorporated into the everyday educational process in each district.

As the transition project drew to a close, the consultant's role focused primarily on helping the core teams plan and conduct transition-related training throughout their district. Consultant interaction with the school administrators also increased as the project wound down. This increase was needed to plan for the necessary supports that would be required to assure that school personnel and parents would be able to continue transition planning activities in the future.

The primary beneficiaries of this 3-year consultation effort are clearly students with disabilities. An emphasis on creating a positive future for students and putting the necessary long-term supports in place constitutes a major change in the previous short-term, year-to-year focus that had dominated special education services. The key players in this change process are many and clearly extend beyond the boundaries of the public school. Inclusion of parents, the student, and adult service agencies in an accountable planning process are making successful transitions from school to adult life possible.

POTENTIAL MARKET FOR TRANSITION-RELATED CONSULTATION

Occupational therapists are well qualified to work with school districts or other agencies on the complex and challenging issue of transition. The occupational therapist's ability to look at the secondary level student or the adult within the context of current or future home, community, work, and recreation environments greatly enhances planning and the design of comprehensive services that lead to positive outcomes for individuals with disabilities.

The market for this type of consultation includes the public schools and those agencies or programs that serve adults who seek productive and fulfilling roles in the community. As transition planning is gradually integrated into public school systems, programs that serve people with traumatic injuries or chronic mental illness can also be included in the potential intervention market.

KNOWLEDGE AND SKILLS NEEDED

Occupational therapists who wish to begin or expand a consultation practice with agencies or systems that include transition issues must demonstrate some basic consultation knowledge and skills in addition to their occupational therapy expertise. It would be beneficial for the occupational therapy consultant to be familiar with the prevailing environmental trends toward integration and inclusion of *all* people with disabilities in community work, living, and recreation settings. An understanding of consumer-driven services that promote self-determination versus services directed and controlled by professionals is essential. Additionally, knowledge of community-based and community-integrated service options that provide positive alternatives to more traditional facility-based or segregated programs will enhance the consultant's skills. The need for professional accountability for client/consumer outcomes in the form of community living and employment is the key to a successful consultation.

The consultant must be a creative problem solver who looks beyond current options and approaches to create or develop new resources. She must have the ability to recognize the prevailing culture of the system in which she is working and to communicate and work effectively within that culture. The consultant must be results oriented while guiding a change process. Skill in helping others to find a solution that will work for them while fostering local ownership of the result or solution is essential and comes with practice, training, and experience.

Other skills that are needed by the consultant include active listening, verbal and written communication, and the ability to adapt teaching and communication strategies to a diverse audience. The ability to distill the main problem, obtain agreement from the consultee, set goals, and maintain a clear direction and focus in the face of competing or contradictory forces constitutes an ongoing challenge for any consultant.

REFERENCES

1. American Occupational Therapy Association: Standards of practice for occupational therapy services in schools, in *Guidelines for Occupational Therapy Services in School Systems*. Rockville, Md, Author, 1987, pp 4–7.
2. Clark FA, Mack W, Pennington V: Transition needs assessment of severely disabled high school students and their parents and teachers. *Occup Ther J Res* 1988; 8:104.
3. Colorado Department of Education: Fiscal year 1989–1990 state plan under part B of the Education of the Handicapped Act as amended by PL 98-199. Denver, Author, 1988.
4. Education for All Handicapped Children Act of 1975 (PL 94-142), 89 Stat. 773.
5. Everson JD, Moon MS: Transition services for young adults with severe disabilities: Defining professional and parental roles and responsibilities. *J Assoc People Severe Handicaps* 1987; 12:1987.
6. Johnson DR, Bruininks RH, Thurlow M: Meeting the challenge of transition service planning through improved interagency cooperation. *Exceptional Children* 1987; 53:522.
7. Rusch FR, Phelps LA: Secondary special education and transition from school to work: A national priority. *Exceptional Children* 1987; 53:487.
8. Sample P, Spencer KC, Bean GR: *Transition Planning: Creating a Positive Future for Students With Disabilities*. Department of Occupational Therapy, Colorado State University, 1990.
9. Secondary Education Transition Model Project: Proposal funded by the Office of Special Education Programs. Office of Special Education and Rehabilitative Services, U.S. Department of Education, Grant #G008730150, 1986.

10. Spencer KC: The transition from school to adult life, in S Hertfelder, C Gwin (eds): *Work in Progress: Occupational Therapy in Work Programs*. Rockville, Md, AOTA, 1989, p 157.

ADDITIONAL READING

Amendments to the Rehabilitation Act (PL 99-506), 100 Stat. 1807, 1986.

Falvey MA: Community-based Curriculum: Instructional Strategies for Students With Severe Handicaps, ed 2. Baltimore, PH Brookes, 1989.

Rainforth B, York J: Integrating related services in community instruction. *J Assoc People Severe Handicaps* 1987; 12:190.

Spencer KC: Overview of supported employment, in Hertfelder S, Gwin C (eds): *Work in Progress: Occupational Therapy in Work Programs*. Rockville, Md, AOTA, 1989, p 181.

Spencer KC: Supported employment: The role of occupational therapy at the job site. *Occup Ther Practice* 1990; 1:74.

Wehman P et al: *Vocational Education for Multihandicapped Youth with Cerebral Palsy*. Baltimore, PH Brookes, 1988.

SECTION B

Occupational Therapy Consultation in Long-Term Care Settings

Long-term care settings have historically been a major focus area for occupational therapy. Occupational therapy consultation, as a specific method of service delivery, flowered in the 1960s with the advent of the Older Americans Act, Medicare, Medicaid, and mental health legislation, and has continued to grow. Technological advances in health care have contributed to an exponential rise in chronically ill and older persons requiring long-term care. As numbers swell and costs expand, quality of life issues within these facilities have become a major issue. The authors in this section share a concern for quality of life. They present a cross section of consultation practice issues that confront the occupational therapy consultant in long-term care.

Cunninghis traces the evolution of a long-term consultation relationship with one facility that needed services for their activities program. She presents multiple situations and the consultation roles required. Additionally, she provides a picture of a consultation practice that has focused on systemwide training for activities personnel throughout the country.

A systems approach to long-term care consultation is presented by Epstein. Using a needs assessment as the consultation focus, she identifies multiple issues faced by facilities caught between mandated regulatory change and realistic fiscal constraints. A consultant team is utilized in this case example. Facing familiar circumstances, where the facility has never had occupational therapy services, the team proceeds to analyze the situation. The team's assessment methodologies and strategies for change provided the client with information they needed to make informed decisions.

Acting as both an internal and external consultant, Gibson presents a picture of multiple consultant roles available to the occupational therapist employed in a mental health setting. Performing the dual roles of occupational therapy director and consultant, she shares vignettes that illustrate the complexities of such a situation. In discussing the establishment of trust, she points out the similarity in techniques used for consultation and the treatment of psychiatric patients.

The important issue of quality assurance surfaces in every long-term care facility. Weiss describes a consultation that focused on the need for a splinting compliance program. She emphasizes the important knowledge and skills necessary to provide consultation in a large state-run developmental center. Multiple rules and regulations, clinical and programatic requirements, and heavy involvement of caregiver staff are part of the consultation concern.

Long-Term Care Settings

AUTHOR	MODEL	LEVEL	LOCUS	GOAL
Cunninghis	Program Development, Collegial, and Educational	Levels II and III: Educational and administrative/ program	Long-term care facility	Facilitate a broad-based activities program meeting resident needs
Epstein	Clinical, Educational, Process Management, and Systems	Level III: Administrative/ program	Nursing facility	Develop needs assessment as basis for occupational therapy program
Gibson	Collegial, Process Management, and Systems	Level III: Administrative/ program	Mental health facility	Identify internal and external consultation roles for occupational therapy director
Weiss	Educational, Program Development, and Systems	Levels II and III: Educational and administrative/ program	State developmental center	Develop quality assurance splint compliance program

CHAPTER 12

Activities Consultation in Long-Term Care Settings

Richelle N. Cunninghis, Ed.M., O.T.R.

OVERVIEW

Long-term care settings can provide an unending variety of service opportunities for occupational therapy consultants. Possibilities include consultation regarding educational and activity programs, environmental concerns and modifications, resources, adaptive equipment, meal programs and feeding problems, wheelchair maintenance, rehabilitation techniques, and positioning. Additionally, helping staff, residents, and families make transitions may be addressed. Which services are provided, of course, is largely dependent on the needs of the facility as well as the expertise, abilities, and, in some cases, marketing skills of the consultant.

An occupational therapist may serve any number of functions in a facility, including the provision of direct, indirect, or consultative services. This chapter describes a consultation practice whose focus is activities programming. Many of the functions just named may also be addressed, but only through indirect services.

The area of activities consultation is an important one for occupational therapists. The training received in activities analysis and occupational performance concepts enables the therapist to provide an important perspective for the activities coordinator. In earlier times, this role might actually have been filled by an occupational therapist, but in today's marketplace it is often assumed by individuals of varying background and education. Therefore, a consultant is needed to provide expert guidance and training for these key individuals working in long-term care.

The indirect service component is an important consideration because of the differing requirements in orientation, skills, relationships, and the type of insurance coverage necessary. The amount of personal satisfaction and demonstrable results that the consultant may experience, as compared to a direct service provider, are also quite different. A high level of clinical expertise and experience are considered to be among the most important qualifications for the consultant. The abilities to be self-directed, risk taking, flexible, effective at negotiation, and to survive with a high degree of professional isolation are also very important.[3]

Given the current emphasis on quality of life issues and the need for accountability of service providers, the consultant's sphere of influence may not be limited solely to activities personnel. Administration, social service, nursing, and other long-term care team members may also become part of the consultative process.

ENVIRONMENT AND SYSTEM INFLUENCES

The author's consulting practice in the field of aging began in 1971 with a return to the work force after an absence of more than ten years. New regulations had recently been enacted that required all long-term care facilities to have trained activity personnel, and occupational therapists had been identified as qualified professionals to provide this training. Therefore, what began as a traditional treatment-oriented consultation quickly expanded to include the training and supervision of the newly formed activities department. And, in time, the concerns and responsibilities of the personnel of this department became the major focus of the consultancy, along with general staff training, particularly in the area of reality orientation and sensory stimulation programs.

The state and national occupational therapy associations worked with the federal Department of Health, Education, and Welfare to identify therapists in each state who were working with the elderly and were potential candidates for a consultant/trainer workshop. The author was one of those selected and has continued to teach a state-approved course for activity personnel under different sponsorships since the workshop's completion in 1972.

The new regulations also stipulated that activity coordinators had to meet specific requirements or work with a consultant until they did (usually for a period of up to two years). A list of these certified consultant/trainers was sent to all long-term care facilities in the state. As a result, referrals for consultation services were received by the author.

Some requests were only to help facilities meet current requirements and did not include opportunities for making any substantive changes. In the role of a consultant, the trainer could only advise and did not have authority for direct intervention. This limitation led to many frustrating situations, as often the consultant's main function was to serve as an advocate for the activities personnel and to help improve staff skills within that department, without impacting on the system as a whole. Because of the two-year requirement for consultation, the arrangement often extended beyond the point where services, given their limited scope, were really needed, or where a legitimate sphere of operation could still be identified. Therefore, it eventually became necessary to limit contracts or take only those where the consultant felt that her presence might make a real difference.

As the consulting practice developed, there were a number of decisions that had to be made. Primary among these were to focus on the elderly, to acquire as much training as possible, and to offer indirect and consultative services only. It was also necessary to make contacts, increase credibility, and develop a network to increase effectiveness as a consultant. These goals were achieved by volunteering for age-related organizations, committees, task forces; becoming a member of the board of trustees of a nursing home; taking training courses, workshops, and institutes; and by offering services as a speaker or resource person for various agencies and groups. Eventually a master's degree in education with a specializaton in gerontology was completed to increase teaching credentials and opportunities.

In the beginning, the practice consisted of a variety of services: consulting to both activity and occupational therapy departments, leading seminars, conducting preretirement workshops, writing training manuals, and teaching courses at community colleges in gerontology, death and dying, and resources for social workers. Eventually, the part-time practice had become more than a full-time nightmare!

In 1979 the practice was formalized and a company, Geriatric Educational Consultants, was founded. Establishing a new company necessitates many steps: designing a logo, printing stationery, establishing priorities, and advertising services. The major decisions at that time included identifying marketplaces, developing marketing strategies, establishing rates for billable services, and restructuring the consultant's time. Allocating more time to the development of the new company also required termination of a longstanding consultancy at a local nursing home, where services were provided two mornings a week. This was a very difficult decision because the relationship developed at that facility provided access to information, group identification, and a knowledge of working with older people that was not available to the consultant in any other setting. It also provided the firsthand experience that was necessary as a background to teach practitioners.

The major long-term care market identified for the consulting practice was activity personnel because of a lack of training courses and materials for this group. The author then began traveling around the country presenting activities-related workshops as well as writing training manuals, developing materials, teaching, and consulting locally in this realm. The area of activities consultation continues to be the major emphasis of the practice. In conjunction with this, the consultant has developed courses and workshops, reviewed books, and served on long-term care and professional committees related to other aspects of occupational therapy. This has included selection as a Role of Occupational Therapy with the Elderly (ROTE) faculty member by the American Occupational Therapy Association (AOTA) and appointment in a university occupational therapy program as an instructor in aging.

Current trends and legislative mandates continue to influence the direction of the practice. Some recent examples of this are evolving approaches for dealing with the increasing numbers of residents with dementia; the emergence of national certification for activity personnel; and changing state and federal regulations.

The first of these has had an impact on the number and type of workshops requested, as well as the development of program materials and publications that specifically deal with appropriate techniques for working with this population.

Requirements for national certification for activity personnel and grandfathering deadlines have resulted in an increased interest in, and demand for, continuing education opportunities. Basic activities courses are now being taught in three states on a regular ongoing basis, and the requests for other workshops have also increased greatly.

Perhaps the greatest changes have resulted from new legislation, such as the Omnibus Budget Reconciliation Act (OBRA 1987). Regulations emanating from this legislation have brought environment and system influences to the forefront.[4] OBRA's focus on quality of care, residents' needs, limitations on the use of physical and chemical restraints, and a comprehensive, uniform assessment system directly affected the delivery of services by activity personnel. This also necessitated a great deal of networking and study on the part of the consultant to keep current with these mandates and their interpretations in order to meet the increasing demands for consultation services and training.

FRAME OF REFERENCE

Activities personnel in long-term care settings must be aware of multiple factors that impact on the resident's ability to participate in meaningful activities. The consultant must help the consultee develop necessary skills to deal with these diverse factors and also assist in working through the problems encountered.[6] The consultant is viewed primarily as an agent of change, provider of resource information, and catalyst for identifying and taking advantage of opportunities.[7]

Using a systems approach, which requires an understanding of the overall organization (nursing facility), and its component parts (activities and residents in particular), the consultant can begin to analyze the situation.[1] Meaningful activities, performed individually by the resident or in groups with the support of activities personnel, must harmonize with established facility routines. Often, poor communication and limited knowledge prevent implementation or successful achievement of activities. Through application of principles inherent in the occupational behavior frame of reference,[8] the consultant is able to help the consultee plan programs effectively and develop the necessary skills for implementation. In this context, the consultant also uses educational and program development skills.

Behavioral, biomechanical, cognitive, and developmental frames of reference[5] also play an important part in shaping the approach to activities consultation. For example, the consultee may have a group of physically disabled male residents whose only interest appears to be television. The consultant may need to help the activities coordinator analyze television programming selected by these residents to help identify interests, related skills, and activities that can then be developed. The need to adapt the activities using specialized devices or task segmentation may arise. The activity itself must be appropriate for the resident's life stage.

CONSULTATION DESCRIPTION

A continuing relationship with a nonprofit long-term care facility, referred to here as Shady Valley, began in the early 1970s when this small residential and nursing facility for the elderly was embarking on the first of many expansions. Services requested included advice on the design of a planned activities room. Most suggestions on the design were adopted, and several months later, the author was asked to consult to the activities department. This consultation relationship was to span almost 15 years. (Refer to Appendix D for a copy of the initial contract and monthly report format used during this consultation.)

Organization

At the time of the initial contact, the facility had a new administrator who was modernizing the existing building to meet the various fire and safety codes, increasing and professionalizing the staff, and bringing the home into compliance with what were the emerging requirements for long-term care facilities. Shady Valley was sponsored by a statewide service organization, and there was a level of commitment to quality care and a concern for residents that appeared greater than average. There was also an openness to new ideas and techniques that was quite different from what was being encountered in other consultation settings.

Support

At Shady Valley, a consultant was not required because of legislative mandates, but rather because the administrator felt that it was important. A good relationship was developed and the administrator was usually accessible and willing to listen to opposing opinions before making up his mind. However, the director of activities had difficulty communicating with the administrator; she found him intimidating and he found her rambling and time consuming. So, the consultant's first task was to work on communication skills with both of them.

Participants

The consultation in these early years followed several different models as the department expanded and the needs changed accordingly. When the consultation began, the structure had just changed from an activity director and an assistant who were responsible for the whole program to two separate divisions with the assistant in charge of the nursing care unit and the previous director responsible for the residential section. This change had not occurred with a great deal of preparation or forewarning to the staff. Therefore, the second task of the consultant was to address the feelings that had been engendered by this move, as well as to help with the organizational changes and the defining of new responsibilities. Subsequently, the consultant provided services to a variety of staff and to new activities personnel. These shifts in services are addressed in the next section.

Services Provided

The consultation model followed at that time was a combination of organizational development and behavioral. As more employees were added and the program expanded, educational, systems, and program development models were also utilized (see Chapter 2). Table 12–1 illustrates some of the consultancy roles and functions that occurred during this period and the models under which they might fall.

TABLE 12–1
Activity Consultation Models and Functions

Behavioral—Addressed such issues as
   Communication skills
   Territoriality
   Problem-solving techniques
   Individual employee concerns
   Time management
   Dealing with change and the continuing expansion of the department

Organizational Development—Advised on the setting up of
   Policies and procedures; job descriptions
   Volunteer program
   Department reorganization and defined responsibilities
   Criteria for, and orientation of, new employees
   Record-keeping systems; budgets

Educational—Identified issues and
   Conducted in-service programs for activity and other personnel
   Interpreted and advised on regulations and regulatory agencies
   Taught process of activity analysis and initiated system of written analyses for
      each activity used
   Trained total staff in reality techniques and set up facilitywide reality orientation
      program
   Taught documentation procedures and content

Program Development—Provided information and guidance on
   Assessing individual needs and interests and designing appropriate programs
   Environmental considerations: site selection for programs, storage, equipment,
      room setups
   Resources: supplies, educational programs, publications
   Addition of new programs, e.g., small group activities, resident council
   Selection of residents for appropriate activities
   Group dynamics and leadership skills

Systems—Worked within the total facility to
   Promote the idea that activities are essential for the well-being of the residents,
      public relations, etc.
   Encourage acceptance and professionalism of activities staff
   Advocate for more personnel, increased salaries

At the end of four years, it was mutually agreed that activities consultant services were no longer required. Good consultants work themselves out of a job,[2] and it had been apparent for several months that it was time to terminate. Almost all of the identified problems had been solved to everyone's satisfaction and the program was running smoothly. In fact, it was considered a model service for other programs in the state. The administrator was reluctant to terminate the consultation, as he wanted his activity personnel to have someone available who understood their concerns. But with assurances that this could be accomplished informally by telephone, he agreed to termination.

Two months later a new type of consultation arrangement was negotiated: an educational model that involved conducting in-service programs. (Appendix D contains a copy of this contract.) These programs were given monthly to two shifts of the total staff and meetings were held periodically with the director of nursing to select the next several topics. This arrangement lasted for 3 years during which such diverse subjects as the psychosocial needs of the elderly and issues regarding death and dying, eating and feeding, sensory changes, aphasia, task breakdown, sexuality, transferring, and safety were covered.

During the next two years only informal contacts were maintained, but then activities consultation services were again requested. The facility, program, and personnel had grown enormously. There were now 12 people in the department and a new activities director. She was a licensed practical nurse and had a strong background in organization and administration, but no knowledge or experience in activities. This led to an unusual situation because the director was also enrolled in the consultant's activity coordinators' training course and it was important that the student-teacher relationship not carry over into the consultation.

This present situation was quite different than it had been two years earlier. Not only had the size of the facility expanded greatly, but the previous administrator had retired, and the director of nursing had become assistant administrator and director of professional services. All administrative contact was now through her, and this presented no problem as a good relationship had been developed in the past. She and the new administrator were very supportive of the activities department and its new director. It was now a more formal arrangement than previously, and almost all communication was through written reports. However, response to any meeting request was prompt and cordial.

This time, although dealing with some of the same issues as before, the focus was on program and organizational development. The first year was spent working almost solely with the director on activity concepts and organizational and personnel concerns. The second year allowed more time to work with other department members, whose number had now grown to 18, with greater emphasis on professional growth and refining of skills.

Another difference in this second consultation contract was that a monthly retainer, rather than an hourly fee, was requested by the consultant and agreed to by the facility. This allowed the consultant to allot the time required for each situation without having to worry about contractual limitations. This arrangement proved satisfactory for all concerned: there were times when several days were spent in the facility in one month and other times when the only contact was by telephone. This type of arrangement, however, required a great deal of trust and flexibility on the part of both the consultant and consultee.

As in most consultations, a complete assessment of the department was done to identify the problem areas and determine where intervention was appropriate. (See Activities Program Evaluation Form and Evaluation of Activities Group Leader in Appendix D.) This set the agenda for the early visits, and the consultant was able to add other issues and concerns as they were identified. Just before the contract was up, two years later, this assessment was repeated to make sure that all the problem areas identified had been addressed and improvement noted.

Outcome

Because of administrative support, the number of available personnel, and the skill the staff achieved, it was very easy to terminate this time, knowing that Shady Hill had an exemplary program. This perception was emphasized in a letter to the assistant administrator that accompanied the final consultation report. The reply received from administration and the facility board of directors demonstrated their gratitude for the help given in achieving their present excellent status.

Although there is no longer a formal relationship to Shady Valley, very close ties are maintained that could be compared to the professional model of consultation. (see Chapter 2). One example is the sharing of resources and information. Staff often call for specific advice or problem-solving help, and they are always willing to field-test the consultant's materials, lend supplies, and host workshops. They also notify the consultant of upcoming meetings and workshops that might be of concern or interest, and send copies of changes in regulations or other pertinent information. Most recently, the author participated in the assessment of several admissions, using the new federally required forms. This afforded an opportunity to actually experience the process and what it entailed, in preparation for teaching other activity personnel.

It is not only the activities personnel with whom there is an ongoing professional relationship, but also administration, nursing, and social service. For example, the consultant collaborated with the director of social services in a project on intergenerational programming, conducted a total staff training series on stress management, and has brought to the attention of the nursing department some new rehabilitation products that were thought to be of value for their residents.

Not only has it been possible for help Shady Valley to respond to changes in the long-term care environment and better meet the needs of its population, but many other benefits to the consultant were derived as well. New materials, tools, and publications were developed and tested during the course of this consultation for use in many other settings and with other older adults. Thus the author's consultation practice grew, and the quality of the services offered was much enhanced.

SUMMARY

The case description presented is only one example of how occupational therapy consultation skills can be used in long-term care facilities. A variety of relationships and methods were demonstrated that can be used to impact on a total system. Through the establishment of a long-term relationship with a facility and its personnel, opportunities existed to change the nature of that relationship as legislative mandates, facility needs, and personnel changed.

The relationship between the consultant and her former consultees has evolved into one that could best be characterized as that of colleagues, with information sharing, advice giving, and opinion seeking flowing freely in both directions. Perhaps that is the best testimony to a successful consultation.

REFERENCES

1. Bennis W, Benne W, Chin R: *The Planning of Change*. New York, Holt, Rinehart and Winston, 1969.
2. Cunninghis RN: *A Professional Guide for Activity Coordinators*. Willingboro, NJ, Geriatric Educational Consultants, 1984.
3. Epstein CF: Consultation: Communicating and facilitating, in Bair J, Gray M (eds): *The Occupational Therapy Manager*. Rockville, Md, AOTA, 1987, pp 299–321.
4. Frank B: Moving ahead with the challenge: Making sense of OBRA. *Provider* March 1990; pp 14–18.
5. Hopkins HL: Current bases for theory and philosophy of occupational therapy, in Hopkins HL, Smith HD (eds): *Willard & Spackman's Occupational Therapy*, ed 7. Philadelphia, Lippincott, 1988.
6. Katcher A: On becoming a consultant to an extended care facility, in *Project for Consultants to Extended Care Facilities*. Los Angeles, Atkins-Katcher Associates, 1969, (Guide Draft).
7. Nackel JG, Jacoby TJ, Shellenbarger MT: *Working With Health Care Consultants*. Chicago, American Hospital Publishing, 1986.
8. Shannon PD: Occupational behavior frame of reference, in Hopkins, HL, Smith HD (eds): *Willard & Spackman's Occupational Therapy,* ed 7. Philadelphia, Lippincott, 1988, pp 142–149.

CHAPTER 13

A Systems Consultation Approach in Long-Term Care

Cynthia F. Epstein, M.A., O.T.R., F.A.O.T.A.

OVERVIEW

Chronically ill and disabled persons have traditionally constituted an area of concern for occupational therapists. A major theme in this consultant's experience has been the older person requiring placement in a nursing facility. Initial experience as a treating therapist in a large community hospital, whose target population included a high percentage of elderly individuals, provided an awareness of the multiple problems faced by patients entering nursing facilities. Later experiences, treating patients in rehabilitation centers, home-care settings, and nursing homes, helped broaden perspective and further an interest in occupational therapy consultation that emphasized health promotion through a systems approach.[4]

Life milestones, including roles as wife, mother, and volunteer leader in professional and community organizations, created a need for flexibility in workdays and hours. Concurrently, significant legislation directed toward long-term care service delivery at state and federal levels mandated increased occupational therapy involvement in nursing facilities.[1]

As demands for occupational therapy service grew in community nursing facilities, it was evident that these treatment services required support through the broader perspective of consultation. Without systemwide intervention, the occupational therapy treatment provided had minimal carryover or continuing effect. Networking through the state occupational therapy organizations confirmed that this problem existed in many facilities, particularly where therapists were part time and practiced in isolation.[4]

In 1979, a New Jersey corporation, Occupational Therapy Consultants, Inc. (OTC), was formed to provide consultative, restorative, and educational services. Starting with four very part-time therapists working in two regions of the state and providing services in six nursing homes, the practice grew in size and scope over the years. By 1991, 45 therapists were employed. Approximately one third were full time, and service sites had expanded to include schools, home care, developmental centers, adult day-care programs, as well as nursing facilities.

Requests for services were generated through satisfied clientele, related professionals, and, most importantly, through the occupational therapy community. This referral base was established as a result of comprehensive, high-quality services, delivered in a consistent and cost-effective manner by a skilled and knowledgeable staff.

The consultation experience presented here was requested by a large (340-bed) state-run nursing facility that had been apprised of OTC's services by a sister facility. The facility (Parkview) was located on a large campus in the midst of a suburban community. It had originally been a retirement home, and therefore its oldest buildings dated back to the turn of the century. The newer buildings had been built in the mid-1960s. Occupational therapy had never been a part of this facility's program. Recent changes in federal and state law[8, 12, 13] had alerted facility administration to their lack of an interdisciplinary team approach that should have included occupational therapy. They were also interested in developing a wheelchair management system.[2] Having heard of the progress made at their sister facility, where OTC had recently begun services, they requested a meeting to discuss their needs.

ENVIRONMENT AND SYSTEMS INFLUENCES

This consultation took place in mid-1990, when the state of New Jersey acknowledged its extraordinary fiscal crisis. A new governor had recently been elected and many changes were taking place. In an attempt to consolidate, the state reorganized jurisdiction for some of its long-term care facilities. Parkview and its sister facilities were among those transferred out of one state department jurisdiction into another. At the time of the consultation, communication lines and funding sources emanating from the new jurisdiction to the facility were still unclear. Rumors abounded regarding possible shifts in personnel. While direct word had not been received, the chief executive officer (CEO) and his assistant had been assured their positions were secure, but they were advised that other lower management shifts might occur.

The CEO and his assistant had recently reviewed new federal and state regulations that were about to be implemented as a result of the Omnibus Budget Reconciliation Act of 1987 (OBRA).[8, 13] Facilities unable to meet these new regulations were at risk of losing major funding sources. Regulation emphasis on quality of life issues and utilization of an interdisciplinary team approach triggered the request for occupational therapy consultation.

Given the existing financial constraints, it was agreed that the focus of the consultation should be a needs assessment. This would determine the scope of occupational therapy services and would suggest a plan of action. Actual implementation of the plan would then be considered, taking into account regulatory mandates, fiscal constraints, and the degree of need identified.

FRAME OF REFERENCE

The frame of reference developed for the long-term care consultation was drawn from several perspectives and considered the needs of Parkview. First, the client wanted to determine if there was a need for occupational therapy services at the facility. Their current operations did not include this service, nor did they utilize an interdisciplinary approach. Second, they wanted to develop a plan that could address ongoing problems with wheelchairs and patient positioning. Third, fiscal constraints only allowed for the development of a plan. Future monies would be sought in the next budget year, should the decision be to implement occupational therapy services.

These objectives required level III, program and administrative consultation, because the system (Parkview) was in need of change. During the course of the consultation, various consultation models were utilized, including clinical, educational, systems, and process management.

The referral had been generated with a specific interest in wheelchair management and seating. Having worked extensively in this area,[2, 3, 5, 6] the consultant and her staff used this specific issue as the key to their system analysis. Wheelchair management required the use of an interdisciplinary team, clearly identified occupational therapy's pivotal role,[7] and was an acknowledged system problem.

While systems theory was the overarching principle in this consultation, the consultant also utilized other frames of reference. Most specifically, occupational behavior and developmental and rehabilitation frames of reference[9] were important when considering patient wheelchair needs.

The occupational behavior frame of reference is based on general systems theory.[11] Its emphasis on the total environment and use of purposeful activity to facilitate adaptation and mastery of skill leads to success in the performance of meaningful occupation. Wheelchair-bound patients in a long-term care facility seek independence in mobility, which is most effectively achieved through a comprehensive wheelchair management system.[2] This approach requires looking at the patient and his or her wheelchair needs, the facility and its ability to support these needs, and the interactive process required to assure that once these needs are successfully addressed, the system can be maintained.

From a more clinical perspective, the developmental and rehabilitative needs of individual patients needed to be assessed. Current and potential function in activities of daily living (ADL) was considered, as was currently assigned wheelchair equipment. The need for change in equipment to facilitate developmental and rehabilitative goals was also an integral part of the assessment process.

The consultants' role was to obtain, analyze, and interpret the data in an objective manner. Communication was crucial and required a planned educational process in order to help the system work effectively with the consultation team.

CONSULTATION DESCRIPTION

Organization

Parkview was a 340-bed facility whose patients were classified at skilled and domiciliary levels of care. The majority of them (300) required skilled nursing care. One wing of 40 beds was the domiciliary, or board and care unit. While the focus was on the 300 skilled beds, residents in the domiciliary unit were reviewed so that the plan could address total system needs.

The organizational structure was traditional in design. Under the CEO and his assistant were the directors of all departments. Rehabilitation services consisted of physical therapy. Contracts were held by outside providers for speech and occupational therapy services, but neither were visible or had active caseloads. Team conferences were held monthly, and the usual attendees were medicine, nursing, and social services. The resident council was dormant and volunteer activities consisted of weekly bingo games combined with monthly outings to community sites.

The physical environment in the main building created mobility barriers. The building, built at the turn of the century, had been modified over the years to accommodate increasing numbers of residents, but its public spaces, such as dining and recreation areas, had not been functionally integrated into the building design. Therefore, some residents were required to traverse the equivalent of three city blocks to reach a communal area.

Two outlying units, each housing 100 residents, had been built in the 1960s, and their design did place public space central to nursing wings. These two buildings were in close proximity, but one needed to go outside to go from one to the other.

Although core staff were assigned to each building, activities, volunteers, social services, and physical therapy staff moved through all units. Because of the fragmentation, communication between disciplines was poor and sporadic in nature. Each building had its own unique characteristics and flavor, which reflected the perspective of the core staff, predominantly nursing, dietary, and housekeeping.

Support

The facility administration sought consultation services to plan for new regulations that required a shift in service delivery. Limited funding was available in the current budget. Fiscal constraints loomed in the future. To analyze their needs and present a convincing argument for increased funding to meet new regulations, the consultation group was asked to perform a needs assessment. A set fee was arranged, days were scheduled for consultant on-site visits, and office space was allocated for the days the consultation team was present. The consultation team was also given access to the facility's computer database to obtain patient demographics. It was agreed that the assistant administrator would be the team's liaison with facility staff.

Participants

The consultation team consisted of the lead consultant and two junior consultant staff. All were occupational therapists. The lead consultant developed the assessment strategies, structured the overall process, and acted as the spokesperson for the team. The team had a general format to follow for data collection. In addition, each consultant was assigned to pay particular attention to one issue. The three issues were environment (human and nonhuman), patient physical status that contributed to ADL functioning, and psychosocial considerations that related to functional performance.

Major support and communication for the consultation came from the assistant administrator. He and his staff arranged to have consultants meet with key department heads. These included nursing, medicine, activities, social services, and physical therapy. The director of social services and her staff were particularly supportive and active in providing information to the consultants. While the directors of nursing and medicine met with the consultants, their support was inconsistent. The consultants, with assistance from the assistant administrator and director of social service, were able to identify a nursing staff liaison in each building. The director of physical therapy was only available for a brief meeting with the consultants. He outlined the maintenance program available, and indicated that little, if any, restorative work was being done.

In general, it was evident that key persons in the facility had different feelings about the consultation. The consultants' strategy was to work initially through those individuals who were supportive and to establish a method for gaining trust with the other key persons during the first days of the consultation.

Services Provided

The consultation team was invited into the system with administrative sanction. An initial meeting, held with the administrator, assistant administrator, and director of nursing, was used to clarify and identify the specific reasons for the consultation request. Groundwork for this initial meeting had been laid through telephone contacts with the lead consultant and administrative networking that occurred between Parkview and its sister facility. In the sister facility, the consultant's organization was providing consultative, educational, and restorative services and had achieved significant recognition for its work.

Subsequent to the initial meeting, a proposal to perform the needs assessment was developed by the consultant. This proposal served as the basis for an agreement between the facility and the consultant group. A sample of the proposal format used can be found in Appendix D. The proposal outlined the consultation goals, identified the consultant team, stated the fee for service, and proposed the consultation time frame. It also stated the obligations of both consultant and consultee, so that each understood their responsibilities in the consultation process.

The needs assessment goals were as follows:

I. Identify and rank critical occupational therapy patient service needs in the following areas:
   A. Activities of daily living (ADL)
   B. Seating and mobility (wheelchair management)
II. Identify and rank critical facility (environment) needs for specialized occupational therapy programs that utilize an interdisciplinary (systems) team approach:
   A. Human environment
   B. Nonhuman environment
   C. Systems approach via an interdisciplinary team
III. Develop recommendations for occupational therapy service implementation.

The first step in the consultation process was to develop a common framework for all facility staff. This would allow for productive communication and provide a basis for the establishment of trust. On the initial visit an orientation meeting was scheduled with all key departments. The lead consultant conducted the 90-minute training session, using a slide presentation, informational handouts to support the lecture, and a question and answer period.

This facility had no experience with occupational therapy services. It did not utilize a team approach to rehabilitation. It had no active restorative programming carried through by nursing staff, and staff had no experience with an interdisciplinary approach to patient care. The 90-minute presentation was keyed to these issues and used the development of a systemwide wheelchair management program[3] as an example. A critical concept, which was reinforced throughout the presentation, was the importance of a team approach and the establishment of specialized restorative programming, such as that utilized in wheelchair management. Figure 13–1 illustrates the concept as it was presented to the facility.

This visual aid enabled the consultant to illustrate the importance of each team member, the interrelatedness of their tasks, and the role played by quality assurance and in-service education to maintain the program. Through this process, it was possible to elicit comments and concerns from each department. These points then helped the consultants to target specific areas for in-depth data collection. For instance, the director of dietary indicated that many residents were not eating in the communal dining room because it required too much staff time to position them functionally at tables. Dietary staff did not see this task as their role. Nursing staff, likewise, did not see it as part of their role. It was therefore easier to provide tray service on the unit for these residents.

The consultation team followed this training session by meeting with key team members on each nursing unit. They were guided to these key persons by the assistant administrator and director of social services. At each unit meeting, the consultants used handouts and experiential learning methods to help staff understand the consultation focus and need for their support and assistance in the process.

Using structured data collection methodology designed for the needs assessment, each consultant then worked with staff and patients on a given unit to

FIGURE 13–1

Restorative Program Team Concept

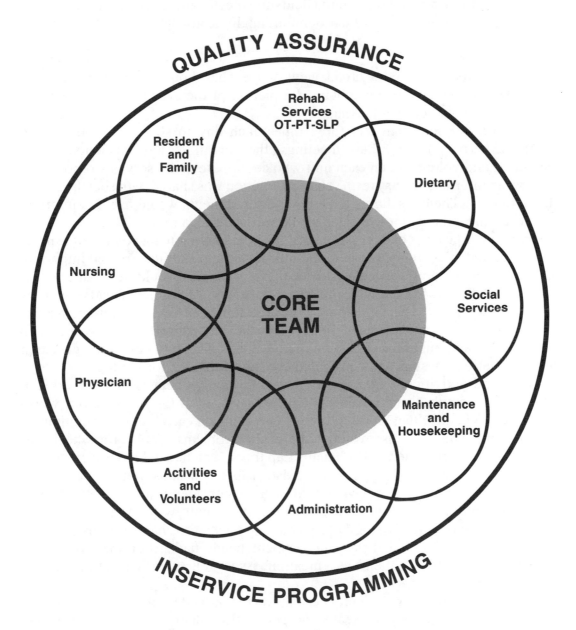

obtain necessary information. The consultation time constraints did not allow the consultant team to perform an in-depth assessment for every patient or problem identified. The team established a set of criteria to identify 20 patients from each nursing unit. The criteria were as follows:

1. Five residents with the longest length of stay who were in wheelchairs or gerichairs.

2. Five residents most recently admitted who were in wheelchairs or geri-chairs.

3. Unit staff identification of (a) five residents who were their most difficult positioning problems and (b) five residents in wheelchairs or gerichairs currently requiring tray service who, in their opinion, might be able to eat in the communal dining room.

These criteria allowed a broad view of the chair-bound patient population. Concurrently, the consultants obtained a picture of the system interactions that supported clinical decision making.

The consultation team met three times each day to share information and special expertise. During these meetings, they identified key residents, family members, and volunteers on each unit who could potentially serve as representatives on an interdisciplinary team. This information was shared with social services and activities. The consultants hoped these departments would use this information when the team met to consider the final consultation report.

During the process of data collection, the consultation team combined aspects of clinical and educational consultation models to help staff understand important out-of-bed positioning concepts. Use of these principles would help patients become more functional. Periodic meetings with key department heads, such as nursing and social services, helped reinforce the need for an interdisciplinary approach on a systemwide basis. In addition, the lead consultant briefly met with the assistant administrator each time the team was on site. These strategies kept communication lines open and provided constant feedback for the team.

Mealtime activities, where positioning and environment issues are critical, were heavily emphasized. Given the concerns voiced at the introductory workshop, the lead consultant chose to observe mealtime in each building's communal dining room. She soon discovered some of the problems. Tables for wheelchair residents were not at the correct height. Lap trays, which could have been used as an alternative table surface, did not exist. Table pedestals were a barrier for wheelchairs with fixed front rigging. Staff had not considered seating patients with positioning problems at tables located close to the entryway. At the entryway, there would be opportunity for dietary and nursing staff to share responsibility for positioning. Nursing and dietary department heads had never met to discuss positioning of problem patients as a mealtime issue. It first surfaced at the consultants' introductory workshop.

The consultant obtained facility permission to take slide pictures of the presenting problems and of patients seated properly after adaptations had been made. These slides were then used as part of the exit meeting presentation.

Consultation evaluation was ongoing. As the consultants established trust within the facility, feedback from staff increased, and collaborative fact-finding between consultants and staff became more common. The facility's informal rhythms and networking strategies became evident. This allowed consultants to utilize an ongoing informal evaluation process. Thus they were able to monitor the effectiveness of their strategies and make modifications as needed.

Closure was accomplished through a series of planned meetings and a final written report. The first meeting was held with the administrator, assistant administrator, director of nursing, director of social services, and medical director. Here the lead consultant, acting as spokesperson for the team, reviewed the assessment findings and the consultant team's recommendations. An exit meeting followed with all departments. The consultants used this meeting to reemphasize the importance of the interdisciplinary team and the coordinating roles that occupational therapy could assume. The meeting served as an open forum regarding the consultation recommendations. A written report followed that again detailed all findings and recommendations.

The report was based on 130 patients rather than the 120 originally targeted. The ten were added through social service referral. This sample constituted 42% of the patients residing in the three buildings. A total of 117 patients, or 90% of those surveyed were found to need some type of occupational therapy intervention. The needs ranged from relatively simple but important aids to independence, such as dressing or eating devices, to complex positioning issues or a need for specialized treatment techniques.

Seventy-two (72%) percent required training in one or more aspects of ADL. Many patients, who were categorized as dependent for such self-care as grooming, dressing, and eating, showed potential for greater independence. These patients, the report indicated, would be identified in the new OBRA survey process. In order to prevent deficiencies, occupational therapy should be involved to provide a functional assessment and plan.

Over 50% of those in wheelchairs/gerichairs required intervention to modify or change their seating environment and/or equipment. Of these, 40% were restrained and required review for compliance with the new regulations. Of particular concern were the large proportion of hemiplegics and amputees and those at risk for pressure sores. The report pointed out that there would be need for special equipment to reduce risk of pressure ulceration and falls; assure stable seating; and improve mobility. A cognitive treatment program utilizing task segmentation, structured learning, and special techniques was recommended for 30% of the population, some of whom also fell into the restraint category.

Sixty-five (65%) percent of the sample were at risk for or had contractures. Of these, 30% required some type of splinting intervention. Specialized programs for range of motion and/or contracture monitoring were also needed.

Many patients (33%) required adaptive/assistive devices to increase their functional independence. Over 50% of the sample had sensorimotor deficits in such areas as postural stability, range of motion, visual-perceptual ability, motor planning, and strength and endurance.

Patients with behavioral problems occupied an extensive amount of staff time and created an environmental "press."[10] They made the unit or dayroom uncomfortable for others. These patients were perceived negatively, and consequently, minimal opportunities existed for positive reinforcement and behavioral shaping. Specifically designed occupational therapy programs and approaches were therefore recommended. It was suggested that task groups and individualized programs that utilize activities to provide positive feedback and achievement could be designed and implemented. As the groups stabilized, the therapist could work with activities staff to help integrate these approaches into their programming. Table 13–1 summarizes the report findings.

When considering the total facility needs, the report recommended utilizing the restorative team program concept presented at the initial meeting (see Figure 13–1). This would involve specialized core teams drawn from the overall interdisciplinary team. Occupational therapy would coordinate programs they designed.[7] Occupational therapy's familiarity with systems theory would help the facility integrate this concept into their method of operation. This approach would facilitate ongoing communication, effective planning, and implementation of restorative programs leading to greater patient independence.

In regard to the nonhuman environment, the consultants suggested that occupational therapy be involved in restructuring communal space in each building. This included multipurpose rooms, dining areas, and wide hallways that could also serve as an area for some meaningful activities.

Development of a wheelchair management system was identified as a strong need. Assignment of proper equipment, well cared for and maintained, would help patients achieve greater functional independence in the facility and community. An eating skills program based on systems theory was also suggested.[14] These two pivotal programs would emphasize teamwork while improving patient and facility functional performance.

In summary, the report recommended that the facility establish an occupational therapy department to address important needs. Given fiscal constraints, a gradual

TABLE 13–1
Occupational Therapy Service Needs

N = 130 patients/42% of population

Patient Area of Need	Percentage*
Requires assessment/ treatment	90%
ADL treatment	72% (4,5)
Seating and mobility (wheelchair management)	50% (1,3,4)
Therapeutic adaptations	65% (2,3,4)
Sensorimotor treatment	50% (1,2,3,4)
Cognitive treatment	30% (4,5)
Psychosocial treatment	30% (1,4,5)

* It is projected that treatment needs of the remaining 58% of the population will not be as great as sample population.
Note: The numbers in parentheses refer to trigger areas that are identified through the Minimum Data Set (MDS)[13] screening tool: (1) = Restraint; (2) = Contracture; (3) = Falls; (4) = Functional independence; and (5) = Behavior.

phase-in was suggested. The department could be started in one building and would gradually expand throughout the facility as money became available. The issues of space, equipment, and supplies for the proposed department were submitted as an addendum to the report.

The consultation terminated with the submission of a final report. It was now the facility's responsibility to consider all findings and determine the feasibility of establishing an occupational therapy department. The administrator indicated to the lead consultant that the major stumbling block to implementation would be the state's financial crisis. He acknowledged the comprehensiveness of the assessment and stated he would advise the consultant group of his final decision.

Outcome

The facility used the consultation report to request funding for an occupational therapy service. Since the consultation took place late in the fiscal year, budgets had already been submitted for the upcoming year. This new request was therefore presented as an emergency need. The request was rejected due to an increasingly bleak state budget. The administrator advised that their only hope lay with the survey process, expected later in the year. The consultant indicated that her organization would remain available to help reinforce the important need for service. As the year wore on, it was evident that the facility faced greater cutbacks. New programs were shelved until the state's financial situation changed for the better.

SUMMARY

A needs assessment format was used for this consultation experience. It illustrates the use of a consultant team, the importance of comprehensive data gathering, ongoing staff education and open communication, and the reality of fiscal constraints.

Recognizing the important role of the interdisciplinary team in long-term care, a systems consultation approach was suggested. Through the needs assessment process, the consultant gained an opportunity to demonstrate occupational therapy's pivotal role in the system. This approach is particularly important for long-term care facilities seeking to meet current mandates. Emphasis on quality of life issues and resident functional independence requires a skilled and well-organized team. This team must appreciate and utilize a systems approach effectively. Occupational therapy consultants, knowledgeable in systems theory and aware of multiple system needs, can help facilities incorporate this approach into their service delivery.

Timing is a critical aspect of any consultation. Changes in a system's climate can directly affect consultation outcomes, as was evident in this case example. While this consultation did not result in the establishment of an occupational therapy service at the facility, the foundation has been laid.

REFERENCES

1. AOTA Government Affairs: Medicare coverage for occupational therapy services. *Am J Occup Ther* 1974; 28:109.
2. Epstein CF: Wheelchair management: Developing a system for long-term care facilities. *J Long-Term Care Admin* 1980; 8:(2)1–12.
3. Epstein CF: Wheelchair management guidelines. Somerville, NJ, Occupational Therapy Consultants, Inc, 1981.
4. Epstein CF: Program model of gerontology services in the community: A written interview, in Hopkins HL, Smith H (eds): *Willard & Spackman's Occupational Therapy,* ed 6. Philadelphia, Lippincott, 1983, Chapter 38, pp. 805–806.
5. Epstein CF: Seating the institutionalized elderly: Keys to success. *Pin Dot News* 1988; 1:6.
6. Epstein CF: Specialized seating for the institutionalized elderly: Prescription, fabrication, funding, technology review 1989, in Gwin C, (ed): *Perspectives on Occupational Therapy Practice.* Rockville, Md, AOTA, 1989, pp 13–16.
7. Epstein CF: Specialized restorative programs, in Kiernat J (ed): *Occupational Therapy for the Older Adult: A Clinical Manual.* Gaithersburg, Md, Aspen, 1991, pp 285–300.
8. Health Care Financing Administration Omnibus Reconciliation Act of 1987: Interpretive guidelines: Skilled nursing facilities and intermediate care facilities. Rev. 232, 1990.
9. Hopkins HL: Current basis for theory and philosophy of occupational therapy, in Hopkins HL, Smith H (eds): *Willard & Spackman's Occupational Therapy,* ed 7. Philadelphia, Lippincott, 1989, Chapter 3, pp. 38–42.
10. Lawton MP: Environment and Aging. Monterey, Calif, Brooks/Cole, 1980.
11. Matsutsuyu JS: Occupational behavior—a perspective on work and play. *Am J Occup Ther* 1971; 24:291.
12. Morris JN, Hawes C, Fries BE, et al: Designing the national resident assessment instrument for nursing homes. *The Gerontologist* 1990; 30:3.
13. Morris JN, Hawes C, Murphy K, et al: *Resident Assessment Instrument Training Manual and Resource Guide.* Natick, Mass, Elliot Press, 1991.
14. Weiss DR, Conyers KH, Epstein CF: A systems approach to eating skills programming in long-term care. *Occup Ther Practice* 1992; 3:2.

CHAPTER 14

Mental Health Consultation in a Long-Term Care Facility

Diane Gibson, M.S., O.T.R./L.

OVERVIEW

Consultation in a large psychiatric hospital, which includes inpatient and outpatient services as well as a variety of varying programs and populations, is a regular and demanding aspect of the occupational therapy director's job. It is defined as a process by which expertise is made available to those seeking assistance in solving problems.[1] Typically consultation involves one or more of the following:

1. Problem identification and solution
2. Program and policy development
3. Conflict resolution
4. Education and training

All of the role functions listed require considerable experience, a high level of interpersonal skills, confidentiality, and an extensive knowledge of institutional norms and structure. In a psychiatric long-term care facility, the major aspects of consultation are those undertaken as an internal consultant. In some cases, the occupational therapy director/consultant may also be asked to provide consultation services to external agencies or facilities, as a part of the overall job or as an independent contractor. This chapter focuses on internal consultation.

Internal consultation, which is defined as consultation inside the hospital, is available to program directors within a matrix model. Typical issues concern staff problems, the role of occupational therapy, or the need for more staff. Specific examples include a physician manager who asked the consultant to determine numbers and qualifications of rehabilitation staff for a new eating disorders unit, and a physician who requested that the consultant discriminate between role functions in nursing and occupational therapy in a neuropsychiatric unit.

Occasionally, the person requesting the consultation, the consultee, is not able to identify clearly the nature of the problem. For example, the problem might be stated, "There seems to be a great deal of tension between the occupational and recreation therapists," or "The borderline personality disorder unit is losing too many staff." The amorphous and perhaps anxious note in the request indicated a potentially complex problem that had generated increasing tension. In dealing with this problem the consultant asked for specific information regarding the issue such as conceptual clarity of staff roles and the mission statement of the treatment unit. Recommendations involved clarification of each discipline's role with resulting reduction in conflict due to territorialism. Other recommendations included a salary survey to provide information regarding comparative salaries and the need for in-service education dealing with borderline personality disorder management.

The dual role of the occupational director and the consultant incorporates role differences that may be both beneficial or counterproductive to the hospital system. As occupational therapy director, the consultant has an opportunity to know the hospital system more completely, thus speeding the process and applying the consultation in a knowledgeable way. However, the potential bias of the dual role might contaminate and reduce the director's impact unless she is astute regarding its impact.

A second form of consultation is external in nature and pertains to recommendations given to occupational therapy departments in other mental health agencies or psychiatric facilities. In some cases, consultation is requested by family service agencies, psychosocial programs, or community support groups.

EXPECTATIONS

The consultee expects the consultant to define accurately and to solve the problem in a manner that will benefit the persons affected as well as the institution as a whole. A series of assumptions exist. First, the consultant will deal with the specified situation in a serious and respectful manner. Second, she will make observations that will elucidate component parts of the problem and tasks in a rational manner. Third, she will provide the information and insight necessary to complete the designated solution.

For example, the medical director asked the author, the internal consultant, to develop a smoke-free hospital policy and program for the entire health care system. In preparation, the consultant studied other hospitals' policies, information available from the American Cancer and the American Lung associations as well as a new state law that prohibited smoking by employees. Second, the consultant formed a small committee comprised of representatives from various departments and the patient population. The committee surveyed the employee and patient body to ascertain the number of smokers, significant attitudes, and need for cessation programs. As director, the author wrote the policy, which can be defined as an administrative function, rather than a consultative service. As consultant, the author assisted in recommending strategies for implementing the smoke-free environment.

The consultant may be asked to use sophisticated education, clinical, or administrative skills in the design of new programs and policies. Consultations to program managers (e.g., the day hospital manager) outside the centralized department may be narrowly or broadly defined. A narrowly defined focus, such as listing the credentials required by the hospital position description, Joint Commission of Health Care Organization standards, or state licensing laws, may be handled easily via awareness of professional standards. However, a broad focus, such as consultation in planning a new halfway house, requires a complex integration of knowledge and skills in many areas in addition to numerous contacts with housing, health, and zoning authorities.

The consultant assumes opinions and findings will be recognized and incorporated into the outcomes sought by the requesting administrator. Success of the consultation is dependent on the willingness and ability of those involved in the project to provide information, to answer questions thoughtfully, and to be willing to change. Usually the consultant must assist the consultee with the change process.

POTENTIAL MARKET

Administrators, program chiefs, and department heads constitute the main market for the experienced occupational therapist consultant in a long-term hospital. Occasionally, lower levels of staff request assistance of a technical nature or an interpersonal nature. Consultation within the hospital enhances the visibility and prestige of the occupational therapy department through the work of the director. Increased system awareness of the director's consultant role expands knowledge and status of occupational therapy practice, thus providing a positive image of the home department. As the competence of the consultant grows, recognition of her expertise grows accordingly, and as a result she may be asked to provide external consultation with agencies and organizations outside her own workplace. Mastery of the consultative processes may open up opportunities in other psychiatric institutions or even far beyond her familiar domain. For example, as a result of her interest in supervision, stress management, and conflict resolution, the author was asked to run training sessions for local businesses, public schools, and the county police department.

Although the perceptive and assertive occupational therapist may be invited to perform a consulting role in identifying and solving problems, she may also tactfully announce her willingness to perform an advisory role. As the competent occupational therapy consultant finds spin-off opportunities opening up for her both within the hospital as well as in the community at large, she needs to take on new assignments with caution and not stretch herself too thin.

KEY POINTS

Necessary Knowledge and Skills

Appropriate, sophisticated knowledge and skills relevant to the area of consultation is an absolute requirement. Both professional competence in occupational therapy and administration are mandatory in most consultations. For example, the psychiatric occupational therapy consultant must possess a high level of knowledge in theoretical frames of reference that can be operationalized in treatment application. Psychodynamic and interpersonal theory are useful in understanding and interpreting patient behavior, whereas cognitive disability theory, the model of human occupation, developmental theory, and behavior modification are employed to guide the treatment of differing diagnoses and age groups. Knowing how to administer assessment instruments and treatment interventions appropriate to each frame of reference is essential in consultation regarding new program development or updating ongoing programs. In an illustrative case, the author was asked to provide consultation in the development of a psychiatric quarterway house for the chronically mentally ill (CMI). The treatment philosophy chosen was a rehabilitation model with behavior modification components. Emphasis was placed on skill acquisition in activities of daily living and community adjustment. Hence, the Bay Area Functional Performance Evaluation (BaFPE) was suggested as an assessment instrument to be coupled with a psychoeducational training program. Patients were expected to learn basic survival skills by practicing them, and as a result of this expectation, the rehabilitation counselors were given training in their role as teachers and supporters of patient efforts. From an administrative perspective, the consultant assisted in planning the architectural design of the quarterway house, reviewing county fire and health codes, establishing the number of CMI clients in the project, and determining a feasible first-year budget. Throughout the consultation the author worked extensively with other disciplines, administrators, and staff of county agencies.

When the consultation involves personnel other than occupational therapists, at least a cursory knowledge of the other professional roles and knowledge bases is essential. Academic course work in administration is valuable in establishing a baseline of needed knowledge; however, the consultant must have experience in everyday problem solving and program development before she is able to choose and implement the strategies with the most positive impact. Bluffing one's way through a consultation without background knowledge or experience leads to disillusionment and disappointment on both sides of the consultation.

Entry Into the System

Not all occupational therapists want to become consultants, given the demanding, stressful, and analytic nature of the consultancy role. The following vignette illustrates an example of entry into long-term care consultation. An occupational therapist veteran with ten years of experience in psychiatry decided to seek the challenge of consultation. She had read widely about the key behaviors involved in consultation and regularly used her experience to promote insight into sophisticated clinical awareness. She had established her professional reputation as one of utmost responsibility, integrity, and competence in psychosocial dysfunction. Knowing that professional dress and behavior were important to securing consultations, she selected tasteful clothing and carried out her duties in a quiet, responsible manner. Interested in making her skills and interests visible, she volunteered to serve on department and hospitalwide committees as well as to assist others in ad hoc problem solving. She made a point of unobtrusively sharing her special interest in group dynamics with her supervisor and with the training specialist, both of whom responded by inviting her to present an in-service on handling the hostile patient in groups. She continued to build entry points into consultancy by sharing her group skills at local professional meetings.

Negotiation with the Potential Client

Prior to entering the actual consultation, the consultant discusses the problem, issue, or need for program development with the client in an effort to arrive at consensual clarity about what is expected. Questions such as, "What outcomes do you expect? How much time do you anticipate the project will take? With whom shall I talk? Where shall I meet with them? and How much will I be paid?" are all basic in the negotiating phase. Frequently, the client formulates a written proposal that describes the agreement in a concrete and formal fashion. Its value rests in prevention of disagreements during and at the end of the consultation.

Within an institution, consultation at the department head level is a formal part of the position description and therefore does not result in extra compensation. Outside the institution, practice varies regarding whether compensation is retained by the consultant or given back to the institution. Hospital policies describe this expectation; if they do not, it is best to discuss this eventuality with a supervisor.

Establishment of Trust

Establishment of trust is a significant part of the consultation's ultimate success. It is created by both parties' belief that each side is genuine in statements of concern and willingness to change. On the consultee's part, trust is engendered by the perceived competence and reputation of the consultant.

In addition, several techniques may be utilized to promote trust; in fact, they are basically similar to ones used for the same purpose in treating psychiatric patients. *First: Listen quietly and carefully to the meaning and reason for the consult request.* In an interpersonal conflict, does the consultee want to calm the conflict by sealing it over or does he or she want to assist the participants in understanding their conflict in an effort to forge an understanding in which both can win? *Second: Determine the overt and covert needs of the consultee*. Ascertaining these needs will allow you to plan the consultation in the most efficient manner and in a way that meets with the least resistance. Is the consult based on a supervisor's power needs, compliance with external standards, or team building expectations? *Third: Empower the consultee* by helping him or her acknowledge personal and professional rights, teaching assertiveness techniques, and assuming that through your actions he or she is capable of solving problems. There is no need for the consultant to assume complete control of the problematic situation. Greater respect and better outcomes will accrue to the consultee if he or she uses your information and support to act on his or her own behalf, particularly in the case of conflict. *Fourth: Use humor to break deadlocks of stress, conflict, and burnout*. Allowing yourself to appear vulnerable and the ability to laugh at yourself is a valuable role-modeling technique in adapting to change. The levity produced through humor reduces anxiety and allows blocked thinking to become more spontaneous and creative.

Consultation Strategies

A decision-making model is useful in planning the stages and structuring a systematic approach to the consultation. Applying the model takes the process out of the intuitive and subjective realms and encourages a calming and rational approach. The stages of the model are as follows:

1. *Identification of problem/issue* includes careful definition, which is arrived at as a result of discussion with the consultee, other significant person, and related reading matter.
2. *Data gathering* is necessary to develop further aspects of the problem and suggest potential options for change. Reports, statistical information, and focus groups are indicated at this stage.
3. *Generating and weighing alternatives for action* is undertaken in order to explore the possible actions along with associated pros and cons. Ultimately a decision or series of related decisions are made and presented to the consultee.
4. *Implementation of the changes* is made according to a plan that outlines who is responsible, what will take place, and when it will occur. Anticipated outcomes are reviewed with the people who will be affected.
5. *Evaluation of the changes* is conducted to determine whether the action was effective. Modifications are made to correct the direction of change and to keep it on target. Outcomes are documented in a final report to the consultee.

A mini case study exemplifies this model. Given unfortunate cutbacks in the hospital salary budget, Mary, an occupational therapy consultant, was asked to determine how patient services were to be provided on the chronic schizophrenia ward. The program administrator asked that the plans be determined collaboratively with nursing staff.

Mary met with the nurse manager on the ward, then with a joint committee of nurses and the ward occupational therapist to clarify the problem and to gather data. She found that members of both disciplines recognized the problem, yet were afraid to collaborate. Mary met with the committee several times in an effort to reach agreement about the common problems and goals. She assisted the staff in identifying the needs of the patient population, objectives for treatment, and eventually which disciplines had sufficient skills to lead different groups. She continued discussion regarding schedules, supervision, and reporting mechanism; the staff reached consensus and implemented the ward-based treatment program. Mary helped the committee draw up evaluative criteria to measure outcomes in terms of quantity and quality of treatment. After periodic monitoring and modification of the changes, Mary terminated her involvement and wrote a final report.

SUMMARY

Consultation in a long-term facility encompasses the same principles as consultation in other settings, despite the variations in staff, patients, settings, or content. The consultant uses technical expertise, such as her knowledge of medical conditions, treatment, and interventions in conjunction with her organizational and administrative knowledge and skill to assist others in solving problems. For example, in mental health, a consultant may provide clinical recommendations such as dynamic understanding of the borderline personality disorder patients' splitting behaviors or means to deescalate an aggressive psychotic patient. Designing new programs and staffing patterns for halfway houses or a smoke-free hospital program are further examples. The role is complex and occasionally difficult, but one for which the occupational therapist is well suited, particularly given her understanding of groups, human motivation, and interpersonal skills.

REFERENCES

1. Epstein CF: Consultation: Communicating and facilitating, in Bair J, Gray M (eds): *The Occupational Therapy Manager*. Rockville, Md, AOTA, 1985.

CHAPTER 15

Quality Assurance Consultation in a Developmental Center

Diane R. Weiss, M.A., O.T.R.

OVERVIEW

Since 1981, quality assurance and utilization review have been mandated as a way to cut health costs and develop criteria and standards for quality care. As a pioneer in this area, the American Occupational Therapy Association, in 1974, included quality assurance as an essential element in its Standard of Practice.*

Occupational therapists practicing in developmental centers and other long-term care settings are particularly concerned about implementation and carryover of care plans that seek to maintain resident goals achieved during treatment. An important example is a splinting program, including the application, use, and maintenance of splints for individual residents. Caregivers who work with residents requiring daily splint application must be well trained, motivated, and committed to carrying out the specific program required for each resident.

As with all medically prescribed programs, splint care-plan compliance is crucial for maximal effectiveness. Consequently, ensuring staff carryover of a splinting program becomes a critical quality assurance issue.

A program development model of consultation was used in a state developmental center to design and implement a splint compliance quality assurance program. The occupational therapy consultant worked collaboratively with direct care staff, nurses, supervisory personnel, educators, related service personnel and other members of the interdisciplinary team. Using case-centered, educational,

---

* References 1, 4–6, and 8–12.

and program levels of consultation, the consultant was involved in assessment, design, implementation, and evaluation of the program.

POTENTIAL MARKET FOR QUALITY ASSURANCE CONSULTATION IN LONG-TERM CARE SETTINGS

Quality assurance within an institution presents a major challenge for rehabilitative service providers. An expected outcome of the rehabilitation treatment process is a maintenance care plan. This plan helps assure carryover of therapy gains into the client's daily regime.[2] Quality assurance is the appropriate vehicle to reinforce this carryover.[3] Rehabilitative personnel are usually a small part of any institution's staffing pattern. Direct treatment services become the foremost focus, with little time available for a quality assurance component, especially one that requires monitoring the performance of other personnel.

An increasing number of nursing facilities and their complex clientele require broader rehabilitation services. The changing emphasis within these institutions, focused on greater client independence and function[7] has created an unlimited market for quality assurance consultation.

Utilization of a consultative model to develop and help implement quality assurance programs is a cost-efficient and effective approach. The consultant brings expertise in the specific quality assurance program area, for example, splints, adaptive devices, wheelchairs, and the ability to help the institution and its multidisciplinary team generate the necessary compliance program. Potential long-term care settings for this type of consultation include developmental centers, nursing facilities, school systems, and group homes. Any facility that requires the incorporation of specialized equipment or programs into a client's daily program may benefit from consultation.

KNOWLEDGE AND SKILLS

The long-term care consultant whose focus is quality assurance must have a broad background in consultation theory, principles, and practice. This must be coupled with an in-depth understanding of quality assurance, its role in long-term care, and its relationship to the regulatory process.

Effective communication skills are critical. Active listening combined with clear written and oral communication that reflects the consultant's findings and observations in a manner supportive of growth and change are important keys. The consultant must help the team to prioritize problems, formulate a cohesive plan of action, implement the program, and then assess its effectiveness. Concurrently, the consultant's talents as a creative problem solver should help identify different approaches and options for the team's consideration. The occupational therapy consultant must also stimulate participant thinking as they negotiate the health care environment to meet quality assurance program needs.[10]

CASE DISCUSSION

Developmental centers throughout the United States form a major segment of the long-term care marketplace. Quality assurance programs form an important part of the centers' ongoing evaluation process. Initial impetus for broad use of quality assurance arose from standards established by federal and state regulatory agencies that oversee developmental centers.[3] The application of splints and the need for splinting compliance was an identified area of deficiency for a developmental center requesting occupational consultative services. The design of a quality assurance program for splint compliance was seen as one possible solution to the problem.

The occupational therapy consultant, hired through a contract agency currently providing direct treatment, was asked to help develop a splinting program for one unit of the developmental center. Working through the administrative sanction of the center's rehabilitation manager, the consultant initially focused on chart and program audits of therapy services in accordance with the institution's quality assurance policies. Compliance of orthotic equipment was minimally evaluated as part of this audit. At this time, no specific audit tool was available to review daily implementation of orthotic equipment and/or programs. An informal splinting compliance program was being used by the therapy and direct care staff without much success.

Findings from chart and program reviews indicated that daily compliance for splint programs was sporadic at best. On a day-to-day basis, splints were lost, damaged, inconsistently placed on clients, or traumatized beyond repair. Staff lacked awareness regarding appropriate methods of splint application, time of usage, and care of the splint. This lack of compliance was identified as an area of concern in program service accountability during an accreditation survey.

The provision of services by all team members, as outlined in each client's individual habilitation plan (IHP), was a crucial factor in service assessment. Program compliance was an essential element used by state and federal regulatory agencies to determine the facility's accreditation and funding. The need for a specialized splinting compliance program to assure effective implementation of clients' IHPs was evident.

The occupational therapy consultant sought input from the staff directly involved in the splint implementation program. Through a series of meetings with direct care staff, educators, supervisory personnel, nurses, and other related services personnel, specific problems that inhibited daily splint compliance were identified and potential solutions were posed for the development of a more effective program.

The team indicated that previous splint programs failed because they were uninformed regarding the following:

1. Purpose and function of a splint
2. Client need for a splint
3. Staff responsible for client splint assessments

4. Staff responsible for initial fabrication and application of splints
5. Notification of splint assignment to a specific client
6. Specific instruction regarding application of the client splint
7. Instruction on splint care and infection control pertaining to splint use
8. Staff responsible for splint application
9. Staff responsible for splint repairs, modification, or replacement
10. Procedures necessary to notify appropriate staff regarding needed splint repairs, modifications, or replacement

This list of issues and concerns clearly identified the problems. Keeping these crucial concerns in mind, the consultant developed an outline for a splinting compliance program, which was then given to team members for review. The outline made the following suggestions:

1. Use of the IHP meeting to communicate splint information to all team members
2. Development of individual splint care plans
3. Daily procedures for splint application, removal, and storage
4. Daily documentation of individual splint application, removal, or lack of use
5. Provision of in-service training to all team members whenever a new splint was introduced, a splint was modified, or care plan was changed
6. Quarterly review/audit of splint compliance programs to determine the program's effectiveness

Team members met with the consultant to develop the final plan. Areas of concern from the team members included site for splint storage; staff responsible for splint application, removal, and storage; daily time frames for splint use; team member responsibilities within the splinting program.

Throughout this process, the consultant kept in mind rules and regulations regarding mechanical supports, individual program plans, program implementation, data collection, placement of splint care plans, staff training, and implementation and documentation as prescribed in regulations governing the center.[3]

The goal of this program was to establish a procedure ensuring that client splint care plans would be carried out daily by team members. Through the use of collaboration and joint decision making in the developing stages, the consultant provided avenues for open communication and acknowledged team member needs. Staff needed to understand that this new program was being established in accordance with regulatory quality assurance guidelines. Accreditation standards had to be met in order to assure funding for the facility.

Involvement of team representatives from the initial stages through development of policies and procedures facilitated its acceptance. Figure 15–1 shows the procedure developed by the consultant and team. Their ownership of the program allowed team members to feel that this new quality assurance activity would not impose more constraints on their already heavy daily work responsibilities. They indicated that the structure might make the splint programs easier to follow on a

FIGURE 15–1

Splinting Compliance Program:
Program Procedure

Step 1: Occupational therapist fabricates splint after receiving medical prescription.

Step 2: Occupational therapist develops individual splint care plan.

Step 3: Occupational therapy personnel provide in-service training on implementation of splint care plan to:
  i. Nursing
  ii. Direct care supervisors
  iii. Direct care staff

Step 4: Splint care plans are posted:
  i. over client's bed
  ii. in client's chart
  iii. in direct care's client program book
  iv. in splint log book

Step 5: Occupational therapy personnel place splint accountability sheet in splint log book.

Step 6: Splint is placed in designated splint storage area.

Step 7: When direct care staff remove splint from storage area, it is checked *out* on client's splint accountability sheet. Staff signs his/her initials in the appropriate space.

Step 8: Splint is placed on client as outlined in individual splint care plan.

Step 9: When splint is removed, it is replaced back into storage area and checked *in* on client's splint accountability sheet in splint log book. Staff signs initials in appropriate space.

Step 10: Direct care supervisor checks splint accountability sheets daily to ensure compliance of splinting program.

Step 11: Splinting compliance program is reviewed and monitored on a regular basis by occupational therapy.

Step 12: Any problems with splints, e.g., in need of repair, adjustment, replacement, or missing splints, are noted on splint accountability sheet and reported immediately to occupational therapy.

daily basis. Previous uncertainty of splint location, staff responsibilities, and daily procedures was now replaced with a consistent routine. Accountability for splints was now shared by all.

In-service training of direct care staff was an important key in the program's success. This training was provided by the consultant and other staff occupational therapists. The sessions provided a learning experience and a forum for caregiver staff to express concerns and observations regarding the program's progress and individual client needs. As new clients entered the program or existing splint plans changed, in-services were scheduled to keep staff updated.

The consultant helped the occupational therapy staff and caregivers develop specific data collection formats to chart client progress. This included a splint accountability data sheet that was used daily on the units for each client. Figure 15–2 shows a sample audit sheet for one client. This accountability sheet provided a concise guide to caregivers regarding use of the splint, the rationale for its application, and precautions. Simultaneously, it clearly showed daily application by the caregiver. If the splint was not applied, the form required an explanation.

Weekly monitoring procedures and quarterly audits were developed, thereby allowing the occupational therapy staff to assess the program's effectiveness on the pilot unit quickly and efficiently.

The team and consultant met to evaluate the program after it had been in place on the pilot unit for three months. The results were positive for all concerned, and the administration requested that the consultant remain to help with implementation throughout the facility.

The consultant then trained the remaining occupational therapy staff so that they could replicate the program in other units. Because of the complexity of fabrication and fitting of some clientele, the consultant also used her splinting expertise on a case-by-case basis upon request. This extended collegial case consultation role helped expand the splinting skills of other occupational therapy personnel and established a strong and supportive relationship between the therapists and consultant. It also enabled the consultant to help the therapists identify barriers to daily compliance and develop creative strategies for problem solving. Primary direction of the splinting compliance program was gradually assumed by the center's occupational therapy staff while the consultant remained available for case consultations and periodic repeat visits to help staff stabilize the program within the total facility.

A successful outcome was clearly seen when the facility was resurveyed 10 months later. Surveyors identified the splint compliance program as an excellent example of quality assurance and complimented the staff on their ability to carry out individualized splint care plans through its use.

SUMMARY

The long-term care marketplace continues to expand. Quality assurance is a critical key in its development and effective service delivery. Occupational therapy consultation that focuses on selective aspects of quality assurance will play an important role in the future growth and utilization of rehabilitative services for this market.

FIGURE 15–2

Daily Splint Accountability Sheet

CLIENT: ___John Doe___

TYPE OF SPLINT: ___® Wrist Support___

WEARING TIME: ___1 hr - 3 times a day___

INSTRUCTIONS FOR USE: 1) Clean & dry hand before applying splint. 2) GENTLY raise hand up while supporting forearm. 3) Place splint into palm of hand. 4) Place forearm into splint. 5) Gently secure straps

PRECAUTIONS: Check for reddened areas or pressure marks. DO NOT place splint near heat or in sun.

PURPOSE: To support wrist; promote hand function; prevent deformity.

MONTH: ___January___   YEAR: ___1989___

Day:	1	2	3	4	5	6	7	8	9	10	11	12	13	14	15	16	17	18	19	20	21	22	23	24	25	26	27	28	29	30	31
9:30–11:30																															
rec'd/on	AF	EV		FS	RS	RS		RS																							
ret'd/off	AW	EV		RS	RS	RS		RS																							
1:30–3:30	1	2	3	4	5	6	7	8	9	10	11	12	13	14	15	16	17	18	19	20	21	22	23	24	25	26	27	28	29	30	31
rec'd on	AW	EV		LM	LM	LM		LM																							
ret'd/off	AW	EV		LM	LM	LM		LM																							
6:30–8:30	1	2	3	4	5	6	7	8	9	10	11	12	13	14	15	16	17	18	19	20	21	22	23	24	25	26	27	28	29	30	31
rec'd/on	RF	RF		LM	LM	LM		LM																							
ret'd/off	RF	RF		LM	LM	LM		LM																							

NOTES/REMARKS: 1/3: Splint to O.T. for repair. 1/7: Patient ill.

INSTRUCTIONS: When you sign your initials in the date box it indicates that you have taken the splint and placed it on the client as indicated in the care plan. When splints are returned, sign your initials in the returned date box.

REFERENCES

1. American Occupational Therapy Association: *Patient Care Evaluation in Action: An Audit Manual for Occupational Therapists.* Rockville, Md, Author, 1978.
2. Epstein CF: Specialized restorative programs, in Kiernat J (ed): *Occupational Therapy for the Older Adult: A Clinical Manual.* Rockville, Md, Aspen, 1991, pp. 285–300.
3. Federal Register, Catalog of Federal Domestic Assistance Program, No. 1-714, Medical Assistance Plan, Rules and Regulations vol 53 (107), 1988, p 20496.
4. Gillette NP: A data base for occupational therapy: Documentation through research. *Am J Occup Ther* 1982; 36:499.
5. Joe BE: Quality assurance and accountability, in Davis L, Kirkland M (eds): *Role of Occupational Therapy With the Elderly (ROTE).* Rockville Md, AOTA, 1986, pp 419–425.
6. Menzel FO, Teegarden K: Quality assurance: A tri-level model. *Am J Occup Ther* 1982; 36:163.
7. OBRA 1987, Code of Federal Regulations. Title 42, Part 483: Conditions of participation and requirements for long-term care facilities, 1989, 483.1–483.80.
8. Ostrow PC: The historical precedents of quality assurance in health care. *Am J Occup Ther* 1983; 37:23.
9. Ostrow PC: Quality assurance requirements of the joint commission on accreditation of hospitals. *Am J Occup Ther* 1983; 37:27.
10. Ostrow PC, Joe BE: Negotiating the environment: Achieving quality care in time of flux. *Am J Occup Ther* 1982; 36:799.
11. Ostrow PC, Kuntavanish AA: Improving the utilization of occupational therapy: A quality assurance study. *Am J Occup Ther* 1983; 37:388.
12. Ostrow PC, Williamson JW, Joe BE: *Quality Assurance Primer: Improving Health Care Outcomes and Productivity.* Rockville, Md, AOTA, 1983, p 14.

ADDITIONAL READING

Joe BE: Efficacy data project. *Am J Occup Ther* 1983; 37.

Law M, Ryan B, Townsend E, et al: Critical mapping: A method of quality assurance. *Am J Occup Ther* 1989; 43.

McColl M, Quinn B: A quality assurance method for community occupational therapy. *Am J Occup Ther* 1985; 39.

Ostrow PC, Joe BE: Quality assurance in geriatric occupational therapy. *Gerontology Special Interest Section Newsletter,* vol 10 (no 1) p 6. Rockville, Md, AOTA, 1987.

Shimeld A: A clinical demonstration program in quality assurance. *Am J Occup Ther* 1983; 37.

SECTION C

Occupational Therapy Consultation in Acute Care Settings

Occupational therapists employed in acute care settings frequently serve as internal consultants. The shortage of occupational therapy personnel, short lengths of stay, and increasing cost of acute care have encouraged the use of a consultation model. Occupational therapists who enter the acute care system as external consultants must assume a more directive role in this clinically oriented environment at times. In such cases, as we have discussed, it is important for the consultant and client to understand and clearly delineate role changes and expectations.

Rogers and Wood describe consultation with a geriatric population in an acute psychiatric hospital. As internal consultants, they provide clinical, research, and educational services. Their primary consultation focus was the functional status assessment of frail elderly psychiatric inpatients. Although the patient was the primary recipient of consultation, the treatment team, family, and caregivers were also involved. More broadly, interaction and collaboration took place with facility staff, students, researchers, and administrators. These authors clearly delineate consultant roles that can be used effectively and efficiently in an acute care setting. Using the functional assessment as their key communication tool, they channel information throughout the system and facilitate client involvement at all levels. They advocate use of consultation as an enabling model for consultant and client, especially in these times of cost containment and limited occupational therapy personnel.

Acute hospital settings present multiple challenges for the consultant, as described by Jacobson. Using three diverse case examples, she illustrates the importance of a broad knowledge base, including extensive management experience. Hospital-based consultation, using external consultants, has not been well documented in occupational therapy literature. Jacobson discusses innovative strategies and important marketing considerations that can be utilized to develop this area of service further.

An occupational therapy consultation practice serving brain-injured clients and their environments is discussed by Giles. Acute rehabilitation services provided by an interdisciplinary team are required for these clients. The case examples presented illustrate some of the problems faced by brain-injured individuals and their team, within the hospital and upon discharge to the community. A high level of consultant expertise is required when working with this population. Giles emphasizes consultant use of ecologically valid assessment tools in order to focus attention on real-world performance.

Health care consortiums are designed to help pool necessary resources and provide effective delivery of care in a geographic region. Devereaux describes mental health consultation services provided in rural West Virginia under this concept. The complex system in which consultation took place included the department of psychiatry in a medical school, community-based psychiatrists, and a community hospital undergoing rapid change while seeking expansion of its psychiatric services, including establishment of an occupational therapy program. Using a systems approach, Devereaux established a multifaceted program for the hospital that required occupational therapy direct treatment and consultation. Her case example illustrates the multiple "hats" consultants must wear when they are faced with limited human and financial resources and a system in crisis. The Section C Acute Care Settings table appears on the following page.

Acute Care Settings

AUTHOR	MODEL	LEVEL	LOCUS	GOAL
Rogers/Wood	Clinical, collegial, educational, and systems	Levels I, II, and III: Case centered, educational, and administrative	Acute geropsychiatric hospital unit	Enable frail elderly to return to community; extend occupational therapy influence through consultation model
Jacobson/Lerner	Collegial, educational, organizational development, and program development	Levels II and III: Educational and administrative	Acute community hospital	Expand occupational therapy services; develop staff management skills
Giles	Clinical, educational, program development, and systems	Levels I, II, and III: Case centered, educational, and administrative	Subacute rehabilitation hospital and client home	Develop behavioral plan for client; train staff in use of plan
Devereaux	Clinical, educational, program development, and systems	Levels I, II, and III: Case centered, educational, and administrative	Acute psychiatric unit of hospital and medical school	Develop occupational therapy services; achieve accreditation for unit

CHAPTER 16

Consultative Models in Geriatric Psychiatry

Joan C. Rogers, *Ph.D., O.T.R., F.A.O.T.A.*
Wendy Wood, *M.A., O.T.R.*

OVERVIEW

This chapter describes the use of consultation with a geriatric population in an acute psychiatric hospital that is a clinical, teaching, and research facility of the University of Pittsburgh's medical school. Factors leading to the transition from external to internal consultation are identified and the influence of the former on the development of the latter is outlined. The interplay between the characteristics of the patient population and the role expectations for the consultants in formulating the frame of reference to guide occupational therapy consultation is highlighted. Implementation of the purchase model of consultation is described in relation to the wide range of consultees served—patients, caregivers, professionals, administrators, students, and researchers. The processes and outcomes of consultation are delineated as well as the indicators used to evaluate its effectiveness. The advantages and disadvantages associated with delivering occupational therapy through consultation in this setting are critiqued with respect to their effectiveness for enhancing the occupational performance of older adults. Consultant qualifications are reviewed in the light of the multiple roles enacted.

Occupational therapy consultation was introduced on the geriatric psychiatry and behavioral neurology module (geriatric module) of Western Psychiatric Institute and Clinic (WPIC) in 1984. Previously, patients requiring occupational therapy were referred to an adjacent, university-affiliated general hospital for outpatient assessment and intervention. Between 1980 and 1984, the bed capacity of the geriatric module increased from 13 to 52. With the fourfold increase in patients, it became increasingly less practical and less cost effective to obtain occupational therapy through outpatient referral. Thus inpatient services were initiated with the hiring of a registered occupational therapist in 1984. A second professional position was added in 1988. From their inception, occupational therapy services were delivered under a consultative model. In essence, services previously provided by external consultants from the general hospital were now provided by internal consultants employed by WPIC.

The two consultants brought a wealth of direct clinical experience to the consultant positions. These included working with physically disabled adults of all ages in acute care hospitals, rehabilitation centers, nursing homes, adult day-care and health programs, hospice, and home care. Indirect service, largely in the form of administration, supervision, and education, was provided in these facilities and services as well as in institutions of higher education. Both consultants had also held substantive leadership positions within occupational therapy, such as president of a state occupational therapy association and membership on the commission on practice. Their postprofessional education was in occupational therapy and emphasized occupational behavior and research skills. Thus their preparation for using a consultation model of practice was grounded in a strong academic background, extensive hands-on experience in diverse clinical settings, and successful performance in guiding others to achieve delineated objectives.

ENVIRONMENT AND SYSTEMS INFLUENCES

While the immediate stimulus for the initiation of inpatient occupational therapy emerged from the practical need to serve adequately the increased patient population, the decision to add occupational therapy to the treatment team emanated from broader economic, political, and clinical trends in health care, particularly in the specialized area of geriatrics. Today, health care providers are challenged to meet the dual, and sometimes conflicting, objectives of providing quality care while maintaining financial accountability within severe economic constraints. To meet these objectives, assessment mechanisms were devised to evaluate the outcomes of specific interventions and health care programs.[3, 9] Programmatic and therapeutic effectiveness can be ascertained by comparing various types of outcomes as well as outcomes of different service providers. Progression toward determining the most cost-effective and optimal health care outcomes is then made by examining relative costs and benefits.

Of major significance for occupational therapy is the increasing recognition of *occupational performance,* or to use the more general term, *functional status,* as a valid index of the effectiveness of medical care, especially in physical medicine and rehabilitation, geriatrics, and long-term care programs for the frail elderly.[7] Evidence from the prospective payment system for hospitals suggests that health care reimbursement derived solely from average costs for treating patients within diagnostic-related groups (DRG) fails to adjust for severity of illness.[4, 5] Inequitable reimbursement is only one possible consequence of neglecting illness severity. Since individual variations in illness and response to treatments are not adequately taken into account, quality of care may also be jeopardized. Because functional status quantifies the impact of disease on the performance of daily living tasks, it is viewed as one way of measuring illness severity. Functional status measurement has been facilitated through large-scale federally sponsored research supporting the development of reliable and valid instruments, such as the Functional Independence Measure (FIM)[6] and the Minimum Data Set for Nursing Facility Assessment and Care Screening (MDS).

Paralleling the developments in fiscal accountability, quality assurance, and functional status measurement was a growing awareness of the increasing numbers of older adults in the American population, and of the need to provide improved health care for the disabling conditions that often accompany aging. Rehabilitation, with its emphasis on reducing disability and maximizing function, currently offers the most viable response to this need.[2, 8] Therapeutic optimism regarding geriatric rehabilitation has been spurred by improvements in the health and well-being of older adults following the prompt identification and treatment of their medical, functional, and psychosocial problems.[12] Rehabilitation philosophy and techniques are increasingly being applied to common functional problems of the elderly, such as falls, reduced endurance, muscle weakness, back pain, visual impairment, confusion, and incontinence.[8, 10] Even when functional independence is not feasible or desired, the quality of life of older patients can often be improved if patients and their caregivers can learn to work synergistically.

Within the context of these trends, the geriatric health services of the University of Pittsburgh, which includes the geriatric module, underwent major expansion in 1984 and 1990. Occupational therapy was a part of this expansion. *Clinically,* occupational therapists were recruited primarily to assess the functional status of frail elderly patients on the inpatient psychiatric service of WPIC. Occupational therapists were to be consultants to treatment teams rather than core team members. Consultation to other components of the geriatric health services, such as follow-up for discharged psychiatric patients, outpatient services for the medically ill elderly seen in ambulatory care, and services to residents of the affiliated teaching nursing home, was an ancillary expectation. With respect to *research,* consultants were obtained who could both initiate research on functional status and collaborate in research requiring functional status measurement. Lastly, consultants were recruited to participate in *educational* programming for undergraduate, graduate, and professional students in the health sciences, WPIC staff, and community-based professionals. Occupational therapy services were thus introduced and developed under the traditional purchase model of consultation.[13] The intent was to purchase expert information and service related to the assessment of functional status and the management of functional disabilities.

FRAME OF REFERENCE

A frame of reference for occupational therapy clinical consultation was developed to meet several specific expectations of the purchaser, namely, the geriatric module. First, consultation was to focus on functional status. No direct responsibility for group programming, such as educational (e.g., hygiene class, relaxation, or assertiveness training), leisure (e.g., use of craft media and games), or psychotherapy groups was anticipated. These were to continue to be the responsibility of social work, nursing, and art, music, dance, and recreation therapy. Second, it was to include the physical aspects of functional status as well as the cognitive and emotional. In other words, expertise was sought to manage functional problems associated, for example, with musculoskeletal or neurological impairments, as well as those involving cognitive and motivational impairments. Third, assessment was to be emphasized. Intervention was to be implemented by core team members. Fourth, it was to include screening for rehabilitation services other than occupational therapy. In conjunction with functional status assessment, the need for consultation from physical medicine and rehabilitation, physical therapy, or speech therapy was to be monitored. Thus the mandate for clinical consultation was that it focus on functional status assessment of the elderly and acknowledge the real and potential impact of coexisting cognitive, affective, and physical impairments on functional status that might require multidisciplinary, rehabilitative services.

In formulating the conceptual framework for functional status assessment, both content and methodology were specified. Functional status is defined as occupational performance in the categories of functional mobility, personal self-care (ADL), and instrumental self-care (IADL). Because the majority of patients on the geriatric module are living independently or semi-independently in the community upon admission, and because functional status assessment is often undertaken to appraise their capability to return to this living situation, occupational performance was interpreted broadly to encompass the skills needed for independent living as well as those needed for basic survival. Functional mobility covers the ability to move in bed, move from a lying to a standing position, walk (or maneuver a wheelchair) on a level surface, manage stairs, and use an elevator. Tasks considered under ADL are feeding, bathing, hygiene and grooming, toileting, and dressing. IADL is comprised of meal preparation, including cold and hot meals; housecleaning, including dusting, sweeping, and cleaning; managing money, including banking and checkbook management; managing medications; using the telephone to obtain information and services; and the capability to pursue leisure preferences.

Information about functional status can be obtained through three basic data gathering methods—interviewing, observing, and testing. On the geriatric module, data about mobility, ADL, and IADL are collected by case managers through patient self-report and/or caregiver report as a part of the admission process. This assessment focuses on the best level of functioning over the past year and functioning immediately prior to admission. Although the same mobility, ADL, and IADL content is assessed by the occupational therapy consultants, this assessment is accomplished through naturalistic observation or performance testing. Naturalistic observation is carried out at the time and place that tasks are normally done in the hospital routine, such as when patients bathe and dress upon arising in the morning. Performance testing requires patients to perform tasks upon therapist request and may be done under standardized or unstructured conditions. Reliance on observation and testing enables consultants to identify reasons for task disabilities and to explore potential intervention strategies for managing them. Thus, while the uniqueness that occupational therapy brings to functional status assessment lies in methodology rather than in content per se, the application of this methodology leads to new information. Furthermore, the points assessed—functioning during hospitalization, at discharge, and functional potential postdischarge—differ from those initially evaluated by case managers.

The findings obtained through observation and performance testing may or may not corroborate those obtained by interview. It is well recognized that asking patients to report their competence can yield highly subjective, and sometimes distorted, perceptions of task or role performance. For example, a depressed woman may report that she cannot cook despite demonstrating competence with cooking when put in a performance testing situation. In contrast, a homemaker with Alzheimer's disease may believe she can cook even though she is observed to burn the eggs and put coffee grounds on her cereal. Similar problems arise regarding the validity of caregiver reports. These may be deliberately biased in the hope of emphasizing illness severity so that more services may be allocated. Or, they may be inaccurate due to a lack of knowledge about the care recipient's skill. Older adults who need assistance for tasks are often perceived by others as being totally dependent, regardless of the extent of help needed. The treatment team depends on consultants to provide *objective* data about functional status and to *interpret discrepancies* in functional status data obtained from patient reports, caregiver reports, performance testing, and observation.

CONSULTATION DESCRIPTION

Organization

WPIC is a regional hospital with a catchment area that spans western Pennsylvania, southeastern Ohio, and northwestern West Virginia. Many admissions follow inadequate response to treatment given within patients' local communities, and hence the clinical needs of the population as a whole are extremely complex and varied. The chief psychiatric modalities are psychopharmacology, psychotherapy, and electroconvulsive therapy.

The typical patient admitted to the geriatric module is over 60 years of age, has a diagnosis of dementia or depression or coexisting dementia and depression, has a chronic medical condition, and requires assistance with activities of daily living. The most common medical conditions are Parkinson's disease, drug-induced parkinsonism, arthritis, diabetes, stroke, cardiopulmonary disease, primary sensory impairments, and osteoporosis. Younger adults requiring psychiatric hospitalization who have physical impairments, such as hemiplegia and blindness, are also admitted to this unit, because it is barrier free and has numerous adaptations including handrails, bedside commodes, and on-unit dining. Staff are also trained to manage medical conditions. While most patients are admitted from private residences, admissions from personal care and nursing homes are also common.

The average length of stay is 7 days for patients with dementing diagnoses and 21 days for those with other psychiatric diagnoses. Upon discharge, the majority resume living alone or with family members. For about 20%, a more supervised living situation is provided at discharge than was present at admission, usually in the form of in-home support services, living with family, or a personal care home.

Functional status enters into both admission and discharge decisions. Psychiatric admission is commonly precipitated by declines in functional status attributable to the onset or acute aggravation of a psychiatric condition. Functional status is taken into account when a psychiatric diagnosis is made, under Axis V of the Diagnostic and Statistical Manual of Mental Disorders (DSM-III-R).[1] The capacity to resume social roles is used as a measure of both mental health and legal competency. Critical points for assessing the functional status of patients seen in geropsychiatry are the point marking the best level of functioning over the past year, immediately prior to admission, during hospitalization, at discharge, and postdischarge.

Support

The consultant positions as well as all equipment and supplies are financially supported by the geriatric module budget. Occupational therapy services are included in the per diem rate. Administratively, WPIC is organized around programs (modules) focused on different age groups and psychiatric diagnoses. Thus the geriatric module provides the administrative and financial support for occupational therapy. One consultant is designated the occupational therapy program director.

Screening for occupational therapy may be done by any member of the treatment team or by the consultants. Common cues precipitating referral are recent declines in functional status preadmission; task performance that is unsafe, inefficient, or variable; history of instability or falls; immobility; chronic physical disability; anticipated or proposed change of living situation upon discharge; and staff perceptions of greater functional capability than is presently demonstrated. Screening decisions are conveyed to a patient's attending psychiatrist or resident, who then writes out the request for consultation (referral). Typically, consultation requests specify "functional assessment," "ADL assessment," "occupational therapy evaluation," or "assess ability to live alone." On occasion, a request is more directive, such as "mobility assessment," "medication management," or "splinting." Most referrals are initiated when patients are psychiatrically stable. Some are requested both before and after psychiatric intervention. Follow-up consultations occur throughout the course of hospitalization as deemed necessary by either consultants or the treatment team.

Participants

In fulfilling their responsibilities, the consultants interact with a number of consultees. Patients are the primary recipients of occupational therapy consultation. On behalf of individual patients, consultation is provided to the treatment team as a unit, to members of the treatment team individually, and to family and paid caregivers. On behalf of the patient population represented on the geriatric module, consultation with staff, students, researchers, and administrators is undertaken.

Services Provided

Upon receipt of the referral, functional status assessment is initiated and is usually completed within three working days. As with other consultation services, occupational therapy appointments take priority over routine, daily activities and are scheduled as they can be accommodated by the consultants. Functional status assessment begins with mobility and ADL and proceeds to IADL, if this progression is warranted by a patient's medical and psychiatric condition and discharge living situation. In other words, all patients are generally evaluated for mobility and ADL dysfunctions, whereas evaluation of independent living skills is more selective and is determined by individual needs after hospital discharge.

The assessment of task competence is based on a test-intervention-retest model. This is a dynamic assessment process designed to reveal a patient's optimal task capacity. The process begins by asking a patient to perform a task that he or she is reasonably motivated to accomplish. If the task is completed independently, safely, and with reasonable ease, task performance is graded as independent. If task performance falters, however, a systematic process to correct or ameliorate task dysfunction is introduced. Potential interventions are encouragement, praise, verbal guidance or instruction, physical guidance, physical assistance, adaptive equipment, modified techniques, and task or environmental modifications. Interventions that provide the least assistance are applied first. Those requiring progressively higher levels of assistance are introduced as needed. Interventions are tried alone and in combination until the patient succeeds with task accomplishment or a determination is made that task performance is not feasible. A task accomplished with the aid of interventions is graded as partially independent. All interventions that facilitated task performance are noted, since they define the conditions under which task performance is possible, that is, they describe the interdependence between the patient, caregiver, and task environment. A rating of dependence is given if task performance is evaluated as not feasible.

The test-intervention-retest process is applied to all mobility, ADL, and IADL tasks deemed to be of concern for a particular patient. Hence at the conclusion of the assessment, a patient's functional status may be described in terms of (1) independence-dependence (including safety and facility) in *specific* tasks—for instance, dressing and meal preparation; (2) competence in each *category* of functional status—mobility, ADL, and IADL; and (3) the amount and kind of help needed to sustain or improve task performance.

Consultation findings are summarized in a written report that becomes part of a patient's medical record. The occupational therapy consultation report includes (1) a description of the patient's functional status, (2) any future actions to be undertaken by occupational therapy, such as a reevaluation of functional status when drug free, and (3) recommendations for managing functional disability and preventing deterioration during and after hospitalization (e.g., referral to physical therapy or driver evaluation). If appropriate, implications of the patient's functional status for discharge planning are drawn. It might be noted, for example, that a patient has the needed skills to resume living alone in the community.

The consultant's expert advice, a substantive proportion of which is contained in the occupational therapy consultation report, provides the foundation for multiple consultant-consultee interactions. The roles enacted by consultants are identified and defined in Table 16–1 and are now discussed in relation to the various consultees served.

Consultee: Patient

Consultation, like occupational therapy, is basically a self-help process. Although patients are not the initiators of occupational therapy consultation, to the extent that they are able, they are its primary recipients. Aiding patients to mobilize resources to deal with their task disabilities constitutes the essence of clinical consultation.

During the functional status assessment, patients are confronted with their task abilities and disabilities. Their independence or dependence in task performance is partially dependent on environmental features. The hospital provides an unnatural context for the performance of routine tasks. It has the positive feature of being a

TABLE 16–1
Consultant Roles

Role	Definition
Diagnostician	Identifies problems and formulates hypotheses about probable cause of the patient's functional deficit
Clinician	Provides intervention for identified problems
Advocate	Persuades consultee to accept particular values, goals, objectives, or actions
Collaborative problem solver	Works with consultee to solve problems
Information specialist	Provides knowledge and technical expertise
Educator/trainer	Teaches consultee attitudes, knowledge, and skills

prosthetic environment in that it is structured to accommodate a variety of impairments (e.g., caregivers supportive of functional independence and large print books and magnifiers for visual impairments). Conversely, it has the negative feature of being largely unfamiliar to patients, and, hence, knowing the location of task objects and understanding the operation of equipment may be problematic. In the testing situation, patients are quick to point out that they could perform "better" or "worse" at home due to these environmental differences.

Hence, the test-intervention-retest method yields an assessment of task performance under conditions that are prosthetic and unfamiliar. In other words, the amount and type of help needed to sustain and improve task performance reflects hospital conditions. To evaluate whether performance would be better or worse in a patient's living situation, information about the actual task environment is needed. Since consultants usually do not visit the home, they are dependent on patients and their caregivers for this information. To assess the impact of the environment on task performance, four features are addressed—space, objects, time, and people.[11] Space refers to the architectural features that promote movement and way finding. Objects refers to the availability of furniture, appliances, tools, and gadgets that promote or hinder task performance. Time refers to the temporal organization and structure of daily tasks and routines. People impact on task performance through their attitudes about caregiving and functional interdependence and their willingness to create an environment conducive for maximizing function. By understanding the similarities and differences in task conditions between the hospital and the home, consultants evaluate the impact of the environment on task performance.

In interacting with patients, consultants initially affirm and reinforce competence. In regard to task disabilities, they collaborate with patients to distinguish aspects of performance that are due to personal factors (e.g., lack of endurance, poor memory, motivational deficit) from those that are environmentally induced (e.g., a chair that is too low to rise from, a spouse who refuses to let the other cook). Typically, task dysfunctions in the elderly have both personal and environmental components, and having identified the relative contribution of each to the identified task disabilities, consultants proceed to discuss reasonable expectations for changing the personal factors and how this might be accomplished (e.g., psychotropic medication, rehabilitation) and the supplemental or alternative environmental changes that may also enhance task performance. Solutions that are most acceptable to patients are identified, as are those that consultants perceive as optimal. The extent to which patients can actively participate in problem solving is moderated by their cognitive status.

Due to time and staffing constraints, direct treatment at WPIC is provided only on an extremely limited basis. Circumstances for which treatment may be given include training in assistive device usage and in techniques for positioning and movement. Thus, in consulting with patients, the chief roles enacted by consultants are those of diagnostician, clinician, advocate, collaborative problem solver, and information specialist; considerably less frequently, the role consists of educator or trainer.

Consultee: Team as a Unit

Several mechanisms are used to disseminate findings from the functional status assessment to professionals responsible for the patient care plan. The written occupational therapy consultation report provides the primary mode of communicating with the treatment team as a unit. The 52 patients on the geriatric module are channeled into 8 treatment teams. Core team members are an attending psychiatrist and/or resident, a case manager, a physician assistant, and a nurse.

Patients are reviewed at a weekly team meeting headed by the attending psychiatrist or resident. Consultation and service requests (e.g., occupational therapy, X ray, magnetic resonance imaging, etc.) are monitored through computerized records and reviewed at this meeting. Occupational therapy consultation reports are a primary data source for information on social role functioning for Axis V of the multiaxial psychiatric diagnostic classification scheme (i.e., DSM-III-R).[1] Consultation reports are used for patient care planning, discharge planning, and determination of competency for legal proceedings. Due to time limitations, consultants attend team meetings only on a selective basis or upon specific request of the team. The chief role served by consultants to the team as a whole, then, is that of information specialist.

Consultee: Psychiatrist and Case Manager

Results of the functional status assessment, including future actions to be taken by occupational therapy and recommendations for supporting a patient's functional status, are discussed with the attending psychiatrist (or resident) and the case manager. The attending psychiatrist has overall responsibility for treatment planning; the case manager coordinates the care plan. Case managers must possess a master's degree, but may have various backgrounds in the human services, such as social work, rehabilitation counseling, nursing, or education.

During this consultation, critical data about a patient's task performance or behavior are emphasized. Conclusions regarding functional status and service needs formulated during the assessment are clarified in the light of information obtained from the psychiatrist and case manager about prognosis and the caregiving situation. Confirmation is also sought that any specific information about a patient's functional status which is required has been adequately addressed. For example, mimicking the living situation, consultants may test elevator use but not the ability to ascend and descend stairs. However, if discharge to a personal care home with stairs is anticipated, stair use would have to be evaluated, and that need would be identified at this time.

Consultants inform team leaders of the actions and resources required to support functional independence during and after hospitalization. Options that appear to be the most acceptable to a patient are pointed out. Various alternatives for obtaining the needed services, such as outpatient rehabilitation, home health services, or supportive living arrangements are identified. Finally, consultants seek to persuade team leaders of the value of optimal functional independence for *this* particular patient. The extent of advocacy and information giving varies with the professional background of team leaders, and differs primarily based on prior experience with rehabilitation services. Thus consultation with psychiatrists and case managers is characterized by advocacy, collaborative problem solving, and provision of specialized knowledge and advice.

Consultee: Primary Nurse

For nurses who serve as primary caregivers during hospitalization, skill training emerges as a salient consultant role. The nursing care model used on the geriatric module is primary nursing, whereby one nurse is responsible for a patient's care. Accordingly, occupational therapy methods for managing task disabilities are taught to the primary nurse, who in turn relays them to other nurses who interact with a patient when the primary nurse is not available.

Consultants typically solicit two types of commitments from primary nurses. The first is a commitment to use intervention techniques that enhance patients' capabilities. If a nurse's repertoire of skills does not include those needed to manage the task dysfunctions exhibited by a patient, that patient's functional independence will be restricted. For example, three people may be needed to get a patient out of bed, whereas one person skilled in transfer techniques could accomplish the task by properly incorporating the patient's residual muscular capabilities into the process. By assisting in executing the transfer, the patient maintains strength while simultaneously deriving the psychological benefits of exerting control over the body. The second commitment is to provide the objects, space, time, and attitudes that encourage patients to use the abilities they have. Environmental facilitators of task performance enable patients to integrate the basic skills that they have into meaningful and effective daily living habits.

Consultant responsibilities include provision of training in rehabilitative methods and techniques for ADL disabilities. Training objectives are highly focused and aim at imparting the knowledge, skills, and attitudes needed to support the functional independence of *this* specific patient in *this* specific task or tasks. For example, a general guideline, such as "Give patient task materials to initiate activity," is related to a particular patient's need, as "Give Mr. Jones his electric razor when his beard needs attention. He can shave himself."

Consultant-nurse interactions are characterized by collaborative problem solving in addition to advocacy, information giving, and teaching. Nurses spend a considerable amount of time with patients and have valuable information to contribute regarding techniques for eliciting positive behaviors, consistency of behavior from day to day, diurnal shifts in behavior, and patient response to interventions suggested by consultants as well as other psychiatric practitioners.

Consultee: Family and Paid Caregivers

To ensure continuity of care, occupational therapy procedures for managing task disabilities must also be conveyed to those responsible for postdischarge care. Consultants serve essentially the same roles for family and paid caregivers as they do for primary nurses—patient advocate, collaborative problem solver, information specialist, and trainer/educator. However, fulfilling these roles may be more complex because these caregivers are not as accessible to consultants as the nurses on the geriatric module. They may also be less knowledgeable about mental and physical illness and the management of ADL disabilities. Conversely, because these caregivers have frequently known or cared for a patient for some time, they have a wealth of information to share about a patient's baseline functional status and successful and unsuccessful techniques for managing ADL disabilities. Depending on a patient's cognitive capabilities, caregivers may be either the sole or a supplemental source of information about the task environment. Their familiarity with a patient enables them to consult about very specific problems in mobility, ADL, or IADL. If these problems are long-standing, they may seek advice about more effective management strategies; if they were exacerbated by mental illness, they may inquire about their resolution.

Consultation with family members may take place on an individual basis or at family meetings set up by case managers to coordinate discharge planning. Case managers frequently assume responsibility for follow-up on consultant recommendations. The discharge summary prepared by case managers furnishes the primary method for communicating with most paid caregivers. When patients are referred for home health nursing or rehabilitation, the home health agency liaison to WPIC reviews the occupational therapy consultation report before discharge. Direct communication may be initiated by either the nurse liaison or the consultant to clarify functional status and care recommendations.

Consultee: Staff

In addition to the education and training that is done in conjunction with individual patients, consultants also periodically hold staff development sessions for nurses and psychiatric residents and interns. In contrast to the case-oriented instruction, this teaching is more general. Favored topics include rehabilitation principles, age-related sensory changes, the use of proper body mechanics, transfer and positioning techniques, and strategies for motivating patients. The material presented is reinforced and individualized when consultants collaborate with staff on the care of individual patients.

Consultee: Module Leadership

As a result of case-by-case consultations, general concerns influencing many patients may be identified. These concerns are dealt with through consultation with leadership of the geriatric module. WPIC is organized around programs, with modules being the basic administrative unit for service delivery. Physically, the 52 beds comprising the geriatric module are separated into two 26-bed units. Module leadership resides in the administrative head, medical head, medical director, nurse clinical manager, chief case manager, and admissions coordinator. This group meets weekly to resolve programmatic issues and plan future directions. Consultants have direct access to this group and are welcome to attend meetings regularly or as the need arises.

From a practical standpoint, consultants have used these meetings to resolve issues related to scheduling conflicts; consolidated, designated space for occupational therapy (e.g., resulting in space for and furbishing of the occupational therapy apartment in 1987); environmental hazards and barriers; and screening and referral procedures. More importantly, consultants have provided input regarding promoting health through meaningful occupation, maintaining patients' functional independence, physical and psychological symptoms of disuse, and alternatives to physical restraints. Consultation with leadership is thus marked by advocacy and expert advice.

Outcome

Consultation aims at initiating, supporting, and maintaining changes in patients, their caregivers, and the systems that provide their care. For patients, the major outcome desired is change in functional status. The preferred result is *improvement* in functional status, which is realized, for example, when patients dependent in transfers at admission become independent at discharge. When improvement is not feasible, change may be reflected in the *prevention* of decline, for example, when patients maintain their residual strength by using it to execute transfers. When decline cannot be prevented, change may be exhibited by a *retardation* of the overall rate of decline, for instance, when patients ward off contractures, muscle atrophy, confusion, and other symptoms of disuse by remaining as mobile and active as their capabilities allow.

For professional as well as informal caregivers, a modification of their behavior, such that patients' task disabilities are managed more effectively and caregiver burden is lessened, is a desired objective. For example, a patient's wife may gain the necessary skills to incorporate proper body mechanics into transfers. Simultaneously, she may experience a decrease in back and leg pain and an increase in self-efficacy with respect to her ability to care for her husband.

At the systems level, a greater acceptance of a rehabilitation approach is a desired goal. As an acute care facility, WPIC focuses on curative interventions. As a rehabilitation profession, occupational therapy focuses on adaptation to chronic conditions in the absence of cure. In geropsychiatric patients, acute psychiatric illness is generally superimposed on other chronic mental or physical disorders. Optimal patient care is thus achieved when the curative and adaptive approaches are mutually reinforcing. An example of a systems change indicative of a rehabilitative perspective would be the incorporation of competence in proper body mechanics in lifting and moving patients into personnel qualifications.

Outcome Indicators

A comprehensive evaluation plan is used to measure the effects of consultation on patients, caregivers, and systems. The principal indicators for measuring effects on patients are functional status and referral rate. Since changes in functional status constitute the essential purpose of occupational therapy consultation, patients' medical records are randomly monitored for documentation of functional stability and gains as well as loses. A steady referral rate, especially when key personnel are replaced, is interpreted as verifying the contribution of functional status consultation to the psychiatric care of older adults.

Measurement of the effects of consultation on caregivers is approached in several ways. One approach involves the incorporation of consultants' recommendations into patient care and discharge plans. After discharge, patient records are periodically and randomly monitored to make this determination. A second approach takes into account informal feedback from family and treatment team members suggesting that consultation has been helpful. For example, following successful implementation of verbal cuing and task modifications to improve nutritional intake, a spouse may recontact a consultant for help with toileting. A third approach uses transfer of learning, or generalization as an outcome measure. Generalization is illustrated when occupational therapy techniques taught in regard to one activity or one patient are appropriately applied to another activity for the same patient or to another patient with similar problems.

System effects are gauged by measuring the extent or range of consultation services. Most immediately, implementation on the geriatric module of policy, procedural, or environmental changes advocated by consultants provides a useful measure. Improved lighting in patient bathrooms and individualized, rather than blanket referrals, are illustrative of these types of changes. Moving more distantly, expansion of *patient-oriented* consultation to health care services outside of the geriatric module and outside of the University of Pittsburgh health sciences complex is evaluated. Outside of the geriatric module, for example, consultation has been provided to the WPIC modules treating adults with depression and schizophrenia; outside of WPIC, consultation has involved the medical and psychiatric geriatric outpatient services. As specialized services for older adults have been introduced into local and regional health care and social service facilities, consultation requests from hospitals, adult day-care programs, personal care homes, rehabilitation centers, and nursing homes have been fulfilled. These requests generally involve consultation with administrators or geriatric practitioners (i.e., health professionals, including occupational therapists) about the development of occupational therapy services or the provision of an accessible, safe, functional, appealing, and stimulating environment for older adults with disabilities. Many of these contacts have been stimulated by practitioners who completed internships on the geriatric module.

Distribution of services to systems other than those directly involved in health care provides an additional index of the salience of occupational therapy consultation. Thus infiltration of consultation to colleagues in both education and research is monitored. As employees of a teaching hospital, consultants are available to health care professionals from other facilities. Occupational therapists, as well as family practitioners, geriatricians, dentists, psychiatrists, social workers, nurses, rehabilitation counselors, hospital administrators, human factors scientists, architects, and educators, have sought advice on topics such as functional status measurement, selection of instruments to measure disability, environmental modifications, rehabilitation philosophy, compensating for age-related and disease-associated changes, exercise, and activities programming. More formal teaching is provided through participation in continuing education programs for state hospital personnel and the general community. Occupational therapy's unique approach to measuring function through observation and performance testing has been sought by researchers investigating the outcomes of medical intervention for dementia, depression, chronic obstructive pulmonary disease, and hip problems.

The expansion of occupational therapy influence is marked by a common theme, namely, it has been stimulated by knowledge of the clinical services provided on the geriatric module. In essence, prospective consultees know or see what the consultants do clinically and purchase consultation services in regard to their own special clinical, educational, or research needs.

Corrective actions are based on trends evidenced in the outcome indicators. For example, one review of medical records revealed that consultants' recommendations were used almost exclusively for discharge planning and placement decisions. Recommendations intended to enhance patients' functioning during hospitalization were less likely to be integrated into treatment plans. To address this deficit, consultants increased attendance at team meetings to articulate more persuasively a rehabilitation perspective and to assist in implementing their recommendations within a psychiatric unit. Quality assurance indicators were then revised to evaluate the degree to which specific interventions, such as falls prevention measures, were incorporated into treatment plans.

Advantages and Disadvantages

Advantages and disadvantages are associated with delivering occupational therapy through consultation in this setting. A major advantage is that a larger patient population can benefit from consultation than would be possible through direct service. The 1 : 26 therapist-patient ratio on the geriatric module precludes extensive direct intervention, and consultees act as service extenders. With the nationwide shortage of occupational therapists, consultation furnishes an effective mechanism for delivering services with scarce human resources. A second advantage, which evolves from using the purchase model of consultation, is that consultation is bought to meet well-defined and very specific needs and expectations. Inherently, there is an openness to occupational therapy expertise. Being internal as opposed to external consultants affords a third advantage. As insiders, it is easier to learn about the intricacies of how the system functions and to cultivate valuable professional liaisons. Consequently, the goal of optimal functional independence for frail elderly persons is promoted.

Among the chief disadvantages associated with consultation are implementation failure, limitations on the kinds of interventions that can be used, and a narrow role allocation. Inherently, consultants are dependent on consultees to carry out their recommendations. Use of the expertise supplied is beyond the consultants' control. Factors such as personal and professional beliefs and limited economic resources for equipment or personal service impinge on the capacity to implement all recommendations. Reliance on consultees also impacts on the number and kind of recommendations that can be made. Consultants must set priorities thoughtfully. Actions that are best for a patient are weighed against those that are less effective and yet more compatible with caregiver capabilities. This often leads to

TABLE 16–2
Occupational Therapy Consultation in Geropsychiatry

Level of Consultation	Consultee	CONSULTANT ROLES					
		Diagnostician	Clinician	Advocate	Collaborative Problem Solver	Information Specialist	Trainer/ Educator
Direct service	Patient	X	X				
Patient consultation	Patient	X		X	X	X	
Case consultation	Team as a unit					X	
	Psychiatrist and case manager			X	X	X	
	Primary nurse			X	X	X	X
	Family member and paid caregiver			X	X	X	X
Colleague consultation	Staff, students, researchers					X	X
Systems consultation	Internal and external administrators			X		X	

the selection of compensatory rather than corrective interventions, for example, the provision of a bathtub bench rather than an exercise program for the underlying mobility impairment. Another factor, and one that limits the possible benefits that could be derived from a purchase model, is that the service purchased as defined by the purchaser may restrict the scope of occupational therapy practice.

Consultant Qualifications

The multiple and varied roles enacted by consultants require a highly flexible and assertive personality. These traits need to be complemented by skills in persuading, cajoling, and motivating others to behave in ways that may be new, difficult, or inconvenient. Fostering a rehabilitation perspective in an acute care setting needs to be viewed as a challenge. Clinically, competence in managing physical as well as emotional and cognitive impairments is essential. To meet the educational and research expectations, a master's degree is required as well as some experience in teaching and research.

SUMMARY

Occupational therapy consultation as organized for an inpatient, geropsychiatric service with the triple mission of treating older patients, educating psychiatric practitioners, and testing psychiatric interventions is summarized in Table 16–2. Consultation is provided on five levels and encompasses both direct and indirect services. The predominating consultant role is that of diagnostician. All other roles emanate from diagnostician, with those of advocate, collaborative problem solver, and information specialist having broader applicability than those of clinician and educator/trainer.

Consultation is an effective and efficient mechanism for helping patients help themselves, helping others to help patients, and fostering a health care system that is more responsive to the needs of the disabled elderly. In times of cost containment and scarce human resources, it provides an efficacious model of service provision. Concurrently, it is an enabling model that promotes the skill development of both the consultants and consultees.

REFERENCES

1. American Psychiatric Association: *Diagnostic and Statistical Manual of Mental Disorders,* ed 3, revised. Washington, DC, American Psychiatric Association, 1987.
2. Brody SJ, Ruff GE: *Aging and Rehabilitation.* New York, Springer, 1986.
3. Department of National Health and Welfare and the Canadian Association of Occupational Therapists: *Report of a Task Force: Toward Outcome Measures in Occupational Therapy.* Ottawa, Minister of National Health and Welfare, 1987.
4. Eisenberg BS: Diagnosis related groups, severity of illness, and equitable reimbursement under Medicare. *J Assoc People Severe Handicaps* 1984; 251:645.

5. Gonnella JS, Hornbrook MC, Louis DZ: Measuring severity of illness: Homogeneous case mix groups. *Med Care* 1983; 21:14.
6. Granger C, Hamilton B, Sherwin F: Guide for use of the uniform data set for medical rehabilitation. Buffalo, Department of Rehabilitation Medicine, Buffalo General Hospital, 1986.
7. Kane RA, Kane RL: Assessing the elderly: A practical guide to measurement. Lexington, Mass, Lexington Books, 1981.
8. Kemp B, Brummel-Smith K, Ramsdell JW: *Geriatric Rehabilitation*. Boston, Little, Brown, 1990.
9. Ostrow PC, Joe BJ: *Quality assurance primer: Improving health care outcomes and productivity*. Rockville, Md, AOTA, 1983.
10. Pynoos J, Cohen E, Lucas C: Environmental coping strategies for Alzheimer's caregivers. *Am J Alzheimer's Care Res* 1989; 4:4.
11. Rogers JC: The occupational therapy home assessment: The home as a therapeutic environment. *J Home Health Care Practice* 1989; 2:73.
12. Rubenstein LZ: Geriatric assessment: An overview of its impact. *Clin Geriatr Med* 1987; 3:1.
13. Schein EG: *Process Consultation: Its Role in Organization Development*. Reading, Mass, Addison-Wesley, 1969.

CHAPTER 17

Hospital-Based Consultation

Sandra L. Jacobson Lerner, O.T.R./L.

OVERVIEW

Very little appears in the occupational therapy literature about hospital-based consultation. As a consultation model, it has been neither conceptualized nor widely used. This chapter details three successful hospital-based occupational therapy consultation experiences utilizing various models of consultation.

- Case study   I: Occupational therapy department in turmoil
- Case study II: Small occupational therapy department with few positions
- Case study III: Institution of a new occupational therapy department

The author is executive director of Comprehensive Therapeutics, Ltd. (CT, Ltd.), who began the corporation with the goal of utilizing consultative expertise to assist hospital occupational therapy departments struggling for recognition and survival. Today it is a relatively large group consultation private practice, comprised mainly of occupational therapists who provide consultation as well as direct treatment to more than 150 hospitals, school systems, mental institutions, long-term care facilities, residential developmental disabilities facilities, and home health agencies throughout Illinois. The practice has attracted many highly experienced therapists, many of whom previously directed hospital departments or managed specialized treatment units.

ENVIRONMENT AND SYSTEMS INFLUENCES

One only needs to read the want ad section of the Sunday paper, occupational therapy publications, or the many letters occupational therapists receive each month from hospitals and health personnel recruitment firms to realize that the demand for occupational therapists is greater than ever before. In addition, a shrinking market for traditional hospital services plus the federal government's prospective payment system have forced hospital administrators to look for new areas of service.

Many hospital service areas exempt from the prospective payment system have traditionally been serviced by occupational therapists. In addition, hospital administrators seek creative community-based programs to bring in more patients and more revenue. Niche rehabilitation programs or programs designed to meet specific identified consumer needs such as work hardening, head trauma, intermediate rehabilitation centers for the elderly, hand rehabilitation, substance abuse and eating disorders, and early intervention programs are mushrooming everywhere, and all of them can utilize occupational therapists.

Administrators and program directors complain of the shortage of therapists with knowledge and experience to establish and manage occupational therapy departments. This plight may be complicated by their search for a single therapist to perform both clinical and administrative duties. Utilizing a consultation model to ensure the success and growth of occupational therapy in hospital settings can be a productive solution to this dilemma.

Although hospitals traditionally have hired administrative, nursing, pharmacy, housekeeping, and other consultants, they have not readily hired occupational therapy consultants. Given current environmental systems and influences, and available dollars in budgets from vacant positions, increased opportunities now exist for occupational therapists to provide hospital-based consultation.

FRAME OF REFERENCE

There are numerous consultation roles that can be utilized in a hospital setting. The consultant can be an *adviser,* a helper, or a facilitator with occupational therapy management expertise who is invited into a system to make recommendations for change. Often the consultant is a *change agent* who, when given the green light to come into a system, can observe and evaluate identified problems, plan short- and long-range goals and approaches, and effect positive changes. A most important consultative role is one of *educator/trainer.* The consultant provides consultees with opportunities to learn skills that will enable them to solve problems and independently carry out department functions in the future.

Another way of looking at an effective hospital-based consultation process is to see it as resembling an occupational therapy treatment plan.[4] This process begins with *assessment* and establishment of *trust.* Appropriate *goals* are then set and a *plan of approach* outlined to effect goal achievement. The consultant can utilize various strategies to assist in goal implementation. These tools may consist of providing policies and forms, in-service training, and/or role modeling. Reevaluations may be necessary to provide feedback and establish new goals. If all the goals are achieved, the treatment or consultation is terminated, although periodic checks may be needed to make sure outcomes are maintained or to determine if there are any additional needs.

Frazian[3] describes a type of hospital consultation in the context of a private practice providing service to the hospital for a set period of time, establishing the department, and then terminating once the department is functioning independently. This is a viable model, and can be utilized when instituting a new department (see case study III).

Given the environmental and systems influences previously discussed, (high demand for services, productivity, profitability, etc.), occupational therapists are being called on in ever increasing numbers to contract their services when there are staff shortages due to vacancies, vacation, sick leave, or maternity coverage. The occupational therapy budget provides financial support for these treatment services. This type of hospital contract is for direct services, *not* hospital-based consultation as described in this chapter.

Hospital-based consultation utilizes four of the models defined in Chapter 2. These are the collegial or professional model, the education model, the organizational development model, and the program development model. Use of these models is illustrated in this chapter. The hospital-based consultant may provide educational, program, and/or administrative levels of consultation depending on the situation.

CONSULTATION DESCRIPTION

Background

Entering a hospital system is usually very difficult. Many administrators lack familiarity with the role that an occupational therapy consultant may play. When all resources have been exhausted and unfinished jobs create pressure from physicians and others, administrators are more likely to seek outside assistance. In other words, a consultant would be called on in a time of crisis.

In one case, for example, a hospital's occupational therapy director had been on maternity leave for some time. Physicians were very unhappy with the minimal service being rendered and complained extensively to administration. An advertisement was placed for a temporary director. The author answered the ad, but offered services as a consultant rather than a director. This solution was perfect at the time, for it enabled administration to demonstrate to the physicians that it was responding to the problem while maintaining the employment status of the original director.

Marketing strategies are vital to success. The way hospitals learn of the consultant's expertise and the manner in which the consultant gains their confidence is critical. A major goal of marketing is to obtain clients who are willing to pay the appropriate fee. The following strategies should be considered:

1. Want ads can identify a pattern of hospitals that advertise frequently. These ads indicate if the need is to fill a slot or to create a new program. A call, with

a follow-up letter to the human resource or occupational therapy department head, can help to gain entry for an interview or proposal (see Appendix D).

2. Marketing occupational therapy consultation services to local management consultant firms may create opportunities for contracting. Generally these firms do not employ occupational therapists. Often, a hospital will first contact these firms for help when a problem surfaces in their occupational therapy department.

3. Networking with local occupational therapists may bring news of a hospital department with a problem. By offering the idea of consultation to the department, an opportunity may be created.

There may be numerous recurring problems in hospital departments that can be addressed through occupational therapy consultation. Commonly occurring crisis situations include the following:

1. Constant staff turnover and shortages.

2. Patient/family/physician/administration dissatisfaction with the quality of clinical services resulting in a decline of department referrals and revenues.

3. Interpersonal departmental problems or poor working relationships with another department.

4. A stagnant department, requesting new perspective, ideas, and vitality in programs.

5. Physicians demand new services. The current director and staff lack the knowledge and experience needed to set up requested service. For example, a new psychiatric unit requires occupational therapy services but the current staff specializes in physical disabilities.

6. A new department head lacks administrative experience.

7. Hospital administration wants to expand occupational therapy community-based programs. Planned focus will be a long-term care facility or work hardening program. The occupational therapy department is not knowledgeable regarding requirements, resources, regulations, and appropriate programming for these community programs.

8. Administrator wants departmental reorganization. Inefficient use of staff, fragmented services, low revenues, and/or needed improvement in the quality and scope of service are seen as problems.

Table 17–1 summarizes the consultation model(s) that may be used when the consultant is first called in to address the specific problem. It should be noted that the process may expand to include other models as identified in the table if the consultation continues beyond the initial focus.

While each hospital occupational therapy department described may have presented a different set of problems, the need for consultation services was identified through similar routes. Potential clients can be identified through networking with local occupational therapists and hospital administrators and by watching for consistent advertising patterns.

TABLE 17–1
Hospital-Based Initial Consultation Issues and Approaches

Problem	Collegial or Professional	Educational	Organizational	Program Development
			CONSULTATION MODEL	
1. Constant staff turnovers and shortages	X		X	
2. Dissatisfaction with service	X	X	X	X
3. Interpersonal departmental problems	X		X	
4. Stagnant department	X	X		X
5. Demand for new service that current staff not qualified to provide	X	X	X	X
6. New department head lacks administrative experience	X	X	X	X
7. Expansion of programs into community		X	X	X
8. Department reorganization needed	X		X	

CASE STUDY I: OCCUPATIONAL THERAPY DEPARTMENT IN TURMOIL

Organization

In one particular case, a competent occupational therapy director at a local hospital with a staff of four had a successful general medicine and surgery and rehabilitation service. The hospital was opening a new psychiatric wing and requested that the director provide occupational therapy for that unit. Although no one in her department had the experience or expertise to develop this type of program, the director did not want to lose the opportunity to get involved and to have this program under her auspices.

The occupational therapy director called CT, Ltd. requesting an experienced psychiatric therapist. It was suggested that she set up a meeting with CT Ltd.'s psychiatric occupational therapist and the administrator of the new service.

The therapist proposed the idea of consultation during the meeting and described how consultation could assure a successful and economical start-up of the service, in addition to training the current staff therapists to provide the service once the framework was in place. She offered to provide a proposal free of charge outlining the consultation goals and objectives, and including time frames and the estimated cost. This marketing strategy (i.e., free proposal and time spent assessing the situation), coupled with the vote of confidence of the occupational therapy department, was used to secure the contract (see Appendix D for a sample proposal).

Support

Before initiating the consultative service, it was essential to negotiate a contract.[2] Besides being a legal document with clearly specified terms, including the cost and the expected time to accomplish the task, the contract also helped the consultant and the key power individuals define and establish the parameters of the consultation services. A job description was provided with the contract (see Appendix D for a copy of a sample contract). In addition to financial support, it was important to have the support and cooperation of key individuals in the consultation process. During the negotiations, honesty was essential. Restricting CT Ltd.'s practice to areas of expertise available within the firm was an important policy. In this case, had an experienced psychiatric occupational therapist not been available, the firm would have turned down the director's request. This assured a track record of success. Good results elicited confidence in the services; mediocrity would have closed doors. References were always provided.

Participants

Decision makers in this case study were the occupational therapy director and the administrator of the new psychiatric program. These participants set goals and established the time frames and the budget parameters for the consultation. They also outlined their problems and needs. The consultant established trust and confidence with these key power individuals. This occurred at the initial meeting and when reviewing the initial proposal and recommendations. A demonstrated understanding of the problem and empathy with the participants was critical. It was essential that the consultant be tuned into their needs.

Services Provided

Consultation service actually began at the time of the initial interview and the writing of the proposal. At that time, problems, needs, and anticipated results were identified. It was important that the consultant analyze the scope of the problems and needs from every perspective, that is, administrator, occupational therapy director, and unit staff. Only then was it appropriate to develop a course of action. If the participants viewed the consultant as a threat, the likelihood of success would have been greatly diminished.

In this case, the consultant was able to develop an organizational framework for the new occupational therapy service. She wrote specific policies and procedures, established an appropriate evaluation tool, developed group protocols, and set up an occupational therapy schedule of activities and groups. A most important function was the educational model of consultation. The consultant provided training and role modeling to the occupational therapy staff assigned to the unit to enable them to function confidently on the unit until the census warranted a full-time occupational therapy position that could be filled by a psychiatric occupational therapist.

Outcome

The consultant stayed on for three months for one to two days a week providing services as just described. At the end of three months, the framework of the program was developed, and the staff was confident and competent in providing the service as needed. The consultant remained on a once monthly basis to evaluate the status of the program, make new program recommendations, and to provide ongoing staff training. Consultation had resulted in successful start-up of the service and a growth in the depth and breadth of the hospital's occupational therapy department.

This hospital-based consultation provided hospital management with greater insight into the occupational therapy department's needs and growth potential; enabled the hospital to develop new services efficiently and economically with a greater chance for success; and improved staff morale by providing support, solutions to problems, and relief of stress. This positively affected the retention of the hospital's most valuable asset, its staff, and improved department function by alleviating problems in a relatively short time.

Consultation was not always effective at every given juncture. It was important to evaluate the outcome and to determine if the problems were fully or partially resolved. Sometimes the problem was not solvable until certain events occurred. For example, as the department was short staffed, it was not possible to initiate a new program until additional qualified therapists were found to carry out the consultant's recommendations. Therefore, the consultant discontinued services for the short term and returned at a later date. What was important to the success of this consultation was that there was a climate of acceptance and sanction by the participants. Timing and outside variables, such as low census, staff on maternity leave, or demands of a student affiliate, could have interfered with the process.

Sometimes a situation may be so complex that it will require a team of consultants with expertise in a number of areas to give the recommendations greater impact and substance. This team concept is an important consideration when examining the problems inherent in reorganizing a multifaceted department.

Once this specific crisis was resolved, the contract was terminated. Yet the consultant's success led hospital management and department heads to utilize consultation for future problems as they surfaced. They did not wait until they became pervasive and almost irreparable.

CASE STUDY II: SMALL OCCUPATIONAL THERAPY DEPARTMENT WITH FEW POSITIONS

Organization

This hospital had a relatively small department with two full-time equivalents (FTEs) budgeted. Demands for service were increasing. Current staff found that they could not keep up with these demands and still provide quality care. Obvious solutions included hiring contract therapists to treat the additional caseload or adding another FTE if warranted. This department had never designated a department head. Current staff were entry-level therapists without administrative experience.

Initially, the hospital-based consultant was called in to provide direct therapy services through a contractual arrangement. During the initial interview and visit, it became clear that administrative support and direction would be more beneficial to the situation than direct contract occupational therapy services. The consultant would provide support, direction, and a foundation to build on in the future. This was particularly important as the increasing demand for service was a trend, rather than a short-term phenomenon.

Support

A proposal was developed and presented to the administrator. The price, number of hours, length of time, and description of services were agreed upon and specified in the resulting contract.

Participants

The participants in this case were the occupational therapy staff and the administrator responsible for the occupational therapy department. Often, the consultant reported progress to the administrator in order to gain trust and confidence and obtain support. The occupational therapy staff were the direct recipients of consultation.

Services Provided

There were many managerial and administrative components to the service delivery system in this occupational therapy department. In this small department the system tended to be informal. As the service grew, the system required more organization, formalization, and sophistication. There was need for a complete policy and procedure manual, departmental forms, an efficient billing system, appropriate documentation procedures for accrediting agencies and third party payers, statistical information, and other elements. As new service areas developed, specific program descriptions, protocols, and schedules had to be delineated. The occupational therapists and other professional staff had to be trained regarding the role and function of occupational therapy in these new arenas.

The hospital-based consultant provided direction and an administrative framework for the staff person designated to become the occupational therapy director. The consultant provided training in handling administrative tasks, acted as a role model, and actually took over some functions until the new director and staff had the time and ability to function independently. The consultant developed efficient systems to increase staff productivity and employed marketing strategies to expand the utilization of the occupational therapy service, thereby justifying additional FTEs.

Hiring occupational therapists can be a very expensive proposition if a hospital relies on advertisements and recruitment firms. Therefore, the hospital-based consultant assisted with the recruitment process, thereby saving the hospital a great deal of money. The presence of the occupational therapy consultant demonstrated the hospital's commitment to the occupational therapy department and to prospective employees. Additionally, the foundation provided by the consultant allowed the prospective therapists to see the position's potential and challenge.

In this case study, organizational, program development, and educational levels of consultation were employed. The models used depended on the tasks to be accomplished, with the major focus on education consultation.

Outcome

The outcome was extremely positive. The consultees were very pleased with the assistance of the consultant. Given the support and direction they needed, their stress levels declined and their morale improved. The organization of the department also improved and administration, physicians, nursing, families, and patients all expressed satisfaction with the service. Increased service brought greater revenue and recognition of the department.

As the department grew, the systems matured and staff became more competent in carrying out administrative functions. Consultation was reduced to one or two times per month to monitor department status, assist in the development of new programs, and support and train staff. In time, with increasing referrals, a confident director, and a broader service base, it was possible to eliminate consultation altogether. This, of course, was the ultimate goal: helping to create a successful, quality occupational therapy department that could function independently.

CASE STUDY III: INSTITUTION OF A NEW OCCUPATIONAL THERAPY DEPARTMENT

Organization

The concept of utilizing a private agency to provide occupational therapy services in hospitals has been widely used. The hospital does not initiate a department per se, but calls on an individual practitioner or group practice to provide service upon physician referral. Thus a small hospital can provide occupational therapy services without incurring the expense of establishing a department and allocating space and budget.

In the model cited by Frazian,[3] the process can begin with a single patient referral leading, within an average two-year period, to an independent occupational therapy department.[1] Her model comes closest to the consultative model that is described more fully in this section.

Although offering direct service initially, Frazian actually provided an administrative and organizational framework, and demonstrated the need for the service through marketing and educational efforts. In other words, although providing direct service, she used the program development model of consultation to establish an occupational therapy department within the hospital.

In this case model, the hospital administrator, physical therapy director, and/or rehabilitation director saw the need for establishing an occupational therapy department, rather than contracting for services through a therapy agency on an as-needed basis. They sought to hire an occupational therapist to fill the newly created position. Due to critical shortages, they were unable to find an experienced and qualified therapist to fill the position and concurrently perform the duties of staff therapist and director.

CT, Ltd. offered to provide the needed direct therapy services on a time-limited basis and to offer consultation services to the rehabilitation director so he could develop the organizational framework of the occupational therapy department. In addition, the firm was to assist in recruiting and training an appropriate therapist.

Support

Developing a contract in this situation was easier than in the other case studies, since the participants had established a need and a budget for the service and were seeking to employ an occupational therapist. The key to success was convincing them that the use of a time-limited consultative/contract model would provide greater benefits than immediately employing a staff therapist. If the consultant worked within the parameters of their budget, providing the consultation as well as the direct contract services needed, support was readily elicited and an appropriate contract ensued.

Participants

The program director, physical therapy director, and rehabilitation director responsible for developing and initiating the occupational therapy service were key participants in this case example. They directed the consultant's efforts, clearly communicating goals, perceived needs, and the result desired of the service. They were pleased with the quality of the service and the flexibility it allowed in obtaining specialized therapists when a case warranted it, for example, a hand therapist for a specialized splint.

Services Provided

In this situation, a consultant was hired to establish the new department and then perform the same types of consultative services as described in case study II. The consultant utilized the program development model of consultation, providing an organizational framework and foundation to ensure successful start-up of the department. The consultant assisted with the recruitment process, and the hospital began employing therapists as soon as the referral base warranted a part-time position. By employing these strategies, staff could be used efficiently and effectively. The hospital paid for expertise only; there were no dollars spent for learning. It also paid for therapy treatment time only when needed. This was particularly important when first initiating the service, as there were not enough referrals or patients to justify the overhead of a full-time therapist.

System entry in this case model required an aggressive marketing approach. Proposing a consultation/direct service model as an alternative to employing staff therapists immediately was a good way to begin. In addition, the expertise of the firm was validated by a local occupational therapist in the community. The hospital had contacted her for the job and she recommended the author's group.

The hospital, with the consultant's guidance, hired a full-time therapist. The current status of the department was then reviewed with the therapist and a written evaluation and recommended actions were presented. The areas evaluated were the therapist's ability to function without consultation, the physician's and other significant professionals' satisfaction with the service, and productivity in terms of revenue and service provided.

Outcome

When all the initial goals and objectives were accomplished and the therapist hired had demonstrated the ability to run the department, consultation was terminated. It was agreed that should new issues arise requiring consultation, hours could be renegotiated.

SUMMARY

Hospital-based consultation is an infrequently used model, and entry into the system may be difficult. Utilization of this option can significantly impact the quality and quantity of occupational therapy services. It enables consultant therapists with previous management experience to impart their knowledge to more than one hospital at any given time, thus helping to address acute staffing shortages where inexperienced therapists may be required to manage a department.

As illustrated in all three cases, positive results were achieved. Departments functioned better and more independently, administration and physicians were satisfied with results, and hospitals paid only for productive services; there was no costly unproductive overhead.

This model of consultation also aids staff retention. Therapists who receive consultation are very pleased to have outside input and a spokesperson for their cause. They feel more supported, which in turn decreases their frustration and stress. Another important by-product is staff recruitment. Most experienced occupational therapy consultants have developed successful recruitment strategies that combine use of their contacts, experience, and knowledge of the field. This expertise can be invaluable as the hospital develops its recruitment plan. In addition, inexperienced therapists will more readily fill positions, given access to a consultant. Experienced therapists also may be attracted to hospitals employing consultants, since the presence of a consultant indicates the hospital's support for the profession.

In all cases presented, consultation was time limited and, in each model, contracts were terminated when results were achieved. However, utilizing consultants on a regularly scheduled basis (e.g., annually or semiannually) could provide hospitals with an excellent quality assurance mechanism and a constant flow of recommendations for upgrading specific areas or developing broader based programs within the hospital as well as in the community.

The longest hospital-based consultation CT, Ltd. provided lasted two years, on a one day per week basis. Consultation was terminated when the department had a competent full-time director, who was then able to build the department to ten full-time equivalents within a relatively short period of time. The consultant stayed on at the administrator's request to establish a student clinical affiliation program and to prepare the necessary documentation for the Joint Commission on Accreditation of Hospitals survey and third party reimbursement.

It is important to note that the author has had calls from and contacted innumerable potential clients over the past 15 years. While proposals were left with most, services have been provided in approximately 10% of those hospital sites. Success has generally varied directly in proportion to the severity of the crisis. The viability of this model of practice has been demonstrated here. Hopefully, this option will be more widely accepted, and hospital-based consultation services will increase.

Occupational therapy managers seeking career options or a more flexible work situation in which to utilize their skills should consider consultation as a viable alternative. In order to develop hospital-based consultations, therapists must be willing to provide free consultation to staff and hospital management to gain entry. Therapists employed by hospitals and in need of assistance must take the risk of asking for consultation when they perceive the need.

In the final analysis, hospital-based consultation is beneficial to the occupational therapy department, therapists, administrators, and the patients needing services. It can also help assure occupational therapy's role in hospitals through the 21st century.

REFERENCES

1. Brown EB: Therapists find clinical career ladders stop short of success. *Advance for Occup Therapists,* 6:8, February 19, 1990.
2. Dutton R: Procedures for designing an occupational therapy consultation contract. *Am J Occup Ther* 1983; 40:160–166.
3. Frazian BJ: Establishing and administrating a private practice in a hospital setting. *Am J Occup Ther* 1976; 32:296–300.
4. Jacobson SL: Group consultation—a private practice model for the 1990's. *Administration and Management Special Interest Section Newsletter,* vol 4, no 1, March 1988.

CHAPTER 18

Occupational Therapy Consultation for Individuals with Acquired Brain Injury

Gordon Muir Giles, DipCOT., O.T.R.

OVERVIEW

The increased demand for services for brain-injured individuals has created many opportunities for occupational therapy consultation. As a result of the rapid expansion of this service area there is a need for all levels of consultation practice. Case consultation may be directed toward the individual patient/client, the family, or the direct service provider. The occupational therapist consultant with a high level of expertise in working with the brain-injured population also may engage in program development consultation. Program consultation may emphasize educational, marketing, or administrative areas of consultation.

No aspect of human functioning is left unaffected by brain injury. As a result, many different agencies may be involved in case management and service provision. Occupational therapy consultation may range from involvement in the legal system, consultation to service providers, to consultation with advocacy groups. The quality of services provided is always a primary concern, irrespective of the type of occupational therapy consultation. This chapter does not focus on treatment issues per se, but on issues surrounding consultation for individuals with brain injury.

The author has had the opportunity to participate in the development and operation of specialized behavioral, acute rehabilitation, and transitional living programs, as well as outpatient and community services. The consultation services described in this chapter highlight some of these experiences. Successful consultation practice in any area of specialization requires that therapists remain within their area of competence. Attempting to provide consultation services for which the consultant is not qualified undermines her credibility and that of the profession.

The consultant should have specific training or experience that qualifies her to provide the services. The consultant should be prepared to state the training and experience on which she bases her recommendations.

The occupational therapist's domain of concern is broad. The occupational therapy consultant should have knowledge of medical, cognitive, motor, and psychosocial disorders in relation to real world functions. There has been a tendency for occupational therapists to emphasize cognitive testing.[1] The quest for objective tests for use by occupational therapists has been stimulated in part by a belief in the superiority of the scientific credentials of other disciplines (e.g., psychology, speech pathology). Many occupational therapy departments in large institutions have developed extensive test batteries, and testing may receive more emphasis than treatment. Assessment procedures not related to real world functions should be avoided by the occupational therapist in work with the brain injured. When providing case consultation, recommendations should always be presented in terms of function.

In consultation practice with individuals who have acquired neurological impairment, the author has found a cognitive behavioral or behavioral training approach the most effective.[2] Severely impaired individuals require highly specific behavior programs. The occupational therapist providing case or educational consultation services should maintain a practical orientation toward the behaviors that individuals need to acquire. Both the environment and the constraints placed on the individual by the neurological damage itself should be considered.[3] Given the occupational therapist's interest in function, the consultant should be interested in the client's normal and customary behavior. Consultation frequently involves an attempt to determine the most appropriate treatment site, the most appropriate placement, or the need for long-term service. Marketing consultation may involve working with facility staff to develop appropriate marketing strategies and training staff in specific marketing techniques. In administrative consultation the occupational therapy consultant may address organizational issues in service provision. The aims of this type of consultation may include reducing the cost and increasing the quality of service provision, the development of procedures required to gain licensing or accreditation, and training in the management of health care staff or other administrative policy development.

ENVIRONMENT AND SYSTEM INFLUENCES

The rapid changes in brain-injury service provision models since the late 1970s have resulted from a combination of factors: advances in biomedical technology, growing recognition of the effectiveness of rehabilitation, advocacy for the brain-injured person, and increasing public awareness of the significance of the public health problem posed by brain trauma. In addition, the legal system is becoming increasingly focused on functional outcome measures with this client population.

Medical rescue services have become more and more efficient with a concomitant decrease in mortality.[4, 5] Klauber and co-workers[6] have reported a reduction in mortality of trauma victims after modernization of the brain-injury service in San Diego County, and similar reductions have been reported in other regions.[7, 8] Brain-imaging techniques and some advances in acute management have also led to a decrease in mortality, particularly in some subgroups of the brain-injured population.[9] Increased survival has led to more individuals with the long-term sequelae of brain injury living in the community.

There has been increasing recognition of the effectiveness of postacute rehabilitation efforts and a growing number of service provision models. The socialization model pioneered at the Rusk Institute, the behavioral model pioneered at the Kemsley Unit in Great Britain, and the psychotherapeutic work of Prigatano and colleagues have all had a significant impact on the conduct of treatment.[10–12] The goal of rehabilitation is to assist clients in the development of behavioral control and independent living skills and to facilitate community integration and return to work. Therapeutic services are being recognized as effective in increasing quality of life and reducing long-term costs to the community. Demands from consumers have also increased. As a result, however, the issues surrounding service provision have become increasingly complex.

Brain-injured individuals and their advocates, through the National Head Injury Foundation, have become an increasingly active lobby for adequate service provision at both the state and federal level.[13] The Glasgow group of researchers highlighted the long-term consequences of brain injury for both the individual and the family and the need for middle- and long-term services.[14, 15]

There has been growing public interest in the plight of the brain-injured adult. The number of books and magazine articles appearing on the problems of these individuals has increased dramatically over recent years. Public agencies are becoming more responsive to the needs of the brain injured. This issue has received federal recognition through a significant increase in funding and by Congress declaring the 1990s "The decade of the brain." A consequence of the greater demand for treatment and care services is that the number of individuals with expertise in treating the brain injured is relatively small. This personnel shortage created a considerable need for expert consultation.

The legal system is becoming aware of the importance of functional assessments. Lawyers require evaluations of brain-injured clients in compensation litigation for two reasons: to determine liability and to apportion damages. Occupational therapy consultation may be required to assess functional limitations as part of the determination of damages. This may involve evaluating the need for future services and the most suitable placement of the client (including estimates of cost). The consultant may be called on to provide expert testimony in court.[16]

FRAME OF REFERENCE

The frame of reference for brain-injury case consultation is based on traditional occupational therapy principles with a behavioral or neurofunctional influence.[3] Occupational therapists are principally concerned with social and functional independence and psychosocial adjustment. In the assessment and treatment of the brain-injured adult, the occupational therapist considers the neuropsychiatric and neuropsychological limitations to new learning resulting from damage to the central nervous system.[2] Functional activities are used to address deficits and to enhance plastic changes in the central nervous system (learning). Interventions selected are based on scientific principles. Occupational therapists may provide a combination of assessment and recommendations for placement or service provision. Recommendations may be requested by family members, public agencies, third party payers, or for legal purposes and are needed to select the optimum type of treatment or placement. The failure of neuropsychological tests to correlate with real world abilities necessitates functional evaluations involving behavioral observations in many of these decisions. The recommendations of an occupational therapy consultant are therefore essential.

Occupational therapists have a central role in assessing the ability of brain-injured individuals to carry out the range of roles required for community living. By analyzing how the individual's performance breaks down, it is possible to determine the type and intensity of assistance required for the individual to maintain the highest level of independence possible. Although there has been a considerable drive to develop tests with good psychometric characteristics among occupational therapists[1] the central role of the occupational therapist in multidisciplinary assessment is to use assessment techniques with high ecological validity.

Ecologically valid tests use real world environments. These tests do not attempt to distinguish impaired core skills (e.g., attention, memory, or judgment); they are more concerned with real world performance. By necessity, tests that consider environmental factors lack normative standards. Ecologically valid tests are required due to the failure of standardized tests to predict important real world competencies. A model for assessment of the brain-injured adult considers the following domains:

1. Assessment of retained functional skills
2. Assessment of deficits limiting independent functioning
3. Identification of environmental factors that support independent functioning
4. Identification of demands placed on the individual by the environment
5. Identification of strategies used by the brain-injured individual in an attempt to overcome functional deficits
6. Identification of methods that assist the individual to relearn functional skills
7. Identification of changes required to enable the individual to function in his or her environmental context[3]

Although formal assessments or rating scales may be used, they often involve substantial loss of data. In addition, attempts to sum scores of diverse functions to produce a numerical score on a hypothetical construct such as "independence" or "degree of handicap" are likely to lead to erroneous results. These types of scales may be helpful in examining a single individual's progress through time but are problematic when applied to patient comparisons or when used to evaluate program effectiveness. Even when the scales are used for comparison of the same subject over time, the points on the scale should never be presumed to be equivalent. Observation of performance of real tasks required for independent living is preferred. In addition, certain agencies may wish to determine an individual's ability to respond to rehabilitative efforts. The occupational therapist needs to determine the ability of the brain-injured individual to acquire and utilize adaptive behaviors in response to specific training.

Rehabilitation efficacy may be demonstrated by administering standardized evaluations through time. An adequate rating scale must be brief enough for clinical application, complete enough to address relevant functional domains, and sensitive enough to capture changes of functional relevance. There are a vast number of scales for use during the acute stage of brain-injury rehabilitation. Scales include Ranchos Los Amigos's *Scale of Cognitive Functioning* and the *Disability Rating Scale* of Rappaport and co-workers.[17] Although not designed for use with the brain-injured, the *Adaptive Behavior Rating Scale*[18] is particularly appropriate for assessing function in the postacute stage of rehabilitation.[19]

CONSULTATION DESCRIPTIONS

The two case examples presented here describe different models of consultation. Case I follows the model of case consultation and interagency collaboration. Case II is an example of the educational and the program consultation models.

Case Example I

Organization

The local Department of Rehabilitation (DR) recognized the need to provide services to individuals with traumatic brain injury and other acquired neurological impairments. The services required by these clients were found to be far more costly and protracted than those required by the DR's general client population. In addition, the agency realized that the complexity of the cases made determining an appropriate case formulation and rehabilitation plan difficult for the DR staff. A relationship was already in existence between the DR and a specialized provider of services to brain-injured persons for whom the author was clinical consultant. The relationship developed through the mutual exploration of resources available to brain-injured individuals attempting to return to work. The service provider proposed that a contract be developed with the DR for client assessment. It was important to determine an assessment model that would meet referral needs, would not duplicate services that the DR could carry out with their in-house staff (e.g., neuropsychological testing), and that could be accommodated within the available funding.

Although the referral question varied from client to client, a central issue was whether, given the resources available to the DR, the patient was an appropriate candidate for vocational return and, if so, how vocational reintegration could best be facilitated. The following case illustrates the initial development of this consultative relationship.

Support

A per client reimbursement was negotiated based on the duration of the assessment and covering report writing and follow-up phone consultation. A provision for a volume discount was included. Assessments were to occur on an as-needed basis. Payment was made per client to the specialist service agency for whom the author was acting as a consultant.

Participants

Client D, a 35-year-old Hispanic female, was involved in a motor vehicle accident the night of the Fourth of July. D, unaccompanied and driving while intoxicated, was thrown from the vehicle and was found nonresponsive at the scene. At the trauma center she was noted to be paraplegic (T6-7) and to have severe lung and cardiac contusions. D required intubation and mechanically assisted ventilation. Her duration of coma was not reported but appears to have been at least 3 days. Previous psychiatric disorders included a history of substance abuse and multiple suicide attempts. Records indicated that 5 weeks following injury, D had made rapid progress and was reported to have achieved independence in all self-care activities. She was seen by the author for evaluation 18 months postinjury.

The DR counselor wanted to assist D but did not know how to proceed. The client's husband was described by the DR counselor as passive, (although invited, he did not attend the evaluation).

Services Provided

Evaluation by the occupational therapy consultant took four hours and involved a review of case notes, a clinical interview (including family and social history), behavioral observations, objective tests, and observations of performance of a range of functional community activities.

D was married with four sons (age range 5 through 18) and a 4-year-old daughter. D reported that her marriage was stable and committed; this view was endorsed by the DR counselor. At the time of the assessment D was being assisted by her family to perform basic self-care activities. She refused to leave the house unaccompanied by a family member. She was able to volunteer at the local museum only because her husband or one of her older sons transported her to and from it. She reported that she could only volunteer for 4 hours twice a week because she was anxious about incontinence. She had been incontinent for both bowel and bladder function at the museum on a number of occasions, and her response to these incidents would be to cry continuously and telephone her husband to come and take her home.

On the formal evaluation, D had marked deficits on immediate and delayed recall of a prose passage, face recognition on the Rivermead Behavioural Memory

Test,[20] and had marked difficulty in following verbal instructions. Her symptomatology was consistent with the sequelae of a severe brain injury. However there also appeared to be elements of exaggeration. For example, she claimed not to remember anything prior to her injury, including her parents and her early family history. (Although cases of almost total loss of personal historical material have been reported, they usually occur following severe psychological stress, encephalitis, or profound anoxia. The pattern of D's symptomatology was inconsistent with these disorders.)

D's initial presentation to the consultant was anxious and childlike. This was particularly marked when her four sons, who had accompanied her to the evaluation, were present. She became tearful on a number of occasions and spoke very softly, making her speech difficult to understand. D was very reluctant to have her sons leave the room and very hesitant to engage in the community tasks suggested by the consultant. Once she was out in the community, away from her family, a marked change occurred. Her speech became stronger and was a total absence of the whiny childlike quality that had previously been so marked. She performed the tasks that she had been assigned in a very competent manner and was safe in maneuvering her wheelchair over the relatively rough terrain of the neighborhood.

Some of D's problems were of long standing. There were some indications that she had a personality disorder prior to her injury and that she was abusing alcohol at a level that affected her day-to-day vocational and social functioning. As a result of the injury, she had genuine cognitive deficits: memory disorder, high level language impairments, and a marked tendency to concreteness. In addition, of course, she had become paraplegic. The combination of these severe stressers and inadequate personality resources, as well as a family that was used to caring for D prior to her injury, led D to exaggerate her level of handicap. Concrete recommendations were made by the consultant to the DR about how the agency could proceed in addressing these difficulties (for a discussion of illness behavior following brain injury see Giles and Clark-Wilson[3]).

Consultation Outcome

Following the occupational therapy consultant's evaluation, recommendations were made to the DR counselor: refer D to a clinical nurse specialist to assist her develop a bowel management program, which would allow her to work at the museum on a more frequent basis; continue the volunteer job with extended hours; and involve D's husband in any intervention. The consultant believed that D would probably be reluctant to give up her symptoms. Since she had considerable secondary gain from the status quo, change in the direction of increased independence was likely to be slow. This was explained to the DR so they did not expect overly rapid improvement. A written report was provided that included the case formulation and recommendations. Follow-up phone contact was regarded as very helpful by the DR and the department representatives were particularly impressed with the construction of relevant functional tasks for the purposes of assessment. A continuing series of referrals from the DR followed as a result of this initial interagency collaboration.

Case Example II

Organization

The author was providing direct treatment in the rehabilitation department of a midwestern university hospital. The author's experience was known to include work with severely behaviorally disturbed brain-injured adults. The department of psychiatry was having difficulty in managing a behaviorally disordered patient, and the clinical nurse specialist on the unit requested consultation with her staff to develop behavior management techniques for working with the patient.

Support

The Department of Psychiatry contracted for 20 hours of services with the possibility of extending the consultation hours.

Participants

The events surrounding the patients injuries were particularly horrific. RB, a 30-year-old husband and father of two, had been involved in a head-on collision when a car traveling in the opposite direction crossed the freeway median. Passing drivers pulled RB from his car into the road whereupon he was run over by a truck. RB was seen 9 months postinjury (coma duration was not recorded but was in excess of one month). RB's wife had been attempting to care for him at home after she had removed him from a nursing home because of her dissatisfaction with his care there. However, she found herself increasingly unable to care for RB. Admission to the psychiatric service was precipitated by RB's repeatedly striking the couple's two young children. RB had suffered multiple system injury and at the time of admission remained severely impaired. He was amnestic: unable to remember information for more than 30 seconds. A right femoral fracture had been treated with an intramedullary nail; the patient was only partially weight bearing. In addition, RB had decubitus ulcers in areas covering both the right and the left trochanters. RB spent most of his day in a manual wheelchair, but was unable to manage this himself and was dependant in mobility, transfers, toileting, bathing, and feeding. In addition, RB was physically aggressive many times per day, striking staff during wound care, transferring, and so on.

Staff on the psychiatric unit were not used to working with patients with the type and severity of deficits demonstrated by RB. They did not know how to manage RB's inappropriate behavior and were becoming increasingly reluctant to work with him for fear of being assaulted.

Services Provided

The author evaluated the client and established appropriate handling techniques. Many of the patient's aggressive outbursts were precipitated by anxiety during transferring. Because the psychiatric staff did not understand the nature of the patient's memory disorder, they were not explaining activities of daily living (ADL) and transferring procedures in a way that RB could understand and remember during the procedure itself. This increased his anxiety and the likelihood that he would be physically aggressive. The consultant described and modeled how to communicate with RB prior to the transferring procedure. Additionally, the consultant discussed with staff during treatment rounds how RB's cognitive deficits (e.g., memory, attention, and initiation) affected his ADL and behavioral functioning. These in-service suggestions led to an immediate reduction in the frequency of aggressive episodes. Prior to the consultation, staff had no prearranged method for handling RB's aggression. Uncertainty as to how to respond to RB's aggressive behavior had resulted in considerable staff anxiety. Establishing a simple set of procedures to be implemented in response to aggression assisted staff to feel more comfortable in handling RB. In addition a training procedure was introduced to help RB learn how to wheel his own wheelchair. This had the effect of helping the staff feel far more positive toward RB. Following this short-term consultation, the psychiatric service staff asked the author to provide them with a series of in-services on brain injury and behavior disorder.

Consultation Outcome

Following the introduction of the procedures just described, there was a considerable reduction in RB's frequency of aggression. Before the consultation, staff were developing an increasingly negative attitude toward RB. By the end of the 20 hours of consultation, staff were no longer negative and felt that RB was making progress. As RB's behavior disorder came under control, it became possible to transfer him to another facility close to his home (which had previously refused to accept him due to his behavior disorder). This move allowed RB's wife and children to visit him regularly. The reputation of the hospital occupational therapy department was enhanced by this successful educational consultation, and there was a markedly increased utilization of occupational therapy services by the hospital psychiatric department.

EDUCATION AND PROGRAM CONSULTATION MODEL

Case examples I and II indicate the complex nature of many of the individual cases and the difficulties that may be encountered in working with brain-injured clients. Work with brain-injured individuals is personally and professionally challenging. Requests for staff education from a consultant are often precipitated by problems with a particular client.

Case consultation II is an example of how an initial consultation to assist staff in working with a difficult-to-handle client became an educational consultation to assist staff in developing skills to work with a client population. The management of physical aggression frequently results in consultation requests. The staff's negative reaction to behavior disorders may affect not only the patient's treatment, but that of other patients on the unit; staff may need rapid and intensive intervention to handle the patient in an appropriate manner. Intrateam conflict around this issue is common. The goals of the staff may not be immediately apparent and it is important that these be established. Education as to what are reasonable goals for the client is often the most important first step.

For example, some staff may regard a behavioral plan as a panacea that will prevent the client from repeating the unwanted behavior. Although consultation requests on technical aspects of client treatment are common, many rehabilitation teams have difficulties understanding the nature of brain injury and its influence on behavior on a more basic level. Untrained or inexperienced teams may attribute lack of effort, poor motivation, and denial of deficit to a preexisting moral weakness in the client rather than to the trauma.

The first goal is often to assist staff in solving the actual problem they are having with the client. Educational intervention is based on information and training, but may develop into a process management approach. While information is a necessary beginning, the most effective type of intervention includes the consultant as a participant in the design and implementation of programs. The consultant helps staff solve practical problems and facilitates the resolution of interpersonal conflicts. Staff conflicts may stem from differences concerning the overall orientation of the treatment team. Conflicts may be particularly marked around whether to function as a multidisciplinary or a transdisciplinary team. In a multidisciplinary team the physician typically retains overall charge of the patient's treatment. Multidisciplinary team meetings provide a focus for the exchange of information and for informing the physician of the patient's progress in what are not strictly medical domains. It may be possible to coordinate simple procedures such as transferring techniques and establish uniformity in simple behavioral interventions, but the multidisciplinary team's ability to coordinate treatment is limited.

In a transdisciplinary team, the team leader is frequently not a physician, but a clinician from a therapeutic discipline who has experience in working with the client population and as a program manager. Team meetings determine goals for each client depending on their needs. This team approach is described as transdisciplinary because only rarely does a client's goal fit wholly within the artificial domain of any therapeutic discipline. Instead, goals are overarching in that they are related to many disciplines.

Although offering many advantages, the transdisciplinary team has disadvantages. Stepping out of role may be stressful for therapists trained in a multidisciplinary team. The approach requires a relatively high percentage of meeting time. Not only must treatments be planned and coordinated, it is often necessary to have staff practice an intervention so that it becomes automatic (for a fuller discussion of the two models of treatment, see Giles and Clark-Wilson[3]). It is often difficulties with specific clients or recognition of avoidable treatment failures that lead to a reevaluation of the whole service delivery model. A number of formal assessment tools are available to assist in program assessment and goal setting.

Two scales of particular interest to the occupational therapy consultant are *The Ward Atmosphere Scale* (WAS) and *The Community Oriented Programs Environ-*

COPES PROFILES FOR TWO TRANSITIONAL LIVING PROGRAMS

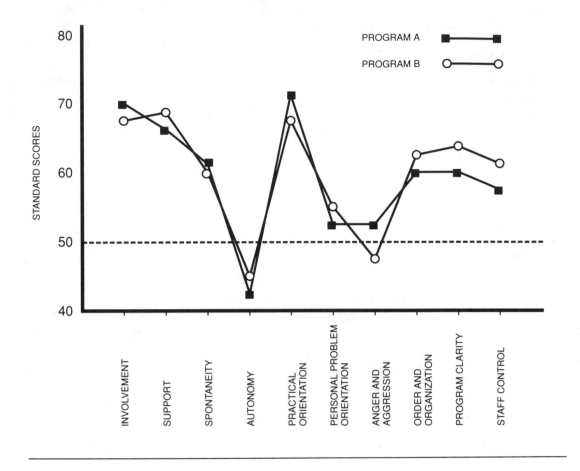

FIGURE 18–1

COPES Staff Profiles for Two Mature Transitional Living Centers.

Involvement: How active clients are in everyday program functioning

Support: How supportive staff are toward members

Spontaneity: How much the program encourages the open expression of feelings by clients and staff

Autonomy: How self-sufficient and independent clients are in decision making

Practical Orientation: The degree to which clients learn practical skills for life in the community

Personal Problem Orientation: The extent to which clients are encouraged to explore their feelings

Anger and Aggression: How much clients argue with each other or staff or display other forms of aggression

Order and Organization: How important order and organization are in the program

ment Scale (COPES)[21, 22]. In both the WAS and the COPES, ten scales are grouped into three domains: relationship, personal growth or goal orientation, and system maintenance. The scales can be used for program evaluation and to stimulate change. Figure 18–1 shows COPES profiles for two transitional living programs with highly functional orientations. Abbreviated scale descriptions and discussion of how these might be interpreted are included (see the COPES manual for a detailed description of the scales and a discussion of its application). Although used here to describe transitional living centers they may also be used in program evaluation of other types of rehabilitation sites[23].

SUMMARY

Occupational therapists have a central role in the rehabilitation of the brain-injured adult. The functional orientation of the occupational therapist is unique in the rehabilitation team and is being recognized increasingly as the key to patient evaluation and treatment planning. The changes in the environment for brain-injury rehabilitation have led to diverse opportunities for occupational therapists in consultation. As the search for cost-effective service delivery models continue, consultation opportunities are expanding. These opportunities include case, educational, program, marketing, and administrative consultation. Community reintegration and vocational return are areas in which the occupational therapy consultant's practical orientation to real world functioning is of great value in developing effective programming. Successful consultation requires that the occupational therapist develop specific expertise in this area of consultation. Developing skills in consultation with this population can provide opportunities for personal and professional growth.

Program Clarity: The degree to which program rules and procedures are explicit
Staff Control: The extent to which staff exercise control over client behavior.

Both of the program profiles (A and B) are staff attitude profiles for transitional living centers for brain-injured adults. Programs are geographically separated and do not share staff. Both programs are mature, although program A is considerably older. The two program profiles are remarkably similar. Program A accepts clients who are more severely handicapped than the clients accepted in program B. This may, in part, account for the lower rating for program A for autonomy as well as program A's greater practical orientation. Program A has approximately twice the census of program B. This may partially account for the lower ratings of program clarity and staff control but it may also indicate a need for these issues to be addressed. The COPES can be used to monitor staff attitudes and orientation to program goals.

REFERENCES

1. Maurer P, Barris R, Bonder B, et al: Hierarchy of competencies relating to the use of standardized instruments and evaluation techniques by occupational therapists. *Am J Occup Ther* 1984; 38:803–804.
2. Fussey I, Giles GM (eds): *Rehabilitation of the Severely Brain-injured Adult: A Practical Approach.* London, Croom Helm, 1988.
3. Giles GM, Clark-Wilson J: *Occupational Therapy for the Brain-injured Adult: A Neurofunctional Approach.* London, Croom Helm, 1991.
4. Baxt WG, Moody P: The impact of advanced pre-hospital emergency care on the mortality of severely brain-injured patients. *J Trauma* 1987; 27:365–369.
5. Becker DP, Miller D, Ward JD et al: The outcome from severe head injury with early diagnosis and intensive management. *J Neurosurg* 1977; 47:491–502.
6. Klauber MR, Marshall LF, Toole BM, et al: Cause of decline in head-injury mortality rate in San Diego County, California. *J Neurosurg* 1985; 62:528–531.
7. Ornato JP, Craren EJ, Nelson NM, et al: Impact of improved emergency medical services and emergency trauma care on reduction of mortality from trauma. *J Trauma* 1985; 25:575–579.
8. West JG, Cales RH, Gazzaniga AB: Impact of regionalization: The Orange County experience. *Arch Surg* 1983; 118:740–744.
9. Servadei F, Piazza G, Seracchioli A, et al: Extradural haematomas: An analysis of changing characteristics of patients admitted from 1980 to 1986. Diagnostic and therapeutic implications in 158 cases. *Brain Inj* 1988; 2:87–100.
10. Ben-Yishay Y, Diller L, Rattok J: A modular approach to optimizing orientation, psychomotor alertness and purposive behaviour in severe head trauma patients, In *Working Approaches to Remediation of Cognitive Deficits in Brain Damaged Persons.* Rehabilitation Monographs no 59. New York, Institute of Rehabilitation Medicine, New York University Medical Center, 1978, pp 63–67.
11. Prigatano GP (ed): *Neuropsychological Rehabilitation After Brain Injury.* Baltimore, Johns Hopkins Univ Press, 1986.
12. Eames P, Wood R: Rehabilitation after severe brain injury: A follow-up study of a behaviour modification approach. *J Neurol Neurosurg Psychiatry* 1985; 48:613–619.
13. Bush GW: The National Head Injury Foundation: Eight years of challenge and growth. *J Head Trauma Rehab* 1988; 3:73–77.
14. McKinlay WW, Brooks DN, Bond MR, et al: The short-term outcome of severe blunt brain injury as reported by relatives of the injured persons. *J Neurol Neurosurg Psychiatry* 1981; 44:727–733.
15. Brooks DN, Campsie L, Symington C, et al: The five-year outcome of severe blunt head injury: A relative's view. *J Neurol Neurosurg Psychiatry* 1986; 49:764–770.
16. Koplan KI: Functional outcome evaluation of the head injured: Its effect on legal rights. *J Head Trauma Rehab* 1987; 2:93.
17. Rappaport M, Hall KM, Hopkins K, et al: Disability rating scale for severe brain trauma; Coma to community. *Arch Phys Med Rehabil* 1982; 63:118–123.
18. Nihira K, Foster R, Sellhaas M, et al: *AAMD Adaptive Behavior Scale.* Washington, DC, American Association on Mental Deficiency, 1974.
19. Benton A: Behavioural consequences of closed head injury. *Central Nervous System Trauma Status Report.* National Institute of Neurological and Communicative Disorders and Stroke, 1979.

20. Wilson B, Cockburn C, and Baddeley A: *Rivermead Behavioural Memory Test.* Reading, Thames Valley Test Co, 1985.
21. Moos RH: *Ward Attitude Scale.* Palo Alto, Calif, Consulting Psychologists Press, 1988.
22. Moos RH: *Community-Oriented Programs Environment Scale.* Palo Alto, Calif, Consulting Psychologists Press, 1988.
23. Cornes P, Horton D: The measurement of rehabilitation centre social climates. *J Occup Psychol* 1981; 54:289–297.

CHAPTER 19

Occupational Therapy Consultation in Health Care Consortiums: Systems/ Program Consultation

Elizabeth B. Devereaux, M.S.W., A.C.S.W./L.,
O.T.R./L., F.A.O.T.A.

OVERVIEW

During the first 15 years of practice, as the only occupational therapist within a 150-mile radius, the author developed important consultation skills that were used to share knowledge and to influence the development of community programs. Consultation was critically needed, as direct service needs could not be met by one therapist in all communities.

A first job, assisting a local Easter Seal Society to start a treatment center, resulted in the author serving as executive director and director of the occupational therapy department. Starting with a small room where occupational therapy services were provided, the program developed to a full service rehabilitation center within 8 years. Hill-Burton funds and much community support helped to build the center. Experiences gained through these efforts formed the basis of the author's consulting skills. In addition, the three consultations described in this chapter expanded the consultant's expertise.

Department of Mental Health

The author's initial experience as an occupational therapist in a pediatric setting required consultation with parents, teachers, and other health care professionals. These consulting skills were transferred to a larger arena in the author's role as the adjunctive therapy director for the West Virginia Department of Mental Health.

This position carried considerable responsibility, but also marvelous opportunities to become involved in system changes and professional growth. Some time was spent working with the central office consultant team representing psychiatry, psychology, nursing, social work, pharmacy, engineering, and fiscal affairs. The majority of the author's time was spent at the various state hospitals and a training center for the mentally retarded. Consultation was provided to the administrator, clinical director, and staffs of the occupational therapy, recreational therapy, industrial therapy, and rehabilitation programs. Program development and troubleshooting for ongoing programs was also a part of the consultation.

Initially the consultant's presence appeared threatening to the adjunctive therapy staffs. There were very few professionals within this group (only two registered occupational therapists in the entire state hospital system). Many staff had been selected from the hospital nursing aides. Those selected for the adjunctive therapies had some interest and skill in arts and crafts. Adjunctive therapy staff jobs were also considered of higher status and more interesting than a nursing aide position. By first developing relationships, a process was facilitated that allowed the consultant and staff to work *together*. This enabled staff to accept recommendations made to enhance patient treatment programs with little or no resistance. The extra time spent in this educational process was extremely important; had change been mandated it could have occurred much more quickly, but staff acceptance would have been questionable. Resentment and lack of understanding of the reasoning behind the recommended changes would have surfaced quickly. By understanding the changes, staff *improved* on them, as they knew their system and patients far better than the consultant. As the consultant and staff worked together, mutual trust was developed. Staff began to realize that the consultant was not interested in having them fired. By helping them learn new skills and gain the administrative support necessary for better job performance and improved patient treatment, the consultant became an ally.

During the seven years spent in this position, the consultant was involved in multifaceted tasks. These included developing many different programs, planning and conducting workshops, developing policy, licensing mental health facilities, writing a manual about the geographic unit system, and implementing this system in all its state mental health facilities. Participation in a series of seminars on organizational design and a week-long workshop sponsored by the U.S. Department of Health, Education, and Welfare with National Training Laboratories faculty facilitated integration of the structures and theories of organizational design and consultation into the consultant's knowledge base. This culminated in a more formalized consultation frame of reference: general systems theory.

The following consultation descriptions are presented to provide an overview of the consultant's varied experiences.

University Administration

A time-limited (two-day) consultation was requested by a university with an occupational therapy educational program. Verbal and written reports answering specific questions were to be provided to designated university officials at the conclusion of the visit, and a written report was to be submitted after the visit. The questions posed by the university administration focused on curriculum, including fieldwork issues, the quality of student preparation, and faculty involvement in research within the occupational therapy program.

Information was gathered from written materials and meetings with faculty, students, administrators, and clinical supervisors. A systems analysis approach was used by the consultant to present an overall picture of what was occurring within the department. Because of a lack of leadership and hierarchical/structural confusion, key department members perceived that they had little power and therefore had resorted to overcontrolling situations. The analysis included recommended strategies for correction.

State Hospital Seeking JCAHO Accreditation

In this example, a slightly different format was followed. Here, the consultant used other consultants on a project for their particular expertise.

The state Department of Health (DOH) wanted a state-of-the-art clinical management system developed for the local state hospital. The primary goal was the development of a clinical service that would enable the hospital to achieve Joint Commission on Accreditation of Health-Care Organizations (JCAHO) accreditation by a specified date. All of the state mental hospitals in this particular state were accredited until the late 1950s, when the American Psychiatric Association (APA) discontinued their accreditation of hospitals. Since then, *none* of this state's mental hospitals had been accredited and this was to be the first hospital to make the effort in nearly 30 years.

The Department of Psychiatry in the medical school where the consultant was a faculty member was asked to submit a proposal for the development of this system. The department was very interested, as they wished to use the state hospital as a clerkship training site for third-year medical students and for psychiatric residents.

The chairman of the department asked the consultant to develop the needed proposals. Subsequently, this proposal was accepted and the consultant was asked to serve as contract coordinator/consultant for the project. The consultant knew the consultation process that would be effective in this situation, but lacked specific familiarity with the preparation of a JCAHO application. Two additional consultants were selected to participate in the project who were very experienced with the JCAHO standards and process on national and state hospital system levels. Equally important was their skill in interpersonal relations, precluding an "expert-novice" relationship with state hospital staff. They brought tremendous expertise to the situation, and both approached the consultation with an attitude of mutual respect. Although they had the JCAHO knowledge, they recognized that the hospital staff had the expertise about their hospital and that the project could be enhanced by a shared knowledge base. The consultants happened to be an occupational therapist and a nurse who were also husband and wife. After much hard work and dedication on the part of all involved, the hospital achieved JCAHO accreditation by the date specified.

The major consultation to be described in this chapter is in the form of a case study. The following is a brief overview of the situation.

Faculty status in the university Department of Psychiatry led to a variety of opportunities for consultation. The consultation to be described arose when a small community hospital sought assistance in upgrading their psychiatric services. This hospital, recently purchased by a national chain, wanted to further develop an already profitable psychiatric unit. To accomplish this, the unit had to obtain the proper Diagnostic Related Groups (DRG) status and meet the standards of all external regulatory agencies, including JCAHO.

Once these goals were identified, the newly appointed community hospital administrator sought consultation assistance from the university's Department of Psychiatry. A sequential plan, comprising direct and consultative services, was then developed by the consultant. This plan included program enhancement and expansion, as well as interfacing faculty from the Department of Psychiatry with the hospital's existing staff. Sanction for the consultation and program enhancement was strong from the top and middle management, with varying acceptance from other program and hospitalwide staff.

ENVIRONMENTAL AND SYSTEMS INFLUENCES

Classes in this medical school began with the January 1978 semester. The school differed from most others in the state-supported universities because it was established as a community-based program. A major goal was the promotion of medical education specifically oriented to practice in rural communities located in the southern part of the state.[7] Few of these communities had hospitals, and other resources for health care were limited. The medical school was organized to reflect the kind of medical practice possible in these rural communities, and thus did not have its own hospital. Instead, affiliation agreements (a requirement of the liaison committee on medical education) were developed with selected hospitals in the community in which the medical school was located.

Political/Interagency Relationships

A large community hospital with the most psychiatric beds and sophisticated programs was selected by the medical school as its primary clinical site for training third-year medical students on their psychiatry rotation and for the psychiatric residency program. Faculty psychiatrists hospitalized their patients on this psychiatric unit.

The small community hospital, recently purchased by a national for-profit chain, had a locked psychiatric unit with 16 beds. This hospital did not have an affiliation agreement with the medical school. When the consultation began, minimal interaction had occurred between the two institutions, and a training program for medical students did not exist at the small hospital. The new owners applied for a certificate of need to convert general medical/surgical beds to psychiatric beds, because they planned to establish a freestanding psychiatric hospital. The large hospital opposed the application, stating that no additional psychiatric beds were needed in the community. There followed several years of hearings and court proceedings until this issue was resolved, and it was during this period that the consultation described here occurred.

Town/Gown Issues

Many area physicians had been active in helping to establish this medical school. They continued their participation in various ways: serving as part-time academic faculty, or clinical faculty, and a few as full-time academic faculty. As various departments in the medical school matured, they resumed or developed research projects, opened their respective clinics, and began to treat patients. Some area physicians appeared threatened by this competition, not only economically but also due to the current, state-of-the-art knowledge of many of the medical school faculty.

These town/gown issues were evident in the psychiatric community. Area psychiatrists became less willing to donate their time for classroom or clinical teaching, to serve on departmental committees, or to participate in other activities supportive of medical education. The split was further apparent at the large hospital where psychiatry section bylaws required five-year staff membership to acheive full privileges, including voting. Thus the town psychiatrists held favored positions for several years. Psychiatry section meetings were frequently chaotic, filled with dissension and obstructionism. It was not an atmosphere conducive to the education and training of medical students and residents. Attracting psychiatry faculty for the school was also more difficult in this environment. In addition, requirements for accreditation of the psychiatry residency program were not met, as the medical school's Department of Psychiatry could not fully implement their educational program without appropriate control of the psychiatry units.

The consultant assessed that the medical school was a convenient scapegoat for some of the town psychiatrists' displaced anger, frustration, and fear. The medical school represented a growing influence in the community at the same time the outside regulations of JCAH and the DRG system were having a powerful effect on how medicine could be practiced. Physician incomes were being affected, as was the usual practice of medicine; they no longer had the freedom to hospitalize patients freely or for long periods of time, and out-of-date treatment methods were questioned. These external forces affecting their practices had very little to do with the medical school issues. But blame was placed on the school for their losses.

Economic Environment

Despite the escalation of health care costs in the mid-1980s, financial support for higher education in many states did not keep pace with inflation. Medical school departments increased their efforts to obtain external funds and medical school deans relied on the indirect costs from grants and a percentage of departmental incomes as their major source of discretionary funds. Much medical care was provided free of charge as patients who lost jobs eventually lost medical insurance coverage. This added to the great number of medically uninsured who continued to need medical care.

The small hospital had less than half the number of beds of the other two major general hospitals in the city, an outdated physical plant, and an average daily census well below 100. The initial contact between this small hospital and the medical school's Department of Psychiatry occurred when the latter was asked to provide, through contract, a seven day a week group therapy program for the psychiatric inpatient unit at the small hospital. The unit had also contracted for limited occupational therapy services during this time. About 6 months later, the hospital administrator requested that the Department of Psychiatry submit a proposal to provide comprehensive programming for the unit, with the hospital continuing to provide nursing services and adding a recreational therapist to their staff. The chairman of the Department of Psychiatry requested that the consultant develop the proposal.

At the time of the proposed program expansion, the Department of Psychiatry was reorganized to add a fourth division, occupational therapy, to the existing divisions of psychiatry, social work, and medical psychology. Occupational therapy would support the contract and begin to respond to the many unmet requests for occupational therapy services within the community. Occupational therapists were successfully recruited over the next few months. In addition to psychiatry, occupational therapy services were contracted to a wide variety of inpatient and outpatient community health care settings.

Interprofessional Relationships and Social Environment

Faculty throughout the medical school functioned in a collegial manner, with many interdisciplinary projects and programs and a team approach to treatment. An active (adjunct) clinical faculty existed within the Department of Psychiatry, and there were numerous outside social contacts within the groups. This reflected one aspect of the social environment, and had its own value when it came to working together.

However, there was another very important aspect to the social environment that could be called a "social conscience." Many of the staff had worked together in research teams and/or made a real effort to keep up with the latest research, and deplored the very antiquated treatment being used by some in the psychiatric community. Whenever possible, the staff provided current treatment programming. This also created a more constructive educational milieu for medical students and residents.

FRAME OF REFERENCE

"The occupational therapist knows the dynamics and process involved in treating the individual client. This same basic model can be extrapolated and built upon in working with groups and in working with the entire community."[4] Working with individuals, occupational therapists perform assessments of abilities/dysfunction; develop the treatment plan in collaboration with the patient/family; and implement treatment and continually evaluate the patient's progress. That same process can be converted to a larger arena, working with groups and the community, and to the consultation process. By gathering all the pertinent information about the larger system and analyzing that data to produce an assessment of functional parts/ dysfunctional parts (problem identification), a program can be developed in collaboration with the consultee to address the situation(s). The consultant can facilitate the implementation of the program and evaluation of the results. Table 19–1 presents a comparison of these processes.

Applicable Theoretical Concepts of Systems Theory

The theory that forms the frame of reference for the consultant's work is general systems theory. It is primarily concerned with relationships, structure, and interdependence. A system is defined as a set of units or components that are actively interrelated and operate within some sense of boundary. The functional components or subsystems that are part of every larger system serve a specialized role

TABLE 19–1
Extrapolation of Occupational Therapy Treatment Planning Process

Individual	Group/Consultation Process
1. Patient assessment	1. Data gathering and analysis
2. Plan treatment	2. Program planning (design)
3. Implement treatment	3. Program implementation
4. Evaluate treatment	4. Program evaluation

in the operation of that larger system. The components of a system are not all parallel to each other, but may be hierarchically arranged, so that the interaction between two components of a hierarchical system is more than a linear cause and effect process. To use an occupational therapy descriptor, it has a "legitimate complexity." The terms *commanding* and *constraining* are used to describe the interaction between the higher and lower components of a system; higher levels are said to command lower levels. Changes at one level of the hierarchy of an open system may resonate throughout several levels due to the intense interconnectedness of these different levels. Attempts to correct or ameliorate problems at one narrow level almost invariably fail if their consequences or impact at other levels are not assessed as part of the process.[1-3,5,6]

The focus is on living, or open systems (as opposed to nonliving, or closed systems), which are characterized as being "open" to internal and external environments. The basic concept of an open system having a cyclic energy and information exchange, described as input→conversion→output, with the outputs of one system becoming available for use as inputs for another system, facilitates the analysis of systems and their interactions at many levels of complexity. The subset of living systems with which we are directly concerned are the individual, small groups, and large groups. This may include a multitude of different combinations or configurations such as interdisciplinary teams, unit staffs, organizations, and communities.[1-3, 5,6]

There are a number of key concepts from systems theory that have particular relevance to this consultation description, some of which are stated as follows:

- Crisis, or disequilibrium, has an accompanying energy that can be used to help the system move to a healthier state.
- The individual (system) and larger systems can become addicted to uproar.
- As a centrifugal force gathers energy, centripetal forces will form as counterforces. Example: The revision of a program (or the initiation of a new program) within an organization will be followed by the formation of one or more smaller groups critical of/in opposition to the program.
- An understanding of the relationships, structure, and interdependencies of one system can be extrapolated to a like understanding of a larger system. Example: Individual→group→community: microsystems, macrosystems.
- An understanding of systems theory can facilitate problem identification through analysis of symptoms and manifestations of the problem.
- Changing the level of inquiry within a system can often assist us to design second-order intervention rather than "more of the same."

Applicable Models of Consultation

The primary models of consultation used in the following consultation description were educational and program development. However, components of other consultation models as described earlier in Chapter 2 were also used because of the complexity of the consultation. The three levels of consultation needed in this situation were case-centered, educational, and program or administrative levels.

CONSULTATION DESCRIPTION: THE PROPOSAL AND THE CONTRACT

Organization

The 16-bed psychiatric inpatient unit at the small hospital provided evaluation, treatment, and discharge planning for patients with a primary psychiatric diagnosis. If other medical problems became primary, the patient was transferred to a medical or surgical service for treatment. Usually, the patient was transferred back to the psychiatric unit upon completion of the needed treatment.

To address the small hospital's goals of meeting the ongoing needs of patients and the requirements of both the Health Care Financing Administration (HCFA) and Joint Commission on the Accreditation of Hospitals (JCAH), the consultant proposed a plan that would provide a comprehensive therapeutic program on the psychiatric inpatient unit. Collaboration with existing hospital staff and personnel from the Department of Psychiatry would facilitate establishment of a treatment program that would be individualized, yet coordinated across disciplines, and would help develop a team approach to patient care.

It was proposed that a position be created for a coordinator of therapeutic programs for the psychiatric inpatient unit. Duties included the following:

- Work with both staffs to further develop a therapeutic program
- Function as liaison
- Prioritize the use of Department of Psychiatry resources
- Continuously assess program needs and make critical revisions to meet these needs
- Provide in-service training program for unit staff in collaboration with the head nurse of the psychiatric unit
- Be accountable to the hospital administrator and the chairman of the Department of Psychiatry

The position required an average of 12 hours to 20 hours per week of the consultant's time, and combined the functions of direct service and ongoing consultation.

Support

All support services for the consultation were provided through the medical school's Department of Psychiatry. These services included typing, copying, monthly billing for the contract services, payroll for all contract personnel, various library literature searches, and videotapes. Medical school media staff videotaped all in-service presentations, and these tapes were made available to those hospital staff unable to be present at the original presentations.

Participants

The national chain that had purchased the small hospital placed one of their own administrators in charge of the hospital to whom the consultant was directly accountable. Key participants in the consultation were the head nurse, the chairman of the Department of Psychiatry, and the hospital administrator. The consultant and head nurse worked together, keeping the administrator and chairman informed about the progress of the program and any unusual events. Using a "management by exception" approach, the consultant and head nurse proceeded with program development, management, and decision making on a routine basis. If out of the ordinary problems occurred, identified options and recommended solutions were discussed with the chairman and/or the administrator.

For example, a space expansion proposal was prepared shortly after the initiation of the consultation and submitted to the administrator. The proposal detailed current use of space, additional needs, lost revenue due to limited treatment areas, and assumptions about program direction. Two expanded space plans drawn to scale were presented. The result was approval for combining the two plans and creation of more functional program space.

Services Provided

In addition to the services of the consultant, important professional staff were provided by the Department of Psychiatry. Three additional faculty psychiatrists, psychologists, psychiatric social workers, and occupational therapists were included. These individuals provided diagnostic, assessment, evaluation, treatment, and discharge planning services.

- *Psychological services*. These services included evaluation, testing, and treatment as indicated, individual/group therapy, participation in treatment and discharge planning sessions, the assessment of patient progress, and documentation of same. Services were available 7 days per week, for a minimum of 10 hours per week.
- *Psychiatric social work services*. Psychiatric social workers conducted daily group therapy sessions. In addition, they participated in the treatment and discharge planning sessions, provided individual, group, marital, and family therapy when indicated, and led special therapeutic topic groups. Their time commitment was 4 hours per day, for a total of 28 hours per week.
- *Occupational therapy services*. Patient evaluation, individual and group treatment, and participation in treatment and discharge planning sessions

were provided by the occupational therapists. Services were provided 7 days per week, for a minimum of 15 hours.

- *In-service training*. In-service training sessions were conducted every two weeks, with topic selection determined by staff and programmatic needs. Initial topics included the following:

  - Treatment planning
  - Developing the team approach to patient treatment
  - Psychopathology
  - Psychosocial rehabilitation
  - Developing skills for conflict management/resolution
  - Opening of Department of Psychiatry grand rounds to staff from the small hospital

- *Evaluation*. Two very concrete measures of consultation effectiveness were the achievement of HCFA/DRG Waiver for the unit and meeting JCAH standards of accreditation. Additional evaluation methods focused on patient census, patient satisfaction, physician referral, and numbers participating on this unit.

This external consultation was maintained for over four years and included both direct and consultative services. Entry into the system was greatly facilitated because the consultant had provided direct group therapy services for this unit during the preceding months. The consultant knew the staff, and a level of trust and a comfortable working relationship had been established previously. In addition, the consultant knew a lot about the environment including procedures, staffing patterns, and the general system.

A discrepancy analysis was performed with the staff during the needs assessment for the proposal. This involved brainstorming under the headings "What We Are Doing Now" and "What We Would Like to be Doing." Planning ensued to figure out how to move items from column 1 to column 2. This was an effective method of involving staff and helping them to prepare for change.

The dialogue and collaborative style of working was continued through the proposal development phase. Meetings between the unit head nurse and the consultant, the unit staff, and nonunit hospital staff kept them involved in the process. During this period of program development and throughout the length of the consultation it was important not to make any programmatic changes without consensus between the head nurse and consultant. This approach continued even though personnel in the head nurse position changed twice during the consultation.

An important bonding was achieved when the HCFA site review occurred early in the consultation. There was enough program in place at that time to receive the DRG waiver. Trust, collaboration, and a feeling of unity took a quantum leap forward.

Treatment Teams

Treatment teams met three times each week, which was often enough to meet HCFA and JCAH requirements and to accommodate the flow of patient admissions and reviews. In addition to the more formal biweekly in-service training provided (to coincide with payday so that shift workers would attend), much informal teaching took place during treatment team meetings by the consultant and two other faculty members, a psychologist and a social worker. With such a small bed capacity, the hospital could not have afforded to hire full-time staff with the credentials and depth of experience they had working with their staff and patients through the contractual arrangement. Much of the teaching was case centered. However, the educational model was used as problem identification and resolution developed in relation to the structure of the program, forms, and procedures. The staff discussed the reasons it would be better patient care to proceed one way as opposed to the other. Either the consultant (or designee) or the head nurse conducted the treatment team sessions, with nursing staff participating on a rotating basis. Psychiatrists, residents, and third-year medical students participated on an irregular basis. The other contract disciplines participated regularly as did the hospital's recreational therapist and medical social workers. The latter provided social histories for the psychiatric patients and were very involved in discharge planning.

Clinical faculty in social work and psychology assisted in providing the services at the hospital on a contract basis. This had many benefits. First, these clinical faculty were delighted to have the opportunity to earn extra money, and medical school faculty were glad to have help in providing these services. Second, since all of the clinical faculty held full-time jobs with other community agencies and hospitals, inclusion in the Department of Psychiatry project helped to upgrade clinical faculty skills and created a widening area of influence throughout the mental health services in the community. This happened subtly, on an informal basis. The relationships developed and the knowledge shared here paid off handsomely many times, particularly during the JCAHO effort described earlier.

Outcome

As stated previously, HCFA regulations were met and the DRG waiver for this unit continued to be granted during the consultation period. JCAH accreditation was also maintained. The space proposal resulted in remodeling of the unit itself and additional space renovation to support program. A recreational therapist was hired by the hospital to complete the psychiatric treatment team.

Many favorable comments about the quality of the treatment provided were received from physicians, patients, and patients' families. The patient census on this unit was maintained at capacity or at near capacity, subject to the usual seasonal waxing and waning of psychiatric admissions. Both the Department of

Psychiatry and the hospital staff generally felt very positively about their involvement in this joint endeavor. The contract was renegotiated each year, with the only adjustments being fee changes and an updating of personnel rosters.

Termination and a New Phase

As planned, at the end of the fourth year, the national chain that had purchased the hospital began assuming responsibility for management, programming, and total renovation of the hospital. The new hospital administrator did not renegotiate the contract, but asked that services continue for an indefinite period of time with an understanding that would include 1 or 2 weeks notice of final termination. This arrangement was acceptable, as the consultant wished to assist the transition.

During the 3- to 4-month overlap it became apparent that many gains achieved through the consultation were seen as inappropriate by the chain personnel. Despite the attainment and maintenance of the DRG waiver and JCAH accreditation, chain personnel requested changes in nearly all areas. However, they could not provide relevant direction for their desired change. Both the consultant staff and hospital staff, who had developed a cooperative and collaborative blending, were taken aback, particularly in light of the success they had achieved. Many adjustments and changes ensued for the hospital staff. The consultation staff tried to be supportive to these colleagues, while realizing, with relief, that their involvement was soon ending.

Such an experience highlights some of the risks of consultation. The efforts of the consultant and the other participants met the goals of the original proposal and contract. It was renewed each year with no changes other than personnel and fee updates. Since the hospital chain brought in their own personnel and programs, no new proposal was prepared to meet their goals. The hospital chain did not directly sanction the original proposal, although it did so indirectly, as the administrator was their employee. When management changes, there is always the risk that expectations, values, and goals will be different or, even if the goals are the same, new management will favor a different process to accomplish them. It was important for those involved in the original proposal and contract to recognize that they did not fail; they succeeded in their efforts. The two different approaches were simply that—different.

SUMMARY

The consultation described is one of much longer duration than usual. It occurred on all three levels of consultation: case centered, educational, and program and/or administrative, and involved several models of consultation. Case-centered consultation was provided each time a case was presented at treatment team meetings, three times each week, and at case reviews every seven days while the patient was hospitalized. It also occurred during the formal in-service training sessions held every two weeks. Educational consultation was exemplified through the in-service training sessions, presented by the consultant and other Department of Psychiatry faculty. An example of program and/or administrative consultation was the development of the space expansion proposal.

A consultant is a change agent. Occupational therapists facilitate change in patients: their behavior, attitudes, and environments. This basic knowledge of occupational therapy concepts and skills can be extrapolated to a larger arena. If we are sensitive to the need to change the structure of the organization when indicated, it is possible for the occupational therapy consultant to achieve this goal.

Understanding general systems theory and using this knowledge as a frame of reference provides direction for the consultant's approach to problem identification, decision making, and change agentry. For instance, the consultant's decision to do informal teaching during treatment team meetings and to ask a psychologist and a social worker to do the same, was based on the consultant's knowledge of general systems theory. As stated previously, changes at one level of the hierarchy of an open system may resonate throughout several levels. The consultant knew that changing the knowledge level, competence, and self-esteem of the hospital staff attending treatment team meetings would resonate throughout and change patient treatment and treatment programs. This was just one way that the quality of the total program was improved.

Becoming a consultant is a process. These experiences, and many more, contributed to the knowledge and skills necessary to function as a consultant in a system as complex as that described.

Each consultation has its own timing, or readiness, to make the needed changes. As consultants, we are sometimes frustrated by the rate and level of change, either too fast or too slow, not enough or too much. But, at its best, functioning as a consultant can be enjoyable and stimulating. Combined with the demands made on the consultant to know more, be more, and do more than in most other jobs, it can also be one of the more rewarding periods of one's career.

REFERENCES

1. Baker F: Paper for Symposium on Systems and Medical Care, Harvard University. Boston, MA, Sept 26–27, 1968, pp 1–43.
2. Baum C, Devereaux, E: A systems perspective—conceptualizing and implementing occupational therapy in a complex environment, in Hopkins H, Smith H (eds): *Willard and Spackman's Occupational Therapy,* ed 6. Philadelphia, Lippincott, 1983, pp. 799–814.
3. Boulding K: General systems theory—the skeleton of science. *Management Sci* 1956; 2:197–208.
4. Devereaux E: Community home health care. 2: In the rural setting, in Hopkins H, Smith H (eds): *Willard and Spackman's Occupational Therapy* ed 5. Philadelphia, Lippincott, 1978; p 664.

5. Grinker, R, Sr: In memory of Ludwig Von Bertalanffy's contribution to psychiatry. *Behav Sci* 1976; 21:207–218.
6. Marmor J: The relationship between systems theory and community psychiatry. *Hosp Community Psychiatry* 1975; 26:807–811.
7. Marshall University: *Marshall University School of Medicine Bulletin: 1980–82* (vol 2, no 1). Huntington, Author, 1979, p 7.

SECTION D

Occupational Therapy Consultation in Community Settings

As discussed in Chapter 7, the mandate for occupational therapists to provide consultative services in community settings was issued in the late 1960s by leaders in the profession (West, Weimer, Mazer, Reilly, and others), when the field of health care consultation was beginning to broaden beyond the traditional medical model. The Community Mental Health Act of 1963 provided the impetus for many of the community consultation activities among health professionals, including occupational therapists. Although several examples of community consultation were provided in the occupational therapy literature of the early 1970s, this area of consultation did not expand significantly. The impact of an economic slowdown in the United States and changes in political and social funding priorities did not provide the reimbursable opportunities for considerable occupational therapy consultation in the community, particularly that with a preventive focus. In the 1980s, public awareness and increased advocacy resulted in greater consumer involvement in community activities and a push for federal and state regulations for social programs. The social and health legislation affecting children and youth, older adults, school systems, mental health facilities, and barrier-free environments created a climate for a resurgence of community occupational therapy consultation. Chapters 20–25 provides models of community consultation in a variety of settings.

Llorens describes a teenage mother project. Although based in an urban hospital, it provided outreach and a comprehensive community health care program to a low-income, high-risk population. Using a collaborative, participatory approach to consultation, developmental and occupational performance frames of reference provided the basis for the consultative strategies to this community population. Consultation was provided to inpatient and outpatient children and their families and to community agencies, including preschools and public elementary schools.

Lang, Klasson, and DuFresne provide models of mental health consultation that focus on the mainstreaming of mentally ill persons into community life. An historical overview traces the influences on and the significant changes in mental health practice as a result of health legislation and social and political trends. The impact of these changes on occupational therapy consultation is also discussed. The authors address the necessity of assessing community needs, coordination of resources, provision of psychosocial and vocational programming, and expanding the use of paraprofessionals in community programs. In both case studies, there is an emphasis on building effective communication networks throughout the community.

Issues of accessibility for disabled persons in community settings are discussed by Samson. The impact of environmental, barrier-free legislation and guidelines for accessible design are described in the two case studies. Consultative activities focused on the legal implications of infractions of these regulations.

Jaffe describes the role of occupational therapy consultants in preventing dysfunction and maladaptation and promoting a healthy environment in an entire community. The case study demonstrates how a school consultation team acted as change agents in a troubled community, providing educational and program planning consultation to community members and elementary school teaching and administrative staff. The process of consultation and progression of levels are discussed, emphasizing a systems approach. Recognition of the external factors that influence behavior and awareness of the political and social climate and needs of the community were identifed as essential to facilitating change. Transition of consultative activities from an initial plan for a school activity program to development of a systemwide community program with a major health promotion and preventive focus is discussed.

Bachner illustrates the multiple issues faced by developmentally disabled clients as they move from institutional to community living settings. Interests in client advocacy, systems theory, and sociological theory influence the consultation approach described. In her case examples, Bachner demonstrates a natural evolutionary process. She was called in to address a case-centered problem and moved into an administrative consultation. This shift allowed her to address the key issue underlying the one that had triggered the case consultation request.

Program development for adult day care in a rural community is discussed by Epstein. Important social, political, and legal issues were encountered during the development of this program, which targeted frail elderly living in the community. Using aspects of social action, educational, organizational, and program development models, the consultant helped a community-based organization restructure its planning. The consultant brought important internal and external factors to light in order to help the voluntary board of directors make appropriate choices as they planned the establishment of the day-care center.

Community Settings

AUTHOR	MODEL	LEVEL	LOCUS	GOAL
Llorens	Collegial and Educational	Levels I and II: Educational and program planning	Hospital-based, community-focused project	Facilitate developmental tasks of adolescence and parenting skills of teenage mothers
Lang et al.	Collegial, Program Development, and Systems	Levels I, II, and III: Case centered, educational, and program	Community independent living residence and community mental health agency	Support development of adaptive, functional skills in community environments
Samson	Collegial	Levels I and II: Case-centered and educational	Community facilities	Assist lawyer with environmental assessment, act as expert witness, and support barrier-free planning
Jaffe	Process Management, Program Development, and Systems	Levels II and III: Educational and administrative	Public school and community	Develop preventive activity program in schools by in-service training, staff development; facilitate communitywide prevention programming
Bachner	Collegial, Program Development, and Systems	Levels I, II, and III: Case-centered, educational, and administrative	Community group home	Facilitate functional skill performance for developmentally disabled clients
Epstein	Collegial, Educational, Program Development, Organizational Development, and Social Action, and Systems	Levels I, II and III: Case-centered, Educational and administrative	Adult day-care center	Develop adult day-care center; community organization

CHAPTER 20

Program Consultation for Children and Adolescents

Lela A. Llorens, Ph.D., O.T.R., F.A.O.T.A.

OVERVIEW

The occupational therapy consultant's role in program development for children and adolescents spans the breadth of the profession. It may involve case finding, evaluation of performance, providing or recommending and monitoring intervention, discharge planning, and/or home programming.

As an occupational therapy consultant, the author has provided services to schools and child-care centers as well as to hospital-based pediatric programs. In the Mount Zion Project described in this chapter, consultation was provided to the health care teams, to individual team members, and to community agencies. The Teenage Mother (TAM) Program of the Comprehensive Child Health Services for Children and Youth Project has been selected for presentation in this chapter as a model of occupational therapy consultation in a community-oriented program that served both pregnant adolescents and their children. Although the TAM Program was initiated in 1967, it is believed that the model for provision of occupational therapy consultant services has relevance for community-based service provision today. Program development for infants and children, including the TAM Program, has been described as a model of participatory consultation.

ENVIRONMENTAL AND SYSTEMS INFLUENCES

The TAM Program provided a vehicle for community-oriented health care for children and adolescents that included a participatory consultation component delivered by occupational therapy. The 1965 Amendments to the Social Security Act, Public Law 89-97, made it possible for the Children's Bureau of the Maternal and Child Health Services, Department of Health, Education, and Welfare to fund comprehensive child health services that included medical care for children and youth, particularly for low income families. The pertinent provision of the law to these programs was Section 532 of Title V, Part 4 of the Social Security Act. The purpose of the grants was to develop programs that would increase the availability and improve the quality of health care services, not replace or reduce state and local community services.[1]

The program for which funds were awarded to Mount Zion Hospital and Medical Center in San Francisco, California, was designed to provide comprehensive health care to a low income catchment area using a community health care model. The grant for the Mount Zion Project was awarded in April 1967. The area served was called the Western Addition of San Francisco, the catchment area in which the hospital was located.[2]

FRAMES OF REFERENCE

Developmental and occupational performance frames of reference were useful in consultation to the project.[3, 4] The developmental frame of reference provided guidelines for selection of assessment tools, development of activity groups, and making activity recommendations to teachers, other staff, and parents. Occupational performance frame of reference provided a guide for determining activity and task assessment in self-care, play/leisure, and education/work occupations and the component skills in sensory, motor, psychological, social, and cognitive development.[3] The occupational performance skills to support the expected life roles of the children and adolescents were the targets for assessment and remediation/rehabilitation as the focus of the consultation.

The consultation frame of reference was one of "participatory consultation,"[4, 5] in which the consultant provides demonstration services in order to create a model that may be carried out by the consultee or other personnel when the consultation is terminated. Leopold[6] described the consultant relationship as one in which the parties are equal, the consultee is not outranked in any way, the consultee is free to accept or reject the consultation recommendation, and either party may terminate the relationship at any time.

Recognizing the boundaries of the consultant-consultee relationship is important to this special interaction. In the Mount Zion Project, the occupational therapy consultant was in the role of demonstrating service provision as well as recommending program development in a special relationship to the health care teams and all components of the project.

CONSULTATION DESCRIPTION

The Mount Zion Project

Organization

The Mount Zion Project was designed to deliver health care using health care teams. Three general health care teams and one teenage mother team were constituted. The general health teams each consisted of one pediatrician, one public health nurse, one social worker, and two community health workers, providing health care for children and youth from infancy to 18 years of age through a combination of home visits, outpatient clinic care, individual counseling, coordination of services with other agencies including schools, and inpatient hospital care as needed. The teenage mother team had one obstetrician in addition to the other health care personnel. The consultants to these teams included three nutritionists, two psychologists, two psychiatrists, and one occupational therapist.

Support

The occupational therapist was an employee, paid by grant funds to provide direct and indirect services. The model for delivering specific services emerged according to feasibility and need. Consultation to the health care teams was a feasible model to deliver some aspects of care. Consultation was provided to primary caregivers: pediatricians, public health nurses, social workers, community health workers, teachers, and parents.

Participants

The occupational therapy consultant provided services to the three regular health care teams, the teenage mother team, the pediatric ward, and other hospital and community professionals; public school administrators and teachers; and parents. Consultation to the primary health teams included participation in team conferences; meeting individually with team members, particularly public health nurses and community health workers regarding issues of stimulating appropriate child development in the home setting based on team discussions and/or specific assessment; and working actively with appropriate team members concerning patients with whom the occupational therapy consultant had primary contact, until such time as other team members caseloads permitted them to take over the case.[2]

Developmental screening was administered by the occupational therapist on a routine basis to all children who received health assessments. Screening served to establish a gross baseline of the child's level of developmental functioning and to identify those children who were in need of more extensive occupational therapy assessment from those who were essentially developing adequately. Relevant social and emotional observations were made that aided in referral for psychological or psychiatric services when indicated.

Through developmental screening of children in the project over one 6-month period, it was found that 48% of the 3 to 5 year olds seen by the project demonstrated developmental deviations suggestive of predictable later learning and behavior problems, if not corrected or modified.[7]

Recommendations for Head Start and nursery school programs for these youngsters were made on the basis of screening information. Recommendations were also made for counseling and home programs. These programs were planned and initiated by the occupational therapist and supervised in collaboration with the public health nurse or community health worker.

More extensive evaluation by the occupational therapist was available upon referral by the team, based on the results of screening and other factors such as diagnosed learning and behavior problems, evidence of mental retardation, known physical disability, or organic brain damage. Appropriate programming for school-age children was developed by the consultant and implemented by the parents following counseling. In addition, the consultant developed home programs and programs for the classroom.

An interdisciplinary group, organized by the project psychologists, worked closely with the Western Addition schools through coordination of school conferences. The conferences were designed to strengthen communication between schools and families, evaluate the overall adjustment of individual children relative to educational concerns, make recommendations, and implement plans to maximize services available to the children. Members of this group, including the occupational therapist, served as school coordinators to provide this service.[2]

The services of the occupational therapist consultant, although available to all schools in the catchment area, were concentrated most heavily in the elementary school that had the largest population of project children. In addition to coordinating school conferences, ongoing relationships were established as needed with teachers of both regular and special classes for consultation relating to issues of behavior expectation, behavior management, growth and development, and techniques to be used in the classroom to facilitate improvement in areas of dysfunction. Programs of specifically recommended supplementary stimulation activities for the classroom were developed with the teachers for individual children.

Within the hospital, the occupational therapy consultant provided direct and indirect services. On the pediatric ward, it was necessary to provide developmental evaluation for hospitalized project children in order to recommend programs of intervention. This information could then be shared in comprehensive care rounds and decisions could be made about needed therapeutic services. Intervention was supervised by the occupational therapy consultant, but care was delivered by child-care personnel.

Continuity of comprehensive health care was extended to project children who were largely served on an outpatient basis when they were hospitalized to minimize the negative effects of illness and hospitalization. A concentrated effort was made by all concerned to provide appropriate stimulation in the form of relationships, toys, and tasks to prevent pathological regression. Additionally, a major effort was made to promote healthy growth within the conditions of hospitalization, recognizing the emotional and psychological damage that can result from separation, isolation, and lack of stimulation. The occupational therapist's role involved evaluation and implementation to facilitate appropriate growth and development, particularly with infants in this setting, as well as with older children and adolescents. Follow-up consultation with the occupational therapist was available to families as needed in predischarge planning and upon the child's discharge from the hospital.[2]

Teenage Mother Program

A specific program within the Mount Zion Project was the Teenage Mother (TAM) Program. It was designed to help pregnant adolescents deliver healthy infants by providing them with optimal prenatal care, continuation of their education, psychological counseling, social work services, nursing counseling, nutritional education, and occupational therapy consultant services.

Organization

TAM was a unique aspect of the Mount Zion Children and Youth Project. During pregnancy, a maximum of 35 girls between 13 and 18 years of age were enrolled in the Mount Zion Service Center at any given time.

Support

The center was jointly sponsored by the San Francisco Unified School District and the Comprehensive Child Care Project to provide the girls with continued education during pregnancy and optimal prenatal, obstetrical, and postnatal care. The infants of the teenage mothers were registered into the project at birth. They were then considered members of the Comprehensive Child Care Project.

Participants

A special team that included an obstetrician, a pediatrician, a public health nurse, social worker, community health worker, and consultants in nutrition, psychology, psychiatry, and occupational therapy served the teenage mothers and their infants.

Services Provided

The occupational therapist provided indirect and direct services to the Teenage Mother Team. Direct service was given to the health education component of TAM in the form of an activity group in addition to evaluative and consultative services. The activity group focused on the developmental tasks of adolescence and impending motherhood. The primary objectives were to help the girls develop more mature relationships, more independence in their functioning in daily life activities, and skills for facilitating their infants' development. The infants of the teenage mothers also were seen by the occupational therapist consultation for developmental screening during well-baby visits at ages 1, 4, 7, and 12 months. Informal counseling and educational consultation regarding mother-child relationships and the importance of creative play and stimulation were provided by the consultant during the course of the activity group sessions.[2]

Consultation Process

The problem-solving process employed in this consultation followed a six-step process as follows:

1. Identification of possible services to be rendered in each proposed area
2. Development of program objectives and a plan of action

3. Implementation of the program plan
4. Review and evaluation at periodic intervals
5. Development of new objectives and plans, as indicated
6. Implementation of needed changes in program

These steps were repeated in a continuing pattern as new service needs were identified.[8]

Program Development

The TAM activity program provided opportunities for the pregnant adolescents to practice productive work habits and skills. They learned to follow directions, make decisions, and complete tasks; practice positive interpersonal skills; and engage in constructive activities to occupy their leisure time.

The focus of the program was to facilitate specific developmental tasks of adolescence while providing psychological support in preparation for impending motherhood, since 98% of the teenage mothers in the project kept and personally cared for their infants. The group was conducted by the occupational therapist and a community health worker.

The primary objectives for the group were to provide opportunities for the girls to (1) practice productive work habits; (2) develop and practice skills in home crafts; (3) practice mature interpersonal interaction; and (4) learn to occupy leisure time constructively as they awaited the birth of their infants. Careful attention was given to helping the teenagers learn to achieve fulfillment of needs for attention, affection, and feelings of belonging in constructive ways. Fifteen to 18 girls ranging in age from 13 to 15 and 16 to 18 constituted each of two groups that met twice weekly.[2]

The activity group personnel included the occupational therapist and a community health care worker. The participants were adolescent girls 13 to 18 years of age, most of whom expected to keep their infants.

The services were provided by participatory consultation. The occupational therapy consultant used activities and tasks to assess skills and to intervene to improve skills and behavior related to occupational role performance.

Outcome

One of the most significant aspects of the occupational therapy component of the Comprehensive Child Care Project was the utilization of the occupational therapy consultant by the overall program of the general pediatric health teams and the special teenage mother team. The primary objective, to facilitate optimal growth and development for the children and for the adolescents and their infants, was achieved. Integration of the focus on physical, social, and emotional areas of development was possible through the contributions of all other staff members.

The efforts of physicians, public health nurses, social workers, community health workers, dental personnel, nutritionists, and psychologists helped to achieve the goals and objectives set by the occupational therapist consultant. Utilization of services was accomplished through appropriate referrals and the inclusion of the occupational therapist consultant in the initial health assessment process. The occupational therapy consultant assisted in determining the functional level of children up to 10 years of age in sensory-perceptual, motor, social, emotional, and cognitive areas of development. Additionally, she helped implement home and ward activities programs to facilitate enrollment in Head Start and nursery schools; scheduled appointments of older children for developmental assessment; assisted with the activity group for teenage mothers; and cooperated in following through with team recommendations.

This kind of cooperation and collaboration was achieved over time. It was fostered by staff education, accomplished largely by demonstration of services that helped to overcome initial suspicions and fears that the occupational therapist would duplicate or replace the services provided by other members of the project. The occupational therapist on this project provided developmental screening and assessment of sensory-perceptual-motor development. She also prepared activity program guides for use in the hospital, home, and/or school to improve developmental functioning of individual children, and she consulted on functional levels of children hospitalized on the pediatric service.[6]

The inclusion of developmental screening as a routine service during health assessment was initially made possible as a result of a pilot demonstration. The demonstration was designed to show the feasibility of administering such a procedure in a limited amount of time, and with findings that would be beneficial as a baseline for continued care and determining whether potential developmental deficits or dysfunction existed. This information was valuable to the health care team as new or corroborating evidence of health status. On the basis of developmental assessment results, specific recommendation were made for Head Start, preschool, nursery school placement, and/or for home programs, as indicated. More comprehensive evaluation of sensory-perceptual-motor, psychosocial, and cognitive development of children with school and behavior problems yielded results that were also useful in program planning for children in school and at home. Through the school conference program, information was transmitted to teachers of the project children.[7, 8, 9]

On the teenage mother program, the results of routine initial evaluation and ongoing activity group observations were useful to the occupational therapy consultant and the community health worker. These observations formed the basis for planning program activities for the teenagers and were also useful to the nurse, social worker, and teachers in the total care planning for the girls.

On follow-up evaluation of the TAM Program, a large majority of the girls reported that they had learned new skills or improved existing skills in the crafts, improved their social skills, and carried over learning from the activity group into leisure activities during pregnancy. Findings from periodic behavior ratings suggested that positive observable gains were made and maintained and that this information was useful to other members of the staff.[2]

SUMMARY

The role of the occupational therapy consultant in program development for children and youth has been described with emphasis on the Teenage Mother Program within the Comprehensive Child Health Services for Children and Youth Project (the Mount Zion Project). Environmental influences brought community needs for services and federal financing together to serve children and youth.

Developmental, occupational performance, and participatory consultation frames of reference were used to guide the consultation process. Occupational therapy program development was based on the consultant's knowledge of growth and development and knowledge of activities, tasks, and relationships to improve occupational performance skills. These include self-care, education, work, and leisure and component skills and abilities in sensory-perceptual-motor, social, emotional, and cognitive functions in children from infants through adolescents. The model of consultation described in this chapter has relevance in today's service delivery climate as the need for effective programs for children and for teenage pregnant girls continues.

REFERENCES

1. U.S. Department of Health, Education, and Welfare, Children's Bureau: *Grants for Comprehensive Health Services for Children and Youth: Policies and Procedures.* Rockville, Md, Author, 1965.
2. Llorens LA: Occupational therapy in community child health. *Am J Occup Ther* 1971; 25:335–339.
3. Llorens LA: *Application of a Developmental Theory in Health and Rehabilitation.* Rockville, Md, AOTA, 1976.
4. Gillette N: Occupational therapy belongs in the community, in Llorens LA (ed): *Consultation in the Community: Occupational Therapy in Child Health.* Dubuque, Iowa, Kendall-Hunt, 1973, pp 127–130.
5. Mazer, JR: The occupational therapist as consultant. *Am J Occup Ther* 1969; 23:417–421.
6. Leopold RL: Consultant and consultee: An extraordinary human relationship. Some thoughts for the occupational therapist. *Am J Occup Ther* 1968; 23:72–81.
7. Llorens LA: The role of the occupational therapist in a children and youth project, in *Proceedings of National Conference of Children and Youth Projects.* New York, New York University, 1969a.
8. Llorens LA: Problem-solving the role of occupational therapy in a new environment. *Am J Occup Ther* 1972; 26:234–238.
9. Llorens LA: The occupational therapist in a community health program, in *Mandate for Change, Proceedings of the Southern and Northern California Occupational Therapy Association Annual Conference.* Morro Bay, Calif, Southern and Northern California Occupational Therapy Association, 1969b.

CHAPTER 21

Occupational Therapy Consultation in Community Mental Health Programs

Susan Lang, M.B.A., O.T.R., A.T.R.
Elayne Klasson, Ph.D., M.P.H., O.T.R.
Georgette DuFresne, M.P.A., O.T.R.

OVERVIEW

In recent years there has been an increase in the use of consultants in mental health practice. Significant social and political trends have provided occupational therapists with opportunities to develop nontraditional careers. Historically, the occupational therapist consultant in mental health practice functioned within the medical model. Program assessment and development within the institution required that the experienced therapist provide assistance to new programs. This expert therapist would function as a resource for the program by training staff and helping to develop policies and procedures. In larger institutions this individual might have moved from one program to another providing new therapists with vital support and guidance in program development.

Community-based consultation has been limited historically due to concentration on hospital-based mental health services. However, the Community Mental Health Act of 1963, which mandated that the National Institute of Mental Health develop community mental health centers, provided the occupational therapist with increased consultancy opportunities. The occupational therapist, especially in day treatment centers, was hired as a consultant to other staff when full-time therapists were unavailable.

Client-centered consultancy was used by occupational therapists to meet the needs of special populations. The occupational therapist would be engaged to consult with an individual who, because of emotional dysfunction, was unable to benefit from a needed service. For example, the learning disabled child would be evaluated by the occupational therapy consultant to identify needs, skills, and interests that might enable a student to make better use of the school setting.

Today we see an evolving service delivery system in mental health as a result of environmental, political, social and biomedical changes. The role of the consultant is widening as an overburdened mental health system attempts to provide quality service. In this chapter, environmental changes and trends that have influenced our mental health systems are discussed. Also described are some of the emerging consultant roles for occupational therapists that have resulted. Frames of reference, which should continue to guide practice in consultancy, as in more traditional practice, are also discussed. Two case studies are presented. One describes a formal, and the other an informal, consultation. Advantages and disadvantages are identified within each consultation.

ENVIRONMENT AND SYSTEMS INFLUENCES

Radical changes in mental health systems in the last half of the 20th century have altered the way in which occupational therapists working with the mentally ill view themselves as well as the ways in which they can practice their profession. The primary influence affecting these changes, and the factor affecting all aspects of mental health service, is the deinstitutionalization movement. Deinstitutionalization has meant the closure of large state hospitals and the movement of severely ill patients from behind hospital walls to the community and sometimes to the street, behind no walls at all. Deinstitutionalization reflects both the shift of responsibility for the mentally ill from state to local agencies, as well as the philosophical notion that mentally ill people will function better away from the confines and protection of the psychiatric hospital.[2, 9, 12]

Because hospital-based care for the mentally ill has become largely short term and crisis oriented, traditional occupational therapy treatment for mentally ill patients has often been limited to assessment and referral for further services. The occupational therapist has become deinstitutionalized, along with the patients once served.[4, 5] Since funds for treating the mentally ill did not necessarily move from hospital programs to community programs, the occupational therapist has had to find creative methods to fund services once provided to the mentally ill as part of a daily hospital room rate. The radical social change phenomenon of deinstitutionalization has affected the occupational therapist's delivery of services.

Many mental health services today are directed toward normalization, or mainstreaming mentally ill persons. The concept of normalization has been used for many years, but increasingly implies that mentally ill individuals are entitled to the same responsibilities and opportunities as the general population. Treatment models are being replaced by psychoeducational models in which clients learn skills in an educational setting and may themselves contract for services when needed.[10] Inherent in this concept of normalization is the idea that the individual has the right to choose when, how, and if services will be received.

An impressive body of research has found that services of any kind are best offered *in vivo,* in the actual environment in which they are to be used.[14] This speaks for occupational therapy that is offered to the client in the home and community rather than in clinic or day treatment programs which can only simulate the environment of the client. In vivo programs would use the occupational therapist as a consultant to the client in his or her home environment, rather than bringing the client to a formal treatment program.

Another influence on the mental health system is the necessity for coordination of services. As the mental health dollar shrinks, careful planning and interagency cooperation have become vital. This climate of coordination has led to the widespread use of the mental health case manager. The occupational therapist as a case manager acts as a broker of services and assists the client in obtaining and using mental health services as they are needed.[13]

As mental health services have moved away from institutionally based care, the classic medical model in which treatment was diagnostically related is evolving to a psychosocial rehabilitation emphasis with a focus on assessing function. This functional assessment forms the basis for a plan of intervention. Functional outcomes can be stated in behavioral terms and become the basis for evaluating a program's relative success. Clients need to demonstrate behavioral gains and functional outcomes that can be measured. The psychosocial rehabilitation emphasis is found throughout mental health care today. It is considered not only the domain of the occupational therapist, but is being adapted into the practices of nurses, social workers, psychologists, and even physicians. However, it is the language of occupational therapists that is now providing the buzz words for mental health. "Insight" is no longer a billable therapy goal, whereas "being able to ride a bus" is more acceptable.

Concurrently, the mental health system finds that decreasing dollars will not stretch to fund long-term programs with reliance on expensive, professional staffing. The treatment-resistant patient, such as the dually diagnosed, cycles in and out of costly inpatient units. Without adequate long-term supports, these individuals tend to decompensate quickly and require rehospitalization. Paraprofessionals are being used more frequently to staff longer term programs. The consultant is hired to provide guidance as needed in community-based programs. The occupational therapist, therefore, may be in demand to consult with the paraprofessional staff in these programs. The therapist may assist in establishing psychosocial rehabilitation programs, reassess benefits of existing services, and meet with staff to problem-solve.

Another influence in the current mental health system is the renewed interest in vocational programming for the severely mentally ill. Increasing evidence exists to support the work potential of mentally ill individuals when appropriate expectations and support systems are in place.[3] The mentally ill individual has a right and usually a preference to work. However, like physically disabled individuals, they may need special adaptations in the workplace. Psychosocial adaptations and supports need to be implemented by professionals who are familiar with job analysis and can consider the needs of the mentally ill worker. The once held attitude of "train and place" is evolving to one of "place and train." In this model, the worker, with assistance from staff, is placed in a job and the needed adaptations and on-job supports are made so that the individual can be successful in the job. This model often requires specialized consulting in the workplace. Although this model may not be useful for all psychiatric clients, occupational therapists, with their knowledge of task analysis, could be valuable consultants in this arena.

Within the increasing number of private sector programs, the occupational therapist is also being recruited to consult in the development of health promotion and employee assistance programs. Decreasing burnout and maintaining productivity are central to these programs and are goals familiar to the occupational therapist.

As America ages, the mental health needs of the geriatric client become apparent. Crowded and sometimes inadequate long-term facilities have resulted in increasing numbers of patients being placed in psychiatric facilities because caregivers are unable to control behavior. Placement of these patients after psychiatric hospitalization is particularly difficult and often not cost effective. The importance of prevention is growing as the hospital seeks to prevent revenue loss. An emerging role for the occupational therapist is consultancy prior to admission. As a consultant, the occupational therapist can provide education to the long-term facility regarding the unique psychiatric needs of the aging patient. In addition, environmental management can be assessed with recommendations for adaptations. The obvious goal is to maintain patients outside the more costly inpatient units.

A recent trend in the court systems of the United States is the use of data from clinicians other than psychiatrists to substantiate functional deficits and the need for ongoing treatment. The consultant can provide timely and efficient reports that will specifically identify capacity to care for self and/or ability to make an informed consent about treatment. Increasing court and hospital costs have elicited an openness to consider the occupational therapy evaluation as a credible method of securing information about an individual's functional capacity.

Additionally, the rise in importance and power of advocacy groups such as the National Alliance for the Mentally Ill (NAMI) directly affects mental health consultation. Organizations such as NAMI are composed of families and friends of the mentally ill and of mentally ill persons themselves. Their goals are mutual support, education, and advocacy for the victims of severe mental illness. Through local and state chapters, self-help organizations have become a powerful force in advocating for rights for the mentally ill as well as in sponsoring creative programs such as supportive independent housing. These advocacy groups have become an important vehicle for change in the mental health system and a source and resource for programs for the mentally ill. They afford yet another arena for creative involvement by occupational therapists.

The environmental influences described have evolved from the deinstitutionalization movement. They include a climate of normalization or mainstreaming of mentally ill persons; the necessity of coordinating scarce resources; an emphasis on psychosocial rehabilitation rather than on a medical model; the use of paraprofessionals with professionals having more limited participation in long-term programs; an emphasis on vocational programs for the mentally ill; increased numbers of private sector programs; expanded needs of the geriatric population; increased use of legal testimony to document functioning; and the rise of the consumer advocacy movement. These influences create new opportunities for occupational therapists in a consultancy role in mental health.

Regardless of the specific arena in which the consultant is involved, a clear frame of reference should guide practice. Although the consultant may not provide direct service, involvement will be more focused and guiding principles more clear if careful thought is given to a frame of reference that will bridge theory and practice.

FRAME OF REFERENCE

Occupational therapy theory guides the direction of consultation decisions and interventions. Regardless of the model of consultation (e.g., client centered, staff focused, organizationally based) some frame of reference should underlie the decision-making process. The value of a frame of reference is not limited to consultation that is strictly clinical or client centered in focus. The case study consultation examples discussed in this chapter have strong administrative components. Even at these levels, the therapist should understand the clinical goals and the organizational structure of the given setting.

The occupational therapist may find that the specific setting in which the consultation is taking place will determine an appropriate frame of reference. For example, if the occupational therapy consultant is establishing a program to promote daily living skills with a brain-injured population where mastery of various cognitive skills is emphasized, the model of cognitive disabilities might be most useful.[1] The following paragraphs describe the frame of reference utilized by the consultants providing case examples for this chapter.

Many occupational therapists in mental health believe that, through goal delineation, supportive planning and, when necessary, skill training, they can assist mentally ill clients to achieve their desired levels of functioning. This process reflects a bio-psycho-social approach that was given clarity and additional definition by Kielhofner in his *Model of Human Occupation*.[8] The two consultations discussed in this chapter, though different in focus, both support a basic tenet described in this model. This model suggests that human beings function as open systems and as such can, with assistance when needed, maintain and/or change their functioning through participation in, and exploration of, three behavioral subsystems: volition, habituation, and performance.

Kielhofner refers to a continuum of occupational behavior with the person being able to participate optimally at a functional end of the continuum through demonstrating competence and achievement. This is opposite to the stress and lack of involvement found at the dysfunctional end. The actualization of occupational behavior occurs through the three subsystems. The volitional subsystem is the energizing component and enables the individual to make conscious choices for occupational behavior in accordance with personal causation (or personal knowledge of self), individual values, and interests. The habituation subsystem serves to regulate and maintain everyday patterns of behavior without ongoing conscious choices. Balancing work, leisure, and self-care activities is part of this habituation. Roles and habits both serve to guide behavior. For example, a worker's role may guide behavior during the day and habits of daily self-care may direct behavior at home. It is the performance subsystem that enables the actual performance of occupational behavior as a collection of images, structures, and processes that are organized into skills. The images are internalized rules about how to act whereas the structure and processes refer to the biologic constituents of behavior.[8]

Together these components ideally serve to move a person toward the more functional end of the occupational behavior continuum. These subsystems can provide structured arenas for intervention in therapy. In consultation, they provide guidelines for the clinical interventions recommended, the structures established, or the educational component offered.

The following sections describe two different settings in which consultation in mental health has been utilized to establish programs, either through direct client involvement, clinical- or staff-oriented education, or program/administrative planning. Consultation at each of these levels promotes behavior, either directly or indirectly, at the functional end of the occupational behavior continuum. Adherence to the model of human occupation allows the consultant to be organized and more efficient in thinking about specific mental health programming.

CONSULTATION DESCRIPTION

CASE STUDY I: A FORMAL MENTAL HEALTH CONSULTATION

Background

A mental health consultation practice was developed based on the concept that occupational therapists should provide services to clients in the actual environment in which they live. As there were few existing positions to provide community-based occupational therapy, a private practice was established. The therapist was philosophically committed to providing occupational therapy to clients in the setting in which they could most use and retain their skills. Additionally, she determined that her skills, expertise, and temperament lent themselves to the structure of a private practice.

This therapist was well established in the network of mental health providers in the comunity and very familiar with the structure of services existing in her geographic area. She conducted informal surveys of the proposed market, gathered information about the business aspects of self-employment, and proceeded to market her services as a clinician and consultant.

Marketing involved making presentations to administrators of state and county programs for the mentally ill and agreeing to do in-service education presentations for the staff of these programs. When the county administrator responsible for in-service education for board and care home operators was planning classes, the occupational therapist was hired to present a program on structured daily activities. The therapist also made presentations on community adaption of the severely mentally ill at meetings of inpatient psychiatry staff at local public and private hospitals. The therapist described and showed through videotapes the role of occupational therapy in the treatment of adult mentally ill individuals living in the community. These presentations helped administrators and mental health workers understand the nature of occupational therapy services as well as the economic and therapeutic benefit of hiring an occupational therapist to consult with programs.

Organization

The occupational therapist leased an office with two other mental health professionals. She determined that the population she would serve, directly and indirectly, would be the severely mentally ill in the community, and she took the necessary steps to finance and equip an office. The therapist spent more than 2 months marketing her services and communicating formally and informally with sources of possible consultative relationships. After this period of marketing and public relations, a clear picture of how to organize her private practice evolved. She realized that she would provide a blend of clinical and consultative work and would incorporate all three levels of consultation.[7] She would perform case-centered consultation when called on to provide evaluations and recommendations for future placement of clients. She would also provide direct service occupational therapy on either a fee-for-service basis or by contractual arrangements. In providing direct service to clients, the occupational therapist functioned as a therapist, not as a consultant. However, because the results of the treatment were then utilized to do long-range planning for the project, she is referred to as a consultant throughout this section. She would perform second level, or educational, consultations when she was contracted to provide in-service education on topics relating to psychosocial rehabilitation. Last, she would provide system level consultation when she worked with the countywide mental health system of supported independent living for the mentally ill.

Support

This case study involved a contract made between the occupational therapist consultant and the local chapter of the Alliance for the Mentally Ill (NAMI). This advocacy organization sponsored a program to provide low-cost quality housing and meaningful support to individuals with a mental illness. The organization did this through a nonprofit corporation called Permahousing and provided a variety of housing options that were alternatives to poorly run board and care homes and short-term transitional placements.

Permahousing was interested in establishing a demonstration program in one of its housing units for the severely mentally ill. The demonstration program was to measure the need for, and the effect of, formal living skills training for mentally ill residents in a supported independent living program. The program, to take place in a home in which six young adult men lived, would use the consultation services of an occupational therapist. The occupational therapist consultant signed a contract to evaluate the current functional levels of the residents and to implement a program of training in daily living skills. After a designated time period, the consultant would make recommendations to other supported independent living units in the county mental health system.

The occupational therapist agreed to provide services as a consultant and to be paid through a special county program to fund demonstration projects. She also agreed to provide all materials, supplies, and personnal to evaluate and train the house residents. The consultant realized that providing occupational therapy to clients in vivo, in their actual living environment, was a model for practice that occupational therapy students might well benefit from observing. Therefore, students from a nearby university occupational therapy curriculum were invited to participate in the demonstration program as part of their practicum in psychiatry.

Participants

The consultancy arrangement consisted of four main participants. The first participant was the occupational therapy consultant. She had many years of clinical work experience, in addition to graduate training and relationships with the local mental health system. This experience seemed to assist in marketing this new concept of consultative occupational therapy for mentally ill persons in their own community. The next participant was the director of the community support subsystem of the county mental health department. Fortunately, this county was progressive in its approach to the severely mentally ill and was receptive to nontraditional approaches for dealing with problems of homelessness and shortages of mental health resources. The county administrator was open to innovative programming and had previously hired consultants to provide services. The third participant was the executive director of the Permahousing projects. She was the writer of the proposal for a demonstration project, and was thus a key participant in the consultative process. The Permahousing director had a commitment to the concept of supported independent living, but was troubled by the problems residents were having in independently maintaining their living environment. The last participants in the consultancy were the residents themselves. These six men had diagnoses reflecting severe psychiatric disorders but were highly motivated to live independently in the community. The demonstration project was explained to the residents and all agreed to participate for the designated period of the contract.

The contract negotiations involved meetings between the director of Permahousing, the county mental health officials, and the occupational therapy consultant. The county offered the consultant a standard agreement for services, in which an amount for the completed consultation was agreed upon. This contract reflected a planned entry on the part of the consultant, with eventual invited entry into the Permahousing program. The total fee for the consultation was based on the consultant's hourly rate and the expected amount of time to be spent on the project. To simplify procedures, all expenses were billed as hourly services to the county and Permahousing. The consultant agreed to complete the contract within 6 months and to provide monthly progress reports to both the county administrator and Permahousing director. She would also provide copies of all the evaluation data collected and would complete a summary report at the completion of the 6-month project. The university agreed to use the demonstration project as a practicum site for occupational therapy students, and the county administrator welcomed this opportunity to form an alliance with the university.

As this was a demonstration project, the explicit goal of all participants was to determine the value of providing this type of programming to mentally ill persons in the supported independent living units. The project would be studied to determine if functional behavior was affected in a measurable and observable manner, and if this approach was cost effective and applicable to other units in the county. As is true of most programs, there was an implicit as well as an explicit goal. In this case, the county was planning to apply for a grant to be a demonstration county and be the recipient of extensive funding to aid the mentally ill. This program would illustrate the progress being made by the county in providing rehabilitation services to mentally ill persons in the community.

Entry Into the System

Establishing trust between the participants in this consultation involved three factors. The first factor was establishing and marketing the consultant's professional expertise. Since the consultant was marketing a new concept, she needed to help the participants in the consultation agreement see both the value of the services as well as the professional expertise for which they would be contracting.

During the months preceding the contract, the consultant presented in-service education sessions throughout the county mental health system. Videotapes showing the consultant at work with mentally ill persons in the community became a valuable communication tool. Brochures and word of mouth from other mental health professionals were an adjunct. The consultant realized that all three levels of consultation (case centered, programmatic, and systemwide) would interplay in her practice. As program directors had problems with individual clients or as individual programs were making changes that would impact on the entire system, the consultant would be available to assist with all issues related to rehabilitation and self-care of mentally ill persons.

The second issue in establishing trust was learning the political power structure of the mental health system and understanding the relationships within the system. In this contract, the consultant needed to understand the workings of the county mental health system, which would be the eventual funding source.

After several confusing meetings, in which the consultant felt like a pawn in various power struggles, she determined that she needed to gain a better understanding of the system in which she was to work. The consultant needed to gather facts and find trusted allies. She scheduled several lunch meetings with county administrators to gain an understanding of the formal and informal structure of the mental health department. As a newcomer, she was unbiased and found she could ask somewhat naive questions about the system and be given straightforward responses.

These meetings helped the consultant understand how the severely limited resources in the county might affect the consultation process. For example, the employees of one program might feel rivalry about a special demonstration project taking place and the attention given to another program. Or, employees might resent money paid to an outside consultant when their own budgets were being curtailed. These factors helped the consultant understand the dynamics of the systemwide meetings concerning the implementation of the demonstration project services for which she had been contracted. The consultant needed to communicate openly with the employees of the system before, during, and after the completion of the contract.

The last issue in trust building can be described as speaking in one's own voice.[6] As a consultant, there is a tendency to promise people what they want to hear or to become so distant and professional that one loses sight of what one started out to provide. The consultant found that she needed to remind herself of both the limitations and scope of her own profession. She did not need to follow every trend in mental health, but to remember the philosophical underpinnings of occupational therapy as well as her own specific frame of reference and method of communicating in her own voice. It seemed that when she remained true to her own philosophical and personal ideology, she was most trusted by those with whom she consulted.

Services Provided

The consultation process began with the planning stage: evaluations were selected, materials for treatment were ordered, and a procedure for record keeping established. The consultant spent about one week orienting the residents of the Permahousing home to the upcoming demonstration project. She received permission and commitments from the residents agreeing to participate in the 6-month demonstration project. After the planning stage, consultation proceeded in the following sequence: evaluation, case management and training of the residents, and reevaluation and recommendations. The evaluation phase lasted approximately one month.

Each resident received a full evaluation of his functional abilities. This included the clients' performance of work, leisure, and self-care skills. A history was gathered for each resident. Additionally, an evaluation was made of how the living unit functioned, including residents' interaction, division of chores and expenses, and handling of crises.

There were no staff persons living in the residence, so the functioning of the house as a unit was considered as well as the functioning of each individual resident. The consultant, with the help of occupational therapy students, administered a battery of tests and interviews of each resident. This included standardized and nonstandardized occupational therapy evaluations and assessments of psychosocial functioning. The consultant also spent time in the house attending house meetings, speaking informally with the residents, and getting to know the neighborhood and community.

From these evaluations, an individualized plan was developed for each resident. The resident received a summary of his functional deficits as well as strengths. Together with the consultant, residents developed short- and long-term objectives. This resulted in a case management approach as well as a group curriculum for skills training within the house. The consultant used a case management approach as issues of problems arose in the daily lives of the residents, and also helped provide ways for the residents to master skills and to learn to solve problems.

Group classes were designed to facilitate cohesiveness in the residence as well as to give the residents opportunities to learn skills in a psychoeducational model. Classes, which occurred in the home and community twice weekly, addressed issues that were problematic for all the residents. Individual case management times were scheduled as needed, usually once a week. The consultant provided the training and used occupational therapy students as tutors. They helped the residents explore community resources and find experts in areas of functional training.

In addition to this case-centered method of consultation, the consultant was also invited into the Permahousing program to provide consultation to the paraprofessional staff of other homes within the program. She became a program consultant as questions arose about independent living, motivation, and in-house activities in other group homes. This was a separate consultation, but related to the Permahousing contract.

Evaluation

Because the project was a demonstration project for other supportive independent living units, documentation was vital. Records were kept on each resident's functional levels and progress within the program. Additionally, monthly reports were submitted to both the county mental health system as well as the Permahousing program. At the end of the 6-month project, an evaluation of the project was submitted to the county mental health department, the Department of Rehabilitation, and the Permahousing program. Also, reports were submitted on the functional abilities of each of the participants in the program. Evaluation of this program was a vital part of the consultation process.

As in any program involving psychosocial disabilities, change is often hard to measure. However, various systems of formal and informal evaluation were used in order to study the impact of a concentrated program of in-house training on the lives of severely mentally ill adults. Formal evaluations involved retesting the residents using some of the same measurements used at the beginning of the project. Other useful data included examining the frequency of hospitalizations, degree of stability and length of stay in the residence, number of crisis calls placed to on-call staff, and quantity of organized activity in the house. Additionally, program evaluations included documenting the residents' ability to procure and retain work, manage their own money and time, and maintain safety and hygiene in the home. Informal systems of evaluation included anecdotal reporting from staff associated with this program and from other programs which the residents attended, anecdotal reporting from the residents themselves, observations of the impact of the program on group cohesiveness and getting along in the house, and general quality of life issues regarding the day-to-day functioning of the house and its residents.

Outcome

The consultation was designed as time limited. Terminating the contract included helping the Permahousing residents say goodbye to the consultant and students. Residents were given the opportunity to evaluate the project, assess their own growth, and plan what they would do to replace the time they had spent with the consultant. Termination of the project also included debriefing the Permahousing executive director and county mental health officials. The final report on the consultation included recommendations for further occupational therapy consultancy.

The final step in the consultation process involves renegotiation. In this case, the consultant proposed similar programs to other supported independent living units. She also recommended that this project be reevaluated after further time had elapsed in order to determine if gains made during the period of consultation effected change over a longer time period. The consultant faced an ethical issue as she reflected on this particular consultation. Because the financial and personnel resources were probably insufficient to support such a long-term project as done in the demonstration project, should such a program be recommended for replication? This remained a dilemma to the consultant.

This six-month consultation resulted in changes for individuals, for a particular program, and for the system. Individual clients received an enriched activity program that helped them gain skills to live more independently in the community. The quality of life in this residence appeared to improve and residents functioned more adaptively in the residence. The program staff gained experience with a structured activity program and became more knowledgeable about psychosocial rehabilitation. Finally, a new model for occupational therapy consultation was introduced to the county mental health system. This county also had the opportunity to experience a demonstration program in which mentally ill residents lived independently, but received the support needed to facilitate successful community adaptation.

Summary

This consultation between an occupational therapist in a private consultation practice and a supported independent living residence for mentally ill adults lasted for six months. Strengths in the design of the consultation included the opportunity for residents to receive assistance in the skills necessary for living independently and for a program staffed by paraprofessionals to learn concepts of psychosocial rehabilitation. A further benefit of the consultation was the exposure of program and system administrators to occupational therapy services. As a result of the consultation, occupational therapy in the community received greater visibility and at least two new positions for occupational therapists were created in community support programs.

The consultation had several problems as well. First, the consultant did almost all of her work in the residence and apart from other professionals. She found a high degree of professional isolation and none of the usual support systems found in more traditional programs. Also, the residents needed to have more opportunities to move on to supported employment upon completion of this program. Most of the residents wanted to work and felt this was the next appropriate step. Another problem with the design was the difficulty in determining if the changes seen in residents' functioning were sustained over time. Finally, the program, as designed, would be difficult to maintain because of shortages in both economic and personnel resources in the mental health system. Despite these drawbacks, however, the occupational therapist found that her role as consultant to a supported independent living program was a rewarding one. The consultation taught all participants more about community programming for the mentally ill and illustrated an exciting new option for occupational therapists working with mentally ill persons.

CONSULTATION DESCRIPTION

CASE STUDY II: AN INFORMAL MENTAL HEALTH CONSULTATION

In contrast to the more orderly entry into formal consultation, many therapists enter the consultation arena in a less planned way through a previous job, structural reorganization, or new program development. This type of entry can be difficult and, if not handled in an organized way, can undermine the potential for effective consultation. The following consultation evolved from an informal one into one with more formal parameters, and is described in two phases.

Phase 1

Organization

The setting for this consultation was a large community mental health service (CMHS) in northern California. This CMHS provided inpatient, outpatient, day treatment, and residential services to mentally ill clients. The occupational therapist became involved in the development of a continuum of vocational services for mentally ill clients in the system. Entry into the consultation was complicated by the agency structure.

In this CMHS, some services were provided by civil service agencies and others by independent nonprofit organizations that contracted with CMHS. Although there had been vocational counselors connected with the system for many years, there had not been any vocational services based in the CMHS. Clients thought to be job ready were usually referred to the Department of Rehabilitation (DR). There were two problems with this method. First, DR was often unable to place clients who were not ready for full-time employment. Second, there were no clear guidelines about how to determine who might best benefit from vocational services. Therefore, many clients were not adequately served, and the relationship between CMHS and DR was less than optimal. Fortunately, collaboration between the two had been improving at that time.

Regular meetings were begun between CMHS and DR. DR awarded a number of grants to mental health agencies to work on improving the referral process and increasing the number of successful placements through the Department of Rehabilitation. Because the supported employment movement demonstrated initial success with the mentally ill population, DR became more actively involved in funding these efforts and in tailoring programs to meet the specific needs of mentally ill clients.

Support

In the past 5 years, there has been an increasing interest in vocational integration for the mentally ill as a broad variety of treating agencies have adopted a more functional emphasis. The term *vocational integration* seems more appropriate than vocational rehabilitation, which implies that the client is going to be rehabilitated, somewhat like a housing project. In fact, there have been problems with provider systems and employer education that have made it difficult for mentally ill clients to choose, get, and keep jobs. It is the integration of provider, consumer, and employer systems that will assist this population in gaining access to the job world.[11]

Current focus on psychosocial models has caused both funding organizations and programs to look at how to develop and fund programs that will assist clients to function in the community. In keeping with this trend toward a focus on functional aspects of rehabilitation, CMHS established two full-time positions to develop a continuum of vocational services for appropriate clients in the system. Both full-time positions were funded as part of a day treatment center that was under the fiscal umbrella of one of the contract agencies associated with CMHS. Eventual consultation by the occupational therapist was the result of the planned development of this systemwide vocational component.

Entry into the system was initiated by the occupational therapist, who had been working for another program when the two positions were established. Learning about such organizational changes is an important facet of networking. At the point the therapist heard about these positions, they had not yet been filled. This was critical, because it provided an opportunity to approach someone in the system and suggest ways in which the occupational therapist could be involved before the structure of the positions was solidified.

The therapist approached an assistant director in the system and expressed her interest in being involved in the process. She did not, however, have a specific proposal at that time regarding consultation. It was clear that there were no provisions for consultation in planning for this expansion of services. The assistant director expressed his interest in having the therapist involved in the program because of her experience in vocational program development, organization structuring, and nonprofit management. At the time, however, it was not clear how this involvement could be structured.

There are many barriers to entering a system with a vague agenda. There were problems with budgeting, personnel, and how to involve the therapist on a part-time basis. In this case, the occupational therapist suggested that one of the incoming staff might want to work 4 days per week and she could work the other day. The occupational therapist wrote a job description based on her experience and understanding of what was needed and submitted it to the director. She was fortunate in that one of the newly hired staff did agree to work 4 days. This structure meant that the therapist was a part-time staff member and not a consultant. Because the therapist was an employee and not an independent contractor, there was no written contract based on reimbursement. The term *consultant* is used to describe the role of the therapist during phase 1. Although she was hired in a staff position, her function was that of a consultant from the beginning.

Participants

There were five main participants in phase 1: the assistant director of CMHS, the director of the agency with whom the contract was placed, the two staff hired to develop the vocational continuum, and the consultant. The organizational structure was extremely complex and, perhaps because of this, lines of authority and communication were not clear. The assistant director, responsible for the addition of the vocational component to CMHS, was the person with the most authority, although the director of the contract agency had ultimate control of the budget and was technically the staff supervisor. The staff were in a difficult position because their relationship with the CMHS assistant director, the contract agency director, and the consultant were unclear.

Although the consultant had considerable experience in vocational integration and nonprofit development, she did not, as part-time staff, have authority to influence the direction of program development. Her ambiguous role in relation to program development made it difficult for her to know when to make program-related suggestions. Communication was not clear and supervisory channels not satisfactorily established. A formal contract for the consultant's services was not negotiated. This lack of role definition created territorial and control issues and a diminished sense of collaborative spirit at the agency. Toward the end of phase 1, the reimbursement pattern was changed so that the consultant was paid on an hourly basis as a formal consultant, no longer as staff in a job-shared position.

Services Provided

The primary services provided by the consultant during phase 1 were in the area of organizational development. The largest problem facing the organization initially was the provision of paid work experiences for clients when no vehicle for payment existed. Formation of a nonprofit organization was a reasonable solution to the structural problem of how to organize vocational services in accordance with all guidelines of the Department of Labor and other agencies.

The consultant drew up and submitted all nonprofit formation papers. She consulted with staff and directors about the formation and functions of a nonprofit organization and board of directors, and secured liability and workers' compensation policies for the organization. She assisted with securing the subminimum wage certificates needed to operate as a nonprofit. These functions followed the model of program/administrative and educational levels of consultation discussed by Jaffe.[7]

The staff and directors were not familiar with nonprofit organizations or board development. Although responsive to learning about these areas, staff was focusing on program development and found it difficult to devote time or energy to nonprofit issues. Although the consultant did develop a prototype brochure for the organization, other areas of fund-raising, public relations, and marketing were not pursued. The consultant might have presented a formal proposal regarding possible involvement in them. However, these functions are very much nonprofit oriented, and introducing nonprofit thinking into a public agency when program development is just getting underway is difficult. In this case, the timing of the consultant's efforts to discuss the importance of marketing and fund-raising was probably premature and should have been delayed until substantial program development efforts were underway.

One of the most important factors in developing a successful consultancy is the building of trust. This is obviously a slow process, but was made more cumbersome because the staff initially viewed the consultant as a part-time staff member. It is important that the consultant not be seen as someone who drops by now and then. This pattern can generate resentment and nullify any positive information given by the consultant.

It should be emphasized that trust building must be mutual. Not only do agency personnel need to trust and respect the consultant, but the consultant must have confidence in the ability of the staff to make informed decisions. The consultant had a good relationship with the director who originally hired her, and his administrative support enabled completion of the structural organizational development during phase 1.

In accordance with corporate procedure, a board of directors was formed, and the consultant was invited to become a member. Although she did so, it became clear that the consultant should not have been on the board while acting as consultant. Because the role of board member frequently does merge into one of consultancy, it is important to keep these two arenas quite separate. In this case, it was almost impossible to act as a responsible board member while knowing a great deal about the inner workings of the organization. The consultant resigned from the board prior to the beginning of phase 2.

To summarize, services provided during phase 1 were organizational due to major problems in structural development. The complexity stemmed from the fact that the consultant was recommending the establishment of a nonprofit organization affiliated with a government agency. There were very few models for this sort of structure. Unfortunately, until the structure was established, there was no legitimate vehicle through which clients could be paid for their work. Since one of the goals of the program was to establish paid work experiences for clients, only a few program elements could be put into place until the structure was determined. Once this occurred, contracts in day treatment centers and work crews could function legally.

Outcome

Phase 1 lasted two years, primarily due to bureaucratic delays. The results of the consultant's involvement in phase 1 were that the organizational structure was successfully established, a board of directors formed, and content for a brochure written. Some clinical programming had begun as a result of staff efforts, such as work contracts in the day treatment centers, as a way to meet some of the vocational needs of the more chronic clients. Mobile work crews had also begun, and a very successful messenger service was developed by the staff. These program components, though not entirely contingent on the consultancy, were able to run more smoothly once the organizational structure was established.

It was evident at this juncture, however, that further work by the consultant would not be helpful unless a clear agreement was negotiated. There were numerous problems throughout phase 1 with delineation of the role of the consultant, communication channels, and supervisory relationships. The role of the consultant in program development, marketing, and fund-raising was never delineated. Program development, of primary importance after the organizational structure had been established, was the focus of staff energies. The staff members seemed uncertain how, or if, they wanted to use the consultant at this time. The consultant became less actively involved at the end of phase 1.

Phase 2

Organization, Support, and Participants

Phase 2 began when several developments in the system caused both structural and personnel changes in the organization. Several day treatment centers were closed due to financial cutbacks. The assistant director was able to negotiate for one of the centers to become a work center affiliated with the vocational effort. One full-time position was retained, already filled by an occupational therapist interested in vocational programming.

Although some staff changes occurred, the two original full-time staff positions remained in phase 2. With the addition of one staff person to develop a work center affiliated with the nonprofit organization, it meant that three full-time positions were dedicated to vocational programs. One of the three staff positions was filled by an occupational therapist. However, the actual contracting procedure was done between the consultant and the assistant director with input regarding consultancy needs from each staff person.

The consultant met with the assistant director and it was decided that if there was any further work to be done by the consultant with the organization, it needed to be clearly delineated first. The consultant discussed her fee, which was different from what she had been paid after her position was switched from part-time staff to an hourly basis during phase 1. She stated that she would draw up a contract to reflect any agreements reached regarding her work, since one was not provided by the agency.

Services Provided

During a meeting with the assistant director and one of the staff, three areas of consultation were outlined: (1) development of an assessment for in-depth evaluation of functional status and vocational potential of clients; (2) development of a vocational information form to become part of an intake packet; and (3) assistance in the development of a research proposal.

During the discussion, it was made clear to whom the consultant would be responsible for each project. A written contract was drawn up reflecting the areas just listed and signed by the consultant and the staff affiliated with the nonprofit organization, whose budget supported the services of the consultant. The approximate time anticipated for each project and the reimbursement schedule were described.

The consultant felt that it was not only the clarity in role and communication channels that enabled phase 2 to be more successful. The organization was now 2 years old and staff more able to clarify their own roles and priorities. In addition, project-based roles for the consultant helped to clarify beginning and ending phases, communication channels, and total anticipated time involvement. Phase 2, ongoing at the time of this writing, has been proceeding more smoothly than phase 1. A formal evaluation component to assess the consultant's involvement has not yet been devised, but this will be important to develop and add to the contract.

Outcome

At this writing, the consultant has developed a Vocational Information Form which, after feedback and refinement, is being piloted by case managers in the system. This will be evaluated and refinements made in three months, after which time it is hoped that the form will be used throughout the system. The consultant also has helped develop a research proposal to assess minority utilization of vocational programming. It is hoped that vocational approaches with minority clients may be more useful than traditional psychotherapeutic approaches. Last, the consultant is working with one of the staff members to develop an in-depth vocational assessment, a long-term project. Each of the three project areas delineated in the contracts are therefore being addressed.

Summary of Phases 1 and 2

The two phases of this consultation provide examples of how important it is to have an organized approach to consultation. When possible, an unwritten, informal situation should be clarified in writing and essentially made more formal. It was when the consultant's role in organizational development was clear during phase 1 that progress was made. In phase 2, the roles were defined, communication lines clarified, and projects specifically outlined. Because of these changes, the consultation experience was more rewarding to the consultant, more useful to the organization, and less frustrating for all concerned.

There are several lessons to be learned from this example of consultation.

- It is critical to put things in writing, even where the consultation involves people with whom the consultant had been working previously. Roles may change, and the consulting role requires new relationships between colleagues. Frequently, these relationships are more difficult than those previously held because of the implied level of expertise of the consultant.
- There must be clear role definition from the outset. The consultant and staff must know when consultation begins and ends and what parameters guide input. A clear picture of what can be offered must be presented to the organization.
- The consultant must know how much information to provide, especially to staff developing new programs. They can handle only so much new material, and consultants must curb their desire to be helpful by telling staff everything they know. Anatole France says it well:

  > Do not try to satisfy your vanity by teaching a great many things. Awaken people's curiosity. It is enough to open minds. Do not overload them. Put there just a spark. If there is some good inflammable stuff, it will catch fire.

- The consultant should realize that she may not always be credited with having generated an idea or line of thinking. If she has, in fact, "put there just a spark," the consultation may be considered successful. The clinicians with whom she is working may not even realize that the consultant had generated an idea when they think of it later. This holds true for written materials that have been shared. The consultant should be in the background and be satisfied that the value of her presence was evidenced by a well-run organization.

SUMMARY

The role of the occupational therapist as a consultant in community mental health programs is growing as more creative, cost-effective, and community-based services are developed. This chapter described the growth and development of consultation in community mental health. Historical trends and environmental influences were presented to clarify these emerging roles. These included the mainstreaming of mentally ill persons and the necessity of coordinating scarce resources, an emphasis on psychosocial and vocational programming, increased use of paraprofessionals, expanding numbers of private sector and geriatric programs, increased use of legal testimony to document functioning, and the rise of the consumer advocacy movement. The model of human occupation, with its bio-psycho-social perspective, was discussed as the frame of reference most suitable to provide guidelines for the consultations discussed in the case examples.

The case studies described both the benefits and challenges of occupational therapy consultation in mental health. Both consultations required personal and professional confidence to assess the needs and resources of the community, gain support from power sources within the organization, and implement and sustain consultant services. Creativity and independence in the work environment were difficult when role blurring, isolation, and limited support and validation existed.

The case examples demonstrated that the occupational therapist consultant needs to develop skills in marketing and networking. Both the Permahousing and the vocational consultation project required that the consultant assess resources, trends, and needs prior to defining the service to be offered. Strategies for entry into the system were devised through formal and informal networking as well as alliances with various key groups in the community.

In both case studies, communication skills and the building of trust were essential in developing successful consultations. Effective communication influenced team members, community board representatives, organizational staff, and clients to respond favorably to the consultant. Mutual trust enabled the relationships to solidify and grow. Simple, clear, and concise communication contributed to the success of the Permahousing project. Lack of this communication led to role difficulties and undefined spheres of influence in the initial phase of the vocational consultancy.

The occupational therapist who is considering the role of consultant faces both personal and professional challenges, as did the therapists in the case examples. Entry into a system as a consultant can be eased by examination of personal and professional resources, skills, and frame of reference. A thorough assessment of environmental influences and constraints coupled with an understanding of organizational needs enables the occupational therapist to develop clear guidelines for the parameters of the consultancy.

REFERENCES

1. Allen CK: *Occupational Therapy for Psychiatric Disabilities: Measurement and Management of Cognitive Disabilities*. Boston, Little, Brown, 1985.
2. Bassuk EL, Gerson S: Deinstitutionalization and mental health services. *Sci Am* 1978; 238:46.
3. Ciardiello J, Bell M: *Vocational Rehabilitation of Persons With Prolonged Psychiatric Disorders*. Baltimore, Johns Hopkins Univ Press, 1988.
4. Dasler P: Deinstitutionalizing the occupational therapist. *Occup Ther Health Care* 1984; 1:31.
5. Fine S: *Occupational Therapy: The Role of Rehabilitation and Purposeful Activity in Mental Health Practice*. White Paper of the American Occupational Therapy Association. Rockville, Md, AOTA, 1983.
6. Gilligan C: *In a Different Voice*. Cambridge, Harvard University Press, 1982.
7. Jaffe E: The occupational therapist as a consultant: A model of community consultation. *Occup Ther Health Care* 1988; 5:87.
8. Kielhofner G (ed): *The Model of Human Occupation: Theory and Application*. Baltimore, Williams & Wilkins, 1985.
9. Klasson E: A model of the occupational therapist as case manager: Two case studies of chronic schizophrenic patients living in the community. *Occup Ther Ment Health* 1989; 9:63.
10. Klasson E, MacRae A: A university based occupational therapy clinic for chronic schizophrenics. *Occup Ther Ment Health* 1985; 5:1.
11. Lang S, Cara E: Vocational integration for the psychiatrically disabled. *Hosp Community Psychiatry* 1989; 40:890.
12. Morrisey J, Goldman H: Cycles of reform in care of the chronically mentally ill. *Hosp Community Psychiatry* 1984; 35:785.
13. Schwartz S, Goldman H, Churgin E: Case management for the chronically mentally ill: Models and dimensions. *Hosp Community Psychiatry* 1982; 37:392.
14. Stein L, Test M: Alternatives to mental hospital treatment. *Arch Gen Psychiatry* 1980; 37:392.

CHAPTER 22

Consultancy Issues Concerning Accessibility

Louise Samson, O.T.R., F.A.O.T.A.

OVERVIEW

Opportunities for consultation regarding issues of accessibility are varied. The author's experiences have included consultation to individuals, architects, builders, planners, school administrators, church expansion committee members, lawyers, city commissioners, and state and federal lawmakers. Consultation of this type may involve all levels of intervention covering the spectrum from specific to global needs. One may be called on to instruct a family member in the building of a ramp or may be asked to review plans and make recommendations for an entire system, such as a total health care complex.

Accessibility issues may appear rather mundane, cut and dry, or black and white on the surface; the author's experiences prove otherwise. Sometimes the issue of an individual's right to get into his or her own home comes into direct conflict with established rules that prohibit additions. Such rules are sometimes found in mobile home park contracts or condominium association agreements. The consultant may spend many hours in negotiation trying to facilitate precedent setting action to gain a special exception. There may be times when the consultant must challenge a large private corporation's policies that allow curb cuts to be built without assuring that federal standards of safety are met, even though the standards may not literally apply due to the private status of the corporation.

Through personal experience, the author is convinced that most people are sincere in their efforts to provide properly constructed and functional areas. Something happens between the standard to follow, the communication, the construction, and the completed environment. It is this major monitoring that experts in adaptation, work simplification, and function can provide—occupational therapists!

Picture this scenario: You are in a rest room that properly displays the wheelchair symbol, proudly announcing that this is an environment that complies with standards for accessibility, but find that the door cannot be closed on the stall with a wheelchair in it. The stall is across from a beautiful mirror, the door to the restroom opens, and anyone is able to see the whole area. (Thankfully friends, or strangers make helpful door watchers.) Then, the wheelchair is moved under the so-called accessible sink—the soap dispenser is low (meeting standards), but it is located at the back of the sink and only those endowed with unusually long arms can reach it. Also there are those instances where grab bars are provided at the proper height, but the commode is low. Did you ever try pulling on a bar that's as high as your head (from a seated position); or had a commode that is high and the grab bar broke off last year; or had the mirror low, but someone decided that the easiest place to attach the soap dispenser is on the mirror (you can see one half of your face at a time)? What happened? Everyone tried—but we have a long way to go. Proper education, along with positive attitudes and expertise, eventually will result in appropriate change.

Every group, at every level, needs to put forth greater effort. The disabled are included in this statement. Clients and their significant others need to be informed, not only of their rights, but of their responsibility. The goal of our democratic society is to provide all citizens with opportunity for the pursuit of happiness, but not necessarily to assure everyone that they can have a fully accessible world. The reality of necessary constraints to some types of environments needs to be addressed as a fact of life for many people, including the disabled.

The recent focus on the aging process and the realization that everyone does grow older is finally beginning to have a direct effect on accessibility issues. A newer trend in housing is the cradle-to-grave home that is actually designed with wide bathroom doors, switches that may be reached from a seated position, and other built-ins that are conveniences for all, but future necessities for some. Cost comparisons by builders have shown that costs vary little when accessibility is considered at the time of construction and are sometimes less. Such community developments are to be congratulated! They provide models for others.

Consultation in the area of accessibility presents an exciting challenge for occupational therapists. Whether one works to solve individual problems, guide planners, or inspect construction with contractors, the opportunity to make positive change exists.

ENVIRONMENT AND SYSTEMS INFLUENCES

Environmentally, issues of accessibility affect society as a whole. Advocacy efforts to advance the rights of functionally limited individuals are being recognized increasingly by members of the media, legislators, and community members. Comparatively recent federal legislation now mandates accessibility of physical structures built with tax dollars for public use.[5] Current legislation (1989) includes the mandated accessibility of a percentage of apartments in housing complexes throughout the country.[2] A climate of heavy controversy prevails with pro and con lobbying rampant. Economic, political, and social considerations are often debated, with outcomes yet to be determined.

The Rehabilitation Act of 1973[4] established the Architectural and Transportation Barriers Compliance Board (ATBCB) as an independent federal agency to ensure compliance with standards issued under the Architectural Barriers Act of 1968 as amended. This serves as the legal authority on which the congressional commitment to the nation's disabled is based. It ensures the disabled the "opportunity to move freely and integrate themselves in society."[4] The original law pertains to federal and federally assisted buildings. Amendments pertaining to the private sector continue to be made, bringing us closer to the accessible environments needed to provide for everyday functioning of physically challenged individuals.

Minimum Guidelines and Requirements for Accessible Design; Final Rule was issued in 1981[3] and provides the enforceable regulation for the nation. The ATBCB worked in close collaboration with the American National Standards Institute (ANSI) and adopted many of its provisions. ANSI standards are not national law; however, they have been adopted by many states and thus have become law in certain circumstances. It is important to note that some states have adopted laws with requirements above the minimum set forth by the ATBCB. Architectural barriers consultants need to be aware of the pertinent laws within the state in which they are working. Also, one must know that the ATBCB Final Rule takes precedence over any accessibility standard that does not meet the national minimum or that is not addressed by the state, but is addressed in the national law.

In 1989,[1] the U.S. Senate approved the Americans with Disabilities Act. This is considered a landmark accomplishment and is termed the Bill of Rights for the Disabled, providing disabled persons the same "protections in jobs, services, and accommodations that currently apply to racial minorities, women, and the elderly."[1] All offices and businesses used by the public are required to provide and/or improve access. The House of Representatives adopted the Americans with Disabilities Act (ADA, P. L. 101–336) and signed it into law on July 26, 1990. Those lobbying against this bill included some Chambers of Commerce, small business interests, and agencies concerned with housing. Cost was the primary concern of those seeking to limit the legislation. However, the advocacy efforts were strong and well organized, leading to successful passage of the act.

There is now a wealth of material available for developers to use as resources for creating living environments. Business interests have discovered the importance of developing particular environments to assist sales, for example, the use of certain colors to reduce work stress or conversational areas equipped with telephones located in bank lobbies so that waiting customers feel less inconvenienced. Large investments of time and money are put into research to create such environments. The issue of accessibility has not been completely left out in planning, but is in its comparative infancy. Planners, developers, and others involved in creating living environments have started to respond to the expressed need and mandates. However, large gaps continue to occur between the planning and accessibility of an environment for the disabled. The concepts of the letter of the law and the intent of the law are often debated and, unfortunately, the absolute minimum is usually addressed.

FRAME OF REFERENCE

Occupational therapists theoretically are uniquely equipped to provide knowledgeable consultation regarding accessibility. The basic philosophy of improving independent functioning with goal-directed activity as the major intervention tool provides the frame of reference for consultation in this area. Also, the generalist approach to occupational therapy education provides the basis for development of expertise regarding issues of advocacy and consultation for the disabled that will positively effect social change. Occupational therapists work to improve the quality of life for those they serve, and consultation can enrich one's professional experience as well as broaden therapeutic skills.

A primary goal in occupational therapy treatment planning should be to assure the availability of environmental supports needed for functional performance. Increased expertise, interest, advocacy, and consultation in service arenas dealing with accessibility issues are therefore needed. In general, occupational therapists are still unable to assure their clients such an environment. Some suffer the stresses and inconvenience of being discharged somewhere other than to their home, because it is not wheelchair accessible. Others may be segregated in an all-wheelchair section of a residential community. This may occur because developers do not want to provide access to the entire complex or because other residents complain about having wheelchairs in their dining room.

Several models of consultation, as discussed in Chapter 2, are utilized in accessibility consultation. When consulting with colleagues or those in other professions such as lawyers and architects, one is using a professional model. A systems model supports the consultant's work with community agencies, school systems, and organizations. Providing assistance to advocacy groups to support the development of accessible community housing would be an example of the social action model.

The case examples that follow demonstrate these models and some of the levels of consultation also discussed in Chapter 2. A combination of case-centered consultation (level 1) and educational consultation (level II) best describes the levels of consultation used by this consultant.

CONSULTATION DESCRIPTION

Organization

The experience chosen for presentation in this chapter is that of the expert witness in accessibility cases. The consultee was a lawyer who had two suits pending for different individuals. One involved a ramp access into a restaurant, the other, a curb cut from a parking lot into a medical complex. The author served as consultant and expert witness in both cases.

As a consultant, referrals come from surprising sources. This consultation experience began with a telephone call from a lawyer's office, stating that he had been referred by a physician with whom the author had worked several years before.

The lawyer had two cases he was defending. In both cases people were seeking damages due to personal injuries resulting from falls. An expert witness was needed to provide an opinion on whether construction of the areas in question met pertinent architectural standards.

Support

After agreeing verbally to provide an opinion, the consultant received a follow-up letter (see Figure 22–1) briefly stating that an hourly fee would be paid upon receipt of a voucher following any services performed. This simple letter, on letterhead stationery, constituted the legal agreement.

FIGURE 22–1

Example of a Consultation Agreement

FORMAT = FORMAL LETTER:

1. Consultant's name and address
2. RE: John Doe
   File No: 0000000
3. Letter:

Within thirty days of receipt of your statement for services rendered, $$$ per hour will be paid. As we discussed (date), your time is to be calculated portal to portal.
Your help is sincerely appreciated.
Thank you.

Sincerely,

John Q. Lawyer

The simple formula was, "I need your service"; "Yes, I'll do it for ?"; a mutual OK, with both parties signing the document; and there was a commitment to consult. Because a signature on anything is considered binding in a court of law, it was necessary to make sure that the signed agreement stated the services the consultant would provide.

Participants

In this consultation model, the consultant assisted the lawyer in building this one area of the case relating to accessibility and safety issues. The lawyer maintained the key power role and was the final decision maker. A legal assistant accompanied the consultant to the actual sites to explain the circumstances surrounding the falls, ask and answer questions, and do needed photography and measuring of the areas in question. (This consultant uses a wheelchair and reaching the areas to be measured in themselves constituted an accessibility barrier!) Those principally involved were two plaintiffs, two defendants, three lawyers, one legal assistant, and the consultant.

Services Provided

Upon finalizing the agreement, the consultant met with the lawyer at his office to discuss each case and share resource information. (Usually, meeting consultees on their home turf is a strategically good move.) He shared his specific plans and asked an opinion of his chosen directions. That initial session ended with the mutual feeling that we would not only assist the two plaintiffs, but would possibly have a positive impact on construction in the area, since approval of substandard items appeared to be a problem.

Case I

The first case involved an individual who fell and sustained personal injuries while assisting a wheelchair-bound relative down a steep ramp. This ramp was used for entry and exit at a restaurant for those unable to maneuver through the front entrance, which had eight 6-inch steps. The ramp was located at the back of the restaurant, was open to the elements, and entered into the back of one of the dining rooms. Usually, an employee would manipulate the individual's wheelchair on the ramp (no one could get up the ramp without assistance; only an individual in an electric wheelchair could possibly go up the first 4 or 5 feet unassisted). However, at the time of the incident, there was no help available.

The individual who fell chose to bring suit against the restaurant to recover medical expenses resulting from the injuries, lost wages, and compensation for pain and suffering. In preparation for the suit, the lawyer felt that a determination was needed by someone knowledgeable about construction of ramps for wheelchairs who could assess the particular ramp in question.

Upon visiting the site, and after further discussion with the lawyer, a statement was provided by the consultant. The critical elements of the statement included citation of the authority used for reference, facts based on assessment and measurement of the site, comparison of the facts and accepted standards, and conclusions reached by the consultant. A diagram of the site was also provided to clarify the statement. Figure 22–2 provides a sample outline used for the consultant's statement.

FIGURE 22–2

Outline for Consultant Statement

STATEMENT OF (CONSULTANT'S NAME)

RE: JOHN DOE
    DATE OF ACCIDENT:
    PLACE OF ACCIDENT:

AUTHORITY REFERENCED:

STATEMENT OF RELATIVE STANDARD:

STATEMENT OF OBSERVED FACTS:

COMPARISON OF STANDARD AND OBSERVED FACTS:

STATEMENT OF CONCLUSION:

ATTACHMENT OF DIAGRAMS IF NEEDED FOR CLARIFICATION:

SIGNATURE

Case II

The second case involved an individual coming out of a doctor's office who tripped over the flared side of a curb ramp leading to the parking lot and sustained a personal injury. This case was brought against the builder/owner of a large medical for-profit corporation.

Several site visits, pictures, and numerous measurements were necessary prior to the statement preparation. However, the length of the written statement did not equal the complexity of the case. The statement followed the same brief format just outlined; however, it also included recommendations for structural change, again clarified through the use of diagrams. Three elements are vital in the preparation of a formal statement: a statement of proper "authority," brevity, and clarity.

One major issue not addressed in the statement was the probability that (at the time of construction) the standards did not have authority over a privately owned parking lot, regardless of the nature of its use. When this concern was brought to the lawyer's attention, he chose to pursue the case on the basis that the intent of the law was that accessibility and safety should be assured, particularly in a medical complex. Additionally, he considered the fact that since funds were received via Medicare for medical service payment, it constituted federal funding.

Outcome

In the world of consultation as an expert witness, you really do "win some and lose some," to use the vernacular. You also gain much wisdom from restrospective analysis. It was not as comfortable for the consultant to be cross-examined in a deposition setting as it was to write consultant recommendations. (The opposing lawyer also had to defend his client and, therefore, was determined to reach this goal.)

The case involving the steep uncovered ramp was settled out of court on behalf of the plaintiff, and the restaurant agreed to take appropriate action to provide safe access.

The case involving the curb cut and the entire parking lot is still pending at this writing (1½ years later). Issues of where the plaintiff actually placed her foot on the sidewalk when she tripped; county versus state and federal public building regulations in effect at the time of the accident; an issue of a parking lot used by the public but built by a private concern without government dollars; and an ethical question of providing curb cuts that do not meet federal standards of safety—all continue at the debate level.

The overall complexities of this case lead the author to speculate that the issues of accessibility will fade and that little, if anything, will be gained. One would think that the issue of safety for consumers would be a vital priority—however, to date, this has not happened. Advocacy efforts on the part of the consumers in this particular case were totally lacking. No group spoke out to support the reconstruction of the parking lot, and those leasing the property were not making their voices heard. Until individuals and groups decide that change is essential and are willing to become involved, such circumstances will remain.

SUMMARY

Personal experience has been shared regarding consultation on accessibility issues. The consultant's occupational therapy educational preparation established a unique base for the use of those skills, interests, and resources needed to effect positive change toward more accessible environments. The generalist approach in the education of occupational therapists provided the background for concern of issues of accessibility. Additionally, the occupational therapist's basic interest in the restoration of the highest quality of life possible for the client includes facilitating the development of independent functioning.

In order to be an effective consultant in this area, pursuit of opportunities to act as an advocate (or build on personal situations if one is physically disabled), and engage in a dialogue with clients about their life experiences will broaden one's knowledge base. A description of the regulations and legal authority under which communities currently function regarding issues of accessibility, as well as current trends of advocacy in this area, have been presented. The two case examples involving the use of accepted minimum standards in the courts described various models of consultation.

Accessibility issues affect everyone, disabled and nondisabled alike. Even though attempts are made to meet standards, environments continue to present unnecessary barriers to independent functioning. Knowledgeable intervention and monitoring are needed. Many groups and individuals are advocates and have prepared numerous types of material available in all formats—print, audiotapes, slides, films, and videos. Occupational therapists can use these materials as resources in their own advocacy efforts. Helping accessibility become part of all environmental planning is the challenge for the occupational therapy consultant.

REFERENCES

1. Americans With Disabilities Act, Senate Bill 933, September 7, 1989.
2. Fair Housing Amendments Act of 1988.
3. The Federal Register, January 16, 1981.
4. The Rehabilitation Act of 1973. Section 502. PL 93-112. 29 U.S.C. 792.
5. The Rehabilitation Act of 1973, Section 504 and subsequent amendments.

ADDITIONAL READING

American Institute of Architects, 1735 New York Avenue, NW, Washington, DC 20006.
American National Standards Institute, Inc, 1430 Broadway, New York, NY 10018.
American Occupational Therapy Association, Architectural Barriers Resource Packet, 1383 Piccard Drive, PO Box 1725, Rockville, MD 20850-0822.
Architectural and Transportation Barriers Compliance Board, Washington, DC 20201.
Governor's Committee on Employment of the Handicapped of each state.
Mayor's Committees are often functioning in cities of all sizes.

The National Easter Seal Society for Crippled Children and Adults, 2023 W. Ogden Avenue, Chicago, IL 60612.

National Park Service, U.S. Department of the Interior, Washington, DC 20240.

Rehabilitation Services Administration, Office of Human Development Services, Department of Health, Education, and Welfare, Washington, DC 20201.

Superintendent of Documents, U.S. Government Printing Office, Washington, DC 20402.

U.S. Postal Service Headquarters, 475 L'Enfant Plaza West, SW, Room 7110, Washington, DC 20260

CHAPTER 23

A Systems Approach to Community Health Promotion Consultation: The Occupational Therapist as a Change Agent*

Evelyn G. Jaffe, M.P.H., O.T.R., F.A.O.T.A.

OVERVIEW

The practice of occupational therapy in community health services is changing from a primarily medical model of treatment and crisis intervention to a more comprehensive approach to health care. Economic, political, and social trends have caused considerable shifts in the health care delivery system, mandating health personnel to reevaluate their service delivery patterns and broaden their focus. These environmental changes are providing increasing opportunities for the occupational therapy consultant to assume a role in community programming and health planning, health education, and health and legislative advocacy.[5] Functioning as a change agent, the occupational therapy consultant in this expanded role is concerned with the community as an overall system and interested in the pro-

---

* This chapter was adapted from Jaffe EG: The occupational therapist as a change agent: A model of health promotion and disease prevention, in Robertson SC (ed): *SCOPE: Strategies, Concepts, and Opportunities for Program Development and Evaluation.* Rockville, Md, American Occupational Therapy Association, 1986, with permission of AOTA.

motion of the general health of the community. As early as 1958, the World Health Organization emphasized that a healthy population is the most relevant and important basic resource of any society.[15] Limited human and financial resources have restricted society's ability to meet the demand for improved health care for all citizens.[4] Occupational therapy consultants can help diminish the professional human resources shortage by involving others in health promotion and disease prevention programs that benefit a large segment of a community.

In the following description of a community system consultation, the role of the occupational therapy consultant is depicted as community health planner, advocate, and change agent in a comprehensive health promotion program. A systems approach to problem identification, analysis, and intervention was utilized. The author and another occupational therapy consultant had been involved in extensive training in community consultation through a county community mental health center. As part of a community mental health team, the occupational therapy consultants were assigned the study of a local school problem. The team was multidisciplinary, consisting of social workers, educational and clinical psychologists, educators, and psychiatrists. The other team members focused their consultations on a variety of community issues, related primarily to the school system. These consultations ranged from individual case consultations regarding children with specific school problems to program consultation with teachers and parents, and administrative consultations with principals and other school officials. The entire team met weekly to discuss the progress of their consultations and issues of concern, including current and potential problems. Ongoing lectures and seminars in consultation theory and process provided the team with the background essential to expand their community consultation skills and knowledge and develop their consultative strategies.

ENVIRONMENT AND SYSTEMS INFLUENCES

The public school system frequently is the social weathervane of a community, predicting its political and social climate and the responses to changes in the environment. Residents of a school district in a small midwestern town were upset by recent city school busing regulations that were enacted to achieve racial integration. The environment of many of the elementary schools in this district had changed as a result of a recent influx of low-income blue-collar workers, hired to work in the new industries developing in the area. Problems arose among students, teachers, parents, the local school board, and the county school administration. Biases and prejudices permeated all facets of this situation. The issues hotly debated in this neighborhood and its schools were indicative of a potential communitywide storm.

The town was a predominantly white middle-class community surrounded by a large university student and faculty population. There had been little industry in the immediate area previously. Although a large automobile manufacturing company employed many blue-collar and unskilled laborers in a neighboring town, there was a division in population between the two towns and interactions were few. The commerce of the town under study, at the time, was dependent on the university population for economic support and employment. However, the interactions between the town and gown communities were not always mutually supportive. Many community agencies viewed the university with distrust or hostility, feeling the university functioned in a vacuum and did not attempt to reach out to the community to share the richness of the resources of a large teaching and research institution.

Many of the local neighborhoods did not feel they benefited from having this prestigious university in their community. They often resented intrusions from university research teams, whom they felt viewed the community only as a population pool for research purposes. Only those neighborhoods of university-associated families, particularly those that had children of lower school age, appeared to recognize the interests of this population in the elementary schools' programs and the neighborhood property associations. Local governmental and educational administrators did not interact with the university as often as either felt could be mutually beneficial. Attempts at outreach to the community and furthering the involvement and interactions between the town and gown populations were being undertaken by certain segments of the university system. The occupational therapy consultants involved in the community system consultation, as employees of the university medical center, were members of the subsystem in the university that was trying to cement relations and enhance interactions with community agencies. They became involved with the community at the mutual invitation of the director of the community mental health center and assistant director of the department of child psychiatry at the university medical center.

Community intervention as a preventive measure by a county agency was a relatively new concept in this county, but one that interested the director of the county community mental health center. Staff at this center studied the trends in the community, the changing nature of some of the neighborhoods, and the basic factors that were precipitating community unrest. They studied these influences, analyzed the issues and concerns of the community, and diagnosed the symptoms as central to the schools. A multidisciplinary school consultation team was formed to deal with problems being manifested in the school system.

FRAME OF REFERENCE

This community health promotion consultation, focusing on the occupational therapist as a change agent, utilized two frames of reference as the basis for the structure of the consultation model. The conceptual frames of reference were based on general system theory and the theory of human adaptation. They provided the framework for the consultation activities and guided the professional decisions and actions of the consultants.

The first frame of reference, drawn from general systems theory, emphasized an open system approach (see Chapter 2). Before the appropriate consultation model could be chosen, it was necessary to review the environmental forces that were influencing community reactions as a result of the rapid changes in the social structure of its systems. It was particularly important to study the entire system, not just the individual problems at the one school to which the consultants were referred. This comprehensive approach to developing a model of consultation facilitated entry into the system and acceptance by the consultees.

The open system theory emphasizes the close relationship between the social system, its supporting environment, and its openness to the influences of the environment.[7] The dynamic events that were occurring in this community and the ensuing reactions of its members demonstrated that the theory of negative feedback, described in Chapter 3, was indeed in play.[9] Longtime community residents strongly rejected the busing of school children and the influx of a new population that were creating a different type of neighborhood. The signals provided to this system by the environmental shifts predicted changes that appeared intolerable. Using this negative feedback, the consultants could develop strategies to help the system correct what it viewed as problems that were creating malfunctioning in parts of the system.

The second frame of reference, based on the theory of human adaptation, was a natural progression of the open system approach. The compatibility of both these concepts helped structure the model of consultation and the intervention process. As Rogers emphasizes, the frame of reference may be ideas drawn from several theories, but they must be internally consistent and not contradictory.[12]

Once the system was analyzed and the problems identified, it was obvious to the consultants that all members in this particular community were reacting to the changes. The parents were very upset by the possibility of busing their children to other neighborhoods and the demographic shifts in their community, the children reacted to their parents' concerns by fighting with the new kids, and the school staff were overwhelmed and very stressed by their inability to control the behavior of the children and get them to attend to schoolwork.

The theory of human adaptation, including the body's adaptive reaction and orientation response to changes in the environment, formed the basis for the second frame of reference and provided the structure for the occupational therapy consultative interventions. This theory is derived from several fields of study including psychology, neurology, endocrinology, and developmental and communications theory. Many scientists have described the relationship of changes in the environment to physical and emotional health. As discussed in Chapter 3, alterations in the environment can cause changes in one's ability to adapt to this new stimuli. The *orientation response* is triggered and may involve complex bodily responses.[14] This orientation response is our key adaptive mechanism and occurs when new information has not yet been processed by the body. It provides the quick spurt of energy that activates physical and psychological reactions, called the *adaptive reaction*. These two processes form the basis for humans' adaptability and functioning in a changed environment.

The adaptive reaction, often referred to as *stress,* can be triggered by shifts and changes in the physical or psychological climate and by anticipation of change.

Overstimulation, including competition, crowded conditions, and physical or emotional violence, can interfere with rational behavioral responses and produce maladaptive behavior and dysfunction.[2] This overstimulation occurs on three levels: sensory, cognitive, and decisional.[14] Disorganized, patternless, or chaotic stimuli, such as were present on the school playground at lunchtime, can cause sensory overload. Cognitive distortions or interference with the ability to think was evident in the degree of conflicting communications between home, school, and the community. Decision stress occurred when these new circumstances in the environment upset the balance of programmed (routine) and nonprogrammed (creative) decisions. These aspects of the human adaptation theory exactly paralleled the circumstances in the school district in which the occupational therapy consultation took place. The situation at home and school combined the effects of decisional stress with sensory and cognitive overload, producing the maladaptive behavior of the children evidenced most blatantly at school lunchtime.

The occupational therapy consultation and intervention also were based on the principles of disease prevention and health promotion. This involvement was intended to serve as a model of occupational therapy community consultation practice in primary prevention and health promotion programs. The inherent goals of the program reflected the following principles of occupational therapy:

> Prevention and health maintenance programs have as their purpose the fostering of normal development, sustaining and protecting existing functions and abilities, preventing disability and/or supporting levels of restoration and change. The central concern is provision of activity experiences which enable the individual to use productively his existing skills, capacities, and strengths; those which provide personal gratification and meet the basic human needs of man for acceptance, achievement, creativity, decision making, autonomy, self-assertion, and social relationships; those which provide opportunities to pursue and develop interests, explore potential, develop capacities, and learn of the resources within himself and within his external world.[1]

This health promotion and disease prevention model utilized an occupational therapy practice model termed "human development through occupation." Reed describes this model as the synthesis of four models: adaptive performance, biodevelopment, facilitation of growth and development, and occupational behavior.[10] As described previously, the situation to which the occupational therapy consultants were referred was chaotic and in peril of further deterioration. The purpose of choosing a model reflecting human development through occupation, emphasizing the adaptive process, was to stem the tide of growing community anxiety, structure the environment to encourage adaptive responses, and provide activities and techniques to facilitate adequate coping behaviors.[11] Expected results of this model of practice also were to prevent inappropriate responses among the parents, children, and school personnel of the community; develop and maintain functions and skills to promote neighborhood cohesiveness; and demonstrate a grass-roots model of community involvement. Further, the techniques developed for this program demonstrated the consultants' role in improving the social climate, which then could foster and promote a healthier community. The consultants also helped train community workers, expanding the human resources pool and enabling these individuals to develop resources so that they could respond effectively to the changes in their environment.

CONSULTATION DESCRIPTION

Organization

The multidisciplinary school consultation team was organized to address specific problems, including individual cases of learning disabilities, student-teacher relationships, parent-school relationships, principal-staff interactions, and special programs. Members of the consultation team worked in groups of two or three in various schools in the district. Each small group dealt specifically with one of these issues. As mentioned previously, the entire team of social workers, psychologists, special educators, and the two occupational therapists met weekly to discuss the consultations and review progress.

The two occupational therapists on the team were consultants to one of the severely overcrowded elementary schools in this rapidly expanding school district. The school, originally built to accommodate 150 children in a predominantly stable, white middle-class community of home owners, had increased enrollment to more than double that amount. The population of students had changed to include a more divergent socioeconomic mix: one group drawn from middle-class families in academic or white-collar positions, the other, newer group from mainly black, transient, low income, blue-collar or service-oriented families living in a new low-cost housing project. Both groups were faced with rivalry, competition, and establishment of an identity in the total community.

The children of all these families could not help but be aware of the pressures in the community and the divisive factions at home and at school. The continued overcrowding of the physical facilities of the school, combined with the emotional and social tensions building among both students and school personnel, led to burgeoning problems throughout the school.

The symptoms of unrest were most evident during the unstructured lunchtime. Fighting and name-calling during lunch occurred daily and the lunchtime problems were escalating. The lunchroom supervisors were overwhelmed with the growing numbers of children in the lunch program and the logistics of staggering the lunchtimes and rotating the groups to accommodate all children during the lunch hour. The children were so overstimulated, either by their direct participation in the negative interactions or by observation of others' activities, that little cognitive functioning was possible in the classroom after the lunch period.

A group of parents, unhappy with the reports from both children and school staff of the fighting and general chaos, met to try to remedy the problems. Although some parents were vocal and committed, they did not know how to organize their efforts. The coordinator of the school consultation team at the county mental health center was apprised of this parent group's endeavors and referred the parent group leader to the team's occupational therapy consultants.

Support

The county community mental health center funded many of the activities of the school consultation team. The occupational therapy consultants maintained their salary as employees of the university medical center, and therefore were external consultants to the community agencies. However, professional and emotional support was an important factor in this new model of interagency consultation. The interdisciplinary team supported one another in the weekly meetings where they worked together to identify and resolve some of the difficulties. The in-service training in consultation techniques and systems analysis was provided to the team by the director and professional staff of the community mental health center.

The school district funded a paid volunteer coordinator position. A community person was hired to direct the activity program that was one of the outcomes of the initial consultation. As the consultation progressed, there was increasing collegial support from the school system and staff, including teachers, lunch supervisors, and administrative officials.

Participants

Central to this consultation was the community mental health center staff coordinator of the school consultation team. Her enthusiasm, interest, and continued support provided the guidance and inspiration to the author for this and many future community consultations. In addition to the occupational therapy consultants and the school consultation team, the participants in this community consultation were many and varied. Initially, the key individuals were the leader of the parent group and the volunteer coordinator.

The players grew as the program progressed. The activity volunteers, teaching staff, lunchroom supervisor, university students, occupational therapy students, and the children themselves were gradually drawn into the intervention strategies.

Eventually, the consultation took a different form and the school principal, school system administrative officials, and community leaders participated in the project. The occupational therapy consultants remained involved throughout the consultation.

Services Provided

Entry
Entry into the system was facilitated by the coordinator of the school consultation team. During the data gathering and analysis by the county mental health

center staff of the trends and issues that appeared to cause concern in the community, the coordinator learned of the interest and efforts of a parent group to address problems in their neighborhood. She spoke to the leader of the parent group to make the initial contact from the county agency. Although this was an uninvited entry into the local neighborhood system (see Chapter 6), the timing was right. The parent group was experiencing the pain of frustration, lack of resources and knowledge of how to proceed. They needed direction and were amenable to help.

Negotiation of a Contract

The coordinator referred the occupational therapy consultants to the parent group. They met with the leader to discuss the nature of the problems and to explore possible alternatives to alleviate the increasing difficulties. A written contract with the parent group was not necessary because the county mental health center had entered into an agreement with the school system to provide consultants to various subparts of the schools that needed help. The occupational therapy consultants were under this umbrella contract, although they had to negotiate a verbal agreement with the leader of the parent group. The direction of the consultation was not evident initially, and the focus or responsibilities of the consultants and the consultee had to be explored.

Establishment of Trust and Diagnostic Analysis

Trust did not come about immediately or easily. Several informal sessions with the leader gradually eased the initial tenuous interactions, which resulted from her stress from the presenting problems. Casual brainstorming helped facilitate the beginnings of a mutually trustful relationship. The consultants used a systems approach to analyze the issues and develop a plan of action. The initial meeting of the consultants and the parent group leader was a fact-finding or diagnostic session, which included assessment of the community issues; discussion of needs; identification of social, cultural, political, and economic factors impinging on the school environment; and brainstorming. The diagnostic analysis revealed that the problems at the elementary school, which was the site of the occupational therapy consultation, were centered on the unstructured lunchtime. A suggestion that more structured lunchtime activities might help diffuse the anxiety and hyperactivity that led to the fighting was positively received by the parent group leader. After several meetings with the parent group and school principal, the consultants helped develop a volunteer-manned lunch and recess activity program. A paid coordinator of the program was hired by the school district.

Goal Setting

The major objective of the occupational therapy consultation was to facilitate the process of problem solving. The paid coordinator became the consultee in the situation, and the consultation was based on an educational/program model of consultation. The consultants provided in-service training in program organization to the coordinator and held weekly meetings with her to help develop program objectives and a specific plan for recruitment of volunteers. The volunteers were called resource teachers, to provide them with an identity and some status within the school system.

Frequent meetings were held by the consultants with the coordinator and the resource teachers, initially to help plan types of services and activities that might deliver a feasible and effective program. Strategies to involve parents, other volunteers, and the paid lunch supervisors were explored. In addition, it was essential to gain the support of the school principal, teachers, and other school personnel to ensure that the program ran smoothly. The program also was presented to the schoolchildren, and their suggestions and ideas for activities were included, whenever possible, in the overall plan.

Once the program was in operation, the consultants held monthly planning meetings with the resource teachers and frequent consultation conferences with the coordinator to review the program, identify problems and/or new areas of service, develop new or modified program objectives as indicated, and help implement needed program changes. The consultants were at the school several times a week to observe the program, consult with school personnel and resource teachers as necessary, and to help with the actual activities when a problem with staffing, programming, or specific children arose.

Evaluation and Analysis of Consultation

The volunteer resource teacher lunch program initially was viewed with guarded and skeptical attitudes by many of the regular school personnel. The concept of a program planned, supervised, and run by people considered outsiders to the school system was new to this district. Entry into the school system by the mental health program consultation team was complicated by the considerable publicity in the media of the unpleasant consequences of busing schoolchildren and by the negative reactions of the community to a new population of schoolchildren.

This school was the target of a variety of outside interests, including college students with special education, sociology, and psychology projects; newspaper reporters; parents; school board members; and the county school administrators. The school, continually overcrowded with too many children, also seemed to be teeming, at times, with outsiders. School personnel resented these intrusions and were less than receptive, initially, to this new lunch program. The staff, especially the paid lunch supervisors, were apprehensive, reluctant to accept ideas from strangers, and even covertly resistant to the volunteer resource teachers. Despite the number of problems they had with the growing school population, they were somewhat threatened by the perceived interference in "their" program. This lack of initial support was confounded by the apparent poor communication from the school administration to the classroom teachers and lunch supervisors.

The consultants worked with the paid coordinator to analyze the problems and also consulted with the school principal. Demonstration of a successful week of activities helped enlist the support of the principal, who, in turn, conveyed his interest in the program to his lunch supervisors and teachers. He gave his permission to hold weekly meetings with the volunteer and paid lunch personnel. These meetings were intended to clarify roles and provide opportunities to exchange ideas and develop strategies to solve the procedural and mechanical problems of moving the children into and out of activities. The meetings also helped to resolve the problems of staffing shortages when program staff were absent. Eventually a cohesive lunch program was developed in which paid staff ran some of the activities. The paid staff developed a collegial relationship with the volunteer resource teachers and even socialized with them outside of school.

Many of the difficulties resulting from the natural resistance to new programs, changes in routines and procedures, reaction to strangers in the system, poor communications, and role confusion were resolved by implementing a problem-solving approach with both volunteer and paid staff. The consultants had to fine-tune their listening skills to hear what was *not* verbalized. They also had to maintain contact with the parent group, the chairman of the local school board, and the school principal.

What started as a potentially explosive situation at the beginning of the school year, as a result of accelerated changes in a community, eventually developed into a positive experience with far-reaching consequences for an entire town. As the program progressed, many positive aspects of this community health promotion consultation were demonstrated. The activities expanded from simple arts and crafts to storytelling, dancing, drama, movies, games, team sports, gymnastics, and cooking. Most satisfying for all those involved was the children's enjoyment of and enthusiasm for the structured activities, which frequently carried over into after-school activities led by the children themselves. The success of the program was reported to the school board and county school administration.

Termination/Renegotiation

The initial educational consultation to build knowledge and skill in program planning and organization through the lunchtime activity program was so successful that this aspect of the consultation was terminated. The continual on-site services of the consultants were no longer necessary.

The pool of volunteer resource teachers expanded to include university students and occupational therapy students. The original consultants supervised the occupational therapy students, who provided direct activity services to the schoolchildren. This was part of the community fieldwork program the author initiated for the Department of Occupational Therapy in the Neuropsychiatric Institute at the university medical center. The consultants continued their employment at the university, but maintained a visible interest by voluntarily attending community meetings.

Outcome

This success story was published in the city newspaper. The publicity resulted in requests by college students and other volunteers to conduct additional activities during lunch and after school. The most positive result for the community was the reduction in the anxiety and stress of children, parents, and school personnel.

The maladaptive reactions to the overload of sensory stimuli by the constant fighting and negative interactions during the lunch period at the start of the school year diminished proportionately as the children increased their involvement in structured activities. The teachers were particularly pleased with the children's behavior when they returned to the classroom after the lunch period. They were able to settle down to schoolwork more easily than they were before the activity program was initiated. The overstimulation and bombardment of continual sensory input was greatly reduced, resulting in increased cognitive functioning, appropriate decision making, and rational behavior.

The initial negative reactions to the rapid and irregularly changing situation in the community environment and to the increased crowding in the school facilities, which had stretched the limits of the students' adaptability, had been modified. The theory of human adaptation, which includes the adaptive reaction and orientation response, was clearly demonstrated in this situation. In addition, rational behavior was restored by the development of predictable and consistent activities that allowed for programmed decisions.

A major consequence of the positive effects of good activity programming at the school was the development of a neighborhood steering committee, which encompassed three housing tracts of low- and middle-income families in cooperative housing projects, townhouses, and single-family dwellings. Initially, the committee was formed to develop a summer recreation program that would continue the positive interactions started in the school activity program. A neighborhood needs survey soon revealed that other community services would be useful. A meeting of the residents was called, a committee formed, and, over a 2-year period, the recreation program expanded into other areas that included child care, health care, transportation services, housing support, a food cooperative, boys' and girls' clubs, and life skills activities for all ages. A new elementary school opened and a lunchtime and after-school activity program were also instituted in this school, with very active and positive support from the new principal.

Throughout the development of this neighborhood venture, the occupational therapy consultants were an integral part of the organization, planning, and programming. The occupational therapy involvement expanded to include fieldwork students and members of the recreational and music therapy staff of the occupational therapy department at the university medical center. The life skills activities, led by the occupational therapy staff and students, included training in babysitting and child-care techniques, prevocational skills, and homemaking hints.

Many county agencies, including the county mental health center and several university departments, were represented on the neighborhood steering committee. The attitude of this community toward the university had changed considerably. The positive involvement of university students from many programs and the high visibility and assistance of staff from the medical center markedly improved the relations between town and gown. Discussions of increased interactions and future collaborative activities between university programs and many of the community agencies were a most positive outcome of this consultation.

SUMMARY

This community involvement demonstrated the role occupational therapy consultants can assume as change agents and advocates to prevent dysfunction and maladaptation and promote a healthy environment in an entire community. It emphasized that a systems approach to adaptation, which recognizes that both external and internal factors influence behaviors in the system, must be the start of any community involvement.

Awareness of the political and social climate of a community, the trends influencing community action and reaction, and the concerns and needs of its residents opened the door to facilitating change. The occupational therapy consultants as health planners, educators, advocates, and change agents emphasized the profession's commitment to delivering high quality health care and improving the quality of life.

As occupational therapists increasingly move into community consultation, they must broaden their perspective to become more aware of the overall systems' needs. They must become knowledgeable about the primary institutions of the community, including the families, schools, local businesses, and even religious organizations. With this appreciation of the cultural and social folkways of a community, in addition to their awareness of the influences of political, economic, and social trends, they can become community change agents and develop strategies that will be responsive to the needs of its systems.[3, 5, 6, 13]

REFERENCES

1. American Occupational Therapy Association: Occupational therapy: Its definitions and functions. *Am J Occup Ther* 1972; 26:204–205.
2. Dubos R: *Man Adapting*. New Haven, Yale University Press, 1965.
3. Finn GL: The occupational therapist in prevention programs. *Am J Occup Ther* 1972; 26:59–66.
4. Fisher AJ: *Health Care in the 70's: A National Crisis*. CPL Exchange Bibliography, no 705. Los Angeles, University of Southern California, 1974.
5. Jaffe E: The role of the occupational therapist as a community consultant: Primary prevention in mental health programming. *Occup Ther Ment Health* 1980; 1:47–62.
6. Jaffe EG: The occupational therapist as a change agent: A model of preventive mental health, in Robertson SC (ed): SCOPE. Rockville, Md, AOTA, 1986.
7. Katz D, Kahn RL: *The Social Psychology of Organizations,* ed 2. New York, Wiley, 1978.
8. Milio N: *The Storefront That Did Not Burn*. Ann Arbor, Univ of Michigan Press, 1970, p 98.
9. Miller JG: Towards a general theory for the behavioral sciences. *Am Psychol* 1955; 10:513–531.
10. Reed KL: *Models of Practice in Occupational Therapy*. Baltimore: Williams & Wilkins, 1984.
11. Robertson SC: Generic frames of reference in occupational therapy, in Kirkland M,

Robertson SC (eds): *Planning and Implementing Vocational Readiness in Occupational Therapy (PIVOT)*. Rockville, Md, AOTA, 1984.

12. Rogers J: Articulating a frame of reference, in Robertson SC (ed): SCOPE. Rockville, Md, AOTA, 1986.
13. Romani J: Consultation Course, Guest faculty, Ann Arbor, Mich, July 1972.
14. Toffler A: *Future Shock*. New York: Random House, 1970.
15. World Health Organization: *The First Ten Years of the World Health Organization*. Geneva, Author, 1958.

CHAPTER 24

Occupational Therapy Consultation in Developmental Disabilities

Susan Bachner, M.A., O.T.R./L., F.A.O.T.A.

OVERVIEW

The author's practice of occupational therapy consultation in developmental disabilities began in the mid 1970s. As legislative mandates for the developmentally disabled began to shift funding and services from institutions to the community, service providers and families of the disabled faced ever-changing challenges. Schools, adult day programs, group homes, occupational training centers, and families became increasingly interested in occupational therapy consultation services.

Many developmentally disabled individuals who had been institutionalized were now required to assume more independence in their daily living skills. Others, who had been cloistered in a sheltered home environment, were confronted by significantly altered daily routines when they became enrolled in day programs, schools, occupational training centers, or supported employment situations. The demands of these new environments, with increased expectations and new relationships, led many developmentally disabled individuals and their caregivers to seek consultative assistance.

Nationwide, chapters of the Association for Retarded Citizens (ARC), established small group homes and supervised apartments for clientele within their communities and jurisdictions. There was a need for a continuum of work activities that ranged from sheltered employment to quasi-competitive employment where job coaching might be provided. Similarly, socializing and teaching the developmentally disabled individual new sets of behaviors required to function as a community resident and participant in meaningful day activity programming, was also an identified need. Trainers required help to develop appropriate strategies and structured protocols in order to meet individual client goals. An increasing demand therefore arose for both occupational therapy treatment and consultation services.

The author's practice included both. In many instances, evaluation and short-term treatment would be followed by consultation. A major focus was case consultation, where recommendations for appropriate goal setting, role-modeling techniques, task segmentation or curricula development were frequently requested. Professional caregivers, family caregivers, and others in the community, such as potential job site managers and co-workers, sought consultation in order to help the developmentally disabled individual successfully integrate in the community.

Homemaker activities, a critical element in supervised residential programming, was frequently problematic for clientele and caregiver. Tasks such as menu planning, shopping for ingredients, and the actual integration of recipes to insure a balanced dinner were important objectives. During consultations focused on these activities, the consultant observed that the staff also had difficulty performing homemaker tasks. Trainers in community residences often were young people, who were themselves neophyte cooks. Thus such daily meal preparation issues as food selection, quantity determination, task organization, integrating the recipes for synchronized completion and clean-up were obstacles shared by trainers and trainees.

In response to this need, the consultant and a free-lance illustrator collaborated to develop a full-color picture cookbook, *Picture This: An Illustrated Guide to Complete Dinners*. It was designed so that the illustrated instructions for the preparation of 12 complete dinners were "user friendly" to the non-reader, the person limited by cognitive deficits, as well as to someone who was simply new to cooking. Also available was a color-coded measuring cup and spoon set that corresponded to the colors in *Picture This*. Each meal was sequenced using the task analysis format. The latter compensated for cognitive integration problems and insured preparation of a nutritionally sound dinner.[2] Since publication in 1984, the materials have been used successfully throughout the United States, the United Kingdom, and Canada. The consultant also frequently lectures to professionals and families on mealtime issues. Topics include meal planning and preparation, the importance of adaptive techniques and equipment, and the psychosocial aspects of mealtime and dining.

The increased visibility resulting from this publication led to a broader referral base and requests for services throughout south-western Connecticut and Westchester County in New York state. At the present time, services include (1) consultation to staff in group homes and day programs; (2) case consultation for individual families; and (3) work with school-age clientele whose families seek transitional employment experiences for their developmentally disabled adolescents.

ENVIRONMENT AND SYSTEMS INFLUENCES

Clinic walls no longer are the boundaries for practice. Most occupational therapists find themselves trying to keep pace with changing needs in the marketplace. Many environmental factors have contributed to these changes. An increasing demand for occupational therapy services cannot be matched with personnel, due to critical staff shortages.[1] Deinstitutionalization, the need for mandated quality assurance in community settings, and self-advocacy programs have created new consumers. Clients, their families, and agencies working with them request a variety of consultation services, ranging from simple trouble-shooting to program development. Outside consultants are called in to help them look more objectively at or redefine their needs to provide assessment expertise regarding client potential for community placement, and, at times, to offer a "second opinion" prior to completing a plan.

As clients, their families, and agencies seek normalized living arrangements, they face community barriers. Unless a knowledgeable and concerted effort is made to educate the community, group homes may be viewed with trepidation and hostility. Rumors abound and challenges are made when a group home seeks to establish itself in a residential area. Once resistance is overcome and the home is established, staff need to be trained. Too often, the staff view the client as dependent, almost infantile. Problems perpetuate or new ones develop as staff take over responsibility for performing client daily living skills, rather than encouraging client involvement.

The thrust and focus of school programs for developmentally disabled students had been toward early intervention, during the first decade of Public Law 94-142 implementation. In the mid 1980s, the developmentally disabled adolescent captured attention: the early intervention recipient had become a teenager! At that time, Madeline Will, Assistant Secretary for the Office of Special Education and Rehabilitation Services, made the transition from school to work a national education priority. She viewed this focus on transition as a bridge from the protective atmosphere of school to the challenges and risks that accompany adult life. Transition plans became a mandated part of educational programming for handicapped students.[12] These plans must be generated when the student is approximately 15 years old. Like the Individual Educational Program (IEP), the Individual Transition Plan (ITP) is a written document that describes goals and objectives for a student. Components of the ITP speak to present and future environments; it attempts to define the student's role repetoire for work, play, and Activities of Daily Living (ADL).

Currently, parents, educators, and professionals concerned with mentally retarded students have more opportunities to help these young adults make their transitions. Enabling legislation created by the passage of the Americans with Disabilities Act (ADA) has opened additional doors.[6] Occupational therapy consultants and others concerned with this growing population now have increasing opportunities to help foster change in the community.

FRAME OF REFERENCE

The author's definition used for occupational therapy consultation with the developmentally disabled is based on the belief that a consultant is someone who provides specialized knowledge. Moreover, ". . . a consultant is an advisor, a fixer, a boss, and a slave; a catalyst, a stabilizer, a listener, and a talker; a specialist and a generalist; a manager and a quasi-employee who works alone or with the client's staff. Consultants act as motivators and monitors; they also serve as work horses and stepping stones."[7, p. 3] This fluid definition emphasizes the multiplicity of consultant roles. It includes the essentials of listening, assessing, sharing, and enabling—all of which are done with professional commitment to the rules that govern the consultative relationship.

While consultation services are usually time limited, they should be adjusted to the needs of the developmentally disabled client. These clients require a longer time frame to develop new skills. Consultants working with this population must recognize the nature of the mentally retarded client's learning curve and allow for this extended time.

Consultation models used in this practice include clinical, collegial, organizational development, program development, and social action models. Within each consultation experience, clients are viewed as part of a social system. Social system theory[3, 5] is used to help analyze how groups of people band together, organize, and operate. Using this information, the consultant is able to address simultaneously the specific needs of a given client and the social system. Each has an effect on the client and his desired goal.

The consultant's analysis considers the developmentally disabled individual's need for new skills and behavior patterns. Realignment of skills and behaviors is often required to help clientele adjust to changed expectations in a new environment. Similarly, providers often need guidance in order to make their reciprocal adjustments. In role theory, the roles of clientele and service provider are viewed as complementary. A re-positioning of one role always impacts on the functioning, expectations and goals of the other.[4]

The practice which then evolved had firm ties to client advocacy, systems theory[9] and social role theory.[4] The case study which follows illustrates a consultation strongly influenced by three components: the organization's needs, the client's needs, and the accepted behaviors commonly associated with the client's role.

CONSULTATION DESCRIPTION

Organization

Individual case consultation frequently brings the consultant into a larger system which, in turn, becomes the major focus. The following case demonstrates how a referral, requesting consultation for a problem client in a group home, became a consultation which later identified problems in the system at large.

A request for case consultation came from an ARC geriatric residential program. Mr. G., a 72 year-old man with mental retardation, had resided in this group home since its opening one year earlier. He still had not been able to assume responsibility for self care. Additionally, several recent incident reports had been filed regarding Mr. G.'s "acting out". These indicated that he had hit staff and physically threatened other residents. The program staff at the home met to discuss his Official Plan of Care (OPC). A referral was generated at that meeting requesting occupational therapy consultation "to identify areas where Mr. G. could increase his independence."

Support

Over the years, the consultant had worked with numerous ARCs and private programs and was approached frequently to provide consultation services for clientele and staff. In each situation, the consultant established an hourly fee for services. When the relationship was to be on-going, service fees were reviewed on a yearly basis. Reports concerning each individual consultation request were sent to key individuals at each consultation site. When appropriate, administrative staff also received reports.

To prepare for this consultation, the consultant requested that all Mr. G.'s records be available to her at the time of her initial visit. She also asked for procedures governing daily activities at the home and requested key staff remain accessible at the time of her visit to facilitate information gathering. In addition, she scheduled her visit at a time when other residents were at home, recognizing that these individuals were also important "players" in the unfolding drama. Further examination of all participants impacting on the system was also planned.

Participants

In an agency-initiated referral, it is important to identify all the people who share the problem. Mr. G. was the central piece in the consultant's fact-finding mission. While his performance was under review, he also provided access to others in his environment. This larger system proved to be a major consultation concern. It included the group home manager, staff assigned to work with Mr. G. and other house residents.

Within the group home, the manager assumed responsibility for scheduling and supervising staff, the development of a positive and facilitory living environment, and linkage with the agency's administrative office. One of the manager's major concerns was the home's resonsibility for and compliance with the regulatory guidelines for quality care established by the State Department of Mental Retardation. Part of the department's oversight function was to review incident reports, required to be on file at the home, including those concerning Mr. G.

Staff assigned to work with Mr. G. had no professional training but did receive on-the-job training in regard to working with mentally retarded adults. The other clients who resided in the home did not seek interaction with Mr. G.—most appeared fearful of him.

Mr. G. had resided in a state institution for the developmentally disabled since the age of 14. Prior to that, he had lived the part of a "sick member" in his family—he did little, and nothing was expected. At the institution, he was given custodial care, and dependence was the by-product. Mr. G. had never had the opportunity to participate in productive work, nor had he been given any consistent responsibility for his self-care ADL. He was de-institutionalized at age 72.

The scenario was reminiscent of 'life begins at 40.' Mr. G., at age 72, like it or not, was expected to identify with that mid-life sophism. In other words, when placed in his new group home. Mr. G. was essentially asked to assume a new identity. This imposed identity or new role was to reflect a "productive" being, someone who was "meaningfully involved" with ADL. The home's staff wanted him to begin a journey towards increased independence, and at age 72 he was to take over responsibility for many of his ADLs. The staff felt ADL self-care was within his ability. Yet, there was nothing in Mr. G.'s medical and social history to support that assumption. This conflict over expectations led to tensions that reinforced and perpetuated the inadequate behaviors that precipitated the consultation request.[4]

Services Provided

The consultant's familiarity with similar group homes helped pave the way for her entry at this site. The initial consultation request, "help to increase Mr. G.'s independence," would require a case consultation approach. Given experience with other group home cases, the consultant anticipated the consultation evolving into a systems consultation model.

Data gathering, the first step in the diagnostic aspect of consultation, was therefore planned to incorporate information pertinent to the specific case and the system as a whole. The consultant's inquiry included information regarding:

1. Mr. G.

   - Prior history, available through past and current records.
   - Current ADL performance levels (strengths & deficits).
   - Behavioral triggers which increased Mr. G.'s acting out.
   - Relationship of other residents to Mr. G. in light of problem behaviors.
   - Staff actions and communications regarding this resident.
   - Staff perceptions and their method of interaction with Mr. G.

II. *The Home (System)*

   - Management expectations.
   - Power individuals in the system.
   - Positive and negative environmental influences.
   - Factors delaying consultation referral until after the OPC meeting.
   - Underlying reason(s) for the consultation request.
   - System flexibility.

- Profiles of other residents.
- Individuals advocating change in Mr. G.

While this outline may appear extensive, one must always get an understanding of the total situation. Wilma West commented "One of our most limiting professional traits is our propensity to seek solutions before gaining a fundamental understanding of the reason for the problem."[14]

Based on prior consultation experience, the consultant's pre-visit analysis was that Mr. G.'s functioning, or lack of it, had perhaps become a management issue for staff, possibly one based on regulatory compliance. The presence of incident reports could trigger investigations by the state and might jeopardize funding.

Clear and open communication was quickly established. The consultant's years of experience and prior success in helping staff and clients from other group homes was an advantage. When a consultant conveys confidence, indicating that she can truly help and that the problem(s) are solvable, she in turn empowers the consultee, and effective dialogue can begin.

At Mr. G.'s home, there was an ease and trust that enabled the sharing of otherwise unavailable information. Staff were eager to use the consultant's expertise and the group home manager had prepared all materials and gathered all the key persons to assure readiness for the consultation.

The information from written and verbal sources was essential as the consultant began her fact-finding process. It allowed evaluation of important relationships, gave perspective in regard to Mr. G.'s past history and provided time for observation of Mr. G.'s interactions and behaviors. Thorough data gathering is an essential part of the consultation process.

A historical review of Mr. G.'s case indicated that he had never been exposed to work activities or given responsibilities which would lead into a work role. Moving from an institutional setting, which fostered dependence, to this home, which sought to develop independence, was seen by the client as a threatening situation.

A thorough evaluation of Mr. G.'s ADL skills was then performed. During this interactive evaluation, the consultant was able to allow some staff observation, and she kept staff informed of strategies used to help Mr. G. perform simple dressing tasks independently. This collegial approach to staff training allowed the consultant to simultaneously evaluate both the client's abilities and the staff's perceptions of his abilities.

Evaluation results indicated that Mr. G. had the potential to dress independently. Given the necessary structure (verbal, physical and environmental cueing), and extended time to perform the tasks, the resident performed well and did not demonstrate abusive behaviors. It was noted that he needed assistance to close his pants zipper, tie his shoelaces, and button his shirt. With alternate clothing choices, these problems could be eliminated. The consultant reviewed these alternatives (i.e. velcro fasteners for sneakers, elastic waist band pants, and pullover shirts) with staff, so that they could plan to purchase these items with the resident on the next shopping trip.

The client's positive response and performance during evaluation served as a springboard for the consultant's major concern with staff attitudes and abilities to communicate effectively with the resident. Meeting with staff to review findings allowed for a discussion of methods which would be effective in promoting Mr. G.'s independence. Role-modeling techniques, used by the consultant during the resident evaluation process, had helped staff understand the need for new approaches and had stimulated their thinking. The consultant encouraged staff to identify and agree upon a unified approach to the resident. The approach should promote Mr. G.'s increased independence and should not cause him to become angry, which would lead to abusive behavior.

During the ensuing discussion, facilitated by the consultant, staff recognized the value of a unified approach. It became evident to them that Mr. G.'s previous living environment, of 52 years, had not demanded any independence. That institution's value system, which he had internalized, prized traits such as compliance and dependence. "Being good" was far more important to the overall ward functioning than independence. The group home's departure from his usual amount of custodial care had created anger, fear, and probable confusion. These significant feelings could be tracked and related to his abusive behaviors.

This open discussion helped the staff to verbalize concerns and share reactions to Mr. G.'s abusiveness with each other and the consultant. Mr. G.'s primary caregiver was able to discuss the problems she had encountered. The resident had hit her on numerous occasions, and the behavior seemed to follow her requests that he do things for himself. This left her fearful and frustrated. Other staff, observing the problems, became equally uncomfortable when required to work with Mr. G. While some staff, as part of their job, made attempts to have him dress himself, others simply wanted to get through a problem-free shift! The approaches were as varied as the number of aides at the meeting.

As the situation was reviewed, staff began to understand how their withdrawal and inconsistent expectations had further bearing on Mr. G.'s recent acting-out. They could then understand his behavior as an attempt to get increased attention and help. They also recognized that Mr. G.'s lack of verbal communication skills could lead to his difficulties in venting his anger and cause even greater confusion. It became clear to them that other residents were taking their cues from staff and avoided Mr. G. entirely. One particular resident, chanted obsessively, "it's not nice to hit!"

The negative implication of staff and other resident behaviors became evident to the group. They were then able to identify and agree upon a structured and unified approach to use in helping Mr. G. reach the staff goal of dressing independence. While the consultant acted as facilitator and advisor to the group, the staff developed the final plan and strategies for its implementation.

The consultant then met with the group home manager to review all findings, and to discuss the content of the final written report and the recommendations which evolved from this case consultation. While the consultation request was specific to Mr. G., and his behavior had been successfully addressed, the consultant's verbal report also pointed out important generic quality improvement issues which had surfaced in regard to staff–resident dynamics. The need for staff in-services was a primary concern. Specific topics that were recommended included roles (the staff's and the residents'), consistency of staff approaches, and residents' behaviors as affected by staff withdrawal and fear.[13]

Since the initial contract had only requested a case consultation, it was then up to the client, specifically the home manager, to determine whether or not there was a need for further consultation services to focus on broader system issues.

The content of the written versus verbal report was also a critical issue. Given the oversight function of the Division of Mental Retardation and the presence of incident reports, it appeared more prudent to discuss other issues, particularly the need for further staff training, on a verbal basis. While the problem could be alluded to in the written report, specific recommendations in the report were focused on the case at hand.

While there is no formula for exiting techniques, the consultant must keep in mind that, when objectives have been realized, the "end" is obvious to everyone. Leopold reminds us that, "The main point is this: once you see that things are going reasonably well when you are not present . . . you should (like a courteous guest who knows when the party is over) pick up your hat; say good-bye to your consultees, and to others in the organization with whom you have developed working relationships; and leave promptly."[11, p. 34] This does not imply that the organization will never again ask for consultation.

The consultant left the door open for possible renegotiation of the contract. The emphasis of future consultation would be on the system need for education and training of staff regarding their interactions with residents and the roles each played in the group home environment.

In discussing these needs with the manager, the consultant also identified sources within the system, such as central office staff, that might be of assistance. At the close of the exit conference, the manager indicated that she would consider the need for further consultation. She and her staff expressed appreciation to the consultant for the comprehensive consultation and successful development of a plan for Mr. G.

OUTCOME

When the consultation is finished, it is time for self-evaluation. Kelley emphasizes the importance of this procedure. It helps the consultant monitor her work performance in an objective manner and acts as a quality assurance mechanism. The self-evaluation is a learning tool and may also help provide legal protection. In addition, it can be a marketing tool. When the consultant analyzes her performance, she may identify more effective strategies for working with a particular target population.[8]

At the end of this consultation, the outcome was measured by considering the following:

- Goals as stated in the consultation letter of agreement.
- Objectives as outlined in the initial data analysis.
- Resident responsiveness to consultant assessment.
- Verbal and written communication:
  a) provided by staff and group home manager in regard to consultation services.
  b) consultation report provided to the manager and team at the home.

In this instance, the consultant had achieved the goals and objectives in regard to the case consultation. While she had been successful in sensitizing all concerned regarding the larger system need for education and training, this did not result in a renegotiation to address this important issue. It did encourage the home manager to seek further guidance from the home office and to plan further training under their auspices. A year later the home reported that Mr. G.'s independence had increased and he was "doing much better". No further incidents were being reported, and the staff appeared to have benefited from the in-house training programs.

SUMMARY

This chapter has described a case consultation concerning a resident of a group home for geriatric developmentally disabled adults. It emphasizes the importance of a broad perspective, looking beyond one specific case to the system as a whole.

The importance of collegial consultation and use of role modeling as an informal training tool was highlighted. A comprehensive and well-planned data-gathering process helped the consultant effectively pinpoint the critical problems underlying this case. Occupational therapy consultants working in the community with a previously institutionalized developmentally disabled population must be knowledgeable regarding both community and institutional environments and the supporting systems.

In this case, the consultant's awareness of these factors helped in the formulation of a successful plan. The consultant used specific occupational therapy expertise to assess a resident who was identified as having problem behaviors and showing excessive dependence in self-care skills. Using the assessment process as a teaching tool, she was able to help caregiver staff and management view the resident from a different perspective. Through the case consultation approach, important system needs were also identified. Since the consultant was not asked to address these training and educational needs, she helped her client recognize their importance and suggested use of alternative agency resources.

The developmentally disabled population and those serving their needs will continue to grow. Occupational therapy consultants can provide important expertise, advice, and information, which will foster greater independence and effective performance. Our rapidly changing world is influenced by ever-changing technology, resource limitations, work situations, lifestyles, and environments. As individuals engage in an ongoing attempt to effectively satisfy their needs in this new world, there will be a continuing demand for consultation services.[10]

REFERENCES

1. AOTA: 1990 Member data survey summary report. *OT Week* 1991; 22: June 6.
2. Bachner S: *Picture This! An Illustrated Guide to Complete Dinners*. Greenwich, Conn, Special Additions, 1984.
3. Bain R (ed): *Sociology: Introductory Readings*. New York, Lippincott, 1962.
4. Broom L, Selznick P (eds): *Sociology: A Text with Adapted Readings*. New York, Harper & Row, 1963.
5. Douglas JD (ed): *Understanding Everyday Life: Toward the Reconstruction of Sociological Knowledge*. Chicago, Aldine Publishing, 1970.
6. Ellek D: Health policy: The Americans With Disabilities Act of 1990. *Amer J Occup Ther* 1991; 45:177.
7. Johnson B: *Private Consulting*. Englewood Cliffs, NJ, Prentice Hall, Inc, 1984.
8. Kelley E: *Consulting*. New York, Charles Scribner's Sons, 1981.
9. Kielhofner G: General systems theory: Implications for theory and action in occupational therapy. *Amer J Occup Ther* 1978; 32:637.
10. Kishel G, Kishel P: *Cashing In On The Consulting Boom*. New York, John Wiley & Sons, Inc, 1985.
11. Leopold RL: The techniques of consultation: Some thoughts for the occupational therapist. *Proceedings from Eastern Pennsylvania Occup Ther Assoc Meeting*. Philadelphia, Eastern Pennsylvania Occupational Therapy Association, 1966.
12. Special Education Resource Center: *Transition from School-to-Work: A Resource Manual for Practitioners and Parents of Children With Disabilities*, 2 vols. Middletown, Conn, Connecticut State Department of Education, 1989.
13. Tudor GE: A sociopsychiatric nursing approach to intervention in a problem of mutual withdrawal on a mental hospital ward. *Psychiatry* 1962; 15:193.
14. West W: Perspectives on the past and future, part 2. *Amer J Occup Ther* 1990; 44:9.

CHAPTER 25

Adult Day-Care Consultation in a Rural Community

Cynthia F. Epstein, M.A., O.T.R.

OVERVIEW

The concept of adult day care (ADC) evolved in England during the late 1950s. Occupational therapists, working in cooperation with physicians and nurses, developed these programs to create a bridge to the community for older, chronically ill patients who had been hospitalized. During the 1960s, adult day care gained increasing interest in the United States.[15] At this time, further recognition was given to growing needs of older persons through the Older Americans Act of 1965, Public Law 89-73. Subsequent legislation in the 1960s and early 1970s led to expanded health services under amendments to the Social Security Act. These included Medicare (Title XIVIII), Medicaid (Title XIX), and Social Services (Title XX) programs.

The 1970s were also a time of change for many rural areas in the state of New Jersey. Farmland was targeted for suburban development, and this was particularly true where the author resided. Many farmers became builders, or retired, selling their land to developers. Community planners and volunteer organizations in her community identified this growing trend and the increasing population of isolated, frail older persons who lived in fear of institutionalization.

A volunteer community organization, committed to helping older persons and supported through a local foundation, was asked to conduct a comprehensive assessment of the needs of older persons residing in the county. The results identified two major areas: adult day care (ADC) and congregate housing. The organization's board decided that the priority was an ADC program, and funding was obtained from the local foundation and the county to develop such a program. program.

The consultant, at this time, was involved outside the county providing clinical and consultative services to long-term care facilities. In this role, she was aware of many older persons who were being institutionalized for lack of ADC services in

419

their communities. Thus, she had intently monitored the progress of the proposed ADC program in her own community.

Since she was also an appointed member of the county board of mental health, she was provided with periodic updates on this project. Involvement on the mental health board also gave her networking access to the county's social service department and office on aging. As an interested observer, she additionally kept up on all newspaper reports regarding the project.

National organizations concerned with aging issues, such as the National Council on Aging and the Gerontological Society of America were promoting the development of ADC programs in the late 1970s. Since the consultant was a member of these organizations, her knowledge base was constantly updated by reading their publications and attending multidisciplinary conferences where ADC was highlighted.

As plans for the ADC program formalized, the community board hired an administrator, using Community Employment and Training Act (CETA) funds. This allowed the board to have a business administrator/planner paid for through federal monies. The administrator, trained in business, had no background in health systems or social services. He was, however, directed to be the spokesperson for the organization and to identify and negotiate space for the proposed center.

Interim reports and newspaper accounts generated at this time indicated that the board had decided to utilize a medical model of day care. This required a certificate of need from the state department of health, and meant that very specific building code requirements had to be met. The model, considered to be restorative in nature, was defined as "intensive health-supportive services prescribed in individual care plans prescribed therapeutic services (should also be) provided."[1, p. iv] Medical model programs were usually located in a hospital or long-term care facility, and were eligible for reimbursement under the state's Medicaid program.

From the consultant's "outsider" perspective, the board had made a wrong decision. Given her current information, and the needs identified in the board study, a social/health maintenance model was the better choice. This type of program could incorporate important aspects of health maintenance, including health monitoring, supervised therapeutic activities, and psychosocial services in the client's care plan. Environmentally, it would emphasize socialization, purposeful activity, nutritional support, and when needed, assistance with daily living needs. These areas of need had been emphasized in the study.

At this point in time, the consultant had no access to the board, nor was she in a position to discuss her observations with individuals she knew on the board's Advisory Committee. While the consultant was pondering this dilemma, an opportunity arose which allowed her to become involved.

The board decided that they were now ready to hire someone to develop the program. They publicized this decision in a newspaper article and listed the job in the classified ads. The consultant decided to apply and try, during the interview, to shift the focus from a position as "director" to one as "consultant".

The consulation experience described here is the result of this strategy. It took place over a period of 10 months, with services starting 1 day a week and gradually increasing to 3 days a week at the height of need.

ENVIRONMENT AND SYSTEMS INFLUENCES

The community organization designated to develop an ADC program for this rural county had an interesting history. The estate of a prominent lawyer in the county, whose family had been early settlers in the area, set up a foundation for the good and welfare of county elderly. The foundation directed local county administration to create an organization to assume this charge and to appoint its board. The composition of the board therefore had political, social, health, business, and legal representation. More than half of the board members were over 65 years of age, and many were from families who had lived in the county for generations.

While the foundation provided major support to begin the project, the board knew they would need increasing financial support from county, state, and federal sources in order to implement the program. This had been a major consideration in their decision to use a medical model. Attendees in the ADC program, eligible for Medicaid, would then be supported through this funding source.

The local hospital, with representatives on the board, appeared interested in the medical model. They had space available and could contract their specialized services to the ADC program. However, the hospital also had a major restructuring plan underway. It was possible that their space, being discussed as the potential site, might be reallocated for outpatient services.

Other community agencies, including the Office on Aging, Department of Social Services, Community Mental Health Center and Community Services Council voiced concern regarding the needs of those older persons who could not qualify under the medical model. The board had responded to this concern through their administrator, who was not knowledgeable regarding health systems, the multiple problems faced by older persons, or the functions of these various agencies in the overall service delivery picture.

This lack of understanding and the defensive posture of the administrator had alienated many of the key persons in power in these community organizations. Since the medical day care program had a certificate of need requirement, it was important to have support from various community organizations. The poor communication between the board and community service organizations had undermined this necessary support. Thus, recent applications, made in regard to the program, had been denied. While various reasons had been given, obvious silence from key organizations was a powerful negative message.

It was at this point that the board felt a more professional voice was needed to speak for the project. Their best strategy, they concluded, was to bring in a director who was a health professional and could plan the program and dialogue with the community.

FRAME OF REFERENCE

Initially, educational and administrative levels of consultation were required to help the system (the community organization, its board, and related advisors) consider a change in focus. During the course of the consultation, various models were utilized. These included systems, social action, organizational development, program development, educational, and collegial models. Toward the end of the consultation, when clients were being assessed regarding their appropriateness for the ADC program, the consultant also utilized a case-centered level of consultation in order to help staff identify appropriate candidates and develop individualized program care plans.

Various frames of reference were utilized during the course of this complex consultation. Viewing ADC as a preventive strategy, the importance of health promotion was emphasized[3] and considered in regard to the clientele to be served. This included both the older persons and their caregivers. Supporting this frame of reference, was the concept of wellness, which Johnson defines as "a context for living, a state of being, a place from which to come as individuals commit themselves to improve life for all humanity . . . "[4, p. 130].

The occupational behavior frame of reference was also used. It emphasizes the importance of the environment and the use of purposeful activity to facilitate adaptation and mastery of skills. This, in turn, helps achieve successful performance in work and play occupations.[10, 14] Similarly, the occupational performance frame of reference integrates the components of sensory, motor, psychological, social, and cognitive functions and the areas of self-care, work, play, learning, and leisure.

In both these perspectives, the environment is viewed as a key factor. Llorens indicates that these frames of reference "operationalize occupational therapy theory in reference to the sociocultural environment and the biological-psychological environment."[8, p. 30] As Kiernat points out, the human and non-human environment play a key role in supporting the independent functioning of the older person.[6]

From a systems perspective, the environment chosen for the ADC program was critical. Thus, a medically focused program would emphasize recovery from illness, while a social/health maintenance program would assume a more proactive stance.

CONSULTATION DESCRIPTION

Organization

This non-profit community organization consisted of 11 appointed board members, a five member professional advisory committee, and one employee, the business administrator who was funded through CETA. While there were no written criteria concerning eligibility for appointment to the board, certain constituencies were evident. Two members were employed by the local hospital (a nurse-administrator and a physician). Three were lawyers, one was the board chairman, another the vice-chairman. The banker on the board was treasurer, and a retired accountant the assistant treasurer. Three were owners of large farm properties (this included two who were also members of the hospital's board of directors) and the remaining member had been the first director of the state's Office on Aging.

The professional advisory committee consisted of 2 family physicians; a social worker from the Community Mental Health Center; the retired director of the county Social Services Department; and the director of the county Office on Aging, who also happened to be a retired nurse.

The administrator was designated as the board secretary. He carried out the day-to-day operations, generated most of the correspondence, handled the bookkeeping and communication with other organizations, arranged for any needed typing, and set up the monthly board meetings. The board rented space in the hospital for their office.

Support

The consultant met first with the board's personnel subcommittee, when she answered their advertisement. The salary offered for the Director's position was less than half of what the consultant earned at the time. She shared this information with the committee and asked them to consider another option, hiring her as a consultant.

At this juncture, she enumerated her qualifications and the advantages her experience would bring to the planning process. Purchasing her services for a limited time would allow the board to stay within budget and the consultant to receive adequate reimbursement.

At the close of the interview, the committee indicated they would consider the proposal while they continued their search. Two weeks later, the consultant was invited to meet with the full board to explain her proposal. Following this meeting, the board voted to engage the consultant to help them develop the program and hire permanent staff. As suggested, the consultant would gradually phase in her time. It was agreed that she would remain with the project until the site was obtained, the program developed and staff hired.

Participants

Key players from the board were the chairman, vice chairman, assistant treasurer, chair of the Personnel Committee and the physician board member. The business administrator for the project was a pivitol figure. Several members of the Advisory Board, who had no vote, were consistent attendees at the meetings and worked behind the scenes, lobbying for their particular perspectives.

The board chairman relied heavily on the business administrator and vice chairman to handle many of the decisions, while keeping him informed. The vice chairman had been more involved in other community organizations and service groups. Since his office was located close to the hospital, he was more available for informal meetings and discussions.

The chair of the Personnel Committee was the nurse-administrator from the hospital. She was most knowledgeable regarding the multiple problems faced by those older persons most at risk. In her position as the hospital's vice president for community services, she had continuous contact with home-care services and other community outreach programs.

The physician, also employed by the hospital, was a senior member of their medical staff. She had practiced in the county for over 40 years, specializing in rheumatology, and had a strong interest in gerontology. She was a very vocal and strong voice on the board.

Among the five members of the Professional Advisory Committee were three very consistent attendees at meetings, who also had important community ties. A family physician (one of two on the committee) with a large geriatric practice, was very anxious to have the ADC become a reality. He had practiced in the county for over 30 years, was widely respected by the medical, religious and general community, and was very active in many community projects.

The director of the county Office on Aging, who had also been a nurse at the hospital before retirement, was a politically astute and knowledgeable member of the Advisory Committee. She knew the consultant from mutual involvement on the Mental Health Board. Her office was the recipient of many inquiries from families and older persons themselves who were anxiously awaiting the ADC program.

The social worker from the Community Mental Health Center (located in the hospital) was also a very committed member of the committee. She too had many clients in need of the service. Since she had attended many Mental Health Board meetings to report on her center's programs, she knew the consultant.

A key figure in this consultation was the business administrator. While he did not have the authority to make major decisions, his was the only consistent, visible community presence regarding the ADC program. He handled the books, correspondence, telephone inquiries, communications with other health and community agencies, and initial site reviews concerning space for the project. As the board secretary, he had been present during all negotiations and dialogue between the board and the consultant.

His background was as a bookkeeper and routing manager for a commercial business. He had no formal training in areas related to ADC, but had read the background materials gathered for the study that had been done 18 months before. He was also thoroughly familiar with the study's final report and had gathered articles regarding ADC programs for an office reference file.

In general, it was evident that everyone was most anxious to see the ADC program take off. How receptive they would be to viewing a model other than medical day care was the question.

Services Provided

The consultants entry into this project did not follow the most traditional route. She had perceived the need and developed a strategy for opening the way. Entry was therefore planned by her, uninvited by the organization, triggered by an opportunistic situation. She was finally invited by the board once they considered her proposal to be in their best interest (see Chapter 6 for a comprehensive discussion on methods of consultation entry).

Her agreement with the board took the form of a board motion to hire her as their consultant until the ADC program became a reality. They agreed to her plan of gradually phasing in time, with one day a week for the first 3 months and 3 days a week thereafter until the project was in place. The consultants responsibilities included:

1. Expanding the Board's knowledge base regarding current "state-of-the-art" ADC programs.
2. Reviewing all previous Certificate of Need (CON) proposals and making recommendations for strengthening the presentation.
3. Meeting with and gathering data from community agencies, organizations and interested professionals who would be potential referral sources.
4. Working with the business administrator regarding identification of potential sites for the program.
5. Developing a program plan for board consideration.
6. Assisting the board in developing referral criteria for clientele.
7. Proposing a plan for hiring staff.

The consultant's first task was to review all prior board deliberations and information regarding their decision to establish a medical day care program. She followed this by meeting individually with Board Advisory Committee members, so that she understood their perspectives. Many informal discussions were also held between the consultant and the business administrator. During this time, it became evident that the administrator had not researched the broader program potential available in a social/health maintenance model. Neither he nor the board were aware of alternative funding sources, outside of Medicaid, that could be used for major support.

With affirmation of her pre-entry diagnosis in hand, the consultant approached the board to request time at their meeting to present an overview of the various models of day care and the implications for the proposed county ADC program. She viewed this educational presentation as a first step in helping the board and its committee consider alternative strategies.

Further information and examples of programs in other rural areas were also needed. At this time, the National Council on Aging (NCOA) had scheduled its annual meeting in the midwest. A highlight of this meeting was to be the formalization of a constituent unit focused on ADC. The consultant felt that this meeting was of extreme importance and could provide the board with valuable, national information.

The consultant therefore requested approval from the board to attend this meeting. She proposed going on her own time, if the board would pay her expenses. Since she was a member of NCOA (the community organization was not), a lower conference fee was available. From the consultant's perspective, this meeting was strategically important as it would provide current data on social/health maintenance programs. This was the more prevalent model nationwide, and successful examples, especially in rural settings, would provide further validation for the board. The board approved her request.

Upon return from this meeting, the consultant had a greatly expanded resource file, extensive national and statewide networking contacts, and solid information regarding alternatives for funding. A meeting of the board and its committee was scheduled to receive the consultant's report. Prior to the meeting, the consultant mailed each person a brief synopsis of her findings and accompanying brochures and information sheets from social/health maintenance ADC programs in other states, along with excerpts from currently published literature.[13]

The information provided, created a more positive view of the social/health maintenance model for all concerned. The consultant followed up on this report with more specific and salient points that helped turn the decision toward the recommended model. The other key points concerned the CON and operating the program on a more limited (less than 5 days a week) basis, in a less formal environment, during its pilot phase.

While a social/health maintenance model could provide access to restorative services, its focus was more preventive in nature. Therefore, it was not classified under the CON process, and no certificate would be required. This model also allowed more flexibility in regard to the number of operational days required. Standards did not exist, and new programs often provided services 1 or 2 days per week. Many of these programs operated in houses of worship or in service organization buildings, where rent costs were either donated or at a minimum.

The presentation resulted in a broad ranging, heated and extensive discussion. Proponents of the medical model were gradually won over by those who saw more potential in the alternative model. Members of the advisory committee were particularly vocal and supportive of the alternative. From their perspective, it would allow quicker resolution of the space issue, and a more immediate response to the community's need. They recommended starting with 3 days a week and saw that as an adequate amount of time for many of the targeted clientele.

The meeting closed with a motion to switch to a social/health maintenance ADC program, which was passed unanimously. The consultant was directed to work with the business administrator to develop the overall plan, help identify space, and propose the program.

The next phase of the consultation focused on identification of space, education of the referral community regarding the model proposed, and development of grant requests and public relations materials.[2] Work progressed rapidly in all areas, and appropriate space was finally identified in a local church which housed many varied community programs.

A major stumbling block then arose. The church board and the ADC board had agreed on all issues, and the program was approved for operation 3 days a week. Since this was a new use, the church board felt it was necessary to check with the Town Planning Board before finalizing the agreement.

The Town Planning Board asked their building inspector to visit the church site regarding ordinance compliance. His report back to this board recommended that they withhold approval as this was a ''medical'' use of space in a community building zoned for social and religious purposes! The consultant and board members met with the inspector (who, at age 82, might have future need for the service) to provide a broader picture of the proposed program and similar programs in other states operating in church settings. The inspector was not to be moved from his recommendation. The Planning Board then advised the ADC board and the church that their only recourse was to request a Use Variance for the church.

Using social actions strategies, the consultant then helped the board activate residents of the town, members of the church, and community organizations, into a unified group advocating for the variance. Letters, petitions, telephone calls to the Planning Board, newspaper articles, and radio interviews alerting the community at large brought the issue to the forefront. The Planning Board then called a special meeting to consider the variance request. Testifying at this meeting were the consultant, board chairman, and director of the Office on Aging. The hearing room was overcrowded with press and many community supporters. The building inspector did not show up to testify, and the variance was granted.

What was initially a stumbling block turned into a very effective piece of publicity. The advocacy generated during the variance hearings also generated innumerable referrals.

At this juncture, the consultant's focus turned toward program planning and working with the business administrator to develop policies, procedures, budgets, and staff requirements. A subcommittee of the professional advisory group worked with the consultant to develop admission criteria and guidelines for a sliding fee scale. A subcommittee of the board worked with her to develop funding proposals targeted to federal and state monies available through the Older American's Act, Title XX of the Social Security Act, and special county funds allocated for low-income older persons.

Once space and program design were approved by the board, the organization was ready to consider hiring a director for the program. The consultant presented various job descriptions to the board for their discussion and review. She helped them identify key skills and experience components needed for the position. With her assistance, they developed a recruitment plan and identified timelines for the process. Once hired, the director would work with the consultant regarding the final phases of program development and start up of the program.

The consultation concluded six weeks after the director was hired. The program had opened its doors, and five county residents were in attendance for up to 3 days a week. During this part of the consultation, the consultant also utilized a case centered consultation approach. The new director, a nurse who had community based experience as the administrator of a county nutrition site, did not have a strong background in functional assessment.[5] Therefore, the consultant provided collegial consultation, helping the director determine specific functional levels for referred clientele. Using her clinical expertise, the consultant identified current needs, which were primarily focused in the areas of self-care and leisure skills and which could be met through the program. She also suggested strategies which might be effective in preventing further decline in particular cases.

As part of the closure process, the consultant met formally with the board and informally with key members to evaluate the consultation. The goals set for the consultation had been achieved. The use of consultation services, rather than employment of a director, had been a cost effective strategy which provided the board with the degree of expertise required during the critical formative period. The board commended the consultant for a job well done and requested that she remain available for possible renegotiation of services, should the need arise.

OUTCOME

This consultation occurred over a decade ago. The ADC program is still housed in what was originally thought to be an interim "first" site. The program now runs 5 days a week, from 7 A.M. to 5 P.M. versus its original 3 day, 10 A.M. to 3 P.M. schedule. The program clientele has expanded from 5 to 30 individuals.

Today's definition of ADC has also changed. Standards have been set by the National Institute on Adult Day Care (NIAD), which is a constituent unit of NCOA. They define ADC as " . . . a community-based group program designed to meet the needs of functionally impaired adults through an individual plan of care. It . . . provides a variety of health, social and related support services in a protective setting during any part of a day . . . ".[11, p. 20] NIAD also views older adults using ADC services as "participants." They view the terms "client" and "patient" as having more of a dependent focus. The term participant . . . "expresses a respect for the individual and an acknowledgement that the person is an active partner"[12, p. 4] in the ADC program.

A day care program may therefore have participants attending who are in need of restorative, health maintenance, and/or social programming. Additionally, funding for ADC participants requiring restorative services may now be obtained in some settings through Medicare as well as through Medicaid.

The ADC program described currently arranges restorative services for its participants on an out-patient basis, at the local hospital. Thus, it is now able to meet the needs of those participants who require a more medically oriented program while providing the necessary maintenance and social programs at the center. While neither the center or the sponsoring community board have used the consultant's services on a formal basis, the consultant has maintained ongoing interest and informal contacts with the program, on a voluntary basis.

From the consultant's perspective, the program's growth and development have more than met initial expectations. From the community's perspective, the ADC program is viewed as an important and necessary part of services provided for older persons in the county.

SUMMARY

Today's functionally oriented and cost conscious society is especially aware of the expanding health needs of older persons. ADC programs are an important preventive strategy for maintaining these frail individuals in the community. Occupational therapy consultants can provide invaluable guidance and expertise to community groups establishing ADC programs. This consultation experience illustrates many varied levels and models of consultation which can be applied to such an experience.

The important contributions of occupational therapy and its roles and functions in ADC, have been delineated by the American Occupational Therapy Association.[7, 9] Occupational therapy consultants can facilitate the development of ADC centers, help assure their maintenance, and provide the case consultation necessary to develop individual plans of care for participants with special needs.

Long-term care has extended its focus beyond institutional walls. Occupational therapy consultants must use their creative abilities in less traditional settings where older persons require health related services. Adult day care programs, nutrition sites, senior centers, and congregate or group living sites are among those to be considered. To improve the quality of life for this population, consultants must develop a diversified knowledge base, expanded resources, and broader system skills. Our aging population, with its multiple needs, will benefit from the expertise that such consultants can provide.

REFERENCES

1. Division of Long-Term Care: *Directory of Adult Day Care Centers.* Baltimore, Md, Health Care Financing Administration, 1980.
2. Epstein CF: The occupational therapy consultant in adult day care programs. *Geron Spec Int Sec Newsltr* 1985; 8:3–4.
3. Jaffe EG: Prevention: "An idea whose time has come": The role of occupational therapy in disease prevention and health promotion. *AJOT* 1986; 39:499–503.
4. Johnson JA: *Wellness: A Context for Living.* Thorofare, NJ, Slack, 1986.
5. Kane RA, Kane RL: *Assessing the Elderly.* Lexington, Mass, Lexington Books, 1983.
6. Kiernat JM: Environment: The hidden modality. *Phys Occup Ther Ger* 1982; 2:3–12.
7. Levy LL: Occupational therapy in adult day care. *AJOT* 1986; 40:814–816.
8. Llorens LA: Changing balance: environment and individual. *AJOT* 1984; 38:29–34.
9. Macdonald KC, Epstein CF: Roles and functions of occupational therapy in adult day care. *AJOT* 1986; 40:817–821.

10. Matsutsuyu JS: Occupational behavior: A perspective on work and play. *AJOT* 1971; 25:291–294.
11. National Institute on Adult Daycare: *Standards for Adult Day Care*. Washington DC, National Council on the Aging, 1984.
12. National Institute on Adult Daycare: *Adult Day Care: A Treatment Program for Persons with Functional Impairments*. Washington DC, National Council on the Aging, 1990.
13. Padula H: *Developing Day Care for Older People*. Washington, DC, National Council on the Aging, 1972.
14. Reilly M: *Play as Exploratory Learning*. Beverly Hills, Calif, Sage, 1974.
15. Weiler PG, Rathbone-McCuan E: *Adult Day Care: Community Work With the Elderly*. New York, Springer, 1978.

SECTION E

Occupational Therapy Consultation in Industrial Settings

One of the fastest growing areas for occupational therapy consultation is in the realm of business and industry. As discussed in Chapters 3 and 7, the escalating costs of health care have had a major impact on employee health costs, resulting in increased prices of many products. Most large corporations and even some small businesses need to reduce costs resulting from employee injury, accidents, environmental hazards, and poor health or lifestyle habits. Loss of employee productivity, high workers' compensation claims, and expensive health benefit packages have resulted in intolerable levels of industrial health costs. Additionally, recent legislation affecting industrial work and hiring policies have caused businesses and industry to seek consultation in adapting the work environment to conform to regulations. Occupational therapy consultants may utilize their skills in environmental and task analysis, remediation of industrial disability, and preventive health education and provide state-of-the-art ergonomic and technical assistance to develop cost-effective industrial programs.

Jacobs provides an example of a self-employed independent consultant to business and industry, utilizing educational, behavioral, and administrative models of consultation. She presents two case studies that emphasize the need for the consultant in these settings to develop business and marketing skills. The case studies illustrate the consultation process in action and the essential phases of systems analysis, identification of the key power individuals, and negotiation of contract in a business setting.

The role of the internal consultant in industry is explored by Ellexson. Diverse consultant responsibilities are described, including consultation regarding appropriate rehabilitation care costs, work station analysis, employee education, program planning for prevention of injuries, and the rehabilitation and return to work of the injured worker. Throughout the discussion there is an emphasis on the consultant's need to assure the support of the system and be aware of the influences of industrial health care costs and legislative regulations.

An employee health education program to improve access to quality care and reduce employee health costs is described by Jaffe. The major external environmental and economic changes resulting from rapidly escalating costs of employee health care are detailed as the impetus for the project. The focus of the program is the health education and health promotion of the employee as the medical consumer. Using an educational and systems approach, Jaffe discusses the role of the external occupational therapy consultant as facilitator of a corporate health education program.

Industrial Settings

AUTHOR	MODEL	LEVEL	LOCUS	GOAL
Jacobs	Program Development System and Educational Program Development	Levels II and III: Educational and administrative/program planning	Industrial consultation business; corporation	Facilitate market analysis for program planning; develop employee health education program to reduce disability from back injuries
Ellexson	Educational Program Development and Systems	Levels II and III: Educational and program planning administrative	Industrial corporation	Develop rehabilitation program for injured workers; Facilitate implementation of program through change agent strategies for system acceptance
Jaffe	Educational Program Development and Systems	Levels II and III: Educational and administrative	Corporations	Improve consumer awareness, understanding and access to health care system; develop cost-effective health education program to reduce corporate health costs

433

CHAPTER 26

Occupational Therapy Consultation in Business and Industry

Karen Jacobs, M.S., O.T.R./L., F.A.O.T.A.

OVERVIEW

As a self-employed, independent consultant, the author undertakes short-term consultations for specific tasks almost exclusively, specializing in work programming with an emphasis on marketing. A broad portfolio of consulting is offered: seminars, in-service training, market research and analysis, product assessment/analysis, and work program development. In addition, services provided are in the area of recruitment, retention, and supervision, and to a limited degree direct client assessment and treatment/programming.

Consultation experiences have been in a variety of settings including rehabilitation hospitals/centers and schools, public and private schools, and an educational collaborative. Additionally, the author has consulted with business/industry and private practitioners.

Initially, there was more diversity in the consultation practice. During the early stages the practice included evaluation, treatment, and in-service training to a geriatric rehabilitation center on a 4-hour per week basis for 2 years. Additionally, evaluations of learning disabled young adults and adolescents for future work potential, supervision of a COTA/L 1 hour weekly at an educational collaborative, and evaluations of severely developmentally delayed adolescents to ascertain appropriate work programming placement in a secondary school environment were provided.

In more recent years, consultation activities have concentrated on in-service training, seminars and lectures/workshops on the topics of work programming, and the development of market analyses. These presentations were offered at educational institutions including universities, public schools, and an educational collaborative; at rehabilitation clinics; at parent and community groups, and at state occupational therapy association meetings. Specific market analyses have been performed for The Work System, a standardized industrial rehabilitation assessment, and for rehabilitation professionals developing and maintaining industrial rehabilitation private practices. Job analyses for various jobs within industry have been additional consultations. Many times these consultations also involve recommendations to employers for compliance with Title I of the Americans with Disabilities Act (ADA).

Another consultation experience included use of the Jacobs Prevocational Skills Assessment (JPSA) for an adolescent head-injured population.[3] On an ongoing basis, consultation is also provided to a large corporation that specializes in crafts and health care products to analyze how clients may benefit by using their product line. This information is incorporated into their catalogues as a marketing device.

Establishment of this solo consultation practice required the development of business skills in finance and marketing. To acquire needed entrepreneurial skills, the author enrolled in a marketing course at a local university and began attending various small business and financial workshops. Various resources by Drucker,[2] Kotler and Clarke,[4] and Von Oech[6, 7] also served to expand this needed knowledge base.

ENVIRONMENT AND SYSTEMS INFLUENCES

Rehabilitation is now seen by corporations and employers as a cost-effective means of returning employees to work quickly. In addition, most employers are now interested in keeping health care costs down with the inclusion of disease and injury prevention and health promotion programs. This has provided a positive climate for industrial rehabilitation programs. For example, one of the greatest causes of economic distress is absenteeism, disability, and morbidity caused by low back pain (LBP) problems.

"It has been estimated that the total cost of all aspects of LBP care, including medical, compensation, legal, vocational, retraining occupational modifications, and lost industrial productivity may be in the range of $40 billion to $50 billion annually."[5]

Work hardening has become one of the fastest-growing industrial rehabilitation treatment services. Competition within this field has become acute, with many types of rehabilitation facilities vying for a market share. Through the use of marketing expertise, occupational therapy work hardening programs can select those program aspects that will help them keep pace with economic trends. These include the shrinking availability of health care dollars and increased costs of care. The application of marketing principles may be a key to survival for work hardening programs.

FRAME OF REFERENCE

Occupational therapy practice inherently deals with the whole person and all facets of the individual's functioning. The author incorporates this basic premise in her role as a consultant. Depending on the type of consultation, the role may be one of problem solver, educator, troubleshooter, sounding board, extra hands and feet, resident sage, adviser, guidance counselor, liaison, expediter, researcher, and marketeer. Marketing philosophy is the basic aspect of this author's consultation practice.

The frame of reference for the first consultation case study (case study I) presented is based on a program development model, which is defined in this text as a service-centered model based on the development of new service programs or modification of existing programs to improve services. Consultation occurred on a level III. That is, consultation was targeted on the specific system (e.g., World of Work) with the focus being centered on that system to promote institutional change by means of administrative or program consultation. See Chapter 2 for consultation models and levels. This case is a 1-day model of consultation.

Case study II is an ongoing consultative intervention that incorporates two models of consultation. The educational model, which is "an information-centered model in which the consultant utilizes activities such as staff development, in-service training, or human resource development where the consultant is an educator and trainer"[4] was used during one aspect of the consultation intervention. During another aspect of this longer type of consultation, a behavioral model, that is, a behavior-focused model in which emphasis is on control, adaptation, modification or change of learned behavior was utilized. Differing from the 1-day model, consultation in case study II occurred on level II. That is, consultation was targeted on the consultee (e.g., employees of Chelsea Fruits & Vegetables, Inc.), with the focus being client-centered to improve functioning, efficiency, and ability.

CONSULTATION DESCRIPTION

ONE-DAY MODEL OF CONSULTATION: CASE STUDY I

Organization

World of Work (WOW) is a free-standing private practice located within a small business park in a moderately sized city in New England. WOW is owned and operated by a physical therapist and vocational rehabilitation counselor who both specialize in industrial rehabilitation. Programming is provided by an interdisciplinary team including occupational therapy, physical therapy, and vocational rehabilitation. The clinical director is an occupational therapist.

WOW had been in existence for a number of years and had a product line that included assessment, job analysis, work hardening, and industrial consultation. It utilized state-of-the-art high and low technical equipment, evaluation instruments, and devices/tools. When established, WOW was the only free-standing, independently operated, industrial rehabilitation program within a 10-mile radius of its city. However, at the time of the consultation, other programs had developed, and competition had increased tenfold. WOW was vying for a viable niche in this market. The owners recognized that WOW was at a turning point. Critical issues of concern were limited space, which prevented increasing caseloads, and limited time for marketing the program. Therefore, the following questions were raised:

1. Should WOW expand its physical space to accommodate a larger caseload?
2. Should an individual be hired to oversee marketing?

The author was hired as a consultant to assist in the decision-making process. The consultation included a one-day interactive market analysis and in-service training on marketing and the field of industrial rehabilitation and a problem-solving session with the three top administrative people (key power players).

Prior to the consultation, the author requested the following information: demographics and statistical data including type and number of referrals, program descriptions, floor plan of the clinic, organizational structure, public relations material, and operating costs.

Support

Consultation services were offered by the day at a daily rate, plus expenses such as travel time, mileage, hotel, meals, and child-care costs. Half-day and hourly rates were also available. In addition there was a rate for development of written material, such as a marketing plan, a list of suggested equipment, and floor plan designs. The company was billed directly by the consultant and payment was received upon receipt of the bill (see Appendix D for a sample copy of the contract).

Participants

The key power players were the two owners of WOW, a physical therapist and a vocational rehabilitation counselor, and the clinical director, an experienced occupational therapist.

Services Provided

Entry to this program was gained through invitation of the clinical director who had attended an educational presentation conducted by the author. The consultant's business cards were distributed to participants at this presentation with a brochure outlining the kinds of consultation services available. This successful personal marketing strategy frequently resulted in new consultation contracts. The clinical director of WOW brought the card to the owners with a description of the consultant's experience in work programming and marketing.

During the initial contact with the consultant, the clinical director of WOW expressed the need for assistance in the area of marketing and for an update on the field of industrial rehabilitation. A fee schedule was discussed during this first contact and the written fee schedule and consultant's curriculum vitae were mailed to the clinical director.

Negotiation of Contract/Fee

Approximately a week following the initial contact, the second contact was made by one of the owners. A 1-day fee with expenses was then negotiated and mutually accepted along with the consultee's expectations for the 1-day consultation. Finally, a mutually convenient date for the initial consultation was arranged. Two copies of the contract, along with a self-addressed and stamped envelope, were mailed to the directors on the following day. The contract included both the responsibilities of the consultant and consultees. For example, the consultant would do the following:

1. Tour WOW to access the program and gain initial information on the overall situation.
2. Provide a half-day lecture/in-service on how to perform a market analysis and the field of industrial rehabilitation.
3. Provide a half day of problem solving, utilizing the market analysis information gleaned during the in-service training period (see Appendix D).

Establishment of Trust

Once the tour of WOW was completed, the consultant and consultees adjourned to a quiet, comfortable office. The milieu was relaxed and free from distractions, including telephone. The next 30 minutes involved an exchange of information that helped both the consultant and consultees understand each other's experiences and frames of reference. The consultant briefly described her various experiences within the field of work programming, and the consultees discussed theirs. This exchange helped the consultees understand and value the resources the consultant could provide, assisted the clients/consultees in developing confidence in the consultant, and provided the consultant with the background and expertise of the consultees.

The consultant provided a packet of material to the three consultees that was used in the market analysis of WOW. This follow along packet was based on the information received prior to the initial day's consultation and was written in clear, easy to follow language.

One strategy that was found useful to assist in the decision-making process was the *force field analysis*. This is the process of having the consultees list all of the positive and negative factors that might have an impact on issues, such as, (1) remaining at the present physical space; (2) expanding the physical space; (3) continuing without the assistance of a marketing specialist; and (4) obtaining outside assistance in marketing. Information learned during this process included each consultee's subjective opinion as well.

Maintenance of the Consultation (Ongoing Phase)

During the interactive in-service on marketing, which incorporated trends in the field of industrial rehabilitation, the consultant served as both an educator and a sounding board for the client's problems. During this consultation one of the best strategies was that of a good listener.

Evaluation

Feedback on whether the consultee's needs were being met was ongoing throughout the 1-day consultation.

Possible Renegotiation

The consultant contacted one of the key power individuals regularly on a 6-month basis for an update of the program. Additional in-service training and formal marketing of WOW may be negotiated in the future.

Outcome

The 1-day consultation provided the catalyst for the owners to hire a part-time individual as a marketing specialist for WOW. The marketing specialist, after performing a formal market analysis, suggested that WOW expand its physical space and target its marketing efforts toward physicians. Six months later, WOW expanded its physical space and was able to double its caseload. One year after increased marketing efforts targeted at physicians, WOW's caseload was again at its maximum capacity in its newly expanded space.

CONSULTATION DESCRIPTION

ONGOING CONSULTATION: CASE STUDY II

Organization

Chelsea Fruits & Vegetables, Inc. is a wholesale distributor of fresh fruits and vegetables in the greater Boston area. It is located in a one-story warehouse building in the center of the produce district. This company employed more than 200 workers.

Recently, the company was purchased and the new management became concerned with the numerous incidences of employee back pain/injuries occurring on the loading dock. The medical director evaluated these injured workers and indicated that there was a need for employee education regarding the use of proper body mechanics.

This consultant was hired to perform job analyses and develop a health educational program. The consultation included the development of a 6-month back injury prevention program.

Support

As in case study I, the consultant discussed her policy of direct billing to the consultee with the manager. Hourly, half-day, daily, and total package rates were provided. In addition, expenses such as travel time, mileage, meals, child care, audiovisual (e.g., videotaping and photographing the job site), the hiring of an assistant to videotape, and an individual to implement a stress management program, were presented. A contract for a customized back injury prevention program was developed and a cost for the total package established.

Participants

The key power players were the warehouse manager and the supervisor of the loading dock. The target population for which the prevention program was designed were 40 employees whose duties were loading and unloading crates of fruits and vegetables. In addition, three of these employees were participants in the job analyses.

Services Provided

Referral to this company came through their medical director. This physician had attended one of the consultant's "Industrial Rehabilitation: State of the Art" workshops held at a local rehabilitation center. The consultant was an invited speaker for a one-hour presentation to an audience of physicians and allied health professionals. At this conference, the physician approached the consultant concerning the increased incidence of back injuries he had noticed within one particular job at the company's warehouse. He expressed interest in the development of a prevention program to help address the escalating workers' compensation costs incurred from an increase of absenteeism due to low back injuries. The consultant suggested performing a needs assessment focused on job analyses. From the results, a prevention program could be developed.

Negotiation of Contract/Fee

One week after the conversation with the medical director, the consultant received referrals for job analyses of three employees. The consultant contacted the warehouse manager the following day. After a brief telephone conversation, arrangements were made for a tour of the warehouse and a meeting with the manager. After the tour, the manager described the increased incidence of absenteeism associated with back injuries for loading dock employees. Through the negotiated contract, arrangements were made for the consultant to perform job analyses of employees working at the loading dock. The consultant requested permission to videotape and photograph these employees. Appropriate permission slips were drafted and signed by both the manager and employees. Having a videotape of a job analysis was found useful in past consultation experiences, particularly in the development of a more personalized employee prevention program. A technician was hired by the consultant to videotape the job analyses.

Based on the results of the three job analyses and interviews with both the manager and supervisor on their perceptions of the job demands, the consultant recommended the development of a prevention program that would include the following components:

1. Lectures on the anatomy and physiology of the back
2. General overview of the principles of appropriate body mechanics
3. Practical application of the principles of body mechanics to the employees, specific to the job demands
4. Lectures on stress management
5. Lectures on the importance of physical fitness
6. Establishment of a 15-minute morning stretching program

The consultant then proposed a 6-month contract, which would be entered into at a packaged rate. This rate was negotiated and a mutually agreeable amount was established. The initial cost of the three job analyses was factored into the packaged rate.

The consultant composed a contract to include both the responsibilities of the consultant and consultee. The consultant's responsibilities included the following prevention intervention strategies:

1. Four 1-hour lecture and slide presentations on anatomy and physiology to groups of 10 employees.
2. Four 1-hour lecture and slide presentations on the principles of appropriate body mechanics and lifting techniques, including printed material. Photographs of employees performing the job were used in the lectures to personalize the program.

3. Establishment of two weekly 30-minute stress management groups for employees to learn effective methods for coping with stress. A COTA/L, hired by the consultant, implemented this program. Employee participation was voluntary.

4. Four 1-hour lecture and slide presentations on the importance of stretching, review of proper stretching techniques, and strengthening and conditioning exercises.

5. Establishment of a mandatory 15-minute stretching program to be implemented daily by the consultant's hired COTA/L. Development of a video-tape of employees in the stretching program to be used in the sessions as a motivator.

6. Daily monitoring of the prevention program by the consultant either in person or by telephone.[1]

Two copies of the contract, along with a self-addressed and stamped envelope were mailed to the manager. One copy was returned to the consultant; the other was retained for the consultee's files. In addition, a billing schedule was agreed upon.

Establishment of Trust

The content for lectures was discussed with the manager prior to implementation. Permission had been granted to videotape and photograph the dock workers at the job site so that a personalized program could be developed. The 2-week process of taking photographs and videotaping along with meeting daily with the manager allowed the consultant to become better acquainted with the daily operations of the company and to become a familiar face to the employees. This visibility assisted in gaining their trust.

Maintenance of the Consultation (Ongoing Phase)

Throughout the consultation experience, the consultant served many roles. During lectures, her role was that of an educator and problem solver, addressing issues such as "When should I ask someone to assist in lifting a crate"? and "How can I tell how heavy a crate is before lifting it"?

When meeting with the manager and supervisor, the consultant served in the capacity of an educator and sounding board. In this capacity, the consultant was an empathic listener and also offered suggestions for solutions.

Possible Renegotiation

After completion of the 6-month contract, the consultant renegotiated for an additional 6 months to provide monthly 1-hour presentations on appropriate body mechanics and lifting techniques for new employees. She also provided a refresher program for those employees needing additional assistance. The morning stretching program was continued; however, the stress management program was discontinued, since similar programs were available within the community and employees were encouraged to attend.

Outcome

Six months after the initiation of the prevention program, there was a 65% reduction in absenteeism due to back injuries/pain for employees on the loading dock. One year after the initiation of the program, there continued to be a reduction in back injuries. This may be due, in part, to an arrangement with the local YMCA to provide a discount fee for Chelsea employees to enroll in physical fitness programs as a result of the consultant's educational presentations and employees' heightened awareness of the need for physical activities.

SUMMARY

Consulting should be a highly personalized service, in which the consultant attempts to see things from the client's perspective, yet remain objective. During the various steps of consultation, the consultant may wear many hats: troubleshooter, problem solver, adviser, sounding board, extra hands and feet, resident sage, marketer, researcher, guidance counselor, expeditor, and liaison. It is only through experience that the consultant can become attuned to which strategies are appropriate during each step in the consultation process.

The acquisition of business skills, including marketing techniques, has become critical for today's occupational therapy consultant. Marketing skills can be developed through enrollment in courses and workshops on the subject, and through application of techniques in one's own practice. Proficiency in this area will allow experienced occupational therapy consultants to incorporate marketing analyses to their product line. Utilizing marketing strategies, the occupational therapy consultant may establish a market niche within the growing field of industrial rehabilitation, injury/accident prevention programs, and industrial health promotion programs. While opportunities for consultation in industrial rehabilitation continue to expand, initiative and creativity are needed to enter into this marketplace.

REFERENCES

1. Bettencourt C: An accident/injury prevention program for occupational therapy employees. *Occup Ther Practice* 1990;1:52.
2. Drucker P: *Innovation and Entrepreneurship: Practice and Principles*. New York, Harper & Row, 1985.

3. Jacobs K: *Occupational Therapy: Work Related Programs and Assessments.* Boston, Little, Brown, 1985.
4. Kotler P, Clarke R: *Marketing for Health Care Organizations.* Englewood Cliffs, NJ, Prentice Hall, 1987.
5. Sutherland R, Counihan W: Functional restoration for the back injured worker: A sports medicine approach. *Occup Ther Practice* 1990;1:1.
6. Von Oech R: *A Kick in the Seat of the Pants.* New York, Harper & Row, 1986.
7. Von Oech R: *A Whack on the Side of the Head.* New York, Warner, 1983.

CHAPTER 27

Industrial Consultation as an Internal Consultant

Melanie T. Ellexson, M.B.A., O.T.R., F.A.O.T.A.

OVERVIEW

During the 1960s and 1970s escalating workers' compensation costs, injury rates, and lost work days forced the industrial marketplace to rethink its strategies for coping with occupational injury. Among the first to develop a nontraditional approach toward controlling these problems were the railroads.

In 1979 the author was hired as a full-time employee of the Chicago, Milwaukee, St. Paul and Pacific (CMSP&P) Railroad. The position required functioning as a consultant and change agent for the operating departments, the legal/claims staff, and management. Many roles were required during this 7-year internal consultancy. One was as a consultant to the legal department on appropriate rehabilitation care, costs, and job accommodations. Another role was to middle management as a partner in restricted work program development, employee education, prevention, job and work station design. Acting as a consultant and case manager for hundreds of employees in 17 states, a program was developed to help workers access the medical/rehabilitation system, cope with periods of disability, and eventually return to work.

Management support was elicited for recommendations concerning program development and education. They helped change work rules that were steeped in labor union tradition once they understood the importance of the recommended changes. In one 18-month period, occupational therapy consultative services were credited with a savings of $1.5 million. Another program reduced back injuries among track laborers by more than 50% over a 3-year period.

This chapter describes many of the ways an occupational therapist acting as an internal consultant can use her unique combination of skills to effect a cost savings to industry and improve the quality of life for industrially injured workers. Initially, the consultant must learn about the company. Information must be gathered in regard to its product, its goals, its perceived status in the marketplace, its view of

445

itself in relationship to others in the industry, its profit motivation, its return on investment philosophy, the strength of its bottom line, its largest problems in production, its injury problems in relationship to the bigger picture of company goals, where its injuries occur and why, its number one injury and the reason for its occurrence, and what workers' compensation system covers its workers.

Most of this information can be obtained from talking with management, reading corporate literature such as annual reports, reviewing injury loss records, and carefully reviewing the prevailing workers' compensation law. Once the consultant is knowledgeable about the company and its corporate structure, she can begin to develop a framework of consultation possibilities. Knowledge about the company helps gain acceptance of a plan of action and the establishment of goals to meet the needs of the industry.

It would have been inappropriate for the author to go into the Milwaukee Road as their occupational therapy consultant and present a program establishing a full service clinic and work hardening program. The company was in financial trouble, they were spread over 17 states, and they were made up of numerous autonomous divisions and departments. Rehabilitation for the injured worker was an idea identified by management personnel who lacked a real understanding of its benefits or possibilities. Knowledge of this corporate structure and culture, financial situation, injury history, and work produced helped the consultant to develop appropriate programs and services that would be accepted, tried, and proven effective.

ENVIRONMENT AND SYSTEMS INFLUENCES

At the time the author was hired by the CMSP&P, railroads were in dire financial difficulties. Bankruptcy had been declared by the CMSP&P, and the lines west of Minnesota were for sale to the highest bidder. Financial stress appeared to precipitate tighter controls, and rehabilitation efforts were employed as stop-gap measures to plug draining leaks on the already threatened railroad cash flow. Utilization of an occupational therapist's services to consult on work injuries was not considered by the railroad until economic conditions forced management to look carefully at where expenses might be reduced. Even then, only those managers understanding the need to spend dollars to save dollars looked at rehabilitation as a possible means of controlling cash shortfall.

In an environment of economic stress it is common to see injuries increase. This phenomenon translates into an increase in financial losses as measured by lost employee time from work. Individuals may be preoccupied with the threat of unemployment and become careless. Layoffs and cutbacks may require individuals to perform more with less help, to work at a faster pace, or to work longer hours. Physical fatigue as well as emotional conflict may bring about less safe work practices. The security of regular workers' compensation wage replacement payment and the often reduced stress of being away from the work site may be more realistic reasons for continued disability after injury than the injury itself. Regardless of why injuries occur or the stress that may increase their frequency, they will happen and continue to be an economic drain on any business.

A look at historical accident records gave the occupational therapy consultant insight into the jobs or activities that related to the injuries. Identification of the type of injuries most often reported, such as the cause and effect of lifting and low back claims or climbing and knee complaints, provided valuable information for planning rehabilitation, education, and ergonomic change programs.

It has been said that it requires 20 years to assimilate change into the job or job environment. This is clear in many manufacturing, material handling, and repair industries. Individuals may be slow to accept new ideas, equipment, or to change lifetime practices, particularly in an industry like the railroad where union rules, long-term employment, and a 100-year practice of patching rather than rebuilding are the norm. In newer industries, such as those producing computers or robotics, the technology may be so new that no thought is given to possible errors in design or methods of practice. An attitude of "it's new, it must be right," or conversely, "it's been done this way since the plant opened, it must be right," is often the prevailing attitude of management and workers.

FRAME OF REFERENCE

There are two major theoretical concepts applicable to occupational therapy consultation in industry. The first was expressed by Hall in 1913 when he described starting a workshop "to fill the dangerous interval immediately after hospital discharge and before regular work can be attempted."[3] This concept of bridging the gap between acute care and return to work is basic to both a company-initiated restricted work program and the work hardening programs available today. The second theory is the "meaning-centered" framework of clinical reasoning described by Mattingly.[4] The role of the occupational therapy consultant is to observe and assess a given situation and put together the interventions necessary to obtain the desired response. The occupational therapist's skills prepare her well to deal with the worker's experience with illness or injury and how that individual perceives and responds to the injury and rehabilitation process.

The meaning-centered concept of clinical reasoning emphasizes the therapist's role of engaging the "patients/clients in a therapeutic process that requires their active participation."[4] Helping both individual and groups or organizations to recognize the injury (ergonomic, safety, education problem) and enabling them to gain control of the situation through responsible, self-directed actions is unquestionably a role for occupational therapy consultation in industry.

Consultation with industry is multifaceted and requires more than one approach and the employment of a variety of consultation models. In the clinical or case management model, the consultant focuses on the worker's problems and ability to develop a specific plan of action for rehabilitation. When the consultant uses an educational or information-centered model, the role is one of educator/trainer to worker, supervisor, and management. A program development model may also be employed to address the design and implementation of a specific project. The systems approach is inherent in the consultation plan. The consultant must have a concise understanding of the industry and the particular setting in order to effect change.

The understanding and acceptance of a company's environment, goals, culture, and mission are essential if the consultant is to help bring about change. Assuming the role of expert without a thorough assessment of the organization and its members dooms one to failure. Recognition of others' expertise allows the consultant to work effectively and to reach the outcomes identified for a successful change. Examples might be to ask a first-line supervisor to teach you how to complete a particular task or to seek the advice of a claims officer in regard to a particular labor rule.

Most commonly utilized by the occupational therapy consultant is the clinical or case management model. In this model the consultation focus is on an individual's problems and abilities. The consultant develops a specific plan of action that allows for the best rehabilitation. In this model the consultant may perform the following tasks:

- Develop a relationship with both the injured worker and the family
- Identify medical specialists, rehabilitation therapies, and providers that are necessary for the particular worker's needs
- Arrange for the services of the medical/rehabilitation professionals
- Obtain any necessary approvals from claims officers, insurance companies, or management
- Explain the plan to the worker, the family, and the company
- Constantly review progress toward recovery
- Plan with the worker and the job supervisor for return to work
- Review and revise the plan as progress is made
- Troubleshoot and anticipate problems or obstacles
- Guide the plan through to completion
- Follow up to assure that a successful outcome continues
- Cut the cord at the appropriate time

The consultant must not become the repository for work or worker complaints that are unrelated to the injury or illness which initiated the case management relationship.

In the educational or information-centered model, there is a role for the consultant as both educator and trainer. Educating management and workers about the value of rehabilitation, the resources available, and the potential outcome in a way that they will both understand and buy into is a very important and valuable contribution for the consultant to make to industry. Training in both general areas, such as injured worker management and technical training in body mechanics, safe work practices, or general fitness, are also valuable contributions.

The assessment, design, implementation, and evaluation of a specific situation and its resultant solution are components of a program development model often employed in consultation. Both new and existing programs may benefit from the occupational therapy consultant's ability to observe, evaluate, and offer alternative solutions. For example, managing the medical care provided and working with the injured worker toward a return to work requires a program that initiates timely contact, includes family consultation, and allows for flexibility.

The occupational therapist who is an internal consultant to industry may identify various levels, or layers of consultation. As stated, the most common, and frequently the easiest to implement, is the case-centered model. Initially, there must be a plan for identifying the cases. There are several ways of accomplishing this.

Industry standards frequently use 30 days of lost time as a benchmark for active intervention. In this model, the consultant must identify those individuals injured and off work for 30 days without a definite return-to-work date. This may be accomplished by prepared lists from claims, operating, or personnel departments. In other situations, it may be necessary for the consultant to track all injuries and establish a system to bring up those individuals off work at the 30-day mark. Another approach may be to use the company physician, claims officer, or manager to identify cases needing intervention. The periodic weekly or monthly department or service area meeting may also serve as a good source. Here, top managers and supervisors from specific areas of the company meet to identify, discuss, and participate in the case management of their injured employees.

Regardless of the method of identification for case consultation, clear assignment of the consultant's responsibilities must be established. Direct contact, record access, and service authorization are essential to good case management. Once a case has been identified, it is important that the consultant establish a relationship with the individual worker and frequently with the family or significant others. Workers may initially be distrustful of the consultant's motives, fearing that they are but one more person checking up on them or trying to disprove their injury. This adversarial attitude of distrust often has been fostered by both past practice, union attitudes, and attorneys specializing in workers' compensation claims. In the case of serious injury, it is not unusual to see a plaintiff's attorney walking out of a hospital room as the consultant and/or claims officer arrive.

A careful explanation of the consultant's role, her responsibility to both the worker and the company, and her experience, professional qualifications, and expertise will frequently help defuse negative attitudes. It will pave the way for the establishment of a relationship of professional trust. Additionally, quick solutions to immediate problems, such as informing the worker of how to collect wage replacement monies, arranging for transportation to physician appointments, and getting medical bills paid or directed to the appropriate source of payment will help establish the consultant as a valuable resource.

The next step is a careful review of the individual's current medical care and understanding of his or her level of satisfaction with that care. It is wise not to challenge an individual's choice of physician or caregiver or the care provider's credentials. Rather, offer several alternatives for a more extensive or specialized evaluation. However, there may be times when the consultant must impose the applicable workers' compensation law that require further evaluation. Most workers' compensation laws allow a company to mandate evaluation, if not treatment, and to require the injured worker to cooperate in his or her own rehabilitation[1, p69] It is the consultant's responsibility to fully inform the worker of the need for any additional evaluation and to explain any treatment recommended. Additionally, it is the consultant's role to explain the worker's job, company's concerns or issues, and problems and possible solution to the physician or care providers so that a potentially successful plan can be established. It is also the responsibility of the consultant to keep the company informed of all medical and rehabilitation plans, the individual's progress, and possible problems. The consultant must educate management, including the claims officer, about the medical or rehabilitation problem and its potential outcome. It is also the consultant's responsibility to seek the assistance, cooperation, and recommendations of the company managers to solve problems and develop a plan to return employees to work.

CONSULTATION DESCRIPTION

Organization

The author was hired as an internal consultant by the CMSP&P to develop rehabilitation programs for its injured workers. When the consultation began, little was being done to address the special needs and circumstances that prevailed in workers' compensation cases. Several other major railroads had attempted to control escalating compensation costs and lost days from worker injury. They utilized internal vocational specialists to work with those individuals unable to return to their former jobs. While this plan was effective in some cases, there remained a vast number of individuals who might have returned to work if timely rehabilitation had been started. Still others were in a limbo situation where they were placed on restricted work activities by their physician, which precluded their return to work, but who could not be declared permanently disabled.

The CMSP&P was in bankruptcy reorganization at this time. The company officers were dedicated to finding creative ways to reduce costs and improve productivity. Due to the uncertain financial situation, injuries were on the increase. This is a situation often seen by companies at time of layoff or cutbacks. The increased tension and stress felt by the workers created situations that resulted in more injuries.

At first, the consultant's task seemed overwhelming. There was obviously no way to provide direct treatment to employees spread over 17 states. Instructions were to do something that would get people back to work and reduce claims costs. Over a period of several months, the author's role evolved into that of a internal consultant to the claims officer, operating managers, labor relations staff, and top management.

The consultation described focuses on internal consultation. The author's definition of internal consultation is when one is employed by the company to provide service solely to the employees of that company. An internal consultant usually has staff, not line, authority for rehabilitation decisions.

Support

Support from the top and the granting of enough authority to make decisions regarding both services and programs is extremely important for the internal consultant role. Facilitating change cannot be done by one person or one idea. The consultant must have enough support to plan and recommend methods that will facilitate the desired change. Winning small battles and developing an army is one strategy. An example of developing support in this manner was used at the CMSP&P. As mentioned earlier, there was an atmosphere of distrust and an apparent need to protect turf among the claims people. Many had been in their respective positions for a number of years and had become somewhat cynical regarding the injured workers. None were trained formally in medical practice, medical terminology, rehabilitation, or counseling. They had enjoyed absolute authority over a case often to the point of directing medical care. The occupational therapy consultant was unknown and perceived as a threat to their authority and a challenge to their practice.

A well-planned, carefully thought out process of education on a case-by-case basis eventually built a strong alliance. Getting an individual claims officer to agree to a rehabilitation plan different from the usual approach and introducing aggressive therapy measures that sometimes required the injured worker to travel or become an inpatient was a very new approach. In each case where the individual was able to return to work and time lost from the job was reduced, a small battle was won. Over time, the claims officers came to depend on the occupational therapy consultant for planning and coordinating the implementation of care. They began to support ideas and programs put forth by the consultant and were indeed an army of voices to push forward the rehabilitation program. The most effective way of gaining their support was by careful documentation of cost-effective rehabilitation plans and the sharing of resources and information regarding injuries and treatment methods. The results were a win-win situation. The claims officers became more knowledgeable and therefore more tolerant of the injured workers. The workers were treated more quickly, effectively, and with better results, reducing not only lost time from work but adversarial relationships and legal action.

Participants

In this internal consultation situation, there were four major concerns: (1) plan the process or program to be implemented; (2) organize the plan around the people involved; (3) lead the people through the plan; and (4) help control the pace of the process.

As information was being gathered about this new work environment, it became clear that not only were there injured workers in need of rehabilitation services, but that the industry itself needed educational programs regarding the potential for employee rehabilitation. Without a basis for understanding the consultant's role and process, work could not begin.

The industry had to be treated first. Claims officers were very protective of their domain and the cases they handled. Rehabilitation to them meant money spent on training and education for job placement outside the industry. They relied heavily on medical reports from treating physicians who may or may not have provided appropriate care. In many instances the medical care was provided in small and/or rural towns where therapy services were not available. Back, leg, and hand injuries were often treated for months with rest and medication. Introducing medical specialists and therapies into this industry meant spending more money without any proof that the end result would be effective. The claims people had to be educated about the benefits of aggressive treatment and the cost savings in the reduction of lost time from work.

The operations managers were very skeptical regarding the provision of restricted work assignments or job site modifications. Their arguments were twofold. One, that they would lose productivity if an employee could not produce 100%. The comment was often heard, ''We cannot run this place with a bunch of cripples.'' The second concern was that if one person was allowed restrictions, then everyone would claim injury in order to get an easier job. There was no understanding of a gradual reentry approach to work. They firmly believed that an individual could be totally disabled for 6 months and return to work at full capacity the first day back. There was no consideration of recruitment, hiring, or training costs for replacement workers because these expenses normally did not come from their budget.

The labor relations staff were concerned that rehabilitation efforts, particularly restricted duty or job accommodation, would conflict with union rules and create contract disputes. There were 26 different union contracts to reckon with, and each had specific rules regarding seniority and the individual worker's right to judge his or her own fitness for work. Fortunately, the consultant had been able to educate top management regarding the benefit of rehabilitation, and they made a commitment to establish a rehabilitation program through the use of an internal consultant.

All of the problems were certainly not one-sided. The author, like most practitioners in health care at the time, came from a traditional medical setting that was mainly nonprofit. Return on investment and productivity were not familiar concepts. If a patient complained of illness or injury, their complaints and motives were believed without question. One learned to be a caregiver and to nurture those cared for. The conflict between traditional health care provision and business practices and ethics had to be addressed and dealt with by the consultant and the company management. Through education, an understanding of both perspectives was gained.

In business there are internal politics and power struggles. Control of one's position, department, and authority within the workplace are always at risk. This may be increased during times of economic hardship. The authority to return an employee to work, modify a job, allow an activity to be carried out differently, share job tasks, or require an individual to seek medical attention may be challenged. In certain situations access to the injured worker, his records (both medical and work related), and even access to his supervisor may be controlled by individuals who are uncertain of the occupational therapy consultant's role and intentions. In the following care descriptions, the claims officer initially allowed the consultant to contact the injured worker in his presence. The department manager limited access to the first-line supervisor or to the job site for fear of losing personal control. Also, the personnel officer questioned the consultant's need to review past work records of the injured employee that were needed to obtain information regarding the use of transferable skills. These internal environmental control issues must be raised and addressed. Clear lines of authority and the consultant's access to information should be established early if the consultant is to be effective and produce the desired results.

Services Provided

The consultant's responsibility to prove the value of the rehabilitation plan to both the injured worker and the company is illustrated here through several mini case studies. These are presented to illustrate the various consultative models described.

Steve was a 23-year-old track repair laborer who had worked for the railroad for two seasons. Track workers typically work 6 to 9 months out of the year and only recently were protected by seniority. Each spring, the Milwaukee Road track employees were rehired with no seniority or protection for future employment.

Steve was loading equipment onto a pickup truck when he lost his balance, stepping back off a 10-inch step and landing hard on his right leg. He complained of some pain and numbness immediately, but continued to work. Later that evening, Steve experienced swelling, loss of sensation, discoloration, and pain in his right foot and leg. By morning he was unable to bear weight.

Track workers like Steve often work away from home and are housed in local motels with fellow workers. One of Steve's fellow workers took him to a general practitioner in the small Iowa town. The physician examined Steve and sent him for X rays. A right calcaneal fracture was identified and a knee length cast applied. Steve was cautioned to be nonweight bearing and was provided with crutches. The track foreman arranged for Steve to be taken home. In gathering belongings and preparing for his return home, Steve applied some pressure to his foot, causing further pain and swelling. After several days at home with increasing pain, Steve sought medical attention in his hometown. The physician who saw Steve determined that the cast had to be removed immediately because vascularity and tissue integrity had been greatly compromised. The fracture was also displaced and required surgical pinning and recasting.

In this particular case, the consultant was asked to get involved prior to the typical indicator of 30 days lost time. The medical problems and questions raised by both the claims officer and the track supervisor caused the early referral. Could this injury have really happened in the manner described, and how could Steve have continued to work on such a foot? The only person present when Steve supposedly injured himself was his friend and co-worker. The injury was not reported until the next day. There was, therefore, a possibility that other circumstances, that is, recreational, were involved in the injury. A question of improper care provided by the original physician was also raised.

The consultant's first task was to contact Steve and ascertain that he was now receiving appropriate care. It was necessary to contact Steve's hometown orthopedic physician to obtain medical records and to arrange for appropriate billing. Next, information was gathered to educate the claims officer and track supervisor about calcaneal fractures and to support the fact that the injury could have occurred as described. The consultant also obtained an opinion from the chief medical officer, external physician consultant, that it was possible for Steve to have continued working for a short time, given the support of his work boots and the area of fracture. It was also noted that the work boots may have prevented a more serious injury and extensive damage to ligaments.

Satisfied that the injury was both legitimate and compensable, the claims officer was able to start wage replacement payments and to cover the medical expenses. The track supervisor, while unhappy that an injury had happened, was more understanding and more willing to discuss future job accommodations for Steve. Due to the nature of the job, Steve was unable to work during the 12 weeks he was casted. He remained off work an additional 2 weeks for daily therapy to strengthen his foot and leg and to improve his endurance. Throughout this time, the occupational therapy consultant was in weekly contact with both Steve and his medical care providers. In late summer Steve was ready to return to work. Some weakness in the right foot and ankle still remained, and Steve complained of pain with prolonged walking. These problems, in addition to those presented by the uneven ground, rocks, climbing, and constant standing or walking required by the job, presented concerns regarding Steve's return to work.

One job available in each track gang was tracking the materials used on a daily basis and ordering more as needed. Some walking was required, but breaks were possible and in some instances a track car could be used. Steve had the necessary skills in basic math, knowledge of the materials and supplies, and writing skills to handle this job assignment. He was returned to work in the accommodated position where he remained for the rest of the season. Steve did return to his regularly assigned job as a track laborer the following spring. The occupational therapy consultant played a significant role in working out the details of the job accommodation, providing the necessary support to Steve, keeping management informed of Steve's condition and his potential for other job tasks, and coordinating medical care. Without this intervention, Steve probably would have remained out of work for the entire season. He might have become discouraged and obtained legal counsel, increasing claims settlement costs and creating an adversarial relationship between himself and his employer.

Education and training programs are another important aspect of the industrial consultant's role. Educating various supervisory and management staff in regard to a particular case was described in the previous case-centered consultation. Education of management, first-line supervisors, and employees concerning general principles of rehabilitation as well as providing specific training in body mechanics, lifting, and exercise may be needed.

Management and supervisory level personnel are not usually well versed in the concepts of rehabilitation. A training session, detailing the benefits of rehabilitation and identifying the role each person will play in the education and rehabilitation process, is therefore a necessary part of the consultation.

Another way of involving supervisory staff and gaining program acceptance is to establish team meetings. With one of the supervisors leading the group, a regular discussion can take place regarding each individual injured worker's progress and the development of return-to-work plans. The consultant's role in this group is to provide information and educational material and to participate in the development of the plan. Areas of general concern, such as an increased number of falls, first aid, or access to timely medical care, may become topics of discussion. Examples of two such programs initiated by the consultant at the Milwaukee Road are presented next.

The first setting was the Mechanical Department repair shop in Milwaukee, Wisconsin. Here, locomotives and railroad cars were repaired and rebuilt and wheels and other parts for both cars and engines were made. Jobs ranged from car repair man, to sheetmetal worker, welder, or painter. Most of the work was heavy and required both skill and good physical fitness. The supervisors, in railroad tradition, were brought up from the ranks without any training to prepare them to supervise men or the jobs. They often were held accountable for injuries that occurred to workers under their supervision. There had even been talk of tying their merit increases to the safety records of the men they supervised. In general, the attitude was that all injuries were questionable and that those individuals sustaining an injury were ruining the team's safety record.

A training session was held with these first-line supervisors to help them learn how to identify potential problem employees, to discuss the appropriate approach to take with an employee who was injured as well as one returning from an injury, and to educate the supervisors regarding the medical and rehabilitation process. Role playing, question and answer sessions, and even scripted dialogue to use in follow-up phone calls to injured workers were utilized in the training. A follow-up session to answer further questions and introduce the concept of a restricted work program was held the following week.

Initial reactions were less than positive. The supervisors did not fully believe all they had been told, nor did they have faith that frequent contact and a positive attitude toward an injured worker would have the desired effect of reducing lost time. Some supervisors did comment that at least they were being given some information and direction as well as some concrete instruction on how to manage an injured employee. This was a first for most of them. Control and support for both the training and the subsequent program activity were paramount to the consultant's success. Left at this juncture the program may not have moved forward. The consultant's successful results with individual case management and a carefully planned program proposal led to top management support. The word came down from the top that the supervisors were to try these new approaches. Some checks and balances were put into place to see that there was compliance.

A second educational approach directed at the employees of the Track Department of the Milwaukee Road was initiated at a later point. A back injury presentation was developed by the consultant to describe what happens anatomically when a back injury occurs. The presentation included the right and wrong way to perform the specific tasks required by track laborers. Slides of current employees and the track equipment of the Milwaukee Road were shown. Decals for the workers hard hats, a popular item, were handed out with slogans reminding the workers of back safety tips.

A third model of consultation is program development for the company or for specific divisions of departments within a company. The occupational therapy consultant must first analyze the work site, the work activities, and the workers to determine what problems are leading to injuries and lost time. At the Milwaukee Road, the consultant identified similar problems in two major divisions. The Track Department and the Mechanical Department both were experiencing a high number of back injuries due to lifting. Both were unable or unwilling to accommodate injured workers.

The consultant developed two programs to address the problem. The first was a restricted work program for the Mechanical Department employees. Contact was made with company-designated physicians and clinics in the area. The consultant designed a form to be used by the physician treating recovering workers. The form indicated the employee's specific physical capabilities and restrictions and was sent to the supervisor. The physicians were assured that careful monitoring of restricted work activities would be carried out by the consultant. In conjunction with the use of the form, additional supervisor training was provided and focused on information regarding job restructuring and accommodation. The union representatives were also informed of the program. The employees were then given a brief explanation of the program, their responsibilities, and the company's responsibilities. A formal agreement for use between the supervisor and the employee was drafted that documented what was expected of each injured employee and the supervisor. This agreement was signed by the employee, the supervisor, and the physician to assure each that the restricted work activity would be carried out safely and in a spirit of cooperation. Initially the consultant played a major role bringing all these individuals together and working with supervisors to determine appropriate job accommodation tasks. After the first year, this program was extended to the Track Department.

A second program was started with the Track Department to address the issue of back injuries. A review of injury records indicated that the highest number of injuries occurred during the second hour of work. The first hour of each day was normally spent transporting men to the work site. It became clear that injury most frequently occurred during the first hour of actual work. To address the problems, the educational back injury program previously described was implemented in the Track Department. Additionally, a warm-up exercise program, similar to that developed for athletes, was designed. Cards were printed with this 6-minute warm-up program and the track gang foremen were given instruction in leading the exercises. This was a mandatory program requiring that everyone from track laborers through management participate. Very soon, the employees themselves began leading the exercise sessions. The employees also then requested time to do these warm-up exercises after lunch because they felt that sitting on the ground during their hour break often caused them to become stiff. This second warm-up was encouraged and most of the gangs participated. This program was extended to the Mechanical Department after the first season.

To summarize, when assuming the role of internal consultant, one must remember that learning about the company and its environment is the first step. Next should be the development of an individual case management system and the establishment of a network of provider resources in the community. Case management also implies analyzing the job tasks and product outcome, the workplace, the equipment, and the physical, emotional, and environmental factors conducive to productivity. Additionally, the consultant must remember that the worker and his or her supervisor remain the experts in the work area. Their input, concerns, and perceptions are essential.

Program development as described in the examples of restricted work activities, educational, and exercise programs may be the next step in the consultation process. Determining the needs of the company and then helping to plan and implement programs will succeed if proper support is obtained and the groundwork for change is carefully laid. Once a program is developed, the consultant should turn the daily implementation back to the first-line supervisors and their managers. Individuals who have responsibility for and a vested interest in seeing a program succeed are likely to work toward the desired change and accomplishment of the goals. The occupational therapy consultant may then continue in an advisory and troubleshooting role. Utilizing this format, the internal consultant maintains contact with key personnel and is alerted to specific needs as they arise.

Outcome

Rehabilitation of the injured worker is the mutually shared goal of the company and the consultant. In establishing a baseline for cost versus outcome at the CMSP&P, the Claims Department was asked to review the first 16 cases serviced by the consultant. They were asked to determine the savings on these serious cases as compared to like number of cases with similar diagnoses and demographics. The Claims Department, which was not sold on the benefits of rehabilitation or the consultant, determined a $1.5 million savings to the company as a direct result of case management services. Nationally it is reported that $30 in savings is gained for every $1 spent on rehabilitation services.[2, p4]

Benefits of educational programs for employees and supervisors may be measured by looking at the reduction in injuries and lost time from work. The educational program at the CMSP&P Mechanical Department in conjunction with the restricted activity program reduced lost time from back injuries by an average of seven days per injury during the first year. This translated into about $1,000 savings per injury. In the first year the savings was over $150,000 for this one department. An additional benefit was the change in attitude of the managers and supervisors. Their initial compliance was mandated by top management. Their faith in the program was nonexistent. After the first year, the first-line managers and several supervisors were such strong proponents of the program that they were asked to present the program at a national railroad seminar.

Prevention programs are measured by reduction in injury. Realistically, to see a permanent trend in reduction this may need to be tracked over several years. The combined education and warm-up exercise program initially started with the Track Department at the Milwaukee Road documented a 51% reduction in lost time from back injuries over a 3-year period.

There are obvious benefits to internal consultation as evidenced by the support, control, and access to information and people demonstrated in the examples. Experts in industrial rehabilitation see this method as a wave of the future. Certainly more and more therapists are being hired by large corporations to develop model programs and act as internal consultants. In today's marketplace, occupational therapy's long-standing involvement on work-related activities has broadened from a medical model to an industrial model of health care.

EXTERNAL CONSULTATION

The principles and steps used to implement external consultation are basically the same as those described in the internal consultation model, but the consultant is not an employee of the company. The first step is to identify the needs of the company. As an external consultant, various possibilities may be offered. What the consultant identifies as a primary need may not be what the company is ready to buy. A restricted work activities program, for example, may have to be integrated slowly after the consultant has provided an educational program or demonstrated case management benefits. Often the external consultant will be successful in introducing one aspect of rehabilitation, but will not have support for further program development.

In external consultation, the consultant needs to determine costs and establish charges that reflect the necessary profit margin when negotiating a successful contract. Time, materials, and the consultant's expertise, as well as the expected outcome, must be considered in establishing a reasonable fee. An hourly charge for consultation services should be established based on geographic and industry norms. Back and other educational programs are usually charged on a per person basis. Some consideration should be given to discounts if a company is purchasing volume service. Program development varies greatly depending on the availability of consultants, level of acceptance by the industrial community, and the expertise and experience of the consultant. Flexibility in regard to available time and type of service is necessary if the external consultant is to be successful in obtaining various types of consultation work. For example, the author was asked recently to discuss development of a carpal tunnel prevention and remediation program. The company, a large and well-known national conglomerate, had already talked with another consulting group that presented a slick, well-polished packaged program with a high price tag. They were unwilling to change the program, to address specific needs of the company, or to negotiate price. The author's approach was to open with a discussion of the company's specific perceived needs and to offer feasible solutions and program possibilities. A price that included reasonable fees for time, materials, and expertise with a very good profit margin was negotiated and the deal was struck.

Developing respect and delivering service in a timely manner builds confidence in the external consultant and develops a demand for further services. The keys to successful external consultation are flexibility, planning, monitoring and correcting, developing realistic expectations of what is to be accomplished and what the company is ready to accept, and establishing goals that can be documented and met. Outcome is the name of the game, and saving the company time and money is the answer. Business is interested in return on investment, whether in regard to producing a product of rehabilitating injured workers. Big business would not stay strong for long if their goals turned from profitability to philanthropy.

As word spread regarding the work being done at the CMSP&P an external consultation was requested. The author was approached by the company physician, representing one of the large steel mills in northwestern Indiana. He and the safety/risk manager asked for consultation on specific cases that required evaluation and job modification in order to return employees to full work status. At that time ergonomic evaluation and work site modification were almost unheard of in this industry. Accidents were looked on as a product of poor personal safety habits rather than a result of a poor work station or inferior equipment design.

SUMMARY

Industrial consultation can provide occupational therapists with challenging, exciting, often frustrating, but very rewarding consultation opportunities. Their training in observation and task analysis, flexibility and creativity in program planning and goal setting, and experience in working as part of an interdisciplinary team make them ideally suited to this emerging area of community practice.

Internal consultation provides a supported environment in which to develop case management, prevention, restricted work activities, and educational programs. Working in one specific industry, the internal consultant studies it in depth and analyzes only one industry and the relevant jobs. As the consultant becomes part of the accepted management team, cooperation is gained from supervisors and workers and top management supports new programs.

Internal consultation does limit the consultant's exposure to the variety of industries, problems, and interests that are available to the external consultant. However, small companies cannot afford and do not need the services of a full-time internal consultant, and can therefore benefit from external consultation in program development. Flexibility in program design and pricing, meeting the current needs of the industry, and attention to outcome are paramount to successful external consultation.

Industrial consultation is driven by rising workers' compensation costs. Changes in workers' compensation laws, which recognize both cumulative trauma and the ergonomic responsibilities of the employer, support industrial consultation services. The benefits of rehabilitation services are increasingly recognized by both insurance companies and industries. This awareness has strengthened the need for industrial rehabilitation consultants.

Occupational therapists are an ideal choice as industrial consultants. They bring knowledge and skills in job analysis, ergonomics, task simplification, physical disability treatment, and management of the rehabilitation process to the industrial setting. By developing programs to bridge the gap between acute care and return to work, they play a vital role in assuring cost-effective health care services. Furthering the goal of health care through prevention programs enhances the importance of the occupational therapist's role in the provision of industrial consultation.

REFERENCES

1. Ellexson MT: Work hardening, in Hertfelder S, Gwin C (eds): *Work in Progress*. Rockville, Md, AOTA, 1989.
2. Farrell G, Knowlton S, Taylor M: *Second Chance: Rehabilitating the American Worker*. Minneapolis, Northwestern National Life Insurance Company, 1988.
3. Kirkland M, Robertson SC: *The Evolution of Work Related Theory in Occupational Therapy*. Rockville, Md, AOTA, 1985.
4. Mattingly C: Perspective on clinical reasoning of occupational therapy. Focus: Skills for assessment and treatment. *Am J Occup Ther* 1988.

ADDITIONAL READING

Benner CL, Schilling AD, Klein L: Coordinated team work in California industrial rehabilitation. *J Hand Surg [Suppl]* 1987; 12A: 936.

Ellexson MT: The unique role of occupational therapy in industry, *Occupational Therapy in Health Care: Work Related Programs in Occupational Therapy*, 2: 35, 1985/1986.

Isernhagen SJ: *Work Injury Management and Prevention*. Rockville, Md, Aspen, 1988.

Tromposh AK: Work related therapy for the injured reduces return-to-work barriers. *Occup Health Saf* 1988; 57: 55.

Mungai A: The occupational therapist's role in employee health promotion programs, *Occupational Therapy in Health Care: Work Related Programs in Occupational Therapy*, 2: 67, 1985/1986.

CHAPTER 28

Health Education Consultation in the Workplace

Evelyn G. Jaffe, M.P.H., O.T.R., F.A.O.T.A.

OVERVIEW

Health care, its cost and quality, has been one of the most important issues in the past decade, and continues to rate front page news as health care costs soar beyond reach of many Americans. Our current system of health care is in turmoil. The universal goal to provide access to quality health care for all has left many Americans in a quandary. A *New York Times* front page article declares that rescuing the nation's health care is one of the most pressing problems facing us today, and may pose the supreme political test of the 1990s. The chaotic and costly system has involved many diverse groups, including insurance companies, corporations, economists, health care professionals, public officials, and concerned citizens. Their plea for sweeping changes in our system leaves Congress with a "herculean task (in) . . . the 1990s."[6] We have not seen such a dramatic political interest in the health care system since the Medicare and Medicaid programs of the 1960s brought some relief to the problem of health care accessibility.

In recent years, large corporations also have been studying the price of health care because of the enormous costs of health benefits to their employees. Corporate health care costs exceeded 55% of before-tax profits in 1989, compared to 8% in 1968.[8] Our present system provides some workers with better care than others. However, millions of Americans, employed and unemployed, have no health coverage. "Three-fourths of the 33 million Americans without health insurance are workers or their dependents . . . and the number is rising."[22] Large companies provide a greater share of employee health care, as they have the advantage of being able to pay more for health without emptying their coffers, putting small companies at a distinct disadvantage to provide their workers with adequate care.

Although corporate America after World War II thought that health care was not a major issue for industry, or that employee health costs easily could be passed on to consumers in the increased cost of products, it is no longer possible to maintain this attitude. Nor is it feasible now to rely on a national health system to absorb the rising cost of health care. Companies are beginning to realize that they must do something internally to stem the tide of the escalating costs. The awareness of an increasing need for health education in the workplace, as a result of the costs of health care, fiscal restraint, and decreased external funds for health service programs, has resulted in some companies seeking other options to their traditional health benefits. The progressive costs, at the same time of the reduction and consolidation of health services, has made it imperative for corporations to address these issues. Internal development of efficient and effective health programs to reduce the costs of employee health services, while providing quality comprehensive care, is now a goal of some corporations. Concepts of both disease and injury prevention and health promotion and wellness in the industry have received increased recognition as alternatives to expensive care.

The occupational therapy consultant in the workplace can make significant contributions to the development and implementation of health promotion and education programs in the corporate world. The Medical Marketplace project described here, is an example of the role that occupational therapists may play in work-site health promotion through an employee education program. The author was the principal investigator of the Medical Marketplace, a federally funded research project designed to assess the effectiveness of health consumer education and training on the reduction of health care costs.[19] This program was developed to help consumers more readily understand the health care system and learn to make wise decisions about their own health care. The ultimate goal of the program was to provide quality health care at the lowest cost to the consumer and employer, thus keeping health care at a cost-effective level. The author provided consultative services to the companies involved in this project.

ENVIRONMENT AND SYSTEMS INFLUENCES

No one will dispute that health care is big business. As described in Chapter 2, the cost of health care in the United States is rising faster than any other consumer service. There have been many studies in recent years that have looked at issues of our health care delivery system. The Bureau of Labor Statistics, the Health Care Financing Administration, the Rand Corporation, the Alan Guttmacher Institute, Louis Harris and Associates, and many others have conducted surveys and done extensive research to document past and current health statistics and analyze trends to predict future use and costs of health care.

Despite the fact that the United States spends 12% of the gross national product (GNP) on health costs, more than any other per capita spending in the world, we are the only industrial country that fails to insure care for all its citizens.[6] The governments of other nations, particularly Germany, Canada, and Japan, have greater national health care coverage and financing than America. For example, the Canadian national health plan, funded by tax dollars, is considered one of the world's most comprehensive health insurance programs. Canada provides health care to all its citizens. In 1960, both the United States and Canada had a GNP of about 5.5%. While that of America rose to 12% in 1989, Canada kept the spending at slightly more than 8% in the same year, with a comparable per capita spending of $2,500 for the United States, and $1,500 for Canada.[17] Of course, there are compromises in the use of the Canadian system. The government is involved in many aspects of the system including maintaining a 4 : 1 ratio of physician generalists to specialists as compared to 1 : 1 in the United States, setting medical fees, and limiting some expensive technological and intensive care services and elective surgery.[17]

It may become necessary for Americans to rethink their traditional demand for unlimited, immediate, and expensive medical care that utilizes the very latest biotechnical and medical services. This change in values and attitudes toward health care utilization will take considerable educating of the American medical consumer. As American health care costs continue to rise at this unprecedented rate, with a prediction that national spending will increase by $50 billion a year, reaching $1.9 trillion by 1999,[13] something must be done.

Additionally, corporate expenses for health care also are rising at an alarming rate, and, if not contained, all profits for the average Fortune 500 companies will be eliminated in less than 8 years. Health benefits are now the second largest cost for service businesses. In 1985 it was estimated that 24% of corporate profits, after taxes, were spent on employee health care and health benefits.[9] Of the total compensation for employees, including wages and benefits, 7% was spent for health care in 1989, as compared to 2% in 1965, or over $60 billion a year spent in workers' compensation.[7, 8, 22] One hundred percent of all companies with over 500 employees provide health coverage for their employees. Smaller companies, which employ more than half of the nation's work force, cannot afford to provide complete coverage, and some do not offer any health benefits. Eighty-seven percent of the businesses in the United States employ fewer than 20 workers and of those that employ over 10, 72 provide some form of health insurance. Many of these smaller companies must compensate for their health packages with lower wages, or not provide coverage. The inequities of job-related health benefits and the uneven pattern in insurance premiums have resulted in the smaller companies, of 50 employees or less, paying $3,000 a person for an annual policy while the bigger corporations may spend less than the national average of $2,500. In addition, unionized workers usually fare better than those who do not belong to a union.

Health promotion, education, and wellness programs in the American corporate world finally are emerging as means to address these shocking facts. Many businesses have active employee health programs, intended to provide opportunities for development and maintenance of the health of their employees. A major incentive for businesses to provide this service is the hope that such programs ultimately will reduce these escalating costs of employee health care.

Companies usually use three main strategies to reduce health care costs:

1. Motivating employees to change their demand for expensive health care by changes in the design and administration of health insurance policies;
2. Changing the structure of the health care system with alternative health delivery systems and participation in business coalitions; and
3. Promoting programs that will reduce the need for health care by increasing the awareness of alternative means of maintaining health through such programs as smoking cessation, weight control, and fitness and exercise.[9]

A fourth strategy was proposed by a private health education firm: addressing medical cost containment by targeting the medical consumer.[19] At the inception of the project, called The Medical Marketplace: The Consumer as a Partner in Medical Cost Containment, there were no books in print that dealt specifically with how the consumer of the medical or health care system could assist in achieving efficient and cost-effective care of high quality.

The author was asked to participate as the principal investigator and project director of the Medical Marketplace and consultant to the companies that would participate as the consumers of medical services. This health education training program, intended to increase the knowledge and skills of employees to make them informed consumers of health services, also provided the author with an opportunity to demonstrate occupational therapy consultant skills in a corporate health promotion and education program.

FRAME OF REFERENCE

The frame of reference for this health project was drawn from the principles of health promotion and disease prevention, using an educational model of consultation. For many years, the author has shared the conviction of some health professionals that appropriate health education can result in improved quality of life, optimal functioning, illness and accident prevention, increased productivity, and even extended longevity.[10-12, 18] This conviction is supported by a basic premise of occupational therapy that comprehensive care, which includes appropriate health education, can lead to optimal functioning. West called on occupational therapists to develop professional consciousness and responsibility in responding to the trends of comprehensive care that include concepts of prevention and health promotion.[23]

Health promotion may be defined as "the systematic efforts by an organization to enhance the wellness of its members through education, behavior change, and cultural support."[15] Health promotion programs, therefore, are primarily educational rather than clinical. Their ultimate goal is to increase the individual's capacity for coping, enabling persons to achieve or sustain appropriate physical, mental, and social well-being. Health promotion programs are aimed at reducing stress; advancing competency, coping skills, and optimal functioning; broadening support systems; and enhancing self-perception. They refer to actions or activities that anticipate problems and foster optimum health and have the basic goal of problem solving. The process is facilitated by information, identification, understanding, commitment, and capable performance.[21]

The Medical Marketplace project was a health education program based on the theoretical concepts of health promotion. The major goal of this Health Consumer Training Program (HCTP) was to encourage individuals to become more responsible for their health care decisions while containing health care costs. The training was designed in concert with the basic concepts of health promotion: enhancing wellness and life satisfaction through attitudinal and behavioral change as a result of increased knowledge and skills.

In addition to an educational model, drawn from a health promotion frame of reference, the consultant used a collaborative model of consultation with the individual consultee in this project, the health benefit officer of each company. This collaborative, or collegial, consultation involved a joint problem-solving relationship, with the consultant, and consultee acting as equal peers.

PROGRAM DESCRIPTION

THE MEDICAL MARKETPLACE: THE CONSUMER AS A PARTNER IN MEDICAL COST CONTAINMENT

Organization

The health education firm, called "Healthco" for this description, applied for a federal grant to explore the feasibility of conducting a research project to assess the effectiveness of health consumer education, motivation, and training on health care cost containment. Healthco received a phase 1 Small Business Innovative Research (SBIR) grant from the Health Care Financing Administration (HCFA) to achieve the following objectives:

1. Refine a guidebook for medical consumers;
2. Develop and pilot test an employee training plan to accompany the guide and enhance its effectiveness;
3. Select a pilot test employer site; and
4. Identify, develop, and pilot-test appropriate measures of cost containment, and evaluate the guidebook and training.

Upon the completion of phase 1, Healthco received a phase 2 SBIR grant from HCFA to evaluate the effectiveness of a health consumer training program with participation of a minimum of 1,200 employees in the greater metropolitan area of a large western city.[19] The evaluation was to measure the success of a 60-minute training presentation by a professional theatre group and a dialogue with the doctor who wrote the accompanying medical consumer handbook, *The Medical Marketplace*.

This federally funded research project was designed to test the effectiveness of an experimental approach to consumer health care cost containment. The intent of this project was to train consumers how to gain access to the health care delivery system in the most efficient and cost-effective manner, thereby cutting down on overutilization. The Health Consumer Training Program (HCTP) attempted to achieve these goals through the following objectives:

1. Increase employee knowledge about cost-effective health care practices and effective use of the health care system;
2. Encourage employees to assume greater responsibility for their personal health and the health of their families;
3. Improve employee decision-making skills to assure high quality health care at the lowest possible cost; and
4. Improve attitudes and encourage behaviors to motivate the passive recipient or patient to be active participants in their own health care.

The research design was constructed to provide empirical evidence regarding the extent to which this approach altered consumer health care decisions, utilization of health services, and health care costs. The technical objectives of this design were to assess the impact of the training on health care knowledge, attitudes, decision-making skills, behaviors, and costs for 1 year following the training or intervention.

The plan was a quasi-experimental research design, as described by Cook and Campbell,[5] which compared pre- and posttraining measures of medical costs, utilization, health knowledge, and behaviors of employees exposed to the training (the test group) with identical measures of employees of the same organizations (the control group) not exposed to the training initially. The primary analytic focus of this study was to compare the test and the control subjects with respect to measures of the following:

- Knowledge of health care and health care systems
- Attitudes toward health care and health care systems
- Decision-making skills in the health care domain
- Actual decision-making behaviors in the health care domain
- Health care expenses

The general hypothesis was that employees who initially received the HCTP (those in the test group) would exhibit significantly greater knowledge of health care and health care systems, improved attitudes, more effective decision-making skills, better health care decisions in their own lives, and have lower cost and health service utilization in the year following the HTCP intervention than the control group.[19]

Support

The major source of financial support for this project was the federal government grant, the SBIR grant from HCFA mentioned previously. Monthly reports were prepared by the consultant and submitted to the SBIR division director, who also made a site visit to meet with the consultant/project director and Healthco administrative staff.

The participating organizations provided in-kind financial support. Although the HCTP was provided to employees at no cost to them and no direct out-of-pocket cost to the employer, each organization was responsible for commiting 5 hours of employee release time for each participant throughout the year of the research project. This arrangement represented considerable commitment from those organizations with over 200 participating employees. Therefore, strong support from top managerial personnel was essential to the success of the project.

Administrative support from Healthco staff was essential to this project from its inception, without which, no doubt, there would not have been a project. Additionally, the cooperation and support of the site coordinators from each of the participating organizations allowed the project to function smoothly. Without their commitment and attention to the many complexities of scheduling and data collection, this project would never have been completed.

Participants

The participants in this project were many and varied. They included the occupational therapy consultant as principal investigator, director, and coordinator of the project, and Healthco staff, who provided administrative support and collated and coded the assessment instruments for computer analysis. The client system included the management personnel, site coordinators (the direct consultees), and employees of the organizations who participated in the project. The HCTP training team provided the direct intervention, and the outside consulting firm of research analysts coordinated the data analysis and provided the final statistical information.

The director of health benefits for each organization, as the direct consultee, was the coordinator and project liaison for the test site and responsible for the implementation of the project for his or her company. This individual is referred to as the site coordinator consultee for the remainder of the description. The consultant developed a collegial and collaborative relationship with these individuals and was in close contact with each site coordinator throughout the project.

Approximately 2,500 employees in five organizations attended the consultant's initial presentations, which included a brief description of the project goals, the projected time lines, the responsibilities of the participants, and the advantages of the HCTP to both employees and the participating companies. Of that number, 1,233 private corporation and public employees agreed to participate in the research project. These individuals were the recipients of the educational intervention.

The HCTP team consisted of a Healthco staff trainer, the physician co-author of the consumer handbook *The Medical Marketplace,* and a very talented, humorous professional theatre group.

The consultant worked with all participants of the research project. Her responsibilities included initial recruitment of organizations, presentations to management personnel at all levels, recruitment presentations to potential employee participants, coordination of the scheduling of the test instrument administration and the HCTP with both the site coordinators and the training team, orientation presentations to the employee participants, administration of the test instruments, and introduction to the training. Throughout the study, the consultant worked with Healthco coding and administrative staff.

Services Provided

This project actually required entry into two different systems: the sponsoring organization and the client organizations. The author was an external consultant in both systems. The consultant became involved in this project initially through the direct invitation of the Healthco executive director, who had heard of the consultant's work from a former employer.

Entry (System 1)

Entry into system 1, the organization sponsoring the project, was considered *invited entry.* A meeting was called between Healthco's executive director, administrator, and training staff and the author. This first meeting was a general orientation to the goals and objectives and the research design of the Medical Marketplace project. It was intended to apprise the author of the ramifications of the project, explore mutual interests, and have the author meet the staff. It gave the staff and the author an opportunity to see if a mutually compatible, working relationship was possible.

Negotiation of Contract (System 1)

The author was offered a contract to serve as principal investigator, coordinator, and director of the project, and consultant to the client systems. For the remainder of this description, the author is referred to as the consultant. The contract was time limited for the year and a half of the research project. Renegotiation was possible depending on the outcome of the project.

A second meeting was held with the research analyst, also under contract from an outside research consulting firm; the author, as project director/consultant; the executive director; and the administrator of Healthco to refine the assessment instruments to be administered in this project and discuss potential evaluation. Therefore, in both outside contracts, that of the project director/consultant and the research analyst/consultant, evaluation measures were considered as part of the initial negotiations.

Entry (System 2)

Involvement in system 2, the client organizations, was more complicated. Initial exploration of possible sites had begun previously in phase 1, during which time Healthco staff had met with health benefit supervisors at general corporate health benefit meetings in the area to discuss the intended project. Several corporation health officers expressed interest in the project.

The recruitment and selection of the employer research sites was the first task of phase 2. The initial exploration had provided the basis for a *planned entry* of the targeted organizations. Specific planned steps were developed by the consultant to recruit companies to participate in the project.

The consultant met individually with management executives from those corporations that had expressed an interest in participating in the project. The proposal to these corporations included the selection criteria. To be a part of the study and have their employees receive the health education, the participating companies had to agree to the following commitments:

- Participation of a minimum of 200 employees enrolled in a co-share or self-funded indemnity insurance plan
- Five hours of employee release time for training and data collection activities
- Cooperation of middle-management, health benefit, and supervisory staff for coordination of the assigned employee group

The tactics for selection of the test sites and commitment from the organizations for phase 2 involved considerable time and energy. Although it was a very time-consuming process, it was critical to the success of the project to obtain, ultimately, an *invited entry* to these corporations. The consultant held many individual meetings with top management personnel from each of the interested corporations to explain the details of the project and the required employer and employee commitments. Additionally, it was particularly important to enlist the support and cooperation from middle managers and the employees' direct supervisors, who would allow the necessary release time.

The consultant designed an employer information brochure and prepared a recruitment packet to be distributed prior to meeting with middle management, the health benefit officers, and the supervisory staff of each organization. Presentations were made at each potential test site, and informal meetings were held individually with each test site coordinator, usually the health benefit officer of the organization.

Negotiation of Contract (System 2)

A number of corporations and two county government centers in the area were finally recruited to participate in this project. The contracts negotiated with each included obtaining a firm commitment to adhere to the selection criteria described previously. In addition, once the test site had agreed to participate, the responsibilities of both the client system and the consultant were outlined. The individual(s) responsible for the process of employee recruitment, scheduling, administration, and data collection for each participating organization was designated. Usually the health benefit officer became the site coordinator and as such was the direct consultee.

Establishment of Trust and Diagnostic Analysis

In all five participating organizations, and three separate sites of one corporation, the process was somewhat different, and each site coordinator had different personalities, different degrees of interest in the project, and varying time that could be allocated to the activities. Some were more amenable to the project than others. Some felt that it was an added responsibility thrust on them by top management; others were deeply committed to the concepts of the project and were willing to devote as much time as possible to its success.

It was essential for the consultant to establish the trust and respect of each site coordinator/consultee before proceeding with the project. The consultant had to do considerable study regarding the structure, functioning, and environmental issues of each organization, including both internal and external influences, in preparing to work with the consultee. To develop a working relationship, the consultant worked with each consultee to analyze the particular values, attitudes, and corporate culture of their organization.

The process of recruitment, data collection, and presentation of the educational program had to be designed around the needs, interests, and functioning of the various client systems. The consultant and consultee explored together, in a collaborative, collegial manner, the most appropriate methodology for their system.

Goal Setting and Planning

Some of the participating organizations preferred a completely voluntary employee sign-up for the project; others felt that a stronger, somewhat obligatory recruitment effort was necessary in their organization. Individual recruitment information, including graphic material, posters, and flyers were designed by the consultant for each organization's employee recruitment campaign. This aspect of phase 2 involved considerable time and effort over a four-month period.

It was essential to work out the details and logistics for each organization before the actual intervention took place. Each organization provided demographic baseline data on their employees that included age, gender, educational level, and job classification. All participants were assigned a code number, which was the only identification subsequently used in the project. Within each organization the participants were randomly assigned to a test group, which received the educational program or HCTP intervention, and a control group, which did not initially receive the training. At the end of the 12th month of data collection, the control groups had the option to receive the HCTP as a courtesy for participating in the research.

During the first 2 months, presentations were made to all eligible employees, those enrolled in the organizations' co-share or self-funded indemnity insurance plans. It had been determined earlier by the consulting research analyst that employees in prepaid insurance plans would be less interested in a health care cost containment effort and less motivated to reduce utilization of health services than those in indemnity plans requiring more out-of-pocket and deductible expenses. By the end of the second month, all potential employee participants had been identified and assigned to either test or control groups.

Implementation of the Intervention

Once the internal process for each organization was established, and the logistical planning and complex scheduling for the administration of the test instruments were determined, the actual training intervention at each site commenced. At some sites, administration of the test instruments and the training program were staggered throughout the day in employee groups of 30 to 70 people.

The test instruments were developed to compare the various outcomes of knowledge, behaviors, utilization, costs, and decision-making skills of the two groups of participants. Additionally, they provided information relative to the dimensions of general health status and demographic characteristics, types of health services utilized, and general health practices. The following test instruments, designed as self-administered questionnaires, provided the data for this project.

1. *Health Care Knowledge Questionnaire:* This questionnaire utilized a 5-point Likert scale and identified the degree to which the participating individuals possessed information and attitudes conducive to both quality health care and containment of costs.

2. *Decision-Making Questionnaire:* This questionnaire presented five hypothetical but realistic case studies in which the respondents were asked what their role as a health consumer would be. They were instructed to answer what they would do or what they would ask in the series of case histories.

3. *Health Care Practices Questionnaire:* This questionnaire was a self-report instrument designed to provide information on the actual health care experiences, choices, and utilization of health services of the respondents.

4. *Health Status Questionnaire:* This rank-ordered questionnaire provided demographic and baseline data and identified changes in health status and utilization during the experimental year.

5. *Health Care Diary:* The health care diary was developed to assess the impact of the training program on actual health-related behaviors as compared to the behaviors of individuals who had not received the intervention. All participants in the study were asked to record their monthly utilization of health services throughout the experimental year on a log specifically prepared to record this information.[19]

During each initial test instrument administration, the consultant presented an introduction to the research project, its meaning to the participants and to their employers, the intent of the questionnaires, and instructions for completing them. In the employee introduction, the employee groups were described as "training" and "comparison" groups, rather than "test" and "control," to diffuse the possibility of a negatively perceived research aspect of the project. Also, during administration of the test instruments, the consultant referred to the assessments as questionnaires, not tests. It was explained that the intent was to provide confidential, anonymous data for the project, not personal information about the individual. The employers did not have access to the information. All questionnaires were sent directly to the coding staff of Healthco.

The questionnaires were administered to employees in both groups as pre- and posttests at specified intervals during the experimental year, according to established research methodology.[1, 24] The pretest instrument administration for the test/training group was conducted approximately a week before the Health Consumer Training Program (HCTP). The training design for the HCTP was developed to achieve the following objectives:

1. Familiarize participants with the consumer guide
2. Motivate them to consult appropriate sections of the guide as needed
3. Teach specific strategies which could affect the quality and cost of medical care.[19]

Initially it was planned to have an 8-hour training period to cover the information in the handbook. However, during the pilot test in phase 1, it proved to be unworkable for employers to allocate that much employee release time.

The consultant introduced the training and stated the objectives of the program. It included assumptions that medical consumers or patients have the right and responsibility to be involved in decisions about their own health care, they can participate effectively in these decisions if adequately educated, and the best quality care at the lowest price will result when health care personnel and the consumer of health services develop a partnership relationship.

The HCTP consisted of a humorous 60-minute performance by a professional theatre group, interspersed with didactic presentations by the principal author, a practicing physician, of the medical consumer handbook *The Medical Marketplace* to elaborate on and reinforce the theatre skits and role plays. Additionally, there was dialogue between the Healthco staff trainer and the physician discussing barriers to active consumer involvement and strategies to overcome these barriers.

Participants had an opportunity to ask some specifically directed questions during the training period, but there could not be unlimited discussion due to employer constraints on the amount of employee release time allowed. Each participant was given his or her own copy of *The Medical Marketplace* consumer handbook at the end of the training period. The book was designed to help readers become more active in their role as medical consumers, be their own best health advocates, and make informed and wise decisions to reduce their health care costs.

This handbook, written in a crisp, readily understandable, and nonjargon style with tips, techniques, and checklists, was to be used when visiting the doctor, considering surgery, having medical tests, or going to the hospital. It was suggested that the test/training group participants take the book with them when using any health services throughout the research year.

The Health Care Knowledge Questionnaire and the Decision-Making Questionnaire were administered again to the test/training group immediately after the training. At specific intervals during the experimental year, postintervention data collection was conducted by the consultant. All participants responded to the four questionnaires again as posttest measures. At the end of the experimental year of training and data collection, the control/comparison groups were given the same health care training that was originally given to the test/training groups and given a copy of *The Medical Marketplace*.

Evaluation

Throughout the project, Healthco staff periodically received the test instruments, which consisted of the four questionnaires described previously. This required many hours of reviewing responses, coding of over 10,000 assessment instruments, and entering the data for computer analysis.

During the course of the data collection, the dropout rates among the research participants were notable. Attrition due to normal changes such as deaths, retirements, moves, changes in employment, and sickness on the day of test administration was accounted for in the original research design. However, there were heavy attrition rates due to unforeseen circumstances in some of the participating organizations. One company experienced a major reorganization during the experimental year, resulting in large-scale employee layoffs at all levels of employment, including two of the site coordinators for the project. Another, a public employee organization, experienced greater than average retirements and terminations of employment with county positions. However, because the sample size was large to begin with, the final participant size was adequate to obtain significant data.

Analysis of the Health Care Knowledge Questionnaire revealed that attitudes and knowledge of the test group were significantly affected by the educational intervention. Overall, the average difference for the test group postintervention was 0.72, compared to the control group difference of 0.07, thus demonstrating a significant knowledge gain for test respondents and negligible difference for control respondents.

Analysis of the Decision-Making Questionnaire also provided substantial support for the effectiveness of the HCTP. Comparison of the test and control group responses showed significant changes in decisions by the test group postintervention and negligible differences in the control group. The mean difference in test respondents was .470, compared to only .032 for control respondents. These results demonstrated that the training program intervention effectively influenced the ability to make better informed decisions and choices about health care situations that can help contain costs and reduce unnecessary surgical or diagnostic procedures.[25]

Evaluation of the Health Care Practices Questionnaire and the Health Status Questionnaire did not exhibit significant changes in either health care practices after the HCTP or in the general health status of test or control groups over time. This corroborates a well-designed study by the Rand Corporation, which also found virtually no difference in health status among participants in a variety of insurance plans.[2, 3]

Also, the health care diary did not show significant differences in utilization of health services in either of the respondent groups. In studying the responses to these questionnaires, analysts felt the reason for the lack of significant differences between groups may have been that the actual level of health care utilization was extremely low for both groups.[25] This also may have been due, in part, to the sample of participants who were chosen only from self- or co-insured indemnity insurance plans as opposed to prepaid programs, whose enrollees tend to make considerable use of health services.

Termination

When all posttests were administered, data collected, and the participants had received the educational intervention, the contract for this project was terminated. As discussed in the original contract negotiation, this was a time-limited consultation for the duration of the project. However, the collegial relationship that developed between the consultant and the Healthco administrator and site coordinators blossomed into a nonprofessional friendship. The consultant met socially with some of the direct consultees (the site coordinators) and the Healthco administrator. This personal relationship was an added bonus to the consultation.

Possible Renegotiation

At the conclusion of the project, the consultant was invited to participate in the marketing of *The Medical Marketplace* handbook for consumers. She attended the initial training session for telemarketing and had the opportunity to be a part of the marketing team. She participated in the program on a trial basis for a month. However, other consultant activities and interests intervened and precluded signing a contract for marketing the book.

Outcome

The successful outcome of this health consumer education project demonstrated the effectiveness of this approach in altering consumer health care attitudes, increasing knowledge of health care systems, and improving decisions about utilization of health care services.

The final responses from the participants who received the training intervention demonstrated by the end of the experimental year that the HCTP had a significant effect on the health care knowledge and anticipated behaviors of these medical consumers. Additionally, a comprehensive review and evaluation of *The Medical Marketplace* consumer handbook by employees of a large electronics company and a sample of physicians indicated that this guide was extremely informative, useful, and well received by both consumers and providers of health services. As a result of these findings, *The Medical Marketplace* was marketed through a nationwide marketing effort to over 250,000 health educators and corporations throughout the country.[25]

SUMMARY

The alarming rise in corporate expenses for health care has made it increasingly difficult for employers to maintain adequate and affordable health care for their employees. The costs described have forced business and industry to confront issues of health maintenance, disease prevention, and, more recently, to study health promotion and work-site wellness.[16] Corporations are beginning to recognize that health promotion and education programs may result in significant financial savings.

However, lack of definitive data in the past had made it difficult to convince corporate management to expend considerable efforts toward employee health prevention activities, when, justifiably, they were preoccupied with their organization's financial health.[18] Recent studies, such as that described, of educational work-site health and wellness programs are beginning to demonstrate the effectiveness of such programs in reducing employee absenteeism due to illness and/or injury and decreasing costs of workers' compensation and medical claims.

Another study, in Des Moines, revealed that educating people about the health care system influenced them to think more about reducing the use of health services. Herzlinger and Schwartz state that, in addition, these changes in attitude must be accompanied by changes in behavior.[9] As seen from analysis of the Health Care Knowledge and the Decision-Making questionnaires, the Medical Marketplace project provided significant empirical evidence that a employee health education program could make a difference in attitudes and behaviors.

A report from the U.S. Department of Health and Human Services revealed that 66% of companies with 50 or more employees now offer one or more health promotion activities.[4] These programs consist of comprehensive health education, health enhancement, and accident prevention activities and also include sessions in weight control and nutrition, exercise and fitness, stress management, smoking cessation, wellness checks, and job safety.

Occupational therapy consultants have the opportunity to be involved in the design and planning of these activities and the training of staff to implement the programs. Additionally, they can participate in program evaluation by measuring individual performance by the active participants in the work-site wellness and health education programs, as seen in the Medical Marketplace project.

The Medical Marketplace: The Consumer as a Partner in Medical Cost Containment was intended to improve the quality of health care by helping consumers find appropriate care more quickly and directly and to reduce costs by eliminating the use of unnecessary or inappropriate services. It is considered a successful example of occupational therapy involvement in a novel approach of health promotion in the workplace. The Medical Marketplace project design included all the elements previously described as essential for a health promotion program: information, identification, understanding, commitment, and capable performance.

Health professionals are becoming more cognizant of the choices consumers face in deciding how and when to use certain health services. "The technological power to cure, treat, and prevent illness is a strong one, but even stronger is each individual's decision to use these medical advances rationally."[20] The pursuit of health is not solely the function of government or medicine. It is a cooperative venture that involves government, business and industry, health professionals, and individuals.[14] Ultimately, wise decisions by informed consumers can help achieve quality of care while stemming the tide of mounting health care costs.

REFERENCES

1. Brogan DR, Kutner, MH: Comparative analysis of pretest-posttest research designs. *Am Statistician* 1980; 34:229–232.
2. Brook RH: Does free care improve adults' health? *N Engl J Med* 1983; 1426.
3. Brook RH: *The Effect of Coinsurance on the Health of Adults*. Santa Monica, Calif, Rand Corporation, 1984.
4. Company health promotion activities. *Weight Watchers International Newsletter*, July–August 1988, p 2.
5. Cook TD, Campbell DT: *Quasi-Experimentation: Design and Analysis Issues for Field Settings*. Chicago, Rand-McNally, 1979.
6. Eckholm E: Rescuing health care: A herculean task for Congress in the 90's, in the *NY Times*, May 2, 1991, pp 1, 16.
7. Gilfoyle EM: Partnerships for the future. Presidential address, American Occupational Therapy Association Conference, Phoenix, Ariz, 1988.
8. Health Care Financing Administration, *NY Times*, May 1, 1991, p A14.
9. Herzlinger RE, Schwartz J: How companies tackle health care costs: Part I. *Harvard Bus Rev*, July-August 1985, pp 68–81.
10. Jaffe EG: Expanding the role of the occupational therapist, Unpublished manuscript, University of Michigan School of Public Health, Ann Arbor, Mich, 1972.
11. Jaffe EG: Prevention, "an idea whose time has come": The role of occupational therapy in disease prevention and health promotion. *Am. J Occup Ther* 1986; 40:749–752.
12. Jaffe EG: Transition in health care: critical planning for the 1990's, part 2. *Am J Occup Ther*, 1985; 39:499–503.
13. Keet RB, Nelson M: *The Medical Marketplace*. Santa Cruz, Calif, Network Publications, 1985.
14. Lee PR, Franks PE: Health and disease in the community. *Mobius* 1981; 1:5–27.
15. Opatz JP: *A Primer of Health Promotion*. Washington, DC, Oryn, 1985.

This chapter has been adapted from Jaffe EG: Medical consumer education: Health promotion in the workplace, in Johnson JA, Jaffe EG (eds): *Occupational Therapy: Program Development for Health Promotion and Preventive Services*. New York, Haworth Press, 1989, pp 5–24.

16. Pelletier KR: *Healthy People in Unhealthy Places: Stress and Fitness at Work.* New York, Delacorte Press/Seymour Lawrence, 1984.

17. Schieber GJ, Pouillier, JP: In Canada, a government system that provides health care to all. *NY Times,* Apr 30, 1991, pp 1, 8.

18. Schwartz RM, Rollins PL: Measuring the cost benefit of wellness strategies. *Business and Health,* October 1985.

19. Small Business Innovative Research Proposal (SBIR): Health Care Financing Administration. Washington DC, U.S. Department of Health and Human Services, 1985.

20. Stein JJ: *Making Medical Choices: Who Is Responsible?* Boston, Houghton Mifflin, 1978.

21. Taylor RL: Prevention in a new key. *Wellness Resource Bulletin* 1980; 1:8.

22. Uchitelle L: Insurance linked to jobs: System showing its age. *NY Times,* May 1, 1991, pp 1, 14.

23. West WL: Professional responsibility in times of change. *Am J Occup Ther* 1968; 22:9–15.

24. Wine BJ: *Statistical Principles in Experimental Design.* New York, McGraw-Hill, 1971.

25. Worth SR, Houchens RL, Englehart LM, et al: *SBIR Research Final Report: The Medical Marketplace: The Consumer as a Partner in Medical Cost Containment.* Santa Cruz, Calif, Keneko Communications, 1987.

SECTION F

Occupational Therapy Consultation in Academic Settings

Consultation to academic programs provides an opportunity for occupational therapy educators to utilize program planning, communication, and administrative skills in a collegial manner with other educators and/or administrators in settings of higher education. This model of consultation demonstrates the effectiveness of faculty consultants in designing strategies to develop, enhance, or expand educational programs.

Zucas provides a description of educational administrative consultation in an international academic setting. Issues of cultural, demographic, social, and health policy differences presented unusual challenges that had to be studied and addressed before consultation strategies could be planned. Consultative activities included assessment and development of an evaluation system for clinical education, facilitation of interpersonal communication to improve relationships between clinical coordinators and academic faculty, enhancement of clinical and academic faculty teaching skills, and suggestions for increasing program effectiveness.

Highlights of possible roles of the higher education consultant are described by Llorens, demonstrating that the key skills in these roles (including observation, communication, problem solving, and analysis) follow the basic consultation skills for all settings. Llorens describes roles of consultation to an academic program, a university personnel department, a university long-range planning committee, and a university disabled student service.

Academic Settings

AUTHOR	MODEL	LEVEL	LOCUS	GOAL
Zucas	Collegial and Educational	Levels II and III: Administrative and educational	Australian school of occupational therapy	Develop system for evaluation of clinical education therapy; enhance faculty effectiveness; Prepare occupational therapy students for clinical placement
Llorens	Collegial and Educational	Levels I, II, and III: Case-centered, educational, and program planning	University	Assess problems of disabled college students; Enhance curriculum planning and management of specific university departments

CHAPTER 29

Faculty Program Consultation Abroad

Rhona Reiss Zucas, M.O.T., O.T.R., F.A.O.T.A.

OVERVIEW

Faculty Consulting

Faculty consulting has been viewed traditionally as an important form of public service in higher education.[3] Many universities believe that faculty consulting enhances both research and teaching, and benefits the institution and society as well as the individual consultant. However, some universities argue that faculty consulting may result in neglect of students and other university responsibilities, abuses of academic freedom, conflicts of interest, and illegitimate use of institutional resources. When viewed as a natural extension and application of professional or scholarly expertise outside the academic institution, faculty consulting relates directly to the intellectual, social, psychological, and economic well-being of the individual faculty member. Additionally, faculty consulting is part of the tripartite mission of most academic institutions (i.e., teaching, research, and service).[3]

Benefits

Studies of faculty consulting have examined the benefits to the individual, to the university, and to society. In addition to supplementing the faculty member's academic salary, which may contribute to economic well-being and morale, consulting also stimulates the continuing education of faculty members by enabling them to test academic teaching and research against real-world experience. Consulting also enhances faculty members' teaching resources, helps them stay abreast of developments in their field, and provides ideas and inspiration for further research.[1]

Faculty consulting benefits the employing academic institution in several ways. By allowing faculty to supplement their base academic salaries, universities with permissive policies are able to attract and retain outstanding professionals. Since faculty consulting complements research and teaching effectiveness, it helps build the professional reputation of the department and university. Because it is an expression of service commitment to the broader community, faculty consulting builds goodwill toward the university. Consulting sometimes results in fieldwork experiences and career opportunities for students, and may provide access to government, private sector, or foundation grant monies to supplement the university's resources.[3]

The benefits of faculty consulting to society are unmistakable. Public and private agencies can draw on the special expertise of faculty and provide solutions to a wide range of problems in a cost-effective manner. Faculty consulting also facilitates the transfer of research findings to the broader community.[5]

Risks

Those who criticize faculty consulting fear the possible neglect of students and other university responsibilities, and view the earning of extra income on university time as "double-dipping."[6] Other potential risks of faculty consulting are abuses of academic freedom and conflicts of interest that may compromise academic objectivity and impartiality.[4] Another potential risk of faculty consulting is the illegitimate use of institutional resources such as university facilities, materials, computers, and staff. The issue of property rights arises when consulting results in the creation of intellectual property for which the patent or copyright may rightfully belong to the university.[3]

In their analysis of the literature on faculty consulting and the National Research Council (NRC) data on a 1981 survey of doctorate recipients, Boyer and Lewis concluded that faculty consulting has been overestimated and underappreciated. The NRC data indicate that only 20.8% of Ph.D. science and engineering faculty and only 12.4% of Ph.D. humanities faculty report having devoted any portion of their professional work time to outside consulting during the academic year. Reported supplemental income averaged only about 14% of base academic salary for the two faculty groups surveyed. This analysis "supports and extends previous studies that showed faculty who consult to be more attentive to society's concerns and priorities and at least as active in their faculty roles on campus as their nonconsulting peers."[3]

Universities need to develop more explicit policies and procedures regarding outside consulting work by faculty. These policies should allow for individual review when the percentage of time spent consulting exceeds a prescribed ceiling. At most institutions, 1 day per week is allowed, but this may vary depending on the individual faculty member's productivity.[7] The literature supports the author's view that faculty consulting should be permitted and encouraged. Policies that impose limits may restrict the productivity of highly active faculty. In the author's experience, the utilization of a consultation model is an important consideration for occupational therapy faculty and educational programs. The university that encourages consultation contributes to the growth of faculty and the development of its educational programs. The mutual benefits permit a greater diversity of roles for the faculty consultant and enrichment of the educational program in which the faculty participates.

Occupational Therapy Faculty Consulting

A 1989 survey of occupational therapy professional and technical educational programs in the United States indicated that 37% of the programs had full-time faculty who were providing clinical and consulting services in settings outside the university's administration.[9] Of those programs responding to the survey, only 17% indicated that faculty were required to provide consulting services; however, several educational program directors commented that faculty were strongly encouraged to do so. About two thirds of the program directors indicated that consulting services have been used for research by faculty, and many involved their students in their investigations. Faculty who included clinical consultations in their role were able to maintain, update, and keep abreast of new information, provide current clinical examples to use in teaching, and also maintain credibility with students. Other benefits of faculty consultation to clinics included the development of level I fieldwork sites, increased research opportunities, improved visibility and image in the community, and supplemental income. In some cases, revenues generated by faculty consultants were used by the educational program for faculty development and teaching resources.

The major problem perceived by occupational therapy educational program directors was related to faculty time constraints. Finding the time to provide consultation services, in addition to fulfilling other faculty responsibilities, was difficult. Another problem was the decreased accessibility of faculty for student needs and departmental meetings. Some program directors perceived consulting activities as competitive with tenure-seeking activities.

Some occupational therapy faculty provided consulting services to more than one agency, and 82% charged a fee for services provided, paid either by the client or the agency. Eighty-one percent of faculty consultants provided their services during regular university working hours, which accounts for some of the revenues being retained by the university or the occupational therapy department. In some cases, faculty were able to retain fees even when services were provided during university working hours. About half of the faculty consultants involved their students in the consultation process by allowing the student to observe either on site or through videos of treatment sessions in clinical consultations.[9]

ENVIRONMENT AND SYSTEMS INFLUENCES

The past decade has brought a significant increase in the nationwide demand for occupational therapy services and significant expansion of third-party reimbursement. Occupational therapy has been identified as one of the most promising careers of the 1990s. Employment opportunities, attractive starting salaries, and an acknowledged shortage of personnel have resulted in increased enrollments for many occupational therapy educational programs. These programs have then encountered greater difficulty in obtaining placements for students on level I and level II fieldwork rotations. This problem has been exacerbated by the shortage of student clinical supervisors given the increased demand for clinician productivity as a result of the Medicare prospective payment system. Numerous opportunities have therefore been created for occupational therapy consultants, particularly those with the expertise and experience of occupational therapy faculty.

Expansion has also occurred in educational programs at all levels. New technical education programs in community colleges, as well as new professional education programs in colleges and universities, have developed. Many programs have expanded their offerings to include professional and postprofessional master's curricula, and several offer doctoral degrees in occupational therapy. This expansion of programs, in conjunction with increased enrollments, has resulted in a serious shortage of occupational therapy faculty.

With cutbacks in government spending for human service programs and limited funding to universities, clinicians and educators have been told they "will have to do more with less." Responding to this mandate in an environment with rising demands for clinical services, research, and education programs, shortages of clinicians and faculty, and pressures for more productivity has created opportunities for increasing use of a consultation approach.

FRAME OF REFERENCE

The process used by occupational therapists to prepare a treatment plan for a client is also useful to the consultant. The clinician gathers information to assess client needs, analyzes this information to identify client problems, plans programs and intervention strategies to solve client problems, implements the program, and provides recommendations for reassessment and follow-up. The occupational therapy educator as a consultant to clinical or educational facilities uses this same process in recommending solutions to the consultee's problems. The consultant must first gather information to assess the consultee's needs. This may be done by conducting interviews with key personnel, attending department meetings, observing in clinic or classroom settings, reading department documents and reports, conducting library research, meeting with clinicians, or meeting with students. The consultant then analyzes the information to identify the consultee's problems and recommend programs or strategies to solve the problems. The consultant may or may not be responsible for implementing the programs but should be available for follow-up when needed.

The recommended programs or consultation strategies may occur on one of several levels as described in Chapter 2. Level I, a case-centered consultation, is targeted on a specific patient or client; level II, an educational consultation, is targeted on the consultee and uses an in-service training or staff development approach; level III, a program and/or administrative consultation, is targeted on the specific system to promote institutional change. Some consultation contracts may require all three levels, as in the case of an occupational therapy educator who provided case consultation for specific children in a private school for multiple-handicapped children (level I), conducted in-service training for teachers and aides on positioning and feeding (level II), and conferred with the school administrator on programs to increase parent involvement (level III).

The following additional examples illustrate the use of occupational therapy educators as consultants to clinical and educational programs indicating the level of the consultation:

- *Problem:* A need for clinical services in facilities with staff shortages
- *Solution:* Level I, case-centered consultation

An occupational therapy educator was invited by her college administrator, who served on the board of a metropolitan children's hospital, to consult to the occupational therapy department of the hospital to facilitate changes in treatment approaches. Change was difficult until the consultant actually provided direct treatment for a caseload of patients. She was then viewed as a peer by the staff, and her treatment demonstrations served as an example for the other therapists. The consultation improved relations between the educational program and the hospital. The faculty consultant also scheduled classes at the hospital and students were able to observe treatment there.

- *Problem:* A need to develop fieldwork programs for occupational therapy students in clinic sites
- *Solution:* Level II, educational consultation

An occupational therapy educator was invited by several clinical facilities to provide in-service training to therapists on clinical education topics, such as writing objectives, designing clinical learning experiences, evaluating student performance, and handling the problem student. The consultations resulted in improved quality of fieldwork for occupational therapy students. Some of the in-service participants subsequently enrolled in the university's master's degree program and have considered academic careers.

- *Problem:* A need to develop the research skills of occupational therapy clinicians and to encourage collaboration between faculty and clinicians on research projects
- *Solution:* Level II, educational consultation

An occupational therapy educator was invited by the director of a clinical facility to provide in-service training to the occupational therapy staff on research design. The consultation resulted in a collaborative research project between the faculty consultant and the staff of the clinical facility with potential for publication and/or conference presentation.

- *Problem:* A need to develop new occupational therapy education programs at all levels
- *Solution:* Level III, program and/or administrative consultation

An occupational therapy educator was invited by the director of a newly developed occupational therapy assistant curriculum to assist with preparation for accreditation by preparing course descriptions, measurable objectives, and evaluation instruments.

An occupational therapy education administrator was invited by the government of a third-world country to consult on the development of schools of allied health and the education of rehabilitation workers.

An occupational therapy educator used her sabbatical leave to consult to an educational program in Canada to assist in the preparation of a graduate-level curriculum.

These consultations improved curricula of technical, professional, and post-professional educational programs, resulting in increased availability of occupational therapists in the United States and abroad.

CONSULTATION DESCRIPTION

Organization

The experience of serving as an educational consultant to academic or clinical education settings can be a challenging and intellectually stimulating opportunity for occupational therapy educators. When the consultation takes place in a foreign country, the challenges and rewards are undoubtedly enhanced. The consultant is expected to bring to the experience an advanced level of academic, clinical, and/or administrative expertise. Additionally, the consultant must become familiar with the culture and environment of the host country, including the customs and lifestyle of the people, as well as a basic knowledge and understanding of the government, economy, health and social welfare systems, and the tertiary education system. If the language of the host country is other than English and one in which the consultant is not skilled, provision must be made for written and spoken translations in order for communication to be effective. Even in English-speaking countries outside the United States, the consultant would be wise to learn the colloquialisms and slang expressions of the region, and make every attempt to avoid using American colloquialisms.

The author was invited by the School of Occupational Therapy of a College of Health Sciences in Australia to serve as a visiting fellow for one academic semester of 17 weeks. The visiting fellowship program was established by the college to attract eminent scholars in the applied sciences to undertake research or program development activity in collaboration with appropriate college faculty. Hereafter, for purposes of uniformity, the author/visiting fellow is referred to as the consultant. Prior to the selection of a consultant, the School of Occupational Therapy at the college had identified a need to improve the clinical education component of their curriculum. The consultant had established a reputation for expertise in clinical education and for several years had been presenting training workshops for occupational therapists and other health professionals throughout the United States and Canada to develop clinical teaching and supervision skills. The consultant also had gained national and international recognition in continuing professional education during the years she was director of occupational therapy education at a large midwestern university rehabilitation hospital. Two occupational therapy faculty members at the Australian college had collaborated with the consultant on several educational projects in the United States and were instrumental in recommending her for the consultancy.

Initially, a letter of inquiry was sent by one of the school's clinical education coordinators to explore the consultant's interest in applying for the visiting fellowship. The consultant expressed interest and was later notified by the college of her selection and asked to come to Australia for the academic semester. After obtaining a leave of absence from her job, the consultant and the college agreed on a contract. The terms of the contract included the salary, paid in Australian dollars, equivalent to that of full-time senior lecturer at the college, as well as round-trip airfare to Australia and a cash allowance for shipping of personal effects. While specific responsibilities of the fellowship were not identified in the contract, it was understood that the focus would be clinical education and program development activity in collaboration with college faculty.

Following acceptance of the position in Australia, the consultant spent 6 months making arrangements for the trip abroad, including application for a U.S. passport and a work visa for temporary residence. The consultant also prepared for this experience by studying the area's geography, demographics, economic and social climate, major industries, government systems, arts and recreation, descriptions of the health and social problems, medical care, and social welfare programs. Arrangements also needed to be made for housing, health care, and schooling in Australia for the consultant's 6-year-old son. International traveler's health insurance was acquired and necessary medical and dental checkups were taken care of prior to departure. The consultant's home in the United States was rented for the months she would be in Australia.

Australia—Land and People

The island continent of Australia is located in the southern hemisphere between the Indian Ocean on its west coast and the Coral and Tasman Seas of the South Pacific Ocean on its east coast. Australia's area is nearly as large as the United States, excluding Alaska and Hawaii, yet the population of Australia at the time was about 15 million. Although Australia has fewer than two people per square kilometer, it is one of the world's most urbanized countries, with less than 15% of the population living in rural areas. Australia's lifestyle reflects the people's predominantly Western origins where the similarities with Western Europe and North America are greater than the differences. Australia is a wealthy country and has the resources to ensure continued prosperity.[2]

Social Welfare

The Australian government's involvement in social security began with the introduction of old age pensions in 1909, invalid pensions in 1910, and maternity allowances in 1912, gaining for Australia its reputation at the time as a pioneer in public welfare. The main components of Australia's social security programs today are pensions for the aged, war veterans, invalids, widows, and lone parents; unemployment and sickness benefits; allowances for families with children; and provisions for health insurance. Men of 65 and women of 60 are eligible for age pensions. Estimated expenditures on social security and welfare at the time of the consultancy was $11.3 million, or 27.8% of federal budget outlays. Most government social security payments are noncontributory and are paid directly to the beneficiary. Invalid pensions are payable to people aged 16 years and over who are permanently incapacitated for work or who are permanently blind. Most pensioners and their dependents are entitled to free medications and free optometrical consultations. An allowance is paid to families to help meet the exceptional costs of bringing up a severely or substantially handicapped child and to encourage the care of these children at home rather than in an institution. A benefit is paid for children under 16 with long-term disabilities who must be accommodated and cared for in approved residential facilities. Benefits are also available to people who, through unemployment, sickness, or injury, are temporarily unable to work and have lost income because of sickness or injury. Most sickness beneficiaries and their dependents are entitled to free medication and free optometrical consultations. Disabled people employed in sheltered workshops may be paid an allowance equal to the invalid pension. Free medical treatment and free accommodation and treatment at public hospitals is available to the unemployed and special beneficiaries whose income is below certain limits.

In addition to the federal government's role, the six Australian states are constitutionally responsible for the administration of many welfare services, including education, housing, public health, and maternal and child welfare. Departments of health and social welfare in individual states share responsibility for services for the aged, providing domiciliary and community-based services to enable old people to live more comfortably.

The Commonwealth Rehabilitation Services (CRS) was set up in 1948 to help handicapped people become economically and socially independent. Teams of medical specialists, therapists, tradespeople, teachers, and vocational counselors work toward developing each person's maximum physical, mental, vocational, and social potential. The service is free to virtually any disabled person in the working age group who can benefit from it. Other social services provided by the Australian government include social workers and welfare officers to help people with personal problems arising from sickness or other unexpected crises, services to aboriginals, and services to migrants and refugees. The government also provides grants-in-aid to four major national welfare organizations: the Australian Council of Social Services, the Australian Council for Rehabilitation of the Disabled, the Australian Council on Aging, and the Australian Pre-School Association.

Other programs of financial assistance include grants to community welfare agencies; grants to approved local government bodies, volunteer, and charitable organizations to establish homes for the aged or disabled; regular subsidies paid to organizations offering approved personal-care services for residents who are frail but not in need of full-time nursing care; and government subsidies to build nursing homes for aged people. Government funds are also available for meals-on-wheels programs of home-delivered meals to aged people and invalids; home-care services for aged people living in their own houses; and to organizations that provide training centers, activity therapy centers, and sheltered workshops for handicapped children and adults. Under the Homeless Persons Assistance Act of 1974, nonprofit organizations and local governing bodies may receive grants to help meet the costs of providing accommodations, food, and care for homeless people.

Children's services are provided by the state governments and include infant and baby health centers, special services within the education system for handicapped children, preschool services (supplemented by Australian government grants), welfare housing, and recreation services for children. The Office of Child Care in the Department of Social Security supports preschool services, day care, vacation and before-and-after school care, neighborhood centers and play groups, and work-related day care.

Health Care

The health costs of eligible pensioners, migrants, unemployment and special beneficiaries, and people on low incomes are covered by the government and include free public hospital accommodation and treatment. All other people must meet their health care costs either through health insurance or by personal payment.

Sixty-nine percent of Australian hospitals are public, excluding mental hospitals and nursing homes. Australia has an average of 6.4 hospital beds per 1,000 population, with about 25% of beds in private hospitals or repatriation (veterans) and armed services hospitals.

Of the 67,912 nursing home beds approved for financial support in 1,344 institutions primarily for geriatric care, 22% are in state-operated nursing homes. There are approximately 4.6 nursing home beds per 1,000 population. The Australian government pays benefits for all qualified patients in nursing homes, but all nursing home patients are required to make a minimum contribution to the cost of their care.

Other government-funded programs include health program grants to organizations providing health services to patients in special need who are not insured; domiciliary nursing care benefits for nursing care provided in the home; public health services for family planning, aboriginal health and arbovirus disease control; and community health programs offered by 15 national organizations. The government's program of aids for disabled people provides a range of aids for daily living for people with permanent disabilities ineligible for assistance under other government-funded programs. The primary aim of the program is to increase the level of independence of disabled people in the community.

Alcohol and drug abuse is a significant health problem in Australia. Until recently, most treatment programs for alcoholics were directed toward people suffering mental disturbance or social incompetence. Apart from Alcoholics Anonymous, most treatment and care was provided in mental hospitals. The Australian Foundation on Alcoholism and Drug Dependence (AFADD) is funded by the government as a national project under the community health program and is aimed at promoting and implementing alcohol and drug dependence intervention, rehabilitation and prevention programs, identifying problem individuals at an early stage.

Tertiary Education System in Australia

Prior to 1988 the Australian system of higher education had three major components: universities, colleges of advanced education, and colleges of technical and further education. While universities and colleges of advanced education provided courses in a number of similar tertiary disciplines, college courses had a greater vocational emphasis. Colleges of advanced education were either multivocational with courses in several disciplines, or single purpose institutions such as agricultural colleges. The School of Occupational Therapy was within a college of advanced education offering courses in several health disciplines. Australian colleges of technical and further education offered training in all the major industrial skills and in a wide range of commercial, artistic, and domestic occupations. Generally, these colleges are concerned with apprenticeship, trade, post-trade, and technician courses. The Australian government financed tertiary education with no tuition fees at universities, colleges of advanced education, and colleges of technical and further education.

In 1988 the federal government initiated a process of change that led to the demise of the tertiary system. Colleges of advanced education were subsumed within the university sector or combined with other colleges to form a university, moving toward what is called a unified system. Along with this change, fees were introduced and the older system of scholarships was brought back to assist students.

At the time of this consultancy there were five occupational therapy schools in Australia, four in colleges of advanced education in New South Wales, Western Australia, South Australia, and Victoria, and one at the University of Queensland.

College of Health Sciences

The college was organized with two departments and seven schools, including the Department of Behavioral and General Studies, Department of Biological Sciences, School of Communication Disorders, School of General Health Studies, School of Medical Record Administration, School of Nursing, School of Occupational Therapy, School of Orthoptics, and School of Physiotherapy. The majority of the courses offered were available on a full-time basis only. A feature of most courses was the requirement for a period of clinical experience to supplement the laboratory and lecture room instruction.

The college also had a center for continuing education to coordinate the continuing education programs offered for its graduates and other practicing professionals. The center for continuing education provided an administrative framework and support for short courses, seminars, lectures, and workshops designed in collaboration with the health professions and funded by participant fees.

The educational services unit provided services related to teaching and learning at the college by assisting college faculty in course development and evaluation, acting as a clearinghouse for information on teaching and learning, carrying out surveys and investigations in areas related to college teaching and learning, developing teaching packages, and providing consultancy services to health professionals in developing countries. The unit provided feedback to college faculty on their teaching, and offered workshops and discussion groups to improve faculty skills.

The administrative officers of the college were the principal, assistant principal, registrar, and bursar. Each of the college's departments and schools was comprised of a head and academic staff (faculty) in a hierarchy of levels that included senior lecturers, lecturers, and tutors, somewhat comparable to the American system of professorial ranks. The schools also employed clinical coordinators who were responsible for the clinical education component of their programs. Clinical education was viewed by the college as an essential and major component of all undergraduate and some postgraduate programs and was aimed at the development of clinical competence of students. This supervised clinical practice was provided in a variety of health care settings and institutions throughout the state.

The School of Occupational Therapy

The philosophical base of occupational therapy in Australia parallels the profession in the United States. Services are provided to individuals or groups whose abilities to cope with activities of daily living are threatened or impaired by developmental deficits, the aging process, physical injury or illness, and psychological or social disability. The primary focus of occupational therapy is the development of adaptive skills and performance capacity in order that the individual may complete activities and tasks essential to life roles at home, work, and leisure.

At the time of the consultancy the School of Occupational Therapy presented a 3½-year full-time course leading to a bachelor of applied science in occupational therapy, and a 1-year full-time course leading to a graduate diploma in occupational therapy, following a specified bachelor of science course at the university. The bachelor of applied science in occupational therapy included courses in the behavioral and biological sciences, occupational therapy theory, psychosocial processes, and sensory-motor processes for the first 3 years, with special investigations and selected studies offered in the third and fourth years.

Clinical education was scheduled throughout the 4-year program and included 145 hours in year 1, held during and following the academic semester, similar to level I fieldwork in occupational therapy programs in the United States. Year 2 included 225 hours of clinical education held at the end of the first semester and during the intersession. Year 3 required 450 hours of clinical education held in 6-week blocks at intersession prior to the start of each academic semester and during the second semester. Students in their fourth year of the program completed 240 hours of clinical education prior to and during semester 1.

Graduate diploma students completed 638 hours of clinical education held prior to semester 1, during the intersession, and following semester 2.

In 1984 the School of Occupational Therapy was staffed by the head of school, three senior lecturers, six lecturers, two tutors, and three clinical coordinators. The student body included about 350 students in the bachelor of applied science program, and 14 students in the graduate diploma course.

Support

Financial support for the consultant was provided, as detailed earlier in the terms of the formal contract. During the initial weeks of the consultation, the consultant enlisted the support of various people within the School of Occupational Therapy and other divisions of the college. The head of the School of Occupational Therapy provided valuable information about the curriculum, faculty issues, student concerns, and clarification of the mission and scope of the college and school. The consultant had access to curriculum materials, course syllabi, and other printed documents, and was invited to attend faculty meetings, fieldwork site visits, and meetings with clinical supervisors to uncover critical issues and problems requiring intervention. The support of the college's administrators allowed the consultant a great deal of freedom in identifying target populations and program strategies. A senior lecturer from the Department of Behavioral and General Studies assisted with the design of a research project developed during the consultation. Additional personnel resources are included in the description of the key individuals that follows.

Participants

Since the School of Occupational Therapy had identified a need to revise the clinical education component of their curriculum, the initial target population for this consultation included the three full-time clinical coordinators of the School of Occupational Therapy and the clinicians who supervised occupational therapy students on their clinical education placements. The school's clinical coordinators were responsible for identifying appropriate clinical sites, scheduling students, monitoring student progress during the clinical placements via telephone and site visits, and serving as a liaison between the clinics and the school. Those therapists who worked in large clinical settings and who had major responsibility for students were designated as student unit supervisors (SUS) or clinical unit coordinators (CUC) and attended several meetings and in-service training sessions at the college each semester.

Later in the semester the consultant interacted with the clinical coordinators in the School of Physiotherapy and their counterpart clinical supervisors. She also attended meetings of the college's clinical education committee, comprised of clinical coordinators from each of the seven schools, and met with the director and staff of the educational services unit (for faculty development) and the coordinator of continuing education. Through meetings additional target populations were identified, resulting in a broader provision of service than originally anticipated. This was the first time that a visiting fellow at the college had extended consultation services and programs beyond the school or department in which they were contracted.

The key power individuals who provided the climate for innovation and change for the consultation were the head of the School of Occupational Therapy and the college's two chief administrators, the principal and assistant principal.

Services Provided

A variety of methods were used to gather information and assess needs of various constituent groups within the college community. Interviews and one-on-one meetings with key personnel as well as attendance at School of Occupational Therapy faculty meetings, SUS/CUC meetings, and various college committee meetings enabled the consultant to identify several problem areas. Additional methods of data gathering included participation in clinical site visits, meetings with occupational therapy students, and library research. The consultant's office was located in close proximity to other occupational therapy faculty, allowing for frequent informal encounters and exchanges.

Within the early weeks of the consultation, multiple problem areas were identified resulting in the following objectives:

A. To help the head, School of Occupational Therapy:
   1. Evaluate the effectiveness of clinical education in the present system, and
   2. Determine the value of clinical site visits, which are very costly to the school.
B. To help the clinical supervisors of occupational therapy students:
   1. Strengthen relationships between School of Occupational Therapy and clinical supervisors,
   2. Provide clinical supervisors with training in clinical teaching and supervision skills, and
   3. Improve clinician's motivation to supervise students.
C. To help the clinical coordinators, School of Occupational Therapy:
   1. Develop a system for evaluating the clinical education component of the occupational therapy curriculum, and
   2. Develop a method for site selection.
D. To help the faculty, School of Occupational Therapy:
   1. Assist faculty in teaching special topics.
E. To help the students, School of Occupational Therapy:

    1. Assist students in dealing with stress related to clinical placements, and

    2. Improve preparation of students for community placements.

  F. To help the clinical coordinators, all schools:

    1. Develop skills to improve effectiveness of the college's clinical coordinators.

  G. To help the faculty, all schools and departments:

    1. Enhance faculty teaching effectiveness, and

    2. Improve interdepartmental relationships and communication.

Numerous strategies were implemented to meet these objectives using a variety of consultative models. Frequently a collegial or professional model enabled the consultant to interact with Australian faculty and clinicians in an egalitarian problem-solving relationship. During the ongoing phase of the consultancy, an educational model was employed with the consultant providing staff development and in-service workshops to meet identified education and training needs. Several of the consultant's strategies were service centered, illustrating a problem development model based on modification of existing programs to improve services.

The specific strategies to meet identified objectives included the design of a research project to measure the value of clinical site visits and the development of a three-part battery of instruments for assessment of clinical education. This included the clinical educator's self-evaluation of supervisory and teaching skills, the student's evaluation of the clinical educator and of the placement, and a peer evaluation of clinical education effectiveness. The consultant also developed a method and criteria for clinical education site selection. Workshops on motivation and effective clinical teaching strategies were conducted for the clinical supervisors. A certification process for clinical educators was recommended. The consultant assisted School of Occupational Therapy faculty by presenting lectures to students on several special topics. Consultation services were directed toward all college faculty through a workshop on teaching style/learning style and on elements of effective instruction provided under the auspices of the educational services unit. A 1-day workshop, "How to Be an Effective Mediator," was offered for all clinical coordinators of the college's seven schools. The consultant also provided input to the development of a postgraduate diploma course in clinical education. The occupational therapy students attended a lecture by the consultant, "Coping With Problems on Clinical Placements." Participant evaluations were collected at all educational programs provided by the consultant, providing feedback to her and other key personnel.

Prior to termination, the consultant submitted a report of recommendations for future activities to meet identified needs and to continue collaborative relationships between the Australian College and the United States. Suggestions to improve relations between the college and clinical educators included the development of nonsalaried faculty appointments of clinical educators, a clinical educators award, and a certification process for clinical educators. Other suggestions included offering college-based clinical services and community-based clinical services provided by college faculty. To continue collaboration with facilities in the

United States, systems for faculty and student exchanges were explored. In addition, possibilities for fellowships and advanced tutorials in U.S. facilities for college alumni and clinical educators interested in furthering skills in clinical practice, education, research, and administration were discussed. The consultant suggested topics for future clinical education workshops and ideas for collaborative continuing education programs for health professionals.

Outcome

Although the consultation officially terminated at the end of the semester, informal contact was maintained between the consultant, the head of the School of Occupational Therapy, and several college faculty through letters and phone calls. During her visit to the United States, one of the senior lecturers of the college spent some time at the consultant's university and continued to explore opportunities for student and faculty exchanges. Other college faculty have presented continuing education workshops in the United States. The consultant has spoken to several classes of occupational therapy students in the United States about Australia and opportunities for specialty fieldwork and employment there. Arrangements were made by the consultant's university for an Australian occupational therapy student to do a level II fieldwork experience in the United States.

Several changes at the School of Occupational Therapy have occurred subsequent to the consultation, but not specifically as a result of the consultant's recommendations. The three clinical coordinator positions have been removed from the School of Occupational Therapy and are now based in the clinical sites, with their salaries jointly paid by the college and the Department of Health. There are now seven persons in these positions, with the new title of fieldwork educator, responsible for planning the fieldwork experiences for eight to ten occupational therapy students in several facilities. With a significant increase in student enrollment, the total number of faculty of the school has doubled. The school now offers a master's by research and a coursework master's. The curriculum for the bachelor of applied science in Occupational Therapy has been revised and a bachelor's honors program is being offered. A 2-year full-time course leading to an associate diploma in diversional therapy has also been added. A recent significant change is that the college has become part of a major university in Australia, and now has the faculty to offer programs at the doctoral level.

SUMMARY

This chapter has presented a model of consultation for occupational therapy faculty. A review of the literature on current policies on faculty consulting in colleges and universities supported the position that consultation should be encouraged. A survey of occupational therapy educational programs also supported the view that faculty who consult keep abreast of clinical trends and enhance the quality of their teaching and research. Various examples of occupational therapy faculty consulting experiences in clinical and educational settings have illustrated the mutual benefits to consultant and consultee.

The author's experience as a visiting fellow in a school of occupational therapy in Australia presented many challenges and rewards and enriched her personal and professional life in numerous ways. The opportunity to share one's expertise with colleagues on the other side of the globe allowed for an exciting and unique exchange. Clinical and educational administrators are encouraged to seek the services of faculty consultants and to help expand and develop their programs in ways that may not be possible with existing personnel.

REFERENCES

1. Aggarwal R: Faculty members as consultants: A policy perspective. *J College University Personnel Assoc* 1981; 32:17–20.
2. Harrison P (ed): *Australia Handbook, 1982–83*. Canberra, Australia Government Publishing Service, 1982.
3. Boyer CM, Lewis DR: Faculty consulting: Responsibility or promiscuity? *J Higher Ed* 1984; 55:637–659.
4. Dillon KE: Outside professional activities. *National Forum: Phi Kappa Phi J* 1979; 69:35–42.
5. Golomb SW: Faculty consulting: Should it be curtailed? *National Forum: Phi Kappa Phi J* 1979; 69:34–37.
6. Patton CV, Marver JD: Paid consulting by American academics. *Ed Record* 1979; 60:175–184.
7. Watkins BT: Colleges urged to set policies on consulting by professors. *Chron Higher Ed* 1986; 31:23–25.
8. Wilson RC: Improving faculty teaching—effective use of student evaluations and consultants. *J Higher Ed* 1986; 57:196–211.
9. Zukas RR, Miriovsky J: A survey of clinical services provided by occupational therapy faculty. Unpublished study, Texas Woman's University, 1990.

C H A P T E R 30

Roles for the Occupational Therapy Consultant in Higher Education

Lela A. Llorens, Ph.D., O.T.R., F.A.O.T.A.

OVERVIEW

The role of the administrative occupational therapy consultant in higher education involves problem solving in the areas of curriculum and personnel, and securing the resources necessary for the successful development and management of educational programs. Implementation of the role involves observation, listening, questioning, analyzing, synthesizing, and reporting.

Sections in this chapter describe consultation with the following:

1. A university academic program in occupational therapy
2. A personnel department in a large urban university
3. Groups (committees) involved in mission and goal setting, strategic and long-range planning, and policy-making (peer consultation)
4. Disabled students' services

PROCESS OF CONSULTATION

Steps in the consultation process include (1) eliciting or receiving the invitation to consult; (2) engaging in preliminary preparation; (3) developing goals/objectives of the consultation; (4) establishing the length and cost of the consultation; (5) carrying out the consultation; and (6) reporting the results.

UNIVERSITY ACADEMIC PROGRAM
IN OCCUPATIONAL THERAPY

The invitation to consult in a university academic program in occupational therapy may be extended by the president, vice president, dean, chair, or other academic administrator. It is important for the consultant to understand the role of the person who extends the invitation and his or her influence within the organization. Preliminary preparation should include reviewing the appropriate primary documents of the university and of the Department of Occupational Therapy. If the consultation is related to an accreditation review, documents such as the university general catalog, specific departmental documents, curriculum materials, and the accreditation self-study should be reviewed. The preparation for such a consultation may include review of the curriculum and its components; review of personnel, fiscal, space, and other resources; and review of any evaluation reports such as institutional program review or accreditation self-study reports. These documents should be studied with particular focus on the mission statement, purpose, educational philosophy, conceptual frame(s) of reference, course content and structure, fieldwork experiences, faculty development, student development, financial resources, and space availability.

The length of the consultation and the consultation fee should be established at the outset. The cost of travel to and from the consultation site, per diem expenses for food and lodging, when the consultation requires the consultant to live away from home, and the consultation fee are standard costs of consultation. The consultant fee should be calculated to cover the costs of preparing materials by reproduction or other means.

The consultant's schedule should be negotiated with the consultee to maximize the benefit of the consultant's services to the consultee.

The author's experience with academic consultation has been limited to short-term consultation of 3- to 5-day visits. Additional preliminary preparation has included literature review of current and future trends in higher education;[1-3] current and future trends in allied health education;[4] past, current, and future trends in occupational therapy education;[5-7] and review of the primary documents of the institution.

The visit should include interviews or conferences with university administrators to whom the program director reports and those to whom he or she is responsible or with whom collaboration and cooperation are essential. Meetings with the program director, faculty, and students should be scheduled. A tour of the facilities would be in order as well as the opportunity for informal dialogue to assess the climate of the particular environment. The consultant's skills in observation of formal and informal group interaction, understanding of verbal and nonverbal language, and ability to assess findings relative to stated and, perhaps, unstated objectives are critical to the process.

Follow-through in the process involves integrating and reporting the consultant's observations, assessment, and recommendations to the consultee.

Consultant reports should address the objectives of the consultation as determined by the consultee. The report may be introduced with background information on the institution or department sufficient only to place the consultation report into a context. The objectives should be stated with assessment of the components of the program reported giving the strengths and weaknesses or areas that need to be developed, recommendations, and summary. For example, a consultation to a Department of Occupational Therapy could be undertaken to evaluate the program and its development within a research university. Such components as budget, leadership, curriculum, space, faculty credentials and salary structure, current and future student enrollment, and environmental support would need to be studied. Interviews would be held with university administrators, members of the faculty, and students. Strengths may be identified such as highly committed faculty, good quality and quantity of space, unique service offered by the program in addition to educational curriculum, supportive climate within the university for the program, and the like. Problem areas such as lack of visibility of the program within the university, too few doctorally prepared faculty, lack of balance between teaching and research, relatively low faculty salary scale, lack of funds for faculty travel, and lack of opportunities for students to take part in individual study and research may be identified. Recommendations would include but not be limited to (1) increase the congruence between department's activities and university's commitment to research; (2) locate and recruit appropriately credentialed, qualified faculty with demonstrated leadership ability; (3) allocate appropriate budget to increase faculty salaries and provide funds for professionally related travel; and (4) assign/elect faculty members to school and university committees.

PERSONNEL DEPARTMENT
WITHIN A LARGE UNIVERSITY

The invitation to consult may be sought from or extended by the manager of the Personnel Department or Human Resources Division. Occupational therapists' areas of expertise that are particularly valuable to personnel or human resource managers are skill in the development of measurable behavioral objectives for personnel management and environmental assessment of the workplace to prevent vocational dysfunction. To be successful in this kind of consultation, the role and sphere of influence of the person with whom the occupational therapist consults must be understood. This level of understanding is critical in order to assess the likelihood of recommendations from the consultation being implemented. It is well known that consultants recommend, and it is the prerogative of the consultee whether or not to utilize the recommendations.

The length of the consultation and the consultation fee should be established in accordance with the anticipated demands of the invitation. Again, the consultant fees should be calculated to cover materials that may be needed to conduct workshops for personnel or human resource managers. In this setting, the model of consultation utilized usually involves active participation by the consultant and is sometimes called the participatory consultation, or action model.[8, 9] In such consultation, a more interactive role is taken by the consultant, such as teaching, demonstration, or conducting a needs assessment. Participation by the consultant may be most effective when the consultant imparts skills to the consultee that will permit the consultee to carry out the recommendations of the consultation.

In the author's experience, one such consultation was an invitation to assist in solving personnel problems with custodial staff who were expressing considerable dissatisfaction with their supervision. Their supervision was perceived to be influenced by favoritism, and personnel decisions and discipline were seen as arbitrary. Numerous grievances were filed.

Observations of the workers, interviews with the personnel, supervisors, and managers, and inspection of job descriptions yielded information about the working conditions and the problems as perceived by all parties. The consultant recommended instituting measurable behavioral objectives for the positions in question so that supervision could be more objective. Thus problems could be identified as they occurred without personal bias as a factor, and all parties could recognize when an objective was or was not being met.

PEER CONSULTATION

In higher education, collegiality involves peer interaction that may include consultation between departments or within groups, primarily on committees, as the major ongoing work of the university occurs in the activity of its many committees.

Occupational therapists' skills in observation, group dynamics, goal setting, problem solving, evaluation, development of measurable behavioral objectives, and reporting are valuable in these interactions. However, such interactions within one's own institution tend to fall within the realm of the position rather than as a service for fee. The exception to this situation is the type of specific consultation that is often associated with specialized knowledge and expertise, contracted for grant development or execution that involves participation beyond the individual's normal workload and may therefore be provided for a fee.

DISABLED STUDENTS' SERVICES

The invitation to consult with disabled students and their families may be extended by the administrator of a designated program. The consultant will use observation and interview and may use testing and history review as well as the review of relevant documents to gather necessary information. The model of participant consultation is most appropriate because the consultant may be called on to assess the student and/or elements of his or her environment as a part of the problem solving required of the consultation. An assessment may be necessary in order to make appropriate recommendations.

Such consultation may be contracted on a fee for service basis. Appropriate reports would be made to the administrator who requested the consultation. This type of service may be appropriate for students with visual, hearing, learning, physical, and/or emotional disabilities.

SUMMARY

Four examples of consultation by occupational therapists in higher education were described. Key skills used by occupational therapists as consultants in higher education are observation, listening, interview, testing, analysis, problem solving, goal setting, synthesis, and reporting. Steps in the consultation process were delineated.

REFERENCES

1. Brubacher JS: *On the Philosophy of Higher Education*. San Francisco, Jossey-Bass, 1982.
2. Carnegie Council on Policy Studies in Higher Education: *The Carnegie Council on Policy Studies in Higher Education*. San Francisco, Jossey-Bass, 1980.
3. Levine A: *Handbook on Undergraduate Curriculum*. Prepared for the Carnegie Council on Policy Studies in Higher Education. San Francisco, Jossey-Bass, 1978.
4. National Commission on Allied Health Education: *The Future of Allied Health Education*. San Francisco, Jossey-Bass, 1980.
5. American Occupational Therapy Association: *A Curriculum Guide for Occupational Therapy Educators*. Rockville, Md, AOTA, 1979.
6. American Occupational Therapy Association: *Occupational Therapy: 2001 A.D.* Rockville, Md, AOTA, 1979.
7. American Occupational Therapy Association: *Target 2000: Occupational Therapy Education*. Rockville, Md, AOTA, 1986.
8. Gillette N: Occupational therapy belongs in the community, in Llorens LA (ed): *Consultation in the Community: Occupational Therapy in Child Health*. Dubuque, Iowa, Kendall-Hunt, 1973; pp 127–130.
9. Mazer JR: The occupational therapist as consultant. *Am J Occup Ther* 1969; 23:417–421.

SECTION G

Occupational Therapy Consultation in Regulatory Settings

Regulation is often viewed negatively by health care providers. However, the regulatory process can facilitate service delivery. Survey deficiencies can trigger immediate administrative response to problems that have impeded progress. For instance, a strategy for increasing facility staffing may be to document the lack of service. Surveyors can then cite the facility and force increased staff allocations. In this case, the surveyor assumes an authoritarian role. In a consultative role, the surveyor provides advice and education and helps the client use the survey as part of a growth process.

Occupational therapists who assume roles as regulatory consultants have opportunities to facilitate positive change in the health care delivery system, and more specifically, in the delivery of occupational therapy services. The authors in this section provide examples of regulatory consultation that address both broad system and specific therapy concerns.

Harlock, in her role as an accreditation surveyor, describes the consultative nature of this task and the mutual conferring, advice-seeking relationship that can be engendered through the survey process. She points out that accreditation organizations, such as the Commission on Accreditation of Rehabilitation Facilities (CARF), help to define the field and increase recognition of the programs provided. This type of consultation differs from other models in that the client must perform an intensive self-study in order to prepare for the survey and consultation. The goal of accreditation is to improve the quality of services provided, based on established standards. The consultant utilizes organizational development and/or program development consultation models. The case example presented demonstrates the interactive nature of the accreditation process. The consultative approach used helped rehabilitation services address specific problems that were impeding their ability to deliver services.

National health care corporations utilize internal quality assurance consultants to monitor their rehabilitation services. Reimbursement and adherence to regulatory procedures are major concerns. Berkeland describes his experiences as a consultant for such a corporation and for an insurance third-party payor company that required a medical review consultant. He served as an expert witness, claims reviewer, and trainer. He also performed related administrative duties for the insurance company. Working internally, the consultant helped educate members of the review team regarding occupational therapy services. Working externally, he helped occupational therapy providers and their teams understand the review process. Ongoing monitoring of current regulations is a crucial part of the consultant's responsibility. Berkeland concludes with key criteria to consider before entering this type of consultation.

The development of regulations for the prevention, remediation, and treatment of institutional child abuse in state-operated residential facilities for children and youth is the focus of Chang's consultation. As an internal consultant, she used a collegial model to facilitate interagency consensus regarding the implementation of these regulations. This complex and unusual case example provides an in-depth picture of interagency relationships and the barriers that may exist when attempting to help such groups unite under one conceptual and regulatory framework.

Izutsu presents the unique concerns of the international consultant. The broad nature of such consultation, tempered with the realities of understanding a different culture, language, and way of thinking in a foreign land are identified and discussed.

Regulatory Settings

AUTHOR	MODEL	LEVEL	LOCUS	GOAL
Harlock	Collegial, Educational, and Organizational Development	Levels II and III: Educational and administrative	Rehabilitation facilities	Improve quality of services
Berkeland	Collegial and Educational	Levels II and III: Educational and administrative	Third-party intermediaries	Assure quality of services
Chang	Collegial, Educational, Systems, and Social Action	Level III: Administrative	State agencies	Assure implementation of regulations addressing child abuse issues in state residential settings
Izutsu	Collegial, Program Development, and Systems	Levels II and III: Educational and administrative	Developing countries; international health organizations	Help establish rehabilitation services in developing countries

CHAPTER 31

Occupational Therapy Consultation for Adult Rehabilitation Program Standards and Regulations

Sylvia Harlock Kauffman, Ph.D., O.T.R., F.A.O.T.A.

OVERVIEW

Can consultation really take place in the context of regulation or accreditation? Consultation and regulation/accreditation are different but complementary processes.

To regulate means "to control or direct according to a rule, to adjust in conformity to a specification or requirement."[9] Accreditation is a particular form of regulatory process in which an organization or program is surveyed to determine that it meets a prescribed standard.[9] Bell defines consultation as "the provision of information or help by a professional helper (consultant) to a help-seeking person or system (client) in the context of a voluntary, temporary relationship which is mutually advantageous."[1, p 1]

Accreditation is consultative in nature to the degree that one believes the following:

- The accreditation standards are appropriate measures of quality.
- The accreditation process is beneficial in verifying or redirecting one's efforts to provide quality services to one's clients (patients).
- The minimum standards will be met, and it is possible to implement recommendations that result from the accreditation process.
- The whole process is beneficial to society in defining quality services to potential customers and in ensuring availability of and access to needed services.

Without these beliefs, the accreditation process is likely to be viewed as an unnecessary hassle or threat to survival. The tendency in this latter scenario is to hide information from a surveyor rather than to direct the surveyor toward problem or developmental aspects of one's program and to engage in mutual conferring, deliberating, and advice-seeking interaction.

Preparation for accreditation is consultative in that an organization evaluates its readiness for accreditation by comparing its operations with the standards. The standards represent the collective consensus of many experts in the field, in essence, many consultants. The actual accreditation site survey process is consultative in that the surveyors are responsible for verifying that an organization or program meets all required standards. Interactive consultation during the site survey itself is likely to be sought and/or given in relation to only a subset of the standards. Those being surveyed have the responsibility of directing the survey process to maximize the time and attention spent by the surveyors on interactive consultation and of directing the survey team to those issues/standards for which consultation is desired.

To be a regulatory consultant one must be knowledgeable of the norms and future directions of the field being regulated. It is very important that occupational therapists be represented in the development, review, and ongoing revision of standards as well as in the individual facility/program accrediting process to ensure appropriate promotion, understanding, and quality enhancement of the field of occupational therapy. In regard to the regulation of multidisciplinary programs, however, the occupational therapist's consultative effectiveness will be dependent also on the therapist's knowledge of the multidisciplinary field as a whole (i.e., comprehensive medical rehabilitation, chronic pain, or work hardening programs).

The author has had experience in developing hospital and rehabilitation regulatory standards, in surveying rehabilitation programs for accreditation, and in providing consultation to occupational therapy and other health care providers. The example of consultation in the context of regulation that is described in this chapter is drawn from a composite of the author's consultation experiences including those as an accreditation surveyor for the Commission on Accreditation of Rehabilitation Facilities.

ENVIRONMENTAL AND SYSTEMS INFLUENCES

Effective use of the accreditation process for consultative assistance depends on an understanding of its role in society and of the way the process works.

A number of factors must be present to stimulate the development of regulatory standards and of accrediting procedures at any given point in time:

- Critical mass of programs of like type.
- Belief of potential harm to the public in the absence of regulatory standards (quality and/or access).
- Cost; protection or wise use of the public's resources.

- Protection of the industry.
- Advocacy for potential consumers of the program.

There must be a sufficient number of providers who see themselves as similar in type to form a critical mass that supports the development of standards and activities of an accrediting organization. Each provider must also be an organizational unit in order to make accreditation possible from an operational standpoint. There are too few occupational therapy programs as singular entities to provide such a critical mass. There are sufficient rehabilitation agencies or programs, however, to meet this criteria. Occupational therapy is acknowledged as a key component of these programs.

The second and third factors both involve protection of the public. Rehabilitation and occupational therapy are rapidly developing fields. They are sufficiently technical that the average consumer and payor cannot easily judge quality and protection from potential harm without assistance from persons trained in the field. Medical technology and the aging of the population are making it possible for increasing numbers of disabled, the users of these services, to survive. All of these trends support the continued need for regulatory activity. In some cases, third-party payment to a facility is dependent on the facility's ability to show evidence to the third-party payor (i.e., commercial medical insurer or governmental payor) of accreditation of the facility/programs by the Joint Commission on the Accreditation of Hospital Organizations (JCAHO) and/or the Commission on Accreditation of Rehabilitation Facilities (CARF).

The industry of rehabilitation and occupational therapy providers also have much to gain from the regulatory process. The process modulates entry of new providers into the system, making competition more predictable and manageable. The regulatory process helps to define the field and thereby increase the recognition and acceptance by payors and users of given types of programs.

Potential users of the programs also benefit from widespread recognition of given types of programs. Such recognition stimulates geographic and economic availability and accessibility. Insurers in some cases utilize evidence of accreditation as a criterion for payment to a given organization for specified treatment services.

There are dangers to regulation as follows:

- Lack of timely adaptation to technical changes in the field and/or environment; regulation tends to cement the status quo at a given point of time.
- Lack of opportunity to test the need for ongoing regulation.
- Cost of regulation.
- Prevention of access to services that do not meet (or seek) the accreditation for reasons other than quality.

Providers, regulators, and the public all have an ethical obligation to question continually the need for regulatory activities as well as to advocate for them when needed.

The accreditation process involves first the development of standards and then surveys of each given organization to determine whether the organization meets the standards. The standards are usually developed by bringing together experts who are knowledgeable about the field as a whole (not just their own program or particular program component) and representatives of the public. Standards need to reflect up-to-date norms of clinical practice and organizational management. Expectations that reflect concerns of the public good, such as measures of efficiency or accessibility, may also be addressed to the degree that they can be controlled by the organization seeking accreditation.

Initial drafts of standards are usually distributed widely for review and comment. Standards are constantly being reviewed and updated by the accrediting organization in response to developments in the field and feedback from surveyors and surveyees. Such updates involve a process of field input similar to that used in the original development of the standards.

The decision to seek accreditation is voluntary. External pressure to seek accreditation comes through the linkage of such accreditation to payment by third parties or linkage to publicly accepted symbols of quality (e.g., Good Housekeeping Seal of Approval).

FRAME OF REFERENCE

Nature of Consultation in the Regulatory Context

To consult means to seek advice or information. It also means to exchange views; to confer.[9] When the organization seeking accreditation conducts its self-study, it is essentially seeking the advice of (consulting with) experts in comparing its operation with standards set forth by experts in the field. The accreditation site survey completes the consultation cycle by verifying that no further consultation is needed (the organization meets the standards) or by discussing and making recommendations for actions to more fully comply with the standards. The site survey is interactive primarily in regard to methods the organization may use to meet the standards. To a more limited extent, it may be interactive in terms of revisions to the standards per se by communicating the organization's suggestions for changes in the standards to the parent accrediting organization (or encouraging the organization to do so directly). No action may be taken on these suggestions at the site survey level, however. Changes in the standards result from more widespread field input and review under the official direction of the accrediting agency.

To utilize consultation in the regulatory context effectively, then, occupational therapists must spend considerable time reviewing their own operations in comparison to the standards (self-study). The standards are written in general terms. There may be many ways to carry out one's activities to meet the standards. The how-tos are often not defined in the standards. To gain maximum consultative benefit from the site survey, then, it is beneficial for the personnel of the organization (including the occupational therapists) to identify specific standards for which they would like consultation on alternative or better ways to meet these specific standards. Unless the personnel of the organization engage in this kind of homework, they are not in a position to participate in the consultation.

The CARF accreditation process is ultimately designed to improve the quality of services provided to individuals with disabilities.[5] The standards focus on the effectiveness of the operation of the organization as a whole and on the effectiveness and efficiency of programs operated by the organization. Consultation is likely to involve the organizational development model and/or program development model of consultation. The organizational development model of consultation is a management-focused model based on organizational structure in which technological assistance, leadership styles, interpersonal communications, and group relations are a part of the consultation. (see Chapter 2). The program development model is a service-centered model based on the development of new service programs or modification of existing programs to improve services. Assessment, design, implementation, and evaluation are components of the program development model to increase or improve a service delivery system (see Chapter 2). Although representatives of all levels of the organization are interviewed during a site visit, the major emphasis of interactive consultation involves persons holding organizational and program leadership positions under the assumption that these persons have more responsibility, power, and ability to maintain and/or shape events.

Bell describes five phases of the consulting process: entry, diagnosis, response, disengagement, and closure.[1] In the entry phase, problems are jointly explored, perceived needs and symptoms are discussed, relationships are clarified, goals and roles are defined, resource parameters are identified, methodology is clarified, and ultimately a contract is negotiated. The entry phase is very structured in the accreditation process by the existence of the standards and minimum qualifications for accreditation, the self-study process, and the application, site visit, and outcome determination procedures.

The diagnostic phase involves the process of determining by examination the cause and nature of a problem. It generally begins with the understanding of the problem as perceived by the client. It includes an appreciation of the client's goals, resources, and the client system's culture, values, norms, and beliefs. The consultant is charged with identifying the sybsystem(s) in which the problem is perceived to be located and the interrelationships between the subsystem and the other parts of the system. Another important issue is the extent and degree to which the client system is willing to commit its resources to a resolution of the problem. The scope of a CARF survey, the organization and preparation of materials by the organization for review by the surveyors, and the broad sampling of input through interviews from all levels of the organization and its customers facilitates diagnostic consultation.

The response or action phase focuses on the selection of a course of action, redefinition of the consultative goals, and identification of appropriate objectives, strategies, and roles. Plans and structured interventions may be employed to correct the problem or improve the situation that was spelled out in the entry phase. The accreditation process does not lend itself to major involvement in this phase. Suggestions and recommendations are made during the CARF survey process and resources for further consultation may be identified. Extensive, ongoing consultation, however, is not a part of the accrediting process and may not be procured from the surveyors themselves.

The disengagement phase deals with the evaluation of the results to determine whether the response has been successful and is progressing as planned and whether there is a need for further consultation. The closure phase acknowledges a formal end to the consultation. The survey exit conference, the formal evaluation of the accreditation experience that is sought from the organization by CARF, and the report on progress on the survey recommendations that is required by CARF of the organization provide structured disengagement and closure mechanisms.

Effective Consultant Interaction

A consultant's effectiveness derives not only from his or her objectivity, expertise, technical performance, and the legitimacy of the role, but from his or her skills in relating and communicating with others.[1,4,6,8,11] In the accreditation site visit the surveyor can usually spend only about 20 or 30 minutes in any given interview, with the exception of time spent periodically throughout the 2 days with two or three key administrative and program directors. The surveyor (consultant) must have excellent listening skills,[3] have a clear concept of the type of information he or she wants to gain from the interaction,[7] communicate clearly that information shared is confidential,[10] be able to ask probing questions and "test" suggestions and potential recommendations in a nonthreatening way, and acknowledge program, performance, and system strengths.

The surveyor (consultant) may use any or all of the types of interventions described by Blake: acceptant, catalytic, confrontation, prescription, or theories and principles.[2] In the acceptant intervention the intention is to give the client a sense of personal security so that he or she feels free to express personal thoughts without fear of adverse judgments or rejection. The client may thus be helped to sort out emotions in a self-reliant manner and thereby get a more objective view of the situation. Catalytic intervention assists the client in collecting data and information to reinterpret his or her perceptions of how things are. In this way, the client may arrive at a better awareness of the problem and how to handle it. Confrontation challenges a client to examine how the present foundations of thinking—usually value-laden assumptions—may be coloring and distorting the way situations are viewed; that is, the client may screen off one or more alternative options which, if he or she were aware of them, could lead to the selection of more effective actions. In prescriptive intervention, the consultant tells the client what to do to rectify the situation. The consultant takes the responsibility for developing the evidence for the diagnosis and formulates the solution as a recommendation to be followed. The theories and principles approach involves the presentation of theories pertinent to the client's situation. The consultant helps the client internalize systematic and empirically tested ways of understanding. This new knowledge permits the client to view his or her situation in a more analytic, cause-and-effect fashion. Thus the client becomes able to diagnose and plan how to deal with the present and future situations in more valid ways. The accreditation situation most lends itself to acceptant, catalytic, and confrontational types of intervention.

CONSULTATION DESCRIPTION

In the following example of consultation in the context of regulation, the consultation process was used effectively by the organization involved, including the occupational therapy department director.

Organization

The consultation took place in the context of a CARF survey of a hospital seeking accreditation for its comprehensive inpatient rehabilitation program. A CARF survey involves a review of the program and the whole organization's performance in relation to the CARF standards. The standards are broad in scope and are organized into three sections:[5]

1. Standards for the organization, which cover such things as governing body, organization and administration, personnel administration and staff development, program evaluation, fiscal management, and physical facilities and safety.
2. Standards for all programs, which include general standards for such activities as intake and orientation of the client, client assessment and individual program planning, individual client program management, treatment, and training, and assessment of program quality among others.
3. Standards for Individual Programs, which include specific standards for each of 19 different rehabilitation programs—comprehensive inpatient rehabilitation, brain injury programs, work hardening programs, community mental health programs, and others.

CARF accredits the organization as a whole (not the individual program), requiring that the organization be in substantial compliance with the standards for all programs surveyed.[5]

The hospital surveyed was a 200-bed community-based hospital located in an economically middle-class, established section of a large city. The hospital was part of a small for-profit multihospital corporation. The hospital environment was very competitive, as reflected in its 50% occupancy rate. The hospital operated a 35-bed comprehensive rehabilitation program serving patients with stroke, hip fracture, and a variety of other diagnoses. The rehabilitation program operated at

70% occupancy and drew patients from a much wider geographical market base than the rest of the hospital. The organizational structure and staffing pattern were typical for a hospital this size and for a comprehensive rehabilitation inpatient program.

Support

The hospital had successfully completed CARF accreditation of its comprehensive inpatient rehabilitation program 3 years previously and was seeking reaccreditation (maximum accreditation is for a 3-year period). The hospital had completed its own self-study using the CARF standards as its evaluation tool and had reviewed recommendations from the prior survey to assure they had been addressed. It had submitted an application for the accreditation survey to CARF along with the necessary application fees.

Participants

The commission had scheduled the survey and selected a survey (consultation) team composed of an administrative consultant (the author) and a program (clinical) consultant to conduct the survey. CARF surveyors are rehabilitation administrators and clinicians who are actively working in the field. They have been selected by CARF with input from their peers in the field and have received training from CARF to become surveyors. CARF surveyors agree to conduct at least three surveys a year to maintain their skills as surveyors and to maintain a broad perspective of developments in the field as a whole. They continue to be active administrators and clinicians in the field to maintain their perspective of practical, daily operations.

In this example, the surveyors were the author, an administrator of a wide range of medical rehabilitation programs in a community-based hospital, and a physician, the medical director of a range of medical rehabilitation programs for a different community-based hospital. Surveyors are always selected from geographical locations outside the region of the hospital being surveyed to avoid conflict of interest and to protect confidentiality of information.

CARF surveyors interact with staff from all levels and all departments of a hospital when conducting a site survey. The key leadership in this example consisted of the hospital administrator, the rehabilitation program director, and the rehabilitation medical director. Over 20 different people were interviewed by one or both of the surveyors during this survey. Three of the interviews were with outside persons (referring physician, insurer, and patient). Others were with clinical staff, rehabilitation department managers, hospital director of finance, director of personnel, safety committee members, corporate director of marketing, and so on.

Services Provided

A site survey usually takes 1½ to 2 days (more if several programs are to be evaluated). The survey team began by conducting an orientation session with representatives of the governing board, administration, and staff and leadership of the program(s) being surveyed. It is very appropriate for the director of the Occupational Therapy Department and the occupational therapy staff involved in the program(s) being surveyed to be present at this orientation session. In this example the director of occupational therapy was present.

At the orientation session the CARF surveyors thanked the organization for inviting CARF to accredit them, briefly described their own professional backgrounds, explained the purposes of CARF and the role of the site visit, described how the team would conduct the survey, and identified possible outcomes of the site visit and of the accreditation process as a whole. (The survey team reports its findings, but CARF makes the final determination regarding accreditation outcome, communicating this outcome to the organization 6 to 8 weeks after the site visit.) Hospital administration and staff were then asked to introduce themselves and give a brief overview of the hospital and the rehabilitation program. This interaction established an initial rapport, clarified expectations, and set ground rules for further interaction. The orientation session lasted about 15 minutes.

Following the orientation, the rehabilitation program leadership was asked to take the surveyors on a tour of the facility. This oriented the surveyors so they knew where to go to interview people later in the day. In addition, it enabled them to check compliance with many of the physical facility and safety standards while touring. The organization had the opportunity to talk about its program, highlighting strengths and raising issues of concern. The tour took about 15 to 20 minutes.

After the tour, the survey team was taken to the room where all the documents (policies and procedures, committee meeting minutes, charts, etc.) were assembled and that served as headquarters for the team during the site visit. The surveyors and the hospital's rehabilitation program administrator worked out schedules for interviews for the day. The rehabilitation program administrator was readily available throughout the site visit but did not hover over the surveyors.

The two surveyors focused respectively on the administrative versus clinical (program) standards and compared observations frequently to identify major strengths and weaknesses in the organization's performance in relation to the CARF standards. In this example, the author (administrative surveyor) first explored the following in order to identify areas that might need further in-depth exploration:

1. Financial audit of the organization: Was the hospital financially stable or in a position of significant financial risk? If the hospital does not survive, the program cannot survive.
2. Data: patient population served, major payors, major referral sources, trends, and so on. What were the major implications for future patient volumes, staff needs (number and expertise), and financial bottom line?

3. Committee meeting minutes, types and quality of operating reports, program evaluation system reports. How sophisticated was the information on operations, how available was this information to the rehabilitation program managers and staff, and how involved and sophisticated were the rehabilitation managers and staff in utilizing this information for planning and decision making?

4. Staff: numbers, types of expertise, turnover rates, organizational reporting structure, evidence of up-to-date performance evaluations, and so on. Did the organization have the personnel resources needed, and was the staff excited, focused, and working together effectively clinically and administratively?

The author/consultant interviewed the rehabilitation program director, the hospital's administrator of finance, the director of personnel, the chief operating officer, and the corporate director of marketing. Additionally, she scanned the rehabilitation departments' and hospital's policy and procedure manuals and minutes of different rehabilitation and hospital (including board of trustees) committees. By mid-afternoon of the first day, the author/consultant had formulated the following tentative picture:

1. Financially stable organization that was efficiently operated but was facing increasingly serious financial constraints (not unlike many other hospitals and inpatient rehabilitation programs in the nation).

2. Seasoned organization in terms of development and implementation of traditional hospital organizational structure and policies and procedures.

3. Physical plant that was older but appropriately designed for an inpatient rehabilitation program and was well maintained.

4. Midway into development of an inpatient rehabilitation business and promotional plan. Evidence of some initial brainstorming/planning for diversification and development of outpatient rehabilitation programming.

5. Some recent rehabilitation clinical staff turnover, current dependence on agency personnel for some rehabilitation clinical staff, and concern over recruitment problems (common to the city as a whole, not just this facility).

The author/consultant next conferred with the other (clinical program) surveyor to see if her observations were supported by his and to see if he had other concerns. He added the following observations:

1. Seasoned rehabilitation inpatient program in terms of development and implementation of traditional multidisciplinary hospital-based inpatient rehabilitation program for older neurologically or orthopedically impaired patients; well-integrated multidisciplinary team; very traditional programs and hospital focused in rehabilitation treatment planning.

2. Dependent on agency for some clinical staff for more than one therapy service, but success in obtaining long-term assignment to assure consistency

of patient care. Recruitment of significant concern, but recruitment and staffing problems not yet significantly impacting patient care; some signs of initial staff burnout and discouragement.
3. Evidence of increased administrative support over the past year for rehabilitation programs in terms of leadership personnel resources.
4. Internal rather than outreach, community-based focus on the part of rehabilitation staff, department managers, and hospital as a whole. Evidence of need for vision of how things could be different and for some increased personnel support at the staff level to pursue such visions/opportunities.

The major recommendations, then, would center around staff recruitment, staff retention, market-based planning, and community outreach.

Up to this point (first day) the consultation had focused to a large degree on fact-finding, on evaluating whether performance met the standards, and on verifying to the organization whether their own self-assessment was accurate.

The evening of the first day, the surveyors each reviewed the standards in detail to identify whether further fact-finding was needed to verify compliance with each specific standard. The surveyors also wrote most of the report that would be presented to the organization the next day, identifying strengths of the organization and making recommendations.

The second day the consultation was more interactive in nature. Observations and possible recommendations were discussed with the key administrative leadership of the rehabilitation program. Possible ways to meet the CARF standards of concern were discussed.

The two surveyors met with the rehabilitation program director and medical director. The methods the hospital had already tried in regard to recruitment of occupational therapists and physical therapists were identified:

• Local and national advertising
• Recruitment firms
• Salary readjustments

Beliefs about why they were having difficulty recruiting were discussed:

• Shortage of available candidates
• Unrealistically high salary expectation of potential candidates
• Lack of potential candidates with interest in geriatric patients
• Competitive attractiveness of a high stimulus teaching hospital nearby

Alternative ways of perceiving the situation were generated without preevaluation of validity/applicability to this hospital's situation (first step in brainstorming):

• Appeal of incentives other than salary to possible candidates
• Opportunity for this hospital to promote the professional/clinical rewards/ excitement of working with the older patient

- Opportunity for this hospital to promote the rewards of working in a small, close-knit, responsive, community-integrated facility
- Opportunity for staff to be involved in program development and community outreach
- Opportunity for hospital to make contact with prospective candidates before graduation and to perhaps assure employment in return for partial tuition support—preselecting students for interest in and willingness to focus elective training on the older patient

The surveyors shared their experiences and knowledge of what other hospitals had tried. The result of this 15-minute interaction was that the rehabilitation program director and medical director began to get excited about some of the possibilities. They began to evaluate which ideas might work at their hospital, in their city. The medical director then asked the surveyors to meet with the director of occupational therapy and of physical therapy and the rehabilitation program director to further explore ideas.

This second meeting included a discussion of practical realities and possible implementation strategies as well as further idea generation:

- If staff are to become involved in community outreach, do they need additional skills and information such as how to make an effective presentation, how to make a cold call on a physician to promote the program, and facts about the physician networks and referral patterns and about other services offered by the hospital?
- What additional resources (time) would need to be allocated to be effective in outreach/promotional activities?
- How do you measure the cost effectiveness of therapists' involvement in promotional activities?
- How do you convince administration to support promotional and program development involvement of staff when you cannot guarantee success up front?
- How can I lead my staff when I have never done anything like this myself? Where do I find mentoring resources?
- Do I need to revise staff selection criteria to include risk taking/entrepreneurial interest or experience?

With this discussion and idea sharing, the rehabilitation program director, medical director, and therapy department directors were able to incorporate the concepts and examples needed to continue to generate ideas and pursue them successfully with administration. This was the extent of consultation appropriate for surveyor involvement. If the rehabilitation administration or hospital had felt significant additional consultation had been needed, the surveyors would have discussed resources for further consultation. As CARF surveyors, they could not have pursued an ongoing consultant relationship with the hospital themselves. That would involve a conflict of interest.

Consultant interaction in these two sets of interviews involved acceptant, catalytic, and confrontational types of intervention.[2] Through the interaction that took place during the first day, the hospital and rehabilitation leadership felt safe in discussing with the surveyors their concerns, frustrations, and dead-end attempts to recruit therapy staff (acceptant interaction). This climate of trust had been generated through clear communication of mutual expectations, through validation of the many things they were doing right, through communication of a genuine desire to be helpful, and through the initial offering of suggestions that were perceived as helpful and new ways of perceiving the situation.

The surveyors were able to highlight and relate bits of information gathered from documents, interviews, and outside sources in ways the hospital and rehabilitation leadership had not previously focused on or viewed such information (catalytic intervention). This enabled the leaders to generate new views of the problems and possible alternatives for themselves.

Confrontational intervention was also used when the leadership prematurely cut off consideration of the new view or possible solution. The leadership was asked to withhold their objections until more information was gathered. For example, they were convinced initially that salaries were *the* primary incentive in recruiting new therapists and were discouraged that their 85th percentile competitive salary package was not enough. It was suggested that they might want to consult the literature and professional organizational resource persons for information on nonmonetary incentives commonly used in recruitment and retention programs, to conduct a survey of new graduates/therapists in the local area regarding prioritization of a variety of incentives (both monetary and nonmonetary), and review their recruitment messages in terms of promotion of nonmonetary incentives.

The exit conference had been prescheduled for early afternoon of the second day. Basically, the same group of people attended the exit as the opening conference. The hospital was informed of its right to tape the exit conference. This helped them ensure that what they heard in the exit conference was the same as what they would receive in the final accreditation report.

The surveyors opened the exit conference by thanking the administration and staff of the organization for their hospitality, their cooperation and participation in the site survey, and so on. Then they explained, as they did in the opening conference, the scope and limitations of their role as the site visit team. Their role was to communicate findings regarding the organization's performance in relation to the CARF standards. The commission in turn reviews the findings to make sure they address the standards, and only the standards, and to make a determination regarding accreditation outcome. This outcome would be communicated in writing to the hospital 6 to 8 weeks after the site visit.

In this example, the surveyors identified many strengths in the hospital's performance and made some recommendations for areas of performance needing improvement. One of the primary recommendations was as follows:

It is recommended that the organization develop and implement short-term and 5-year recruitment and retention plans to assure that the organization is staffed appropriately in number and qualifications to carry out current rehabilition service delivery programs and program development plans for the future.

The surveyors invited questions and comments from the hospital's administration and staff. The exit conference closed with thank-yous by both the surveyors and hospital staff for the participation and assistance provided.

Outcome

In this example, the perspectives of both the surveyors and the hospital administration and staff were similar. The hospital personnel felt they had received a fair assessment and valuable suggestions for new ways to address their concerns. This hospital did obtain a 3-year accreditation. They were determined to be in substantial compliance with the CARF standards.

If the perspectives differ, the surveyors have the obligation to explain the basis of their findings and recommendations but to "call it like they see it." The organization seeking accreditation has the right to appeal the decision rendered by CARF after receiving the decision in writing. CARF identifies clearly the appeal procedures in the CARF Standards Manual.[5]

After receiving the accreditation report from CARF, the organization has 90 days in which to respond in writing to CARF identifying how they have or are in the process of addressing the recommendations. In the example portrayed, the hospital submitted a short-term and 5-year rehabilitation therapy staff recruitment and retention plan. The plan showed that administration and staff had utilized some of the ideas presented by the CARF surveyors, and more importantly had gone beyond to generate ideas and solutions for themselves and to contact other resources for additional ideas.

SUMMARY

Consultation is an integral part of effective regulation. Preparation by an organization for accreditation, as one form of regulation, stimulates the organization to assess its operation in relation to standards that represent the collective consensus of many experts in the field, many consultants. Interaction with accreditation surveyors and effective use of the recommendations resulting from the survey complete the consultation process.

Occupational therapists and other personnel of the organization benefit most from regulatory consultation by thoroughly studying the standards before the site visit and by identifying the specific standards for which they would like consultation on alternate or better ways to meet these standards. It is also important for the occupation therapy profession to be represented actively in the development, review, and ongoing revision of standards to ensure appropriate promotion, understanding, and delivery of quality services.

Occupational therapists are encouraged to explore possibilities for serving in regulatory consultant roles such as that of an accreditation surveyor. Preparation for such a role involves the development of expertise in the field of occupational therapy and acquisition of a broad knowledge of accreditation program arenas including medical rehabilitation and/or work hardening. This knowledge must include an awareness of the practice norms nationwide as well as an awareness of cutting edge developments and probable future trends in the field, practice, and regulatory environments.

REFERENCES

1. Bell CR, Nadler L (eds): *Clients and Consultants*. Houston, Gulf, 1985.
2. Blake R, Mouton JS: *Consultation*. Menlo Park, Calif, Addison-Wesley, 1976.
3. Callanan J: *Communicating: How to Organize Meetings and Presentations*. New York, Franklin Watts, 1984.
4. Cohen W: *How to Make It Big as a Consultant*. New York, American Management Association, 1985.
5. Commission on Accreditation of Rehabilitation Facilities: *Standards Manual for Organizations Serving People With Disabilities*. Tucson, Commission on Accreditation of Rehabilitation Facilities, 1992.
6. Epstein C: Consultation: Communicating and Facilitating, in Bair J (ed): *The Occupational Therapy Manager*. Rockville, Md, AOTA, 1992, pp 299–321.
7. Frank MO: *How to Get Your Point Across in 30 Seconds or Less*. New York, Simon & Schuster, 1986.
8. Lippitt, GL: The Trainer's Role as an Internal Consultant, in Bell C, Nadler L (eds): *Clients and Consultants*. Houston, Gulf, 1985, pp 73–83.
9. Morris W (ed): *American Heritage Dictionary*. New York, Houghton Mifflin, 1975.
10. Nock S, Moore AL: Managing the Consultant, in Bell C, Nadler L (eds): *Clients and Consultants*. Houston, Gulf, 1985, pp 268–272.
11. Rogers CR: The Characteristics of a Helping Relationship, in Bell C, Nadler L (eds): *Clients and Consultants*. Houston, Gulf, 1985, pp 49–62.

CHAPTER 32

A Model of Medical Review Consultation: Insurance Criteria

Rondell S. Berkeland, M.P.H., O.T.R.

OVERVIEW

The author has had two primary consultation experiences with major corporations: one, a provider of long-term care services and the other, a major insurance company. Both companies had highly defined organizational structures calling for consultants with specific knowledge in quality assurance, rehabilitation services, and reimbursement. In addition, it was necessary to possess the management skills that would facilitate implementation of the knowledge bases within complex organizational structures.

National Health Care Corporation

The author's consultation experience with a national corporation that owned and operated long-term care facilities throughout the country was essentially as a general consultant for the establishment and administration of specialized rehabilitation services in skilled nursing facilities. The consultant was employed full time by the corporation. The focus of the consultation varied depending on current issues, reimbursement and regulatory problems, and management goals for rehabilitation services. The consultant also was responsible for identifying relevant issues, bringing them to the attention of management and facilitating appropriate action. The scope of responsibilities fell into three areas: quality assurance, education, and program assistance and development.

Quality assurance criteria were established for provision and documentation of specialized rehabilitation services. A comprehensive system was established for long-term care facilities to evaluate their services in light of the predetermined criteria. The consultant conducted reviews of facility services at the request of company management and facility administrators. Independent reviews were also conducted at the discretion of the consultant. Results of the reviews were documented and shared with the facility administrator, rehabilitation personnel, and the corporate management.

Educational services were implemented through workshops and on a one-to-one basis. The one-to-one experiences were generally between the consultant and either an occupational therapist, physical therapist, or a speech language pathologist. The primary focus of the one-to-one sessions was to assist therapists in meeting the company standards for therapy services and third-party payor requirements for coverage and documentation. Workshops were provided for various levels of personnel including administrators, certified nursing assistants, office and bookkeeping staff, professional nurses, and therapists. Workshops were directed to some aspect of rehabilitation compatible with current case management problems, for example, feeding problems. Workshops were also conducted on basic regulatory and reimbursement issues such as Medicare and medical assistance coverage and documentation.

A third area of consultation was program consultation to assist in establishing therapy services, such as occupational therapy, in unserved areas. Assistance was also provided in planning and carrying out projects, implementing new company policies and procedures, and promoting new programs.

Insurance Company

The remainder of this chapter is based on the author's position as a medical review consultant for an insurance company. This model of consultation was chosen for several reasons. First, rather than being as global as the consultation with the national health care corporation, the responsibilities of this position were clearly defined and for the most part were measured by a single outcome, payment recommendations. Second, the services provided through this position could be applied by virtually any third-party payor. The transition from a global consultation role to a more focused set of responsibilities had certain advantages. Providing a more singular service allowed a level of skill development not possible with the open position description. It also was realistic to provide these services on a part-time basis. Although there were advantages to a more narrow focus, it was necessary to recognize the limitations of the scope of influence and to keep in mind the services the consultant had specifically contracted to provide.

The consultant role with the insurance company spanned several categories of consultation responsibilities. The range of activities included serving as an expert witness, reviewing claims for occupational therapy services, and making recommendations as to whether or not they should be paid, presenting workshops and in-services, and participating in special projects such as documentation form development. Each of these activities is discussed in detail later in this chapter.

ENVIRONMENT AND SYSTEMS INFLUENCE

One of the fortunate environmental factors that created consultant opportunities in the immediate geographic area of Minnesota was the proportionately large number of therapists in the state. Additionally, a supportive medical assistance fee for service payment system and Medicare reimbursement had created a strong market for occupational therapy services and a large network of provider organizations. The active professional organizations, professional education programs, and progressive health and human service policies all contributed to a broad awareness of rehabilitation services and subsequent demands for occupational therapy services. The heavy utilization of occupational therapy services led to the development of peer review systems and the use of rehabilitation specialists for the medical review of service claims. An efficient method of peer medical review is through the use of consultants. A strong demand for rehabilitation services, a subsequent heavy volume of system claims, and progressive attitudes of the major payors have contributed to an environment amenable to consultation services.

The insurance company served by the consultant had utilized rehabilitation consultants since the early 1970s when a physical therapist was hired to review Medicare claims. An occupational therapist consultant was added in the late 1970s and a speech language pathologist in the early 1980s. The acquisition of these therapists closely paralleled the changing philosophy of the health care financing administration as intermediaries were encouraged to utilize therapists to review peers' claims. The position held by the consultant was an established position that was vacated by the original job holder, also an occupational therapist. Much credit must be given to the insurance company for their foresight and commitment to providing accurate claim resolution through the concept of peer review.

The insurance company had supported the concept of peer review for many years. The medical review staff, in particular, were strong advocates for the use of peer review for therapy services. A typical pattern for a third-party payor would be to use another medical specialist such as a nurse or physician to review therapy claims. The insurance company in question, however, has supported a complete consultant network of physical therapists, an occupational therapist, and a speech/language pathologist.

FRAME OF REFERENCE

There were eight primary concepts that defined the frame of reference or philosophy used by the consultant to meet the responsibilities of the consultation contract successfully.

Client Centered

Though often repeated as a basic concept of consultation, the process must be approached from the perspective that the consultant is providing a specific service for the consultee. It was necessary to identify clearly what services were desired, the extent of authority the consultant was granted in representing the consultee, and the specific results expected with respect to the contracted services.

Goal/Outcome Orientation

The consultant's relationship with the insurance company was based on receiving a fee in return for a definable service. It was important to provide a service that met the client's time lines, standards of performance, product outcome, and volume expectations. The consultant reviewed his performance whenever a payment request was submitted and asked, "What services were provided for this money, what was the cost per reviewed claim, and how did the consultant's activities benefit the consultee?"

Application of Corporate/Program Criteria

The most important component of decision making with respect to insurance claims was to have a clear understanding of the company's criteria for coverage. The criteria then became the basis for each coverage decision. Decisions were a reflection of how closely the evaluation and treatment services provided by the occupational therapist were in compliance with the insurance policy's list of covered services and the conditions for covering those services.

Rationale

Each decision regarding payment for therapy services was accompanyed by a stated rationale. The rationale outlined coverage criteria met or unmet and served as the basis for the decision. Focusing on a specific rationale lent objectivity and consistency to the payment recommendation and provided a sound base should any decision be challenged.

Education Through the Decision Rationale

In addition to writing a rationale as the basis for the coverage decision, it was an excellent vehicle to describe occupational therapy services, projected outcomes from the therapy modalities and methods, and model criteria for interpreting similar cases in the future.

Collaborative Decision Making

One of the distinct advantages of this consultation experience was working with the skilled staff in the medical review department. Employed staff consisted of one physical therapist and two physical therapy assistants. Claims were first reviewed by either the physical therapist or one of the assistants and then forwarded to the consultant if the staff had questions about a claim or simply wanted another opinion. An effort was always made to discuss decisions and come to an understanding as to the rationale behind any given coverage recommendation. Another important communication avenue was between the consultant and the provider. Frequently, providers called directly and sought advice with regard to individual cases. An important element of these discussions was to utilize a collaborative decision-making process whereby the providers were asked a series of questions about their cases that allowed them to come to their own conclusions about whether or not the case was appropriate for Medicare coverage. Providers were then left with a system for reviewing similar cases on their own.

Communication Style

In consultant relationships it has been the most effective to engage in what Gibb[1] defined as nondefensive communication postures. A defensive reaction in the consultee is more likely to be prompted by certain styles of consultant communication; an attitude of superiority, for example, is likely to trigger a defensive response whereas an attitude of equality lessens defensiveness. Gibb identified six postures that tend to elicit defensive responses in the message recipient: superiority, control, evaluation, strategy, neutrality, and certainty. He also notes the corresponding attitudes that tend to lessen defensive responses. They include equality, problem orientation, description, spontaneity, empathy, and provisionalism. To approach the consultant relationship from a perspective of equality versus having all of the answers, to solve mutual problems versus taking over, to describe situations rather than labeling or evaluating them, to be up front rather than presenting an air of hidden or ambiguous messages, to understand and respond to others' feelings regarding a situation, to approach situations with an openness rather than certainty or dogmatism—all facilitated a cooperative working relationship amenable to solving problems. Gibb's categorization of communication attitudes or postures has been one of the most useful guidelines the consultant has encountered. Whenever an element of defensiveness in an interaction was sensed, the consultant could frequently identify the probable basis for the antagonistic interaction as stemming from one of Gibb's defensive postures.

Base of Knowledge

There were two knowledge base sets that were necessary for the medical review consultant: first, an overall knowledge of occupational therapy with a functional outcome perspective, and second, a knowledge and appreciation for reimbursement systems based on objective coverage criteria. These two knowledge bases were applied within both educational and clinical/treatment models of consultation. On occasion, special projects necessitated a program or administrative level of consultation. This approach was used, for example, in coordinating the development of a new certification form for occupational therapists. Whatever the model or level of consultation, the consultant's knowledge base had to incorporate a functional outcome perspective of occupational therapy with established coverage criteria of the insurance plan.

CONSULTATION DESCRIPTION

Organization

The insurance company served by the consultant was one of many companies that held contracts to serve as fiscal intermediaries for Medicare beneficiaries. The chain of command, beginning with the Department of Health and Human Services and ending with the intermediary is illustrated in Figure 32–1. The insurance company, in turn, managed the contract through their government programs section. All of the therapy consultants worked within this section. The network included a physical therapist and speech language pathologist. These individuals

---

FIGURE 32–1

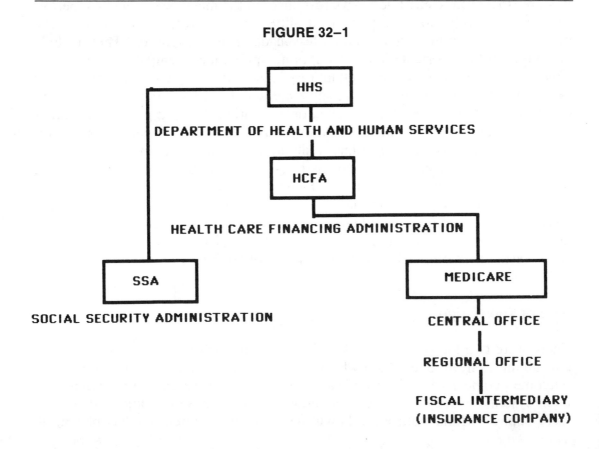

served in the same capacity as the occupational therapy consultant and were excellent resources for interpreting company policies and procedures.

The Health Care Financing Administration (HCFA) had subtly, but distinctively presented a philosophy that it would be preferable if medical claims were reviewed by professional peers. This philosophy had been reflected by, and in many respects, progressively initiated by the insurance company. The company had utilized peer review for approximately 10 years for occupational therapy and was one of the few intermediaries in the country that utilized an occupational therapy consultant.

Support

Financial compensation for consultation activities was delineated in the formal agreement or contract between the consultant and the insurance company. Payment was based on an hourly rate established on a yearly basis. The consultant completed a bimonthly time worksheet that included the hours worked and a brief description of the services performed. The worksheet was submitted to the consultant's immediate supervisor for approval and then forwarded to accounting. Payment was sent directly to the consultant.

The insurance company had a standard contract for consultant services. The contract outlined mutual responsibilities, terms for continuation and termination of service, and support services provided to the consultant, for example, liability protection and financial compensation. There was virtually no negotiation involved in establishing the contractual terms, since it was a standard contract and the terms were acceptable to the consultant.

The contract used by the insurance company contained two sections outlining consultant responsibilities and one section describing the insurance company's responsibilities. The two sections outlining the consultant's responsibilities included statements regarding the following general provisions:

1. The consultant would consult with appropriate medical review personnel to establish the appropriateness of occupational therapy treatment;
2. The consultant would be allowed access to materials and records necessary to carry out his or her responsibilities;
3. In a more general sense, the consultant would consult to the insurance company on matters within his or her area of expertise; and
4. The consultant would report the results of all consultations in a format mutually acceptable to the insurance company and the consultant.

The section of the contract delineating the insurance company's responsibilities contained two major points:

1. The insurance company had the authority to make all final decisions regarding recommendations for payment of insurance claims; and

2. The insurance company would inform all beneficiaries and/or providers of results of claim review determinations.

The agreement between the insurance company and the consultant also contained a liability clause that relieved the consultant from any "claim, injury, damage, or judgment including any legal and incidental expenses incurred by the consultant in connection therewith, resulting from the review of any claim of a specified patient or provider."[2] This provision essentially protected the consultant from any patient or provider actions subsequent to a review decision. The insurance company assumed the liability unless negligence on the part of the consultant could be determined.

The contract was effective in terms of allowing significant autonomy and flexibility for involvement in projects as directed by the insurance company as well as clearly indicating what the primary consultant responsibilities and consultee expectations were. Remaining portions of the contract described the processes for amending the contract, maintaining confidentiality of beneficiary records and related data, and the support services provided to the consultant.

In addition to support in the forms of financial compensation and legal protection, there was a strong element of professional respect and staff support from the medical review department. When a medical review decision was returned by the consultant, the recommendations were typically carried out as such. This consultant enjoyed peer relationships based on mutual respect and an attitude of collaborative decision making between himself and the medical review staff. The intermediary also provided excellent support in terms of job-related services and supplies such as duplication and preparation of materials for workshops and miscellaneous supplies needed for carrying out the claim reviews.

Participants

There were four key participants in this consultation process: the insurance company supervisory personnel, the medical review staff, therapy providers, and the beneficiaries. The supervisory personnel allowed the consultant maximum autonomy in terms of reviewing claims, representing the company at workshops, and responding to provider inquiries. Interaction with supervisory personnel primarily focused on policy and procedure issues, approval of time worksheets, and contract renewals.

The consultant's day-to-day interaction was with the medical review staff. As noted previously, the medical review staff consisted of nurses, physical therapy assistants, and a physical therapist. Any of the medical review staff could request that a claim for occupational therapy services be reviewed by the consultant. Once the claim was reviewed, the decision was typically discussed with the individual who referred the claim and a written rationale was submitted. The relationships between the consultant and the medical review staff were integral to an effective consultation process.

Services Provided

Entry into the System

The consultant position was previously held by an occupational therapist who had initiated the service. A debt of professional gratitude is owed to this individual for sharing her experiences and offering insights as to how to best meet the needs of the insurance company while serving the provider and beneficiary. The opportunity to interview for the consultation position came about primarily through the personal recommendation of the previous therapist as well as a physical therapy consultant. The circumstances surrounding entry into this system are a strong endorsement for professional networking.

Closely related to professional networking, is a concept termed by the consultant as related involvement. *Related involvement* simply refers to a professional activities through one's job, professional association, or with colleagues whereby one participates in activities involving quality assurance, reimbursement, regulation, peer review, documentation, and policy development. As professionals, it is important to involve oneself consistently in tasks, activities, and projects to enhance a range of skills that could potentially be marketed and offered as a set of consultant services. The purpose of related involvement is not necessarily to prepare for a specific position, but to keep one involved in a general area of interest in preparation for a new opportunity when and if it should arise.

Establishment of Trust

In addition to the formal work agreement established and defined by the contract, it was necessary to develop the fiduciary or trust component of the work relationship. In the opinion of the consultant, there were six basic facets of trust vital to this type of consultation agreement.

Nondefensive Communication.—The messages likely to elicit defensive responses have been previously described. Consultation relationships have the potential to be sensitive depending on the content and dynamics of the interaction. Consciously using language that minimizes defensive responses facilitates an atmosphere of trust.

Timeliness.—The medical review staff worked under time lines for completing case reviews and either denying or paying a claim. It was important for the consultant to be aware of those time lines and to complete case reviews in sufficient time to allow the medical review staff to process the claim.

Work Completion.—Work completion was closely related to timeliness, but was more encompassing. Each week the insurance company's medical review staff forwarded claims to the consultant. The staff counted on the consultant to maintain a consistent flow of completed claim reviews and recommendations. In addition, the consultant maintained a work volume commensurate with the hourly compensation.

Project Performance.—Another tenet of trust was performance on assignments and projects. The primary projects associated with this consultation experience were professional presentations. Thorough preparation, cooperative working relationships with the intermediary staff, and positive audience response all contributed to a sense of mutual trust and confidence. It was important that the staff of the insurance company had enough confidence in this consultant to delegate projects and assignments freely. This level of confidence was typically based on a past history of successful project outcomes.

Company Representation.—On almost a daily basis, an occupational therapy provider called the consultant to seek advice regarding a specific patient's coverage or interpretation of a Medicare policy or guideline. The consultant frequently was put in the position of being a company representative for the consultee. The consultant had to be clear about the extent of his or her authority and clearly indicate the basis for any information or decisions rendered. The consultant could not, for example, grant prior authorization for payment for occupational therapy evaluation or treatment. In order to establish trust between the consultee and consultant, the consultee had to have confidence in the consultant's response to provider and consumer questions or inquiries.

Responsible Decision Making.—When called on to make a coverage decision, it was extremely important for the consultant to stand by each decision and be clear that he would support the consultee's medical review staff who came to the consultant for assistance. Most of the case-related decisions were not clear-cut and hence required a careful rationale and a sense of confidence on the part of the consultee that payment decisions would be supported by the consultant.

Services Provided

This consultant's first experience with the insurance company was as an expert witness for a multicounty demonstration project whereby medical assistance funds were being distributed on a prospective payment basis. The hearing required a decision and opinion as to the reasonableness of occupational therapy services rendered to the disputing client. Occupational therapy services subsequently were reviewed in several cases under the demonstration project but none resulted in hearing processes. This activity was limited in duration, as the demonstration project subsequently ended.

The primary responsibility of the consultant was to review claims for occupational therapy services under the provisions of Medicare. The insurance company served as a fiscal intermediary for administering Medicare benefits. Claims were routinely routed to the consultant who reviewed them, made a decision as to whether or not to recommend payment for the claim, or portion of the claim, and developed and recorded a rationale for the decision.

Each claim was subjected to a four-step process: first, it was necessary to determine if the claim met the criteria of medical necessity. That is, was there evidence of a critical event or set of circumstances such as a new diagnosis, exacerbation of symptoms of an existing condition, or a recent decline in the patient's functional abilities? A patient may have had ongoing functional problems related to a previous medical diagnosis such as a cerebral vascular accident (CVA), but, unless there had been a recent decline in function or a change in the patient's condition that could affect functional abilities, the services would be questionable. In addition, it must be reasonable that the skills of an occupational therapist were necessary to intervene in the documented condition. The basis for this decision was the current standard of practice as related to the condition in question. In order for the service to be "skilled," elements such as "evaluation," "changing" treatment in accordance with the patient's response, utilizing a "complex" modality or documentation of a "complex patient" needed to be evident. The second step in the claims review process was to assess whether or not the treatment was "reasonable and necessary."* To be reasonable and necessary it had to be determined that occupational therapy services could reasonably be expected to facilitate significant practical improvement in the patient's condition within a generally predictable period of time. Significant practical improvement could be defined in several ways, but the most common indicator was for the patient to improve in terms of assistance level, for example, from moderate to minimum for a given functional skill, such as dressing. The third step in the claims review process was to check the documentation for the following information: the initial and current evaluations, treatment goals, treatment plan, and progress as expressed in functional changes. The fourth step was to make a coverage decision based on review of the preceding information. The most typical reasons for recommending that payment for a claim be denied included the following: medical necessity had not been established, the services being provided did not require the skills of an occupational therapist, treatment was being rendered on a maintenance basis, or there had not been significant practical improvement within a reasonable period of time. On occasion the claim may have been denied because the provider did not include sufficient documentation to make a proper determination. Once a claim determination had been made, the consultant wrote a rationale and submitted the recommendation to the insurance company's medical review staff who made the final decision.

Another major role for the consultant was to provide educational services. Educational services encompassed several levels. Formal workshops were conducted for therapists throughout the state to facilitate an understanding of the review process, including revised coverage criteria, data elements necessary to include in one's documentation, and suggested formats and forms to use in documentation. A second form of education was small group in-service training for facility staff. These sessions were tailored to the clientele of a particular facility and were scheduled as part of their normal in-service or staff meeting schedule.

Additionally, the consultant's responsibilities included special projects such as the development and implementation of a revised certification form for occupa-

---

* Quotation marks denote key words and phrases common to HCFA documents describing the conditions and criteria for Medicare coverage.

tional therapy services. The form was used by providers who submitted claims to the insurance company for Medicare coverage. The form was designed to collect the data elements required by the Health Care Financing Administration (HCFA) in order to evaluate whether or not a claim for occupational therapy services was coverable.

Although the bulk of the consultant's responsibility was to review Medicare claims, a separate contract was negotiated for the normal business side of the insurance company. Under terms of this contract, the claim of any insurance beneficiary for occupational therapy services could be referred to the consultant for review. Business side claims frequently involved children or other clients who had long-term rehabilitation needs. These cases presented difficult decisions whereby a balance had to be struck between effective utilization of the health care dollar and insuring maximum benefit to the patient to the extent allowed by his or her insurance policy.

Maintenance of the Consultation

This consultation agreement continued on a somewhat routine basis, as there was a constant flow of claims to review, unlike some experiences, which depend on the development of new projects or tasks and are somewhat sporadic in terms of workload. The contract was formally renewed on an annual basis and unless either party, consultant or consultee, had a specific issue to renegotiate, the terms were simply extended for an additional year. The contract contained a provision whereby either party could terminate the agreement within a set period of time.

Evaluation

As a fiscal intermediary for Medicare, the insurance company, was subject to a review process known as the Contract Performance Evaluation Program (CPEP). The CPEP process covered several elements of intermediary contract provisions, some of which were referred to as critical elements. Many of the critical elements in the CPEP reviews, which were carried out by the HCFA regional offices, were in the area of medical review. Claims, for example, were reviewed for accuracy of decisions. The CPEP reviewer may have selected a number of random claims and compared his or her decision with the intermediary review. Key results would include patterns of over or under coverage, soundness and consistency of rationale, and degree of agreement with the CPEP reviewer's decisions.

The consultee did not have a formal review process for the therapy consultants. There were, however, several components of the consultant's responsibilities that logically served as key factors for determining his level of performance. One of the most evident performance factors was the number of claims completed and the timeliness of those claims. In addition, the number of claims subject to reversals and/or disputes could have been an indicator of the consistency of claim decisions and the appropriateness of those decisions. Since presenting workshops was a primary task of the consultant, workshop evaluations also served as a source of information concerning consultant effectiveness. In a general sense, the outcome of any assigned project was a reflection of the quality of work. Finally, the primary determinant of the consultant's effectiveness was the personal resolve of the consultee's medical review staff and the medical review supervisor. It was the consultant's responsibility to establish a cooperative working relationship with the medical review staff and the therapy providers served. Complaints, positive feedback on services provided, and the quality of work completed all contributed to how the consultant's services were evaluated.

SUMMARY

This consultation experience was both personally and professionally beneficial to the consultant. The process of claims review and association with the government programs section of a major insurer forced the consultant to keep up to date with current legislation. A part-time consultant position such as the one described could also enhance one's primary employment. An important factor to consider before pursuing a consultant relationship, if already employed in another capacity, is the attitude of one's primary employer and compatibility of the consultation process with the goals and missions of that organization. This consultant served as the director of the occupational therapy program at a large research university. Fortunately, serving on the faculty of a university was an exceptional fit for involvement with a health care corporation; the university had the advantage of enhancing its public image and, as the faculty member, the consultant had the advantage of expanding his knowledge and skills in areas of reimbursement, regulatory legislation, and contact with the clinical sector through documentation review. The university administration approved all such outside agreements to ensure compatibility with the mission and goals of the university.

Establishing a consultant agreement for a regulatory or insurance company such as the one described could easily be replicated given a few conditions and key criteria. First, it would be necessary to find the right environment. As noted earlier in this chapter, it was important to have an environment that was supportive of rehabilitation services and a reimburser who enlisted the concept of peer review.

A second criterion for a successful consultant/consultee relationship was to establish a payoff for the consultee. One must be able to present a clear financial benefit for the consultee.

A third important criterion was for the consultant to have clear expectations, including what services were to be provided, time lines for completion of tasks, specific reporting forms or processes to be used, and the chain of command. Additionally, the consultant should know the appropriate process for accessing support services from the consultee.

Finally, it was the consultant's responsibility to have a clear picture of his parameters and authority, which included decisions within his purview of power and what questions should be deferred to one of the consultee's resources, for example, a particular department or staff person.

Given the right environment, clear definition of roles, a sound base of knowledge, and a thorough understanding of interpersonal communications, a consulting arrangement with a third-party payor, such as an insurance company, can be a rewarding, successful part-time position that results in significant benefits to both consultant and consultee.

REFERENCES

1. Gibb JR: Defensive communication. *J Communication* 1961; 141–148.
2. Blue Cross Blue Shield of Minnesota: Standard Consultation Agreement. 1990.

CHAPTER 33

Interagency Regulatory Consultation for Children and Youth

Christine Chang, M.P.H., M.P.A., O.T.R.

OVERVIEW

This consultation experience was a part of the author's assignments as a full-time employee of the New York State Council on Children and Families. The council is a unique state agency, mandated to coordinate services across systems for children and their families. While the agency does not formally refer to its activities as consultative, in practice it follows the models and levels of consultation described in Chapter 2. For instance, case consultation is offered regarding the placement of children considered hard to place. Technical assistance is given through a program development model of consultation regarding school-age child-care programs. In addition, policy analysis and data gathering are performed on a regular basis, as described in the social action model, to facilitate the coordination and development of improved services to children and their families.

The consultation experiences selected for this chapter involve the author's role in the development of model regulations for the prevention, remediation, and treatment of institutional child abuse in state-operated residential facilities for children and youth. This consultative task used several models of consultation, but primarily used a collegial or professional model with an interagency group convened to reach consensus on a specific task.

Entry by the consultative team, consisting of council staff, was uninvited by the consultees themselves. Instead, it was mandated by the state legislature in the Child Abuse Prevention Act of 1985 (CAPA). The consultees were representatives of other state agencies mandated by the same law to develop regulations related to institutional child abuse. The regulations were to be coordinated "to the extent possible" by the council so that confusion regarding the implementation in dual

533

licensed or regulated facilities would be minimized and equal protection to children in residential care would be provided regardless of agency auspices.

Unlike most consultees, the representatives of the other state agencies were not previously functioning as a single entity. The legislation, however, required the agency representatives to temporarily function as one group, yet return to their roles within their separate state agencies at the end of each interagency meeting. As in other consultations, the consultees did not have to follow the recommendations of the consultative team. While there was a strong incentive to cooperate, the extent of compliance with the group's recommendations was determined individually by each agency. Since CAPA also mandated a subsequent evaluation of the final plan, should the agencies fail to succeed in the implementation of the recommended regulations, amendments or new legislation could then be passed to mandate compliance.

This chapter describes the processes involved in the consultation project, describing the models of consultation used. It is important to note, however, that the consultants did not always consciously apply specific consultation theory to their interactions with the consultees. Instead, as with the application of occupational therapy theory as a clinician, experience in both the application of consultation strategies and knowledge of each other as consultation team members became the basis for an intuitive flow of consultative interactions.

ENVIRONMENT AND SYSTEMS INFLUENCES

Before examining the actual process of the consultation, it is important to consider the historical background. In 1980, a study of child abuse and neglect in foster care institutions was initiated by the New York State Temporary Commission on Child Welfare.[6] As a result of the study, it was learned that more than 80% of all alleged incidents of child abuse and neglect were never reported, despite the legal requirement to do so.

Consequently, the subcommittee developed and field-tested a comprehensive administrative response system model. In addition, Cornell University developed a comprehensive child-care worker training curriculum to enhance the capacity of workers to work with children. By training them in alternative ways of managing behavior and by teaching them about child development, it was hoped that workers would be less likely to become perpetrators of child abuse incidents.

The next phase of the study involved the comparative analysis and evaluation of other child-caring systems within the state, including the Division for Youth, State Education Department, Office of Mental health, and the Office of Mental Retardation and Developmental Disabilities. As a result of this additional study, it was felt that many of the same problems relating to institutional child abuse and neglect existed in these systems as well, thereby providing justification for the subcommittee's recommendation that a statewide system for the protection of children in residential care be created.

Following the release of the subcommittee's report, the Child Abuse Prevention Act of 1985 was passed.[3] The act extended the responsibilities of the

Department of Social Services related to registering and investigating incidents of familial abuse and neglect to include the reporting and investigating of incidents of alleged abuse or maltreatment in its residential care facilities, as well as those regulated by the Division for Youth and the State Education Department. The department also was directed to establish training standards for investigative staff, to approve or disapprove standards for investigative staff, to approve corrective action plans, and to prepare annual statistical and analytic reports of child protective services.

The Commission for Quality of Care for the Mentally Disabled, an agency whose primary functions included the monitoring of the quality of care in all mental hygiene facilities, was also mandated to submit an annual report to the governor and legislature on the protection of children in residential care in mental hygiene facilities (Office of Mental Health and Office of Mental Retardation and Related Disabilities). The commission was to establish training standards for their staff to conduct investigations of institutional child abuse and neglect and establish investigatory procedures to assure the effective investigation of such incidents.

The specific focus on institutional child abuse and maltreatment was not new for the commission, since they had the authority to investigate any such incidents under their agency-specific mandates. While the commission would conduct the investigations, however, the Department of Social Services maintained the authority to make final determinations in all institutional child abuse and maltreatment incidents. In other words, the Department of Social Services would serve as another cross-check before any incident would be considered indicated.

The Office of Mental Health and the Office of Mental Retardation and Developmental Disabilities were to cooperate with the commission's investigations and to provide for the development and implementation of corrective action plans when there were indicated reports. Procedures were to be established for effective investigation of all patient abuse or maltreatment allegations. Prior to the act, the Office of Mental Health and the Office of Mental Retardation and Developmental Disabilities facilities had investigated incidents internally, reporting the results to their regional and central offices. This was felt to present a conflict of interest situation, which the act was intended to correct by using an outside agency as the investigatory body.

The State Education Department and Division for Youth had to cooperate with the Department of Social Service's investigators in a similar manner. Before the passage of the act, these agencies also had maintained their own internal systems of investigations and corrective actions. Neither agency had a previous relationship with the Department of Social Services in terms of investigating institutional abuse allegations.

The council, which was established under the state executive law to ensure the coordination of services to children and families and achieve the most rational and effective system of services possible, was mandated by CAPA to contract with a nonstate agency to conduct an evaluation of the implementation and effectiveness of the act. Additionally, it was to "facilitate cooperative efforts among state agencies having responsibilities for operation and supervision of facilities and programs providing residential care for children toward the promulgation of standards for the prevention, treatment and remediation of child abuse and maltreatment which, to the extent possible, shall be uniform and consistent with one another.''[3]

An important element of the contract (in this case, the legislation itself served as a contract) between the other state agency representatives and council staff was the mandated time frame. The coordinated regulations or standards were to be promulgated and operationalized within 6 months. An evaluation report on the implementation of the act was to be submitted to the governor and the legislature in 3 years, with a sunset provision for the act 2 months later.

Beyond the confines of the consultation itself, public fears related to child abuse in day-care centers and within treatment facilities were an ever present political pressure on the interagency representatives (the consultees). The respresentatives were personally invested in protecting children under the care of their agencies. However, they were well aware that if the tasks were completed in a manner that would not ensure effective implementation, it would be extremely bad press for their commissioners or directors, the governor, and/or the board of regents. Should the evaluation reflect poorly on their efforts, it would become a public document in an election year.

FRAME OF REFERENCE

As described in Chapter 2, this consultation was a level III (programmatic or administrative) consultation, where the focus is centered on a system to promote institutional change by means of administrative consultation. It was specifically targeted on children and youth in residential care operated by specific state-level human services agencies.

The legislative directive established the parameters of the project for both the consultant and for the consultee regarding which areas of care needed to be addressed. These included qualifications and screening procedures for staff and volunteers, staff supervision, safety procedures, removal of children, corrective action plans, and training. General standards were also to be agreed upon related to the definition of maltreatment in the act, including standards for food, shelter, and clothing; medical, dental, optometric, and surgical care; restraint and isolation; supervision of children; and custodial conduct.

As each topical area was addressed, the representatives had to ask the questions, ''How can this be applied to our system of care? In what way will this have to be modified in order to work in my system? Will this provide the level of protection intended once it is implemented?'' As consultants, the council staff had to be acutely aware of when compromise was needed without impeding effective implementation; when the group process became less effective or more effective; and whether or not the original goal was met or in need of revision.

Technical questions also had to be addressed, such as, ''Should model standards take the form of regulations, statutory change, administrative directives, memoranda of understanding between agencies, informal agreements, or policy changes? Would it take an amendment to the legislation to implement effectively the directions to which the group agreed?'' In other words, how much clout would be needed to make the implementation match the rhetoric?

In addition to the questions related to resolving the problem at hand, other aspects of the consultation had to be considered. As Berzine points out in *The Fifth Estate: Consulting in the Public Sector,* consultation in the public sector is increasingly used for problem analysis that is distinct from the usual work within government. The types of tasks consultants might be assigned include[66] (1) acting as scientific justifiers of reasonably firm, though unarticulated political decisions; (2) bypassing restrictions of civil service; (3) aiding in identifying and securing federal funds; and (4) stimulating constituent demands for spending or policy changes favored by the contracting bureau, but opposed by the administration's top level policymakers.''[2]

Berzine's categories, while not perfectly descriptive of this situation, do point out the need to consider the hidden agendas of contracts or assignments that develop in public sector work. In this case, the intent behind the legislative mandate had to be considered. Of course, any challenges to what was actually produced would be based on a variety of legal interpretations of the act. For the purposes of this project, the referral back to intent was essential. For instance, was the intent to interpret the act literally so that all agencies would have to create new regulations, or would policies suffice for the Office of Mental Health, which traditionally worked through policies rather than regulations? How should "to the extent possible?" be interpreted?

Answers to these questions were readily provided by the various agency legal counsels, but frequently their interpretations of the legislation were conflicting. Opinions from the legislative staff who helped to draft the legislation were helpful, but lacked the weight of the legislative wording itself. In the end, representatives had to draw on their own knowledge, tempered by the information presented by the other members of the committee, to contribute to the direction of the final model regulation package.

CONSULTATION DESCRIPTION

The first order of business in this consultation was to reach a common understanding of the mandates contained within the legislation. Consequently, in preparation for convening an interagency committee, the legislation was summarized, outlining the various agency responsibilities. In addition, the reports from the senate subcommittee were reviewed and discussed with council staff who had contributed to that report. This provided a common basis of information to share with the interagency committee.

A letter was also sent from the executive director of the council to relevant agency commissioners and directors, requesting that they designate representatives to work with the council and stating the nature of the assignment and the importance of the issue. By sending a letter to the highest administrative level, the commissioners would be aware of the project and select a staff representative who would treat the assignment with the proper respect. In addition, such a procedure leaves the door open at a later date for the highest ranking person in the convening agency to contact the commissioners directly should difficulties arise.

Once the designees were known, the arduous task of coordinating schedules for the first meeting began. For the first meetings, agencies sent not only program staff, but also legal representatives. Each was armed with documentation of existing agency regulations that would need to be considered as an agenda was established for addressing institutional child abuse and maltreatment.

Initially, the committee reviewed the legislation together, sharing varying interpretations of what needed to be done. While in some respects the agenda seemed very clear, the committee also felt there were gray areas that had to be discussed at length. These included the level of specificity that should be attained within standards that would be simultaneously useful to incident investigators (staff hired specifically to investigate alleged incidents of institutional child abuse or maltreatment) and easily understood when implemented by facility staff. At all times, the group members had to maintain loyalty to their own agencies while trying to work cooperatively within the group.

The committee meetings occurred in the conference room of the council, which was perceived as a neutral forum for interagency meetings. Usually, four council staff attended, in addition to the executive director who chaired most of the meetings, and a counsel (legal representative) on an as needed basis. By having the executive director chair the meetings, the assignment was symbolically given status as an important task. Within state government, the importance of an interagency gathering to the convening body can often be measured by the level of staff they invite from the other agencies—commissioner level, senior staff, program staff, or technical staff. Senior staff were delegated to this task.

The process of developing custodial conduct regulations, one of the more controversial regulations, is described as an example of the group process that evolved. The process readily demonstrated that what appeared superficially to be straightforward issues in this consultation were almost never straightforward.

When custodial conduct became the agenda item for discussion, each representative shared information regarding his or her agency's existing regulations and policies that related to the topic. In most cases, the existing terminology never used the term *custodial conduct,* therefore, the first task was to reach consensus on a definition. Lack of previously accepted definitions made this a relatively easy task; the committee readily agreed to *staff behavior related to job performance.*

Beyond the purview of the agencies, however, consideration had to be given to civil service requirements. What restrictions would be considered an infringement of employee rights? For instance, if the recommendation would be that employees not carry firearms, would this be extended to carrying firearms in personal cars? This seemed wise for situations where staff parked their cars on facility grounds where children could potentially get into the cars and gain access to firearms. On the other hand, this could be a personal infringement of the right to bear arms. If firearms were ill-advised, then it seemed sensible that other weapons should also be banned. However, when is a knife a weapon versus a pocketknife kept on a key ring for whittling? Should the regulations be applied to security officers on duty? In some Division for Youth facilities, police officers regularly arrive on campus for a variety of reasons. Should they be forbidden to carry firearms?

The discussions often sounded like philosophical debates. It almost appeared that anyone in the room could argue strongly on either side of each issue. Difficult decisions had to be made that could be unpopular with segments of each agency's constituency. Wording had to be carefully selected in terms of the impact on all members of the service system, from consumers to the multitude of providers.

It was helpful to reach the decisions as a group because of the breadth of experience the committee members represented. Frequently, once draft language for a regulation was shared, the members would then present hypothetical or real situations from their agencies and raise questions regarding implementation of the wording on the staff and children in each situation. If the committee members did not do so, the consultative team would initiate discussion by directly asking various members how the wording would affect their agency. Sometimes this was done with full knowledge that certain agencies would find it problematic; other times this tactic was used as a means of getting all members to participate. In either case, it always served as a reminder that the issue was a real one, and not merely a paper exercise.

The compromise language that evolved after hours of discussion was, "Clients shall not be exposed to the dangers of firearms or other weapons on the grounds of residential child care programs. The facility must have policies and procedures governing the presence of firearms or other weapons in the facility or on the grounds."[4] This would make facilities address the issue while recognizing that various settings would need to assess independently what steps should be taken.

Other staff behaviors that the committee easily agreed should be forbidden, such as the use of corporal punishment, were not so easily agreed upon when specific definitions were sought. If a hit on the wrist is corporal punishment, how do you allow for behavioral modification techniques, such as wrist slaps as a negative reinforcer? At what point would the hit be too hard, and could this be determined in an objective manner? What if the child was in a fight with another child and the staff had to use some degree of force to protect the children from each other or to protect themselves? At what point could a restraint be considered a punishment? In most systems, use of handcuffs or anklecuffs were clearly inappropriate. The Division for Youth, however, routinely used anklecuffs for transporting youths that were known for their potential for escaping and, in some cases, for violent behavior. These youths had been ordered under their custody by courts that expected the maximum security to be provided to protect the community.

Language for any model regulation, therefore, had to be flexible enough to accommodate the general treatment philosophies of the other service systems, yet allow the Division for Youth to meet their court-ordered responsibilities. The answer seemed to be similar to the determination of pornography. It could not be defined, but, if seen, it could be recognized. As a result, the model regulations never added a definition, but simply forbade the use of corporal punishment.[4]

The interagency deliberations on the various regulations did not end the process. After model regulations were formally accepted by the agency commissioners, each agency had to redraft the language to fit the idiosyncrasies of their traditional agency regulations or policies. In the case of the State Education Department, draft regulations had to be presented to the board of regents, as well as to the commissioner.

All agencies then had to have regulations printed in the *State Register*,[5] a publication released routinely to the public. This permitted a period of public comment prior to finalizing the regulations. Public comments are not always incorporated, but agencies usually issue statements regarding why they accept or reject suggestions. Revised final regulations or policies are then released with effective implementation dates.

Should the legislature feel strongly that individual agency regulations and/or policies are incompatible with their original intent in passing the legislation, the option exists to amend the legislation to include a definition that is acceptable to them. This is true in both state and federal regulatory settings. Whenever agreement could not be reached, council staff asked the representatives if a mandated definition was the preferred solution. Sometimes this moved the committee to reach consensus, but other times it was agreed that there needed to be more specific directives via legislation. As consultants, it was important to focus discussions to address not only the difficult task before the committee, but also to serve as a reminder that the final decision or lack of decision would have repercussions in the future.

In the issue of corporal punishment, for instance, where it was decided not to include a definition in the model regulations, a problem arose in implementation. Fair hearing officers were overturning child abuse indications because of the lack of ability to determine objectively what was punishment versus what was an acceptable restraint. Although the State Education Department was able to adopt language defining the term, other agencies never defined it further in their regulations or policies. The interagency group has continued to struggle with this issue and has yet to resolve it to everyone's satisfaction. This consequence points out that no matter how carefully regulations are designed, there is almost always a need to reevaluate them after a period of implementation.

Similarly, the Office of Mental Health chose to develop policies in some instances, which were then released to their facilities in the form of policy bulletins. It was the opinion of the agency that policies were more flexible and more easily changed if implementation efforts proved problematic. The disadvantage to this approach has been that fair hearing officers seem to prefer to rely on regulatory language rather than policy statement regardless of the agency's common practices, thereby resulting in overturning some of the indications against staff on technicalities.

Support

All individuals serving on the interagency committee were paid staff from the relevant agencies, assigned by their commissioners to attend committee meetings and to work with the council staff. However, allowing the representatives to make institutional child abuse and neglect a priority was clearly important. Not only did the primary interagency representatives need the sanction to attend meetings over other assignments, but also the commissioners had to support the assignment of other staff as needed to complete the task.

During the course of the consultation, there were no major legal or ethical issues about the financial or administrative support given the council staff, as is possible in a more typical consultation setting where a fee for service or confidentiality issues might be more pertinent. Probably the greatest difficulty was in the constantly changing interagency representatives (consultees) assigned to work on this issue. This occurred through unavoidable natural attrition, which made it difficult at times to maintain the group focus on issues.

Participants

Members of the consultative team included the executive director of the council, whose position would be similar to that of a commissioner of a small agency in other states; the director and one staff member from the Bureau of Research and Information Services whose primary responsibilities dealt with the contracting for the evaluation; a legal representative, or counsel, from the council; the director of the Bureau of Program Planning and Policy Analysis within the council; and the author as a member of the same bureau.

Relevant backgrounds of the council staff assigned to the project included a variety of experiences and academic preparation. The director of the Bureau of Research had served as staff for the senate committee report that led to the passage of CAPA. The other member of her bureau had been assigned to overseeing the internal investigations of institutional child abuse and neglect in his previous employment with the Office of Mental Health. Both members of the Bureau of Policy Analysis had extensive experience in policy analysis on a variety of legislative, regulatory, and programmatic issues.

The clinical background of the author as an occupational therapist in a children's psychiatric facility gave invaluable experience in group process, which was a basic element of this consultation. In addition, vivid memories of how easily ward staff could be inadvertently drawn into abusive situations with seriously disturbed youngsters gave a reality-based perspective to the task at hand.

Graduate work in both public health and public administration helped to integrate the occupational therapy theory, experiences, and knowledge into a broader, more systematic approach to this consultation. An awareness of the long-term impact of regulatory change and the working knowledge of policy analysis at a macro level were essential to the successful completion of this project.

In addition, involvement with state and national association political endeavors, such as lobbying for state licensure, provided experience in developing political allies, compromising, knowing the constituency, and thinking in a broader arena than the clinic. The sensitivities to client needs honed through practice as a therapist were invaluable for involvement in the development of human services regulations, but were insufficient to gain entry without further academic and practical experience. The most helpful aspects of the author's background as an occupational therapist included work as a staff therapist and director of occupational therapy in pediatric facilities serving children with emotional and developmental deficits, serving on a facility behavior modification protocol review committee, and being a member of a quality assurance review team for intermediate care facilities for the federal government.

The interagency representatives had equal status (primarily as middle managers), if not equal histories in terms of their involvement in the area of institutional abuse and neglect. Some were very experienced in the area of regulations development; others had greater experience in advocacy. All provider agency representatives came with extensive knowledge of programs of residential care provided by their agencies. Directors of residential programs, child-care staff, union representatives, and quality assurance officers were important constituents of the agencies represented, although they were not official members of the group.

While some of the representatives had worked together before, the total combination of individuals had not worked together. Some staff were new to their jobs; others had years of working within the system and knowing exactly what would or would not succeed in their agency.

Services Provided

Entry into the system and the negotiation of the contract were previously addressed. There was no negotiation by the participants, only among legislators in the passage of the act. The next phase of the consultation, the establishment of trust, was probably the most difficult to achieve.

The initial strategy was to present an outline summarizing the content of the act, delineating each agency's responsibilities. Initial meetings of the group were punctuated with formal protests of the minutes, with some members asserting that the committee should go beyond the mandates of the legislation and standardize all regulations for residential care for children. Equally strong assertions were also made that only the minimum requirements of the law should be met.

In addition to the usual group dynamics that take place in any group situation, each representative came bearing the philosophical attitude their individual agencies followed. At times it was difficult to discern whether personal opinions were being expressed, or whether statements reflected agency positions. Past interagency and personal relationships from outside this group also influenced the interactions, although the consultative team could only hypothesize about this factor.

Prior to each meeting, the team from the council prepared an agenda, briefed the executive director if he were chairing the meeting, and had minutes from the previous meeting delivered to all members. Initially, meetings occurred once a week. At the request of the members, minutes were hand carried to members so that they would have time to review them prior to their arrival at the meeting.

Due to the sensitivity of the issues, the principal staff also chose to address creature comforts. Each meeting had coffee provided, and, as often as possible, other refreshments. Interestingly enough, the provision of food became a symbolic matter, which was evident in the conclusion of the initial tasks, described later.

The role of the consultative team was primarily that of mediators when disagreements occurred; clarifiers when it seemed a valid point was being made, but was not understood by the group; moderators that established the agenda; and information sources when the committee needed more information. Following each meeting, the consultative team met without the executive director to have an informal debriefing. Besides an initial cathartic reaction regarding the process, the meetings focused on identification of emerging issues and any outside influences on the process.

As a result of these discussions, there were occasions when it was decided that meetings should be arranged with individual commitee members outside of the group. This was arranged in order to avoid deadlocking, or sometimes to provide a better understanding of the extent of their concerns. These meetings were extremely important, because the representatives could be more straightforward regarding their reasons for taking certain positions on issues. In addition, compromises were discussed, and information was sometimes shared in confidence. It was then up to the consultative team to find a way to bring the same issues to the whole committee in a way that was more comfortable for all concerned.

For instance, during the early sessions, when personal hostilities began to be problematic, the consultants concluded that it would be helpful to meet separately with the staff who seemed to be the most unyielding in their positions. The objective was to discuss how they might be able to make their points in a more positive manner. When this did not work, a phone call was made by the director of the council to the head of the agency involved to discuss diplomatically what could be done to break the impasse. It was critical not only to have a director with the administrative clout to influence changes in attitude, but also to have that person highly skilled in exerting that influence in a way that allowed the other agency to save face. This time, the strategy was effective.

As time went on, committee members became comfortable with seeking each other out between meetings and then reporting on their collaboration at the next meeting. This level of trust, however, took a long time to build. For at least 2 months, it seemed that it would not be possible to ever reach agreement just to begin drafting model regulations despite the legislative mandate.

Many times, the author was reminded of Saul Alinsky's advice while seeking the motivating force for the group. The more pertinent Alinsky "rules"[1] for this consultation may be summarized as follows: (1) In order to understand the politics of any situation, one has to set aside the idea that any approach is either positive or negative; (2) Compromise is a critical means of being able to move forward; and (3) Be flexible enough to accept other approaches to resolving a problem, even if you are sure your own approach is correct.[1] In this consultation, it was desirable to get the committee members to acknowledge validity in opposing viewpoints so that they could then be motivated to reach a compromise. Sometimes this meant asking the person presenting an unusually worded regulation to explain the rationale behind the regulation, or reminding each other of the differences in the populations served by each agency. Often strategies developed prior to meetings would change when the group convened, due to new information or because committee members had been able to negotiate a compromise outside of the meeting.

One of the hardest things to do as a consultant is to let the process play out. An analogy that may help the occupational therapist understand this difficulty is the tendency for inexperienced therapists to feel they must have all the answers in treating a client. With experience, it becomes evident that the habilitation or rehabilitation of any patient involves not only what you know and bring to the therapy session, but what the patient knows and is capable of creating.

It took the representative from the State Education Department, an agency which had no regulations related to institutional child abuse in place at the time, to suggest that the committee should stop debating and try to draft one of the regulations and see what would happen. Everyone at that stage appeared ready to try a new approach. All members had explained their viewpoints extensively. No new information was forthcoming, so the committee finally had to move.

In drafting that first regulation, and the other regulations that followed, all agencies were asked to present their current regulations so that areas of conflict or deficiencies could be identified. The draft regulation was then written on a large flip chart in the front of the room, a useful tactic for neutralizing conflict. By focusing the group on words on a paper, a slower, more thoughtful reaction resulted. This may be due to the fact that eye contact now was directed toward a neutral object, rather than toward a person with whom the speaker disagreed. As the facilitator, it also provided confirmation of the discussion, which made the task of taking minutes much less controversial.

The task orientation also was helpful, with the group now focused on areas of agreement. Specific areas of regulation that had to be addressed as outlined in the law were selected as a first priority of action. Other areas less clearly mandated by the legislation were to be addressed as time permitted. As in occupational therapy theories of task analysis, breaking the task into component parts made it far easier to find the solution and/or reach consensus.

Through working on the first component, the committee grew to understand and trust each other enough to risk working together on the second component, which also happened to be the most controversial part. It was equally important for the committee to feel they had defined the parameters of the task, so that they could take justifiable pride in the end results.

Evaluation

As previously mentioned, another aspect of this consultation was the evaluation of the project. The council was mandated through CAPA to submit an evaluation report, which was to be conducted through a contract with a nonstate agency. This resulted in the provision of consultation to the contracting agency by the Bureau of Research staff, using the technical assistance model of consultation. The evaluators needed assistance with negotiating the various agency bureaucracies to gain access to data essential to completing their task. In addition, the data collectors needed training to explain what aspects of institutional child abuse and neglect were able to be documented and what were the important characteristics of the investigatory process.

Although the contents of the final evaluation were of interest to the interagency committee, by the time it was completed, the committee already was discussing possible next steps to improve implementation of the act. Since the evaluation occurred during the developmental stages of implementation, corrective actions were taken on an as needed basis, without waiting for the results of the evaluation.

Termination

After 5 months of intensive negotiations, the committee finally reached agreement on the model package. The arduous task of reaching consensus developed a sense of camaraderie and genuine respect for one another among the participants. At what was thought to be the last interagency meeting, everyone spontaneously brought food to celebrate their accomplishments. It was surprising, and gratifying, to witness the extra effort made by the commitee members, which included bringing home-baked goods and festive-looking dishes. Even more surprising, 1 month after the package of model regulations was completed, the members reconvened to go to lunch together as a purely social function.

Two months after the package was submitted to the agency directors and commissioners, it was formally accepted by the members of the Council on Children and Families. This body consisted of chief executives of the involved agencies, as well as other agencies serving children and families. While the committee members were aware of the meeting and the vote, it seemed almost anticlimactic, since the agencies were already at the point of implementing the regulations or policies. Nonetheless, it was a technically important step because it signified the formal acceptance of the package across systems.

Possible Renegotiation

Although the mandates of the legislation had been met by the committee, the interagency committee spontaneously reconvened at the request of various members to discuss problems that arose during the implementation of the regulations. Often the member agencies would try to work out conflicts independently, but when impasses were reached, they would request the council to reconvene the full committee.

In addition, a sunset clause was built into the act that would commence shortly after the submission of the evaluation to the legislature. Consequently, the committee was reconvened, with additional representation of legal staff from each agency, to recommend amendments and extension of the act. Once again, consensus was hard to reach. Some felt the act should be moved from familial law to penal law, but others felt it should remain the same. Most agencies felt the act should be extended to other residential facilities serving children and youth. Agencies operating such facilities, however, were unsure if they agreed. Such debates will no doubt continue in the future. A sunset clause provides a timetable for this dialogue, but even without the clause, periodic amendments could be submitted to the legislature by anyone concerned about the implementation of the act.

Due to the nature of the council's enabling legislation, renegotiation of the consultation can occur at any time if assistance is needed to resolve interagency disputes. Unlike traditional contracts, there are no fiscal barriers to such a renegotiation.

A difficult personal issue, which the consultant must consider in renegotiating the consultative relationship, is whether there is real need for continuation or whether the enjoyment of the consultative relationship and comfort in working with the familiar are the determining factors. This is an important issue, since consultants can be persuaded into staying in the consultative relationship beyond the point that they are needed. There is nothing more seductive than success, but the true test will be if the agencies continue to work together despite the lack of a legislative mandate.

Outcome

The outcome of the consultation was successful in terms of meeting the original goal of coordinating regulations across systems. In addition, the evaluation was completed on time and recommendations were submitted to the governor's office regarding the extension of the act. Member agencies have continued to work with each other on problem areas related to implementation. Abuse and maltreatment incidents are being investigated and corrective action plans are being developed and implemented as intended by the act. While qualitative issues still exist, it appears that they will be addressed by the relevant agencies.

Positive results from the committee efforts have been documented in the evaluation, as well as informally reported among the committee members. Agreements also have been reached regarding the acceptance of recommendations between agencies.

SUMMARY

In summary, some basic guidelines to consider when consulting on regulatory issues, regardless of whether the consultation is contracted or atypical as the one described in this chapter, are as follows:

- Be well versed in relevant existing legislation, regulations, and/or policies. Analyze them in terms of potential conflict or overlap, as well as the effect on all concerned parties (consumers, providers, unions, agency operations, etc.). Be aware of what other states or the federal government have done related to the same issue.

- Understand the historic involvement and philosophical attitude of the agency or agencies involved. Be familiar with their mission, whether mandated or informally established, and the bureaucratic structure of the agency. These factors will have a strong influence on what can be accomplished.
- Define the goal for the consultation. This should be done as part of the contracting process, or, in an atypical case such as the one presented, know what goal has already been preordained.
- Determine the process that will most likely accomplish your goal. Select the administrative structure that will facilitate your desired outcome, such as regulations versus legislation. While this may seem to be in reverse order, it is more effective to fit the structure to the process than vice versa. Be flexible in your approach, as consulting is a dynamic process.
- Build in an evaluation component at the beginning. This will provide objective feedback regarding your success and help you to make necessary course corrections as needed.
- Once the mission is accomplished, try to determine objectively whether there is a need to renegotiate. Whether the motivation is fiduciary, altruistic, or personal, the consultant must be clear as to why the contract should be renewed.

Occupational therapists can make useful contributions to the regulatory process, either as consultants to regulatory agencies or as individuals providing public comment or technical assistance during the development of regulations. Credibility as consultants in such settings, however, will be enhanced by further academic and experiential undertakings, such as course work in systems analysis, public policy, or public administration and participation in legislative or regulatory activities.

REFERENCES

1. Alinsky D: *Reveille for Radicals*. New York, Vintage Books, 1969.
2. Berzine R: *The Fifth Estate: Consultation in the Public Sector*. Unpublished paper for the John F. Kennedy School of Government, Harvard University, Cambridge, Mass.
3. Chapter 677 of the Laws of New York, 1985, S 31.
4. New York State Council on Children and Families: Unpublished model regulatory guidelines, approved May 16, 1987.
5. *New York State Register*, published monthly by New York State.
6. New York State Senate Subcommittee on Child Abuse: *Protection of Children in Residential Care: A Study of Abuse and Neglect in Child Care Institutions in New York State*. National Center on Child Abuse and Neglect Grant Project #90-CA-802A, September 1983.

CHAPTER 34

Program Consultation to Agencies in Developing Countries

Satoru Izutsu, Ph.D., O.T.R., F.A.O.T.A., F.A.A.M.D.

OVERVIEW

Occupational therapy is relatively unknown in most developing countries. During the last decade, however, the World Federation of Occupational Therapists (WFOT) and occupational therapy associations from more developed nations around the world have promoted the value of occupational therapy services in the delivery of health care to the developing countries. Additionally health leaders from some developing countries, while visiting the United States and Europe, have observed occupational therapy programs with keen interest. They often return to their countries with a desire to implement similar programs in their homeland.

To establish occupational therapy programs in developing countries, knowledgeable consultants will be required. Health workers in these countries, independently or through international agencies, will seek consultants to help design and plan health care programs. The United States could be a valuable resource. The role of international consultant offers American occupational therapists exciting opportunities to provide much-needed health care services. An extensive background in direct patient care, training and education, counseling, program development, administration, and previous establishment of occupational therapy programs internationally provided the author with the variety of experiences necessary to gain entry and credibility in health agencies of developing countries.

POTENTIAL MARKET FOR INTERNATIONAL CONSULTATION

Opportunities for occupational therapy consultation in developing countries are becoming increasingly available. There may be individuals with experience and

548

expertise living in these countries, who usually have been educated and trained in the United States or Europe, however, the indigenous expert is not always recognized by his/her own country. This creates a greater market for the outside consultant. The potential consultant should be innovative, flexible, imaginative, conscientious, and highly professional, with specialized expertise. The areas of expertise most sought include curricula development for new academic programs, organization and development of treatment programs, and financing and management services. In many instances, the request for consultation is to garner support to present or promote new program ideas to administrators.

KEY POINTS

Entry Into the System

Usually the international consultant must sell himself. There are two avenues of entry. One is for the consultant to become known in a circle of other health care leaders, also sought for their particular expertise. To gain entry to these countries and achieve success as an effective international consultant, the potential consultant should obtain some prior experience working abroad. This may be possible through international volunteer positions, such as those offered by the Peace Corps or similiar overseas volunteer organizations and by church mission volunteer programs, or by volunteering in the country's own agency programs. This initial experience can provide a base of knowledge regarding problems and issues in developing countries. Consultation in these countries demands a special understanding and awareness. Early volunteer experiences give the potential consultant a basis for understanding different cultures, habits, and health practices and can put him in touch with key individuals in the country's health system.

The second entry to developing countries is to create a reputation as a health consultant, with specific expertise in an area known to be of interest in these countries. Presentations at international conferences and seminars and publications in international journals are invaluable. Academic titles, attendance at or graduation from prestigious American universities, and references from well-known leaders are considered important in many developing countries. Letters of introduction from mutual acquaintances and well-prepared resumes are another way to develop initial rapport and reputation.

Knowledge and Skills

Basch states "The international health worker must develop a keen awareness of: (1) the place of health among other factors in the total scheme of national development; (2) the relationship of health services to health status; (3) the place of curative medicine within health services; and (4) the likely consequences of establishing, or of not establishing, the particular health program under consideration. Inconsistencies and contradictions abound. The advanced creations of science and technology must be carefully weighed for appropriateness in the local context." (1, p402) These criteria appear particularly applicable to the international occupational therapy consultant.

In addition to the knowledge, skills, and attitudes inherent in any consultation, the international consultant must have a strong sense of self. Working in a foreign country can be lonely and frustrating, especially when the culture, language, and way of life are completely different from one's own. Emotional and physical health are important attributes. The ability to accept new situations as adventures, not obstacles, will enhance the consultation experience. Maturity and varied life experiences enrich the background of the consultant and help prepare him for the challenges of consultation in countries where resources, knowledge, and basic health services may be limited.

The international consultant should have some understanding of the language of the country and be able to communicate with other health workers and administrators. Presentations in the country's own language have a more powerful impact and convey a message of respect and caring for the host country. If interpreters are necessary, they should be screened by the consultant. Although there may be individuals proficient in English, specific technical terminology or nuances and subtleties may be lost. It would be efficient and cost-effective to orient the interpreter prior to the presentation. The ability to analyze, organize, and present thoughts in a simple, clear, and comprehensive manner are essential. It may be necessary to devise simple visual aids quickly, without the benefit of advanced audio-visual techniques. The consultant should be aware that audience participation in these countries is not common. However, if an audience does not pose questions, it does not necessarily mean that there is immediate acceptance of the consultant's views or the content of his material. Many listeners to new or outsider presentations will review the material silently, yet critically. Acceptance of foreign veiws does not come easily. The consultant must possess patience and resilience.

Understanding the System

A major consideration of international consultation is knowledge of the culture, habits, practices, and values of the country. The consultant should study the geography, demographics, economy, and political climate of the country. Examination of works by anthropologists and sociologists also would be helpful. If possible, a study of the country's 5 year health plan and interviews with local experts and residents would enhance understanding of the country.

Consultants in developing countries may not receive written contracts as standard procedure. Many countries operate on verbal agreements and a handshake. Specific amounts of money for services may not be discussed openly. The consultant must determine how to negotiate a contract and outline the terms, objectives, expectations, and fees in the specific country. If possible, written agreements prior to entry to the country is advisable. It is important to understand the administrative and bureaucratic structure of governmental agencies and the standard operating procedures of the system.

Needs of the Client

It is essential for the international consultant to accept the client. The level of understanding of health program development, technology, and utilization of resources may differ from the consultant's usual experiences. The consultant's most difficult task is to refrain from imposing his own culture and values, national standards, and usual approach. Awareness of the need to address the client's concerns and interests, regardless of one's own prejudices, political or religious beliefs, will enhance the client/consultant relationship, as in any consultation experience. However, due to the major differences between life styles and health practices in highly developed nations and those of developing countries, this factor is especially important.

Development of sensitivity to the particular folkways of the host country may be facilitated by spending some time in the new country prior to the consultation. Learning about and adjusting to the time zone, climate, people food, and language before starting professional activities is invaluable. It is important to remember that *the consultant is a guest*.

Considerations for Program Development

The initial impression the consultant makes on the host country is crucial, especially as a foreigner. Formal appointments with the leaders and administrators of the system should be made at the beginning of the consultation period. Presentation of the consultant's scope of activities, role responsibilities, and expectations should be verified with the key people for accuracy and mutual understanding.

The consultant should study the mission, goals, and organizational structure of the system in which the program is to be developed. Analysis of the clientele (number and type of patients served), budget, locus of the services, human resources, and in-service training requirements are all considerations for program development. A complete environment and systems analysis is essential, especially in systems new to the consultant.

Issues of disease prevention and health promotion are crucial in developing countries. Health education for patients and clients is usually of prime importance in the planning and design of health programs. Occupational therapy activities may include instruction in nutrition, home safety, home health care, and parenting techniques, all at appropriate levels for the particular culture and local folkways.

Planning for the delivery of home health services also is important, as 80% of the population in developing countries live in rural communities. Inversely, only 20% of the health personnel practice in those rural areas. Because of this uneven distribution of available health personnel, and the usually depressed economic state of these rural areas, the consultant should include training of caregivers in the home as part of the program development services. Additionally, local individuals without formal professional education, can be trained as adjunctive health workers to assist the few professionals in the area.

The physical environment of the particular country also should be considered in the development of the program. Indigenous materials and resources should be studied, for example, use of bamboo for splinting or warm ocean currents and waves for substitutes for whirlpools.

When the consultation period has terminated, the consultant should provide an exit interview for the leaders and key individuals and present an oral report and evaluation of the consultation activities. This should be followed by a carefully written report, preferably in the language of the host country.

CASE EXAMPLES

The following brief vignettes are presented as case examples of occupational therapy consultation in developing countries. The author's experiences in international consultation have been varied. A background in specific areas of clinical practice, including work with cerebral palsied children, adult prosthetic training, and a sheltered workshop for a geriatric population, provided the clinical expertise required. Advanced training in psychology, health planning, and public health and a position as a health planner in the Pacific provided additional expertise. These vignettes describe the author's involvement as a program consultant and health planner in Yugoslavia, Thailand, and Romania.

Yugoslavia

Consultation in Yugoslavia was initiated by the American Friends Service Committee. The request was for an American occupational therapist to initiate an occupational therapy training program. The economic and political changes of the fifties gave an impetus to provide training for a cadre of occupational therapy technicians. Yugoslavia, in 1959, had a socialist government with strong overtones of communism. Recovery from the ravages of World War II resulted in a young population moving from an agrarian society to an industrialized one. Cities were expanding at a rapid rate as new industries developed. In the rush to keep pace with the rest of the world, there were many industrial accidents resulting in loss of limbs.

The occupational therapy consultant was requested to develop a prototype training course. The objective was to train 11 occupational therapy technicians in 6 months to function independently as members of rehabilitation teams in hospitals in various parts of the country. The goal of the technicians was to return injured workers to the workplace as quickly as possible. Their course work included training in anatomy, physiology, kinesiology, principles of occupational therapy, use of therapeutic activities, and construction and fitting of prostheses.

The consultant, in collaboration with staff at a rehabilitation center, established the training program and worked with staff to develop subsequent classes for occupational therapy technicians. It was essential for the consultant to have a firm foundation in anatomy, neurology, kinesiology, and the principles and practice of occupational therapy. Extensive experience in the disability area provide the clinical expertise required. Knowledge of the language and strong communication and interpersonal skills enhanced the consultant's ability to develop rapport and a collaborative relationship with coworkers. The author has kept in contact with the program he helped to develop over 30 years ago. Although no school of occupational therapy has been established, several training courses have been provided since the author terminated the consultation. Upon return to Yugoslavia several years ago, he discovered that three of his original colleagues still worked at the rehabilitation center where the first course was conducted.

Thailand

In 1972, the American Public Health Association (APHA) received a grant from the United States Agency for International Development (USAID) to initiate a project entitled the Development and Evaluation of an Integrated Delivery System in three countries. [4] The countries targeted for this project were in Africa, South America, and Asia. As a result of varied international consulting experiences in Yugoslavia, the Pacific Basin and the Far East, the author was invited to be a member of the fact-finding team to determine which Asian country would be selected. The author's positions as director/planner for the Regional Medical Program of the Trust Territories of the Pacific Islands, Guam, and American Samoa and faculty member of the University of Hawaii School of Public Health provided additional qualifications for this team.

The team's mission was to assess three Asian countries and recommend the one most suitable to host the development and evaluation of an integrated health delivery system. This project was to include maternal and child health services, sanitation and family-planning programs, review of epidemiological and biostatistical data, and the training of multiple levels of health workers. Thailand was selected because of its stable government at the time, its friendliness toward the United States, its commitment to change, and the willingness of the government to finance the recommendations.

Delivery of health services in Thailand was a major problem. Seventy-five percent of the population lived in rural, agricultural communities where health services and personnel were limited. The majority of health workers, including physicians, practiced in more urban centers. Because of the dearth of health personnel in the villages, the provincial hospitals, where fewer doctors practiced, were overloaded.

The author, as a planning consultant for this project, collaborated with the Ministry of Public Health to develop a multiple-year health service delivery plan for Thailand. The plan, submitted to USAID for funding, included the following considerations: development of a health personnel base, establishment of a data system to be used for research and evaluation of the project, and a focus on the problems of maternal and child health care. Services were to be delivered by *multi purpose* health workers, trained to provide villagers with primary health care and health education, including information about prevention of disease and injury and activities related to health promotion.

The outcome of the author's consultation was a planning proposal, accomplished in a 6 month period, for a multimillion-dollar grant. The project, known as the Lampang Project, after the province in which the pilot activities were instituted, had a sweeping impact on Thailand's health delivery services. Drastic changes in the delivery of health care were demonstrated in terms of how health services could be delivered, by whom, and in the involvement of the people affected (including villagers in remote regions). The villagers even assisted with suggestions for alternative ways to provide adequate health care for their region.

The positive outcome of this project, which was conducted from 1974–1979, resulted in the prestigious Medal of the White Elephant, a distinctive honor for foreigners from the Royal Thai Government, awarded to the USAID and APHA team. Concepts from this project are still in use, including the replication of some of the service delivery to rural areas in other Southeast Asian countries and the model of training *physician extenders,* used throughout the world in other developing countries.

Romania

In the last decades of the twentieth century, dramatic political changes have occurred, especially in Europe, which have had a direct effect on the delivery of health care. After the 1989 political revolution in Romania and the downfall of its communist dictator, it was revealed that there were approximately 100,000 abandoned children in large government institutions. The world responded with help for these children, many of whom were mentally and physically handicapped.

World Vision International, a non-government voluntary organization, established the Romanian Orphan's Social and Educational Services (ROSES) Project in 1990, directed by an American physician. The goal of the ROSES Project was to develop a 5 year program to provide direct professional care for up to 15,000 orphans. The project was to include teams of child development specialists and counselors to Romanian professionals, para-professionals, and volunteers to set the standards of care for these children.[3]

World Vision International requested that a consultant team of therapists, representing the American Occupational Therapy Association (AOTA), American Physical Therapy Association (APTA), and American Speech-Language-Hearing Association (ASHA) assess the needs of the Romanian institutionalized orphans. The author, as the United States WFOT Delegate and member of the AOTA Executive Board, was selected to represent occupational therapy on the team. The goal of the team visit was to determine the feasibility of developing a partnership between the ROSES Project and these three American professional organizations.

The task of the occupational therapy consultant was to estimate the prevalence of disorders in the target population that could benefit from the services of occupational therapy and then develop a collaborative service delivery plan, in addition, determine the material and equipment needed for identification and intervention, and finally, to develop a service and training delivery plan compatible with existing programs and to plan for dissemination of current pediatric rehabilitation literature.[2]

As there were no services or treatments considered as occupational therapy in Romania at the time, additional expectations of the occupational therapy consultant included identification of Romanian health professionals as counterparts to occupational therapists, assessment of how occupational therapy services could be administered to these institutionalized children, and recommendations on the role of AOTA in assisting establishment of an occupational-therapy professional program in Romania.

Upon return from this visit, the author submitted the following recommendations: "that a short-term relationship be established with the ROSES Project to (a) provide educational material to include pediatric continuing education, (b) identify teaching materials for training supportive personnel, (c) link AOTA members interested in short-term service in the ROSES Project with World Vision, and (d) establish short-term mentoring experiences in the United States" for Romanian health workers. Further recommendations include sending a master occupational therapy pediatric clinician/teacher to Romania as an itinerant consultant to the ROSES Project for a minimum of 6 to 12 months. The therapist would teach occupational therapy modalities to Romanian health professionals for the treatment of infants and children. Additionally, the value of occupational therapy would be demonstrated to multi-disciplinary teams. "In time, occupational therapy, as a profession, (could) be established in Romania." (3, p14)

SUMMARY

The role of the occupational therapist as an international consultant is challenging and varied. Descriptions of program development, educational consultation, and systems analysis for administrative planning have been provided to demonstrate the ways in which the occupational therapist consultant can be involved in developing countries. The skills, attributes, and knowledge that will enhance the consultation activities and interactive relationships and lead to successful outcomes are based on mature professional and personal life experiences. The international consultant is not born overnight. Development of specific expertise, broad knowledge of health policy, environment and systems analysis, program planning and administration, and an awareness of the issues and needs in developing countries are essential.

The rapidly changing world scene, uncovering increased health problems in formerly supressed societies, will provide greater opportunities for international occupational therapy consultation. Roles and responsibilities appropriate for consultants to developing countries may include in-service staff training; training to indiginous, unskilled workers; caregiver and family health education; health planning; skill development in administration and program implementation; and advocacy and change agent functions.

The author's experiences in Yugoslavia, Thailand, and Romania were different in time frame (each occured in a different decade, under different political, social, and economic conditions), location, culture and needs. The roles, responsibilities, and functions of the consultant also were different. However, the common thread in these international consultations was the overriding emphasis on the consultant's need to be prepared for the issues specific to each country, with an awareness of the unique life styles, health care practices, and cultural differences in each country. Consideration of consultation in developing countries involves a strong commitment to humankind, with internal fortitude, willingness to learn, ability to take risks, and acceptance of new challenges to achieve improved health care and quality of life for the peoples of the world.

REFERENCES

1. Basch PF: *International Health*. London, Oxford University Press, 1990.
2. Izutsu S: Project ROSES, Romania. Submitted to World Vision International, March 1991.
3. Izutsu S: AOTA representative explores partnership with orphan project in Romania. *OT Week* 1991; 2g:14
4. *Lampang Health Development Project, 1974–1981*. 6 vols. Thailand, Ministry of Public Health.

SECTION H

Technology in Occupational Therapy Consultation

Assistive technology has opened new vistas for disabled individuals who have trouble seeing, hearing, walking, talking, and even breathing. Occupational therapy consultants are key members of the assistive technology team. They work to develop a consumer-responsive technologically supported environment that enables individuals with disabilities to expand and enrich their lives.

The term *assistive device* has been one of occupational therapy's hallmarks. Today's multifaceted and expansive array of assistive technology devices demands that the knowledgeable occupational therapy consultant and her team work together closely. They must maximize their information base to provide optimal equipment for each client in a given environment. The client/consumer is viewed as an important team member. The contributors in this chapter provide illuminating examples of technology in occupational therapy consultation.

Post provides a comprehensive picture of a technology team's evolution within a state system. The client base, developmentally disabled individuals and their caregivers, required extensive technology assistance in the areas of seating positioning and mobility. The case examples provided illustrate the multiple roles required of the consultant at case-centered, program, and administrative consultation levels. The important role of the caregiver and the need for active listening on the consultant's part are emphasized. Without this relevant input, sophisticated and expertly designed technological devices, which are potential enablers, may be ignored or rejected.

Environmental control units (ECUs) have become an accepted part of daily life. People enjoy remote control of their TV, and the tired commuter appreciates the garage door opener on a rainy night. Bain, working with physically challenged individuals and their caregivers, highlights the importance of ECUs for clients with severe disabilities. The consultant brings her expertise to the given situation, providing comprehensive evaluation and client education, which helps to develop the necessary base for informed decision making and eventual utilization and maintenance of the unit. In today's world of technology, she points out, the ECU consultant is a key resource.

557

As we encounter increasingly sophisticated and varied assistive technology, technology resource centers become a central source of information and consultation for the consumer. Grady presents a teamwork perspective that maximizes the information base and collaborative approach necessary for the prospective users and their support team. Collaboration among user, caregiver, consultant, and technology team creates an interactive environment that encourages creative problem solving.

Technology Consultation

AUTHOR	MODEL	LEVEL	LOCUS	GOAL
Post	Collegial, Educational, Program Development, and Systems	Levels I, II, and III: Case centered, educational, and administrative	Client home; nursing facility	Develop functional seating and positioning program for clientele
Bain	Collegial and Educational	Levels I and II: Case centered and educational	Client home	Facilitate client use of ECUs
Grady	Collegial, Educational, Program Development, and Systems	Levels I, II, and III: Case centered, educational, and administrative	Technology resource center; client home	Enable client to make informed choices

CHAPTER 35

Technology Consultation: The Leading Edge

Katherine M. Post, M.S., O.T.R./L.

OVERVIEW

Occupational therapy's focus on the use of tools and devices to help people achieve functional goals has naturally brought the profession into the forefront of assistive technology.[10] Consultation roles may be found in such varied environments as industry, acute health care, rehabilitation, schools, long-term care, research, community health, and individual client homes. In each of these settings, the occupational therapy technology consultant works as part of a specialized team.

The growing complexity of available technology and the rapid changes occurring in the field require a cohesive team with representatives from many different specialty areas. In addition to the client or consumer, the team may include rehabilitation engineers, physical and occupational therapists, speech and language pathologists, social workers, medical equipment salespeople, and others. The team's diverse but related concerns and knowledge can successfully blend important baseline data with state-of-the-art information to address the often complex and multifaceted needs of the person requiring rehabilitation technology services.

The author's technology consultation experiences over the past 14 years include work in a variety of environments and with diverse teams. The occupational therapy consultant adds to the team expertise in evaluation, a broad background in adaptive equipment, ergonomics, activity analysis, group process skills, and an understanding of the occupational performance factors that impact the specific technology need. As a consultant, the author has helped initiate and develop technology services in varied settings, serving as an internal consultant in some cases and external in others.

The two case examples presented in this chapter occurred while the author was a clinical consultant for Adaptive Design Services (ADS) at Belchertown State School. The ADS team designed and fabricated specialized equipment for people

560

with developmental disabilities in western Massachusetts. They also consulted with caregivers and community service providers to ensure successful integration of the equipment into the users' daily routines. These examples are particularly relevant for occupational therapists contemplating consultation as part of a technology team because they emphasize the importance of the caregivers, the client's environment, and the service delivery system. Rather than highlighting successful outcomes, they identify some of the pitfalls one may encounter, evaluate the strategies used, and suggest alternatives to be considered when consulting in this complex market. While the cases focus on seating and positioning, similar concerns and issues arise with other technologies, such as robotics, augmentative communication, environmental controls, architectural design, and personal transportation.

ENVIRONMENT AND SYSTEMS INFLUENCES

Dramatic advances in medical technology have allowed many children and adults to survive severe traumas such as premature births, high spinal cord injuries, and traumatic brain injuries. This has been paralleled by the development of new devices that allow people with physical challenges greater independence in mobility, communication, and control of their own environments.[1] These devices are far more complicated than adaptive eating utensils and splints, and the number of new devices and the speed with which they enter and leave the market is staggering. Consultants with advanced training and experience in the application and use of technology are needed to ensure that people obtain the most appropriate devices, and that increasingly limited financial resources are spent wisely.[2]

Many occupational therapists are well suited for jobs in assistive technology. State programs receiving federal funding to provide technology services have sought occupational therapists to act as consultants and administrators. In school systems, occupational therapy consultants help teachers utilize technical devices to integrate students with disabilities into classrooms. Some colleges and universities utilize consultants in their resource centers for students with disabilities. Occupational therapy consultants help commercial manufacturers and vendors design, market, or sell equipment. Centers providing habilitative and rehabilitative services to people with severe disabilities have also sought this service to address adaptive equipment and assistive technology needs.

A growing number of assistive technology organizations provide advanced training, continuing education, advocacy, lobbying support, and forums for the exchange of information for consumers and professionals. These include RESNA, Closing the Gap, the President's Committee on Employment of Persons With Disabilities, and the International Society for Augmentative and Alternative Communication. Occupational therapists are well represented in their membership and leadership. The American Occupational Therapy Association has also increased its focus on technology. Members may join the Technology Special Interest Section, call the technology program manager for information, read publications highlighting the use of technology in practice, and attend many technology-related papers and courses at the annual conference.

People with disabilities and their advocates have labored long and hard to achieve the right to free choice in treatment, place of residence, education, and employment, and much of the legislation guaranteeing these rights specifies the use of technology. One of the provisions of PL 94-142, the Education for All Handicapped Children Act,[5] is that schools include assistive technology needs in the individualized education plan (IEP) of students receiving special education and related services. The 1986 Amendments to the Rehabilitation Act, PL 99-506,[6] extended rehabilitation technology services to individuals receiving vocational rehabilitation services. PL 100-407, the Technology-Related Assistance for Individuals With Disabilities Act,[7] was passed in 1988. It was designed to help states develop or improve services for information, referral, and delivery of assistive technology to people with disabilities. With the passage of the Americans With Disabilities Act in 1990,[8] private industry has a greater responsibility to provide access to employment, education, transportation, and other activities of daily life. Technology will certainly play an important role in that process.

PL 100-407 was the first piece of federal legislation to introduce the phrase "consumer responsive" to the provision of technology services.[11] While it fails to provide a concise definition of what makes services consumer responsive, the bill clearly communicates the notion that people with disabilities must be included in all phases of the assistive technology process. This includes not only assessment and selection of specific devices for use by an individual, but the design and evaluation of new or custom products, the development of service delivery systems, and the formation of policies and practices.

In 1972, advocates for people with developmental disabilities in Massachusetts sued the state over deplorable living conditions in the institutions and the lack of services and facilities in the community.[9] The resulting consent decree identified adaptive equipment services as an important part of the residents' treatment, necessary to get people out of bed and into programs and functional activities. The state established adaptive design programs at each of its five residential institutions, and purchased whatever equipment was needed by residents. Title XIX of the Social Security Amendments of 1971 allowed public institutions like Belchertown State School to be reimbursed for these and other services by Medicaid, as long as they ensured that residents were receiving "active treatment."[4]

Adaptive Design Services continued to provide consultation, design, and custom fabrication services at no charge when clients moved out of Belchertown and into the community, but commercially available equipment was then paid for directly by Medicaid. As commercially available technology became more sophisticated, the design consultants focused increasingly on evaluating clients, determining their needs, and recommending suitable equipment from commercial vendors. Custom design and fabrication was reserved for severely disabled clients requiring highly individualized devices.

The occupational therapy consultant brought skills in physical assessment and knowledge of seating and positioning with an emphasis on functional outcomes to the job. Using a collegial model, the consultant helped the team identify design features necessary to enhance the client's functional abilities and ease the caretakers' job. Most of the professionals referring clients for services recognized the importance of proper seating as a prerequisite for many other skills, including feeding, communication, mobility, and vocation. Using a clinical treatment model, the clinical consultant often assessed these skills while fitting and adjusting the seating system. A collegial and educational consultation model was then used with the primary therapists to develop a training program for caretakers that incorporated the new equipment.

The success of the consultant depended on listening and leadership skills to focus participants on identification of needs, setting priorities, making decisions, and reaching compromises. Group process training proved valuable to the clinical consultant in work with diverse groups, including professionals, technicians, caretakers, families, and clients. A collegial or professional model of consultation was usually employed, emphasizing problem-solving relationships where all group members were peers. Training and education of participants was also required at times. When outside resources were needed, the clinical consultant helped identify appropriate referrals for other types of intervention. This required some knowledge of funding systems and services available in the client's community.

FRAME OF REFERENCE

The technology consultant who specializes in seating and positioning people with severe developmental disabilities may utilize a neurodevelopmental approach, incorporating principles of sensory integration. The extensive skeletal deformities and age of many of the ADS clients also required a biomechanical focus. Equipment design often incorporated goals for maintenance of range of motion, accommodation of existing deformities, and prevention of skin breakdown. Consistent with the principles of normalization,[12] there was a strong emphasis on age-appropriate equipment. Thus adult clients used adapted switches to control radios or kitchen appliances in their homes or day programs, rather than to control toys. Biomechanical principles helped determine both caretaker needs, such as seat height for transfers and feeding, and client needs, such as wheel position for independent propulsion of a manual wheelchair. High priority was given to medical needs, such as positioning the head to minimize the risk of aspiration or having the ability to adjust the seating system's orientation in space to vary weight distribution and prevent pressure sores. A broad view of occupational performance as determined by the client's skills within the physical and social environment helped in formulating realistic goals and approaches. Collaboration between the consultant, primary therapists, client, and caregivers was critical in determining appropriate solutions to problems.

CONSULTATION DESCRIPTION

A CLINICAL CONSULTATION: CASE 1, LISA

Organization

Adaptive Design Services at Belchertown State School grew out of the physical and occupational therapy department, becoming a separate department in 1975. By 1982 there were six designers on staff, four concentrating on seating and mobility systems, one specializing in environmental design, and one spending more than half his time managing the department. The designers also worked with communication systems, adaptive switching devices, and protective devices like helmets and gloves. Two additional full-time employees were responsible for most of the upholstery and repair work. The work flow had been organized so that each designer worked on two or three projects at once, allowing them to keep working on other projects while waiting for parts, materials, or a scheduled fitting for a particular project.

The region was divided into five areas, and the institution had been divided into units that represented the clients' areas of geographical origin to facilitate community placement. ADS provided one major project slot for each area or unit in the institution and one slot for each area office in the community. As a project was completed, the designer and clinical consultant met with the team to begin the next project. It was the responsibility of the area office contact person or the primary treatment team at the institution to decide priorities and the order of the waiting lists. There was some flexibility within this system, since minor projects could be squeezed in between other projects, but there was generally a long waiting list for custom wheelchairs and seating systems.

Most referrals came from therapists who had previously worked with the department. They usually had some idea of the type of equipment they were interested in obtaining for the client. The clinical consultant and a designer met with the client and referral source first to perform a screening. Commercially available equipment could be recommended at this preliminary evaluation. For example, the team might select a wheelchair or mobility base on which the seating system would be built and then submit the paperwork necessary for funding and ordering. The equipment would thus be available when the designer was ready to begin the project.

Support

As noted previously, support for this program was mandated through legislation designed to restructure services for people with developmental disabilities. The long-term goal of providing appropriate equipment was to help clients reside in community settings whenever possible. When funding for special equipment could be obtained from other state or private sources, such as Medicaid, private insurance, and so on, this was sought.

Participants

Lisa was a 19-year-old girl with severe cerebral palsy and mental retardation who lived with her parents in an old mill town in the western hills of Massachusetts. She attended a special classroom program in one of the town's two elementary schools. Her physical therapist, Nancy, contacted Adaptive Design Services at the suggestion of a wheelchair vendor who felt she could benefit from a customized seating system and a large wheelchair. The teachers and therapist wanted equipment that provided better postural support, and they were concerned about Lisa's safety during transporting in her old wheelchair. Lisa's mother was the primary caretaker at home, and she took great care to involve her in family activities.

Services Provided

When Nancy contacted the ADS clinical consultant, she was advised to submit a referral form to the appropriate area office. The contact person at the area office determined Lisa's eligibility for Department of Mental Retardation services and placed her on the ADS waiting list. After about 4 months, the clinical consultant called Nancy and scheduled an appointment for the evaluation.

Most adaptive equipment evaluations were scheduled in the client's own environment—at school, home, day program, or wherever the most caretakers and service providers could gather. This was essential not only for getting all the information needed to determine the problems, but to involve the people who would be using the equipment with the client in developing the solutions. Lisa's initial evaluation was held at school, with Nancy, Lisa's teachers and aides, and her mother attending. The discussion was dominated by Nancy, the teacher, and the classroom aides. The mother seemed very shy and quiet, leaving the discussion several times to go sit on the mat with Lisa. The design team noted the accessibility of the classroom, with wide doorways and a large open area with tabletop work areas, floor mats, and adequate space for maneuvering wheelchairs of any shape or description.

The consultant evaluated Lisa with the rest of the team. Lisa's motor skills, developmental level, reflexes, tone, abnormal movement patterns, and other characteristics helped determined the physical parameters of the equipment related to her need for support and function. The care providers described how her tone and alertness varied from day to day, at different times of day, with different people, and from home to school. The consultant observed transfers, feeding, dressing, and mobility activities to determine the caregiver's physical needs.

Before completing their recommendations, the designer and the consultant visited Lisa at home. Her mother talked more freely there, sharing how Lisa spent her time at home and what the rest of her family did. The meticulous care she gave Lisa was quite evident in her description of feeding and bathing activities and in Lisa's clean and neat appearance. The designer noted areas of the home that might cause problems in handling the equipment as follows:

- The narrow hallway from the back door to the kitchen.
- The furniture and gas heater crowding the door of the dining room, which served as Lisa's bedroom.
- The steepness of the driveway and street.
- The flimsiness of the temporary ramp built from the driveway to the back door.

The designer took measurements to determine the maximum width of the finished equipment and suggested some simple changes that might make things easier. The method of transporting Lisa and her equipment to and from school was also reviewed, since her accident on the school bus in the old travel chair was a great worry to everyone involved. One issue of particular concern to her mother was getting Lisa out of the house and down to the street, particularly in bad weather. The school van could not be driven up the driveway, and the driver could not help them from their door, since the van had to have an attendant inside at all times.

To the designer and the clinical consultant, these factors all pointed to the need for equipment that would provide adequate support of Lisa's trunk, head, and extremities to maintain postural alignment, with adjustment for growth and change in condition. Many clients with Lisa's general condition had benefited from custom chairs that allowed periodic adjustment of orientation in space, shifting weight from the buttocks to the back and relieving the superincumbent effects of gravity on the spine and head. This type of chair would be larger and heavier than Lisa's current chair, but the team had said her chair was too small for her size and weight, as evidenced by its tendency to tip over in the school bus. With larger wheels and a longer and wider base, the chair would traverse uneven terrain more safely and easily. The clinical consultant shared these recommendations with Lisa's mother, showing her pictures from wheelchair catalogs and the ADS portfolio to illustrate the features. The mother's reaction was reserved, but she seemed willing to try a chair with the promise of greater comfort for Lisa and more safety in handling.

The designer and the consultant left Lisa's home confident that their recommendations would meet everyone's stated needs. After substantial work on the wheelchair, the consultant called the mother and Nancy to schedule the first fitting at school. Nancy and the school staff were very pleased with the support the chair offered Lisa, the way it tilted back in space, and the adjustability of the components. Lisa's mother, however, was again quiet and seemed afraid to offer her objections. "It's awfully big," she said. "I don't think it will fit in my house." The ADS staff then took the chair to the home, meeting Lisa and her mother there after school. Since the designer had used the measurements of the hall and doorways in modifying the chair, it fit through, but it was a tighter fit than the travel chair had been. Lisa's mother looked uncomfortable as the consultant showed her how to operate the chair. She explained the importance of the trial period before the chair was completed and upholstered. A return appointment was scheduled in 2 weeks. Lisa's mother agreed to try the chair during that time, and understood that further modifications could be made if there were problems. The suggestions made earlier about simple changes in furniture arrangement or door casings were repeated, and Lisa's mother said she would talk it over with her husband.

Sensing some difficulties in acceptance of the equipment, the consultant called the social service agency to see if Lisa's social worker could be present for the next fitting. When they all arrived at the house 2 weeks later, Lisa was sitting in her old travel chair and the new wheelchair was in a corner of the kitchen. Lisa's mother hesitantly described the problems she had faced during the trial period. The clinical consultant slowly realized that, even with further modifications, the chair was not going to be accepted. While the larger wheels and casters made the chair roll over rocks and bumps more easily, the chair was too heavy for Lisa's mother to control going down the driveway or the sidewalk. She liked the idea that the chair could be tilted back, but found it took up more space in that position. She said the headrest positioned Lisa's head well for feeding, but the footrest made it more difficult to pull up to the table at meals. While the chair just fit through the doors and hallway, she had to be very careful not to hit the walls. She also had to move the coats hanging on hooks by the back door in order to get the chair in and out.

The clinical consultant and the designer talked with the whole team about possible solutions and the compromises involved with each, and finally came to the conclusion that the chair was not going to meet the family's needs. After some negotiation, they decided to repair the old travel chair so that it provided better postural support and was more durable. The new wheelchair was taken back to ADS and stored. It was hoped that Lisa would need the new equipment when she graduated from school and began attending a day program.

A key part of consultation service delivery is evaluation. In this case, the team and consultants learned a great deal from the evaluation process and in-depth learning experience, and developed a follow-up plan for the client. With all the problems and pitfalls of this experience, the evaluation process gave the participants an opportunity to move toward a more positive outcome. They identified the many issues and concerns that should have been assessed more carefully prior to and during the implementation phase.

Interpersonal dynamics and communication were high on the list. Although the clinical consultant and the designer had made some efforts to get information from all the people involved with Lisa, they had failed to take into account a number of subtle issues. These included the dynamics between the school staff, Nancy, Lisa's mother, and the social workers helping with long-range planning. As is often seen, there was some antagonism between home and school. The school staff was impatient with the family's babying of Lisa and the lack of carryover of their programs in the home. The family felt that the school staff did not really understand their needs, and they questioned the value of the changes being demanded of them.

Lisa's mother felt she was contending not just with changes in the chair, but with threats to the whole system she had worked out for Lisa's care. She was afraid these changes would upset the balance in her family's life, or that Lisa would get hurt, or look too disabled. At the same time, she was very timid about disagreeing with any of the professionals, since she was "only" the mother. The structure of evaluation and fitting sessions can have a profound impact on people's willingness to participate in discussion, and, in this case, it had obviously inhibited the mother's confidence in expressing her preferences and making sure she was being heard.

The need for future planning was recognized by the team, but its importance to the family in relation to their equipment needs was not adequately determined. Since Lisa was approaching her 21st birthday and the transition from the school system to adult services, a social service agency had begun working with the family on plans for the future. The agency and family talked about her attending an adult day program and, perhaps when the family could no longer care for her, moving Lisa to a group home. With the prospect of different staff, setting, and transportation systems, there was pressure from the agency to get Lisa out of the old travel chair she had used for 10 years and into a more age-appropriate seating and mobility system. However, the agency, consultants, and team had not provided a strong enough rationale to the family to have this issue override their current needs for the travel chair.

Education and training, both important aspects of the consultation process, are critical when working with technology dependent clientele. An important component of involving people in the design and decision process is teaching them about the equipment so they can make informed choices. This includes sharing findings from the physical assessment with parents and nonprofessionals and having equipment available for demonstration and simulation. Lisa's mother seemed to have some difficulty envisioning what the team was recommending until she actually saw it. Seeing how different options worked and looked would have given her more information on which to base her choices. She might then have been able to express her preferences with greater confidence. Additionally while Lisa was unable to communicate her needs verbally, her physical and emotional reactions to simulated positions and positioning in trial equipment would have revealed something about her preferences and her functional potential.

Understanding the client system must take into account the larger system surrounding the client. As the experts coming in from the outside, the ADS consultant and designer should have been more sensitive to the social history and dynamics of the community. Whatever changes in policy and practice had been made by the state in more recent years, the clinical consultant and design staff came from a facility and an agency with a very unflattering history of intervention with the mentally retarded. Particularly among the older communities in the hill-towns, the state's reputation of intruding on the families' care of their children remained. Lisa's family was one of many that had decided long ago to keep their children and care for them at home instead of locking them away and forgetting them. The clinical consultant and staff were state representatives telling them what was best for their child, part of a larger group pushing for changes in their lives. The mistrust and fear that this engendered made it difficult to obtain honest answers about their needs and preferences from the family.

The consultant and designer established a monitoring communication process with the team at the time the new chair was stored at their facility. The consultant remained available for telephone consultation. Equipment problems did not arise during Lisa's last year and a half in school. Over this period, the team, parents, and social service agency worked out a plan for Lisa to attend a day program. The designer then worked with the day program staff to complete the chair so it could be used there and during transporting on the van. Lisa has continued to use her travel chair at home.

Outcome

A long-range solution was eventually achieved for Lisa, her caregivers, and the multidisciplinary team. However, the complexities of technology consultation made for a bumpy road along the way. The so-called wonders of technology cannot solve all the problems of real life. The consultant and team identified many issues that had prevented initial acceptance of more sophisticated equipment. Important factors were listening skills, interpersonal dynamics, and other communication abilities; training and educating the client and caregivers; and understanding the client's environments or systems.

The consultant and designer also recognized that they had been too quick to impose their own values on the situation. To them, a wheelchair that tilted in space with large rear wheels, a longer wheelbase, and a better balanced center of gravity was safer, more convenient, better for Lisa, and the best choice. They were accustomed to how these chairs looked and how much more they weighed. They assumed that they would have been willing to make the changes necessary to accommodate this type of chair. By ignoring Lisa's mother's quiet protests, they were not respecting her individual preferences and needs and her right to live her life the way she wanted. She stifled her disagreement because she want to please them, and they heard only what they wanted to hear.

Since that time, many new wheelchair frames that might have offered better compromises have become available, but the lesson in working with clients and their families remains. Part of a technology consultant's role is to respect and support family concerns and establish a solid relationship from which effective communication can occur. This sometimes means allying more closely with the family than with the other professionals. It also means casting aside more authoritative models of consultation, and recognizing the rights of the client and the caregivers to share in identifying and solving problems to improve the quality of their lives.

CONSULTATION DESCRIPTION

A SYSTEMS CONSULTATION: CASE II

Technology consultants can also play an important role in larger organizations or systems. Clients who are severely disabled often reside in long-term care settings. Caregivers and professional staff in these settings may not have had exposure to or an understanding of the technology advances applicable to their clients. Through the use of specialized adaptive equipment, clients in these facilities may require less care and can live with greater independence. This case consultation is an example.

Organization

The Commonwealth of Massachusetts stopped admitting children to its large institutions for people with mental retardation and developmental disabilities soon after the consent decree was issued. However, some children with severe disabilities and long-term medical needs required residential care. Four long-term pediatric care units were established in nursing homes across the state, with one in ADS's catchment area. The pediatric unit at this nursing home had 40 beds filled with children with multiple disabilities, some requiring respiratory support and fed through gastrostomy tubes. These children ranged in age from 2 to 20 years, and some had lived there more than 5 years awaiting foster or group home placement.

Support

Medicaid paid the nursing home to care for most of the children needing skilled nursing care and therapy services, but funding for equipment was a problem. As a skilled nursing facility, the home received an all-inclusive rate and was supposed to provide whatever was needed for residents, including wheelchairs. However, staff had been unaware of a clause in the Medicaid regulations that allowed payment for equipment which was so customized as to preclude its use by other residents.[3]

Because they resided in the region and were diagnosed with developmental disabilities, the children in the nursing home were eligible for DMR services, including equipment design and fabrication services from ADS. The first seating systems built for these children used cast-off wheelchair frames found in the storage shed, cut and rewelded to suit their individual needs. Although the design and fabrication services were provided by the state at no charge, these projects were so labor intensive that they ended up costing the state far more money than purchasing commercially available equipment.

Participants

The nursing home employed one part-time occupational therapist to oversee the clinical program on the unit but contracted with a local therapy agency to provide the rest of the clinical staff. Unfortunately, this had resulted in a steady procession of part-time physical and occupational therapists providing the minimum evaluation and consultation services required of the nursing home by funding sources. The ADS staff would start the evaluation of a child with one therapist, but by the time the chair was completed, another therapist would have taken over the case.

The children's therapy programs were generally carried out by minimally trained direct care workers who had moved into therapy aide positions from jobs as nursing assistants. A number of them had been there for years and had seen many professionals come and go. Most of them were fairly emotionally involved with ''their kids.'' There was some antagonism between the aides and the nursing staff as well, with resentment of perceived workload and salary differences.

Services Provided

The clinical consultant and designers at ADS had seen five or six of the children in the home before they realized how much more could be achieved with each child by establishing a closer relationship with the staff. Although this was considered a community placement, the nursing home had many similarities to the state school. The consultant suggested using approaches that had worked at that institution and identified a strategy of conducting staff training and periodic follow-up and evaluation clinics at the facility. Equipment problems at the nursing home revolved around several key issues: communication with staff during evaluation and fitting, proper use of the equipment, cleaning and maintenance, and referral for follow-up when adjustments or further modifications were needed.

While the consultant felt there was little she could do about the overall systems problems at the nursing home, she believed that some changes around equipment issues could be made by working directly with the aides. Dave, the supervising occupational therapist, supported this idea. He had good relationships with most of the aides but he admitted that his own clinical background in seating and positioning was limited. He was helpful in scheduling in-service training time, releasing aides to come to evaluations and fittings with the children, and including the ADS staff in the monthly clinic visits made to the facility by the consulting orthopedist.

Staff training was accomplished in several ways. Principles of positioning and the use of different types of equipment were presented with slides and client demonstrations during in-service training sessions. The clinical consultant involved staff in these sessions by having them select the ''favorite'' children for demonstration, soliciting help with physical handling, asking staff to simulate positions on each other, and encouraging them to share their own solutions to problems. Evaluation and fitting sessions offered more opportunities for individual instruction, though, and staff seemed more comfortable asking questions at those times than with the whole group present. Since the nursing unit was relatively small, most of the staff knew all the children and these meetings could be used for more general discussion of when to make referrals, how to assess needs, and how to use and monitor the completed wheelchairs.

As with the community-based clients, initial evaluation sessions were held at the nursing home. This enabled the clinical consultant and designer to talk with the supervising therapists and nurses as well as nursing and therapy aides, school staff, and involved family members. These meetings were particularly interesting when disagreements arose between professional and direct care staff. It became clear that, while the aides might not understand theories and interventions, they had the most information about how the children were cared for, what they could do in their chairs, and when things got broken (blame the third shift!). Without the full support of these workers, equipment would not be used properly and could not be expected to last.

The consultant focused first on improving communication with the aides. The aides knew how difficult their lives could be without effective equipment, but they did not believe that anyone would listen to them or take their concerns seriously. Treating them like professionals encouraged them to act professional, keeping appointments and promises, and providing accurate and useful information and feedback. They also became the greatest source of referrals; once one child got a new chair that worked well, the aide wanted new chairs for all her kids. Most of the aides seemed to enjoy the responsibility of coming to the fittings, which were held at the shop in Belchertown, 15 miles from the nursing home. This was when detailed decisions about the equipment's operation were made. The aides were the people who most used the equipment, and it was critical that they understand the basic mechanics of the chairs.

One of the most difficult aspects of designing and building seating systems is recognizing when a goal is unrealistic. The children at the nursing home were very severely disabled; most of them had very low cognitive levels and complicated medical conditions. Their muscle tone, reflex involvement, and skeletal deformities made positioning them a real challenge, and it was tempting to try complicated devices to provide better support or control. These required endless fine-tuning and were more prone to breakage. Together, the ADS staff and the aides had to resolve to keep equipment simple and as uniform as possible so that three shifts of workers could cope with them. Most of the nursing home children were assigned to one designer, and he and the consultant worked closely to standardize the equipment. This ensured easier use by staff, quicker replacement of broken parts, and more efficient use of design and construction time.

The staff also had to learn that equipment could not solve every problem. Some problems needed to be addressed through therapeutic intervention; others were staffing issues. Equipment had to be seen as an adjunct to therapy, allowing some carryover from treatment sessions and helping to maintain some of the gains from active treatment. Dave, the supervising occupational therapist, helped keep the lines of communication with new clinical staff open so that the consultant could suggest changes in therapy programs. These might help acclimate the client to the new equipment, achieve some of the goals identified during the equipment evaluation, and address areas of concern not provided for in the equipment.

While fittings could be completed more efficiently at the shop, the designer and the consultant found it important to deliver the finished chairs to the nursing home. A number of staff people could be trained at once, assuring that they agreed with and understood the final product. This training became simpler after the chairs became more standardized. Cleaning was of particular concern, since it was the third shift's responsibility and they could not be involved in evaluation, fitting, or delivery sessions. A videotaped demonstration of the consultant disassembling a chair for cleaning made some difference, but only when it was followed up with some personal contact from Dave and the nursing supervisor.

Being in the nursing home on a regular basis allowed the consultant and the designer to monitor most of the chairs that had already been completed. The aides usually made referrals to the team when there were serious problems, but relatively minor repairs were often ignored until they became big problems. The designer spent time working with the volunteer who maintained the nursing home's chairs and periodically supplied him with boxes of hardware and fasteners so that he could easily replace missing bolts and broken parts. This volunteer was another person who felt undervalued by the system, and the time spent listening to him and his suggestions was well spent.

Outcome

While ADS continued to provide services for those children with severe deformities who had poor funding resources, a growing number of needs could be met with the availability of more sophisticated commercial products. Teaching staff how to apply for Medicaid funding under the custom clause opened the door for obtaining adjustable equipment with a variety of support components. However, selection and application of these devices required close work with a commercial vendor and thorough knowledge of the equipment being recommended. The consultant worked with the nursing home's own therapists to evaluate children for commercial seating systems, and trained the therapists to do more of their own assessment and prescription. This was a combination of client-centered, professional, and educational consultation, depending on the needs of the individual child and the skills of the particular therapist.

SUMMARY

Occupational therapists clearly have a great deal of skill and expertise to offer in the field of assistive technology. The increasing focus on the use of technology to improve the quality of life of people with disabilities requires the involvement of experts in the selection and application of devices. Occupational therapists will find a growing number of opportunities for consulting in this field in the next decade and beyond: teaching, listening, evaluating, recommending, training, and sharing their knowledge and experience with professionals and consumers alike.

REFERENCES

1. Blackman A: Machines that work miracles. *Time*, February 18, 1991, pp 70–71.
2. Christiansen RC, Smith RO, Fox LB: Technology specialization for occupational therapists, in *Technology Review '90: Perspectives on Occupational Therapy Practice*. Rockville, Md, AOTA, 1990.

3. Medical Assistance Program: *Durable Medical Equipment Manual*. Commonwealth of Massachusetts, 1981, pp 4-12–4-13.
4. Public Law 92-223, Social Security Amendments of 1988, 53 Federal Register 20496, June 3, 1988.
5. Public Law 94-142, Education for All Handicapped Children Act, 42 Federal Register 42411-12, August 1977.
6. Public Law 99-506, Rehabilitation Act Sections 501-503, 40 Federal Register 54718, November 25, 1975. Redesignated at 45 Federal Register 77369, November 21, 1980.
7. Public Law 100-407, Technology-Related Assistance for Individuals With Disabilities Act, 54 Federal Register 32771, August 9, 1989.
8. Public Law 101-336, Americans With Disabilities Act, 56 Federal Register 7452, February 22, 1991.
9. *Ricci v. Greenblatt,* 72-469-T, Federal District Court (Massachusetts, 1972).
10. Trefler E: Technology applications in occupational therapy. *Am J Occup Ther* 1990; 41:697.
11. Williams R: Consumer responsiveness: Knowing it when you see it. *Assistive Tech Q* 1990; 1:1.
12. Wolfensberger W: *The Principle of Normalization in Human Services*. Toronto, National Institute of Mental Retardation, 1972.

RESOURCES

American Occupational Therapy Association, 1383 Piccard Drive, Rockville, MD 20850-4375.

Center for Special Education Technology, Council for Exceptional Children, 1920 Association Drive, Reston, VA 22091.

Closing the Gap, P.O. Box 68, Henderson, MN 56044.

International Society for Augmentative and Alternative Communication, P.O. Box 1762, Station R, Toronto, Ontario M4G 4A3, Canada.

President's Committee on Employment of Persons With Disabilities, Work Environment and Technology Committee, 1111 20th Street NW, 6th Floor, Washington, DC 20210.

RESNA, An Association for the Advancement of Rehabilitation and Assistive Technologies, 1101 Connecticut Avenue NW, Suite 700, Washington, DC 20036.

CHAPTER 36

Environmental Control Unit Consultation

Beverly K. Bain, Ed.D., O.T.R., F.A.O.T.A.

OVERVIEW

In today's world of expanding technology, increasing numbers of environmental control units (ECUs) are being developed to facilitate society's everyday activities. One can use a remote control device to turn on the lights before entering a dark house, or press a button on a bedside control box to turn on the coffee in the kitchen, or change the TV channel from a comfortable chair. These are but a few technological aids that enable people to control their environment. For physically challenged people with limited hand skills, ECUs may be the *only* way they can interact or control parts of their environment.

The author defines an ECU as a system that enables individuals to interact purposefully with their surroundings by means of a mechanical or electronic assistive device. Each ECU system is composed of four parts: the input or switch, the throughput or the processing unit, the output or peripheral (usually an appliance), and the feedback or display.

Historically, occupational therapists have treated clients who are dysfunctional in the performance of activities of daily living (ADL) and as a part of their work have assessed their clients' needs for adaptive equipment. Today, therapists need to consider the potential benefits a client may derive from the use of various technological assistive devices. Consideration should be given to the variety of environments in which the client lives, works, and spends leisure time. The technology consultant can assist therapists providing direct treatment as they determine a client's needs.

Potential Market

With the passage of the Americans With Disabilities Act,[1] an increasing number of people with disabilities now seek employment, use public transportation, attend public functions, and generally participate in the mainstream of life. Through the use of environmental control systems, they are able to conserve their energy, perform instrumental ADLs, and take advantage of the increasing opportunities in the world around them.

The evolution of medical technology during the past decades has saved many lives. Concomitantly, many of the survivors are individuals with multiple problems including very limited ability to control their environment without the type of assistance available through ECUs.

The expanded use and availability of personal computers has also had an impact. Today's computer can be designed to incorporate ECU functions, thereby providing a comprehensive and efficient tool that allows physically challenged individuals greater independence while using socially acceptable and familiar equipment.

The consultant can help expand the use of ECUs in a variety of health care and related environments. ECUs are needed in schools and developmental centers to facilitate client independence and assist caretakers in conserving energy and simplifying work patterns. In acute hospital settings they can help individuals gain a sense of control over their environment. A study conducted on young spinal cord clients found that those who received ECUs and were properly trained were more inclined to attend college, work, and become independent than a control group who did not.[6] In nursing facilities, a resident's room is his or her personal space, yet many times it is shared with another person whose problems are very different. For example, one resident may have a hearing problem and the other a hip fracture; each wants to control more of their environment for their own needs. Through consultation, it may be possible to identify two separate, safe, low cost, easy to assemble and maintain ECU systems to meet the residents' disparate needs. The blind and hearing impaired benefit greatly from ECUs, which can increase their safety and independence. Systems can be programmed and controlled by blind computer users, and hearing impaired individuals may utilize ECUs for visual feedback, which is critical to their independence and safety.

In the area of educational consultation, professional and continuing education programs are vital for therapists working with this technology. Similarly, caregivers and other health professionals need guidance and educational programs when these devices are placed with a given client.

KEY POINTS

Necessary Knowledge and Skills

The assessment process encompasses the client, any current assistive technology devices in use, ECUs under consideration, and the environments. A holistic physical evaluation of the client may be performed. Many alternative access approaches are considered, such as head, neck, tongue, or toe motions; eye and breath control; or voice activation. The psychosocial and cognitive aspects of the evaluation are crucial if the technological device is to be effective. What does the client need? Can they follow two- or three-step directions? How does the client feel about being dependent on a machine?

A knowledgeable consultant is

- Familiar with state-of-the-art devices, from the simplest to the most complex
- Experienced in adapting, modifying, and adjusting the equipment
- Able to assess client potential to utilize ECUs
- Aware of related technology that interfaces or can utilize ECUs
- Capable of educating and training the client, caregivers, and treating therapist in regard to operation, care, and maintenance of ECUs.

The ECU consultant's role includes case centered, educational, and program development levels. Performance components relative to the occupational therapy domain should be considered during client evaluation, training, and selection of the ECU. For example, most switch activation includes sensorimotor involvement and the cognitive skills of sequencing and following instructions for the use and maintenance of the ECU system. Psychosocial components also must be considered if the client is to accept and fully utilize the system.

The consultant also educates the treating therapist regarding the potential uses of ECUs. They may be used in a variety of environments, including bedside, within a health care facility, and/or at home, school, work, and community. It is imperative that present and possible future environments be considered in the selection of the ECU system and in the training of the client. A structured procedure for assessment of the client, the assistive technology device, and potential environments is the key to success.[2]

The client, caretakers, and treating therapist must also be instructed in the care and maintenance of the devices, as well as sources for any needed replacements. Most ECUs have electrical parts needing periodic checks to assure client safety, which is always a priority.

Important theoretical foundations[3] that provide a basis for the application of ECUs with any given client population include the following:

- The biomechanical approach; specifically, the work simplification/energy conservation principle
- The acquisition frame of reference[5]
- The developmental frame of reference
- The rehabilitative frame of reference.

Major theories of learning, classical conditioning, operant conditioning, and social learning also need special mention. As society moves toward a push button age to control the environment, the physically challenged person becomes socially integrated by performing everyday tasks as others do.

The biomechanical model is useful when considering such factors as energy conservation needed to perform ADLs. The ECU can augment the physical strength necessary to participate in many functional activities.

The acquisitional frame of reference as defined by Mosey, "provides a structure for linking learning theories, the reality aspect of purposeful activities, and the process of acquiring specific skills needed for successful interaction in the environment."[5] This frame of reference should be considered when suggesting the use of ECUs.

The developmental frame of reference can be considered when the disability is congenital or when function is lost through the aging process. Use of an ECU may help develop or maintain autonomy and prevent learned helplessness. In a rehabilitative approach, the ECU may be a precursor to learning higher level skills. For example, clients can learn to control their personal living environment prior to learning the use of a power wheelchair. Learning to activate a single ECU switch also serves as an introduction to the more complex tasks required for the operation of a computer or augmentative communication device.

Case Study

The following case consultation, concerning a physically challenged student (Arlene), her family, and school, illustrates how an ECU consultation encompasses the needs of client, caregivers, and environments.

Arlene attended a special school where she received a full complement of related services. However the therapist's technology skills were limited to those needed to determine the most efficient and reliable control site for switch access to a communication device used at the school. The school's child study team also noted that Arlene's constant demand for attention and her learned helplessness were detering her school progress. Additionally, home problems had been noted that were contributing to Arlene's school behaviors. These included the physical layout of the home and the availability of caregivers when Arlene needed assistance. The school occupational therapist requested consultation from the ECU consultant, whom she had heard lecture.

The consultant and school administration then negotiated a contract specifying the need for client, caregiver, and environment assessment in the home setting. It was agreed that the consultant would identify the needed ECUs; recommend their placement in the home; develop operational plans; provide training to Arlene, caregivers, and the primary therapist; and help identify funding sources for the necessary equipment.

A meeting was then held with the family, primary therapist, and Arlene, to introduce the idea of and need for ECU implementation in the home. The family consisted of Arlene, a 7-year-old cerebral palsied student with quadriparesis who was the youngest in this family of five, her parents, grandmother, and two brothers, ages 10 and 12. Responsibility for Arlene's care fell primarily to her mother and grandmother, as the father traveled 2 to 3 days a week. The mother also worked 3 nights a week so that she could be available for Arlene and her brothers during the day. The grandmother, who was most consistently at home, is hearing impaired. The family lives in a split-level home. Arlene's bedroom is upstairs, as is her parents' and brothers' rooms. The grandmother's bedroom is on the ground level.

The consultant and all concerned identified Arlene's major needs as follows:

- Communicate her need for assistance, especially while in bed
- Control her room environment when she is in bed, that is, the TV, fan, lights.

The caretakers' major needs were as follows:

- Quick illumination of the outside ramps/walkways at night, in order to push Arlene's chair or carry her into the house
- Remote monitoring of Arlene's respiration when in bed
- Energy conservation remote control strategies to help the grandmother. She needed to be available to control Arlene's lights, monitor her breathing, and answer other problems. Due to the home configuration (split level) and the location of her room, the task of caregiving was exceedingly draining for her.

To meet these varied needs, the consultant evaluated parts from several different ECU systems, and developed the following configuration:

- Sensitive switches to be mounted for Arlene's bedside use
- Portable control units that could be used as needed by Arlene and/or her family
- A visual feedback component to allow the grandmother to respond to Arlene's communications
- Establishment of the number of appliances or outputs required.

Once a sample unit was configured, tested, and determined to be appropriate, the consultant trained the client, caregivers, and therapist. Written instructions and literature were provided regarding use, care, and maintenance of the system. Each member of the home team demonstrated their understanding of the unit operation as part of the training process.

The final issue was identification of funding resources necessary to purchase the equipment. Since most state and federal agencies and few insurance companies pay for these systems, other sources had to be found. The consultant suggested a method she had found to be successful, "the collaborative extended family method." This involves asking members of the extended family, such as aunts, uncles, and cousins, to buy parts of the system. One might buy the control unit, another the remote unit, and so on. All the parts are then wrapped as gifts and given to the client and family as a special holiday present. Other possible sources were discussed with the family. Possibilities could be explored through special technology funding. The consultant offered to teach Arlene's father and her therapist how to fabricate several of the switches. This helped them learn the basics of switch control, prepared them to make minor repairs, and provided encouragement for them to modify battery-operated toys that Arlene could then operate. The use of these toys would enable Arlene to interact further with her environment and also learn to play independently.

At the close of the consultation, it was agreed that the treating therapist would send periodic reevaluation reports to the consultant. In this way, the consultant could monitor the effective use of the environmental control system by Arlene and her caretakers.

Additionally, the ECU consultant was asked to review the case in depth prior to the development of Arlene's next IEP. This would then allow all concerned to agree on any needed changes or additions to the system.

SUMMARY

The ECU consultant can make important contributions in many settings and with many age groups. Given the increasing importance of health care technology in today's world, occupational therapists must develop greater knowledge and skill in this area. The ECU consultant should be a key source for those lacking these abilities. The consultant can provide important training and information to occupational therapy students, practicing therapists, clients, and caregivers, utilizing specific occupational therapy (theoretical bases) and consultation models.

In today's marketplace, the ECU consultant is a key resource. Appropriate use of these special devices provides the therapist with another tool to help address a basic occupational therapy rehabilitation principle, "restore the disabled to a life that is purposeful and satisfying, one that allows each individual the opportunity to function . . . as a member of society with the capabilities to meet the responsibilities of that society."[4]

REFERENCES

1. Americans With Disabilities Act, PL 101-336, Washington, DC, July 1990.
2. Bain B: The assessment of clients for technological assistive devices, in *American Occupational Therapy Association: Technology Review '89*. Rockville, Md, AOTA, 1989; pp. 55–59.
3. Hopkins H, Smith S: *Willard and Spackman's Occupational Therapy,* ed 7. Philadelphia, Lippincott, 1989.
4. Licht S: *Rehabilitation and Medicine*. Baltimore, Waverly Press, 1968.
5. Mosey S: *Psychosocial Components of Occupational Therapy*. New York, Raven Press, 1986.
6. Yudin M, Dickey R, Seil G, et al: Instrumentation for the severely disabled: An update. *Spinal Cord Digest* 1980; 16:2.

CHAPTER 37

Technology Adoption: Linking Through Communication

Ann P. Grady, M.A., O.T.R., F.A.O.T.A.

OVERVIEW

The consultation process in an era of increasingly advanced assistive technology applications for persons with special needs brings together the expertise of the technology program consultant and the needs of the provider or consumer of assistive technology services. Effective communication between the persons involved in the process is essential. Anytime two or more persons come together to talk things over, deliberate, seek opinion or advice to decide or plan a course of action, communication provides the means by which they proceed. One of the functions of interpersonal communication is linking with other people to share information and meaning.[1] Communication promotes transfer of ideas, creation of new ideas, understanding of values and perspectives, expression of feelings, identification and resolution of differences. Linking with persons who have information about technology and understand the meaning it may hold for others is particularly important to consumers or providers who are considering adoption of technology as part of their lives. Although use of technological solutions in occupational therapy for persons with special needs is not new, the use of advanced, complex, electronically-based technology does represent a significant innovation or practice, in the field.[9] The most significant departure from the usual ideas of occupational therapists about technological adaptations is the complexity of the equipment, which differs sharply from the simpler devices adopted in the past. For example, a pencil holder was used in the past and now a computer is used for producing written communication. The complexity of electronically-based assistive technology sometimes produces uncertainty in both the provider and user of equipment. Uncertainty over whether a person feels he or she can do it, fix it, teach it, or live with it can act as a barrier to the adoption of new technology.[5] Reducing uncertainty through communication is the key to adoption of innovation and therefore the key to successful consultation.

In the course of linking technical knowledge with others by sharing information and feelings, each person reveals something about himself to the other person. Telling someone how you feel, or sharing information that might be challenged, or stating your position on an issue involves risk. At risk is a person's concept of himself as someone who is knowledgeable, competent, angry, sad, or whatever is appropriate for the situation.[1] In presenting new technological information to a client, whether another professional, a consumer of therapy services, or a family member, the knowledge or feelings offered via communication may be accepted by verbal or non-verbal responses that signify agreement. If the person sending the communication feels that what was said was accepted, then he or she will feel accepted as a person as well. The sender's image of himself as knowledgeable, or as someone whose feelings are justified is confirmed by the positive response from the receiver of the communication. If the information or the feeling shared is rejected, either verbally or non-verbally, for example, if the other person shakes his or her head "no" while listening to a new idea being expressed or interrupts frequently, then the person sending the message feels rejected. At stake is the person's self-concept as an expert on topics being discussed which means that from the expert's perspective both the idea and the expertise are being rejected.

As Director of the AccessAbility Resource Center, this author functions as a consultant to adults and children with differing abilities, their families, and the professional service providers who work with them. In addition, the author consults with organizations, professional and consumer groups in the areas of technology and consumer/family-centered care. As a consultant, the author may be considered an expert in these areas. If ideas proposed are rejected, it is easy to become defensive. Many situations of misunderstanding and conflict are predicated on personal feelings of rejection that occur during interpersonal discourse. Most successful relationships are built on positive confirmation, like eye contact, or encouraging words, or clarifying questions that occur during communication and indicate acceptance of the information or feelings being expressed. These basic components of acceptance–rejection, or confirmation or failure to confirm relate to all interpersonal communication situations, regardless of the nature of the relationship. Since communication is a vital aspect of consultation, ideas that enhance acceptance or minimize rejection of recommendations and reduce potential for conflict over ideas may be useful to the consultant. The next section describes the essential components of successful technology consultation that links information through effective communication.

POTENTIAL MARKET

The need for consultation in provision of consumer-responsive technology services is growing rapidly. Several factors are affecting the emergence of new opportunities:

1. Proliferation of electronically-based technology for typical everyday activities that can be adapted as assistive technology for persons with differing abilities.

2. Complexity of available technology, which makes learning and adoption of technology operations challenging for consumers and providers.

3. Need for consumer-responsive and consumer-driven services in area of assistive technology.

4. Legislation, such as the Assistive Technology Act, which funds states to develop assistive technology programs and policies, and the American with Disabilities Act, which sets regulations for assessibility of all environments to all citizens.

Occupational therapy's long tradition of creating and adapting equipment for persons with differing abilities as well as individual therapist's concern for focusing on consumer-identified goals means that occupational therapists are well suited for leading the provision of technology-based services in collaboration with interested consumers. However, uncertainty over the role of electronically-based technology in therapy, growing complexity of equipment choices available, and increased interest in technological applications by the broader community, such as employees, educators, and consumers themselves, create a rapidly growing market for assistive technology consultants. In addition, moving from a service-provider–centered system of service delivery to a consumer-centered model of service requires specific consultation for building collaborative relationships.

KEY POINTS

Necessary Knowledge and Skills

This author's consultation activities occur within various types of interpersonal relationships, for example, between colleagues, within supervisory relationships, between providers of services, such as occupational therapy service, and recipients of services, or their family members. Regardless of the nature of the relationship, interpersonal communication is an integral part of the transaction. Consultation usually results in generation of new ideas or recommendations to change the ways things are done. In consultative relationships, like all interpersonal relationships, communication serves as means to share both information and the meaning information holds for both the sender and receiver of the information. During the consultation process, acceptance of new ideas, recognition of differences in perspective or position, resolution of conflicts, adoption of ideas by a greater number of people, and further development of the consultative relationship are all accomplished through communication.

In consultative relationships, information is offered to solve an obvious problem or to create a plan that solves or prevents a number of problems. In any case, information offered probably represents new ideas or an innovation that may provide an acceptable solution to the recipient. Adoption of a new idea is affected by ways in which information is shared and knowledge of recipient's perspective on the proposed change inherently contained in the information. For example, if a colleague is seeking expert information in order to change service delivery patterns, commitment to change has been made and information dispels some of the uncertainties about how to make the change. If a consumer seeks consultation because an accident or illness has changed his or her abilities to function, the consumer may be more interested in returning to original ways of functioning than in seeking new ways for performing activities. Uncertainty on the part of the consumer over whether old ways of functioning are possible means that a consultant's information needs to be communicated with concern for addressing the consumer's questions and priorities about the future while perhaps introducing new ideas or innovations, such as adaptive equipment, in ways that are acceptable to the client. The key to acceptance of new ideas is communication that includes creating and sharing information in order to reach mutual understanding.[8]

There are some factors that influence acceptance of new ideas. If the person perceives an idea as having a *relative advantage* over the old method, whether financial, social, personally convenient or satisfying, the new idea will be more quickly adopted. Acceptance depends more on a *personal perception of better* than on objective evidence that reports the advantages of the new ideas. A consultant can promote acceptance of recommendations by understanding the other person's perspective, including values and attitudes about present situations, and by presenting new information in ways that address personal rather than global advantage of proposed change.[8]

A factor related to relative advantage is *compatibility*. New ideas that are perceived as being consistent with existing values, past experiences, and current needs by potential recipients are more easily adopted. For example, new ways of functioning that are compatible with the roles people play in an organization or a family are likely to be accepted more quickly than ideas that change fundamental roles. *Complexity* is another factor in acceptance. Complexity describes the degree to which an innovative idea is viewed as difficult to understand or use and is seen to require acquisition of new skills to be successful. Even in our current information age, use of electronic technology, such as computers for performing work and assisting with restoring lost function, may be viewed as too complex and too difficult to learn to be acceptable. If a consultant recognizes the complexity factor associated with a new idea, information conveyed can include plans for learning new technology as well as subjective and specific examples of ways other individuals have managed adoption of complex technology in their practice or everyday lives.[8]

The last two factors in adoption of new ideas are related to experience with proposed innovation. *Trialability* refers to opportunities to try something new on a limited basis. A trial period or implementation part of the times or with part of the operation seems to provide information that reduces uncertainty associated with a final decision with no opportunity to reject ideas that did not work. Again, one's own experience becomes the basis for full adoption of new ideas or technology.

Case Example
Judy T.

When Judy T. came to the Center with her mother, she stated that she wanted to explore possibilities for improving her mobility. Although she was ambulatory with a cane, right hemiplegia caused her to be slow, unsteady, and subject to fatigue. Now that she had entered high school, she was having difficulty changing classes rapidly and safely. She wanted to try a power scooter or power wheelchair, but had also heard about a new one-arm drive wheelchair that might meet her needs as well. After trying all three mobility devices, she decided to try the one-arm drive chair for a month. Since the chair was new to the staff as well, they had little experience with it over time and could not suggest anyone who had used it enough to provide information from personal experience. After the trial period, Judy and her family ordered the one-arm drive chair and intended to use it as her sole chair.

Six months later Judy T. returned for modifications and stated that she was very unhappy with her one-arm drive chair and had reverted to using her old, ill-fitting manual chair most of the time at home. At school, she used the one-arm drive chair, but was usually pushed because the chair was difficult to manipulate in crowded hallways. Her mother found the chair difficult to push or load in the van to transport. What went wrong? A trial period had preceded the final decision. The trial, however, had been inadequate, since it occurred in the summer, mostly outside with lots of space and without much need to transport the chair. Issues like manipulation in crowded places, resistance from carpet inside house and school, frequent loading and unloading, especially in cold, inclement weather, and weight when pushed by another had not been considered. In addition, there had been no opportunity to talk with another user about the pitfalls. Trialability needs to be carefully constructed to simulate all circumstances before final decisions are made.

Finally, *observability,* or the extent to which the results of a new idea are visible to others, influences acceptance. Once others see the results of an innovation, there is discussion of relative merits, and the person who first accepted the new idea becomes a resident expert. More opportunities are created for personal testimony of value, which generally influences other individuals' acceptance more effectively than general objective data supporting success or usefulness of an idea.[8]

Entry into the System

In consultation, as in most interpersonal relationships, a good working relationship is essential for successful outcome. A good relationship recognizes that both the substance or topic under consideration and the relationship with the people involved are important.[3] Attention to both substantive and people issues enhances acceptance and creation of new ideas.

Case Example

Johnny G.

Johnny G. has been receiving speech/language therapy since he was about 18 months old. At 4 years old, he had improved in development of receptive language, but had little expressive language. His speech pathologist recommended an augmentative communication device, but Johnny's parents refused and were viewed by staff as resistive and unrealistic. Staff felt threatened because the recommendation was not accepted. Until this incident, relationships between staff and family had been good, but staff and family became concerned that the relationship would be affected by the conflict. In a parent conference, both parents and staff confirmed their satisfaction with their working relationship and viewed the recent incidents as a difference in opinion rather than a change in the basic relationship. They then addressed their interests rather than their positions on the issue of "communication device–no communication device." Johnny's parents were interested in development of Johnny's ability to use speech for expressive communication, they were concerned that he was too young for a communication device and might "stop trying to speak" and never develop speech. Besides, they always understood what he wanted at home. His speech pathologist was interested in Johnny's development of expressive communication and felt that the communication device would assist development of expressive language and motivate him to verbalize to the extent possible. Parents and speech pathologist shared a common interest in Johnny's development of expressive language but had taken different positions about the means to achieve their interests or goal. Without exploration of interests, they were defending their positions along with their role in the decision as a parent or professional. Continued defensiveness could have led to conflict and negative impact on their relationship, but, once common interests in language development were established, family and staff brainstormed options to meet goals and criteria for selecting options. Ideas came forth like: use a low-tech system first and try to combine with verbalization; use an electronic augmentative system part of the time to work on functional expressive communication or when he is in his preschool where not everyone understands his current communication; etc. In each option, continued work on Johnny's own verbal language was included. Criteria for selecting options were developed and included: must be affordable within current level of reimbursement; must address need for both direct speech/language intervention and introduction of an augmentative system; etc. Family and staff decided together to begin with a low-tech system so Johnny could develop his ability to use symbols and continue direct intervention therapy in conjunction with a low-tech system. A re-evaluation of the potential and the need for a more complex augmentative system would take place at the next family and staff conference.

In any relationship, it is not unusual to discover differences or experience disagreement that may be coming from differences in knowledge or opinion, values or attitudes, or past experiences. Communication is often the means by which differences are discovered as well as the way in which conflict over differences can be resolved.[4] Behind most differences about what to do and how to do it are usually common interests or agreement on goals.[3] Common interests provide the foundation for resolving conflict and often lead to creation of new ideas or ways to proceed that neither individual would have developed alone. Fisher and Ury[2] have developed a strategy that can be used to resolve differences or to begin planning based on common interests before conflict over differences is evident.

Negotiation with Potential Client/Consultee

The first step in the process is to *separate the people from the problem*.[3] Colleagues, consumers, family members are all people first, and then people in roles such as parent, physician, consumer of occupational therapy services, consultant, consultee. Persons involved in a relationship, such as a consultative relationship, are interested in both the topic under consideration and the relationship they have with the person or persons with whom they are working. Relationships and positions or opinions about a subject sometimes get entangled, especially when people involved are acting from different positions. Individuals may have different ideas about how to accomplish a goal or they may sense rejection from the other person's communication style and respond emotionally or defensively. Working with people in any role involves trying to understand as much as possible about their perspectives, values, attitudes, reasons for opinion or emotional response, as well as understanding reasons for one's own perspectives or reactions. Direct communication about perspectives on the problem and the relationship and acting on relationship problems before they escalate often help separate the people from the problem.

Establishment of Trust

The next step in the process is to *focus on interests rather than positions*.[3] Discovering common interests is the key to beginning to work together toward solving a problem or accepting a plan of action.[7] To focus on interests, each person involved needs an opportunity to define the problem and identify his or her own interests, which include concerns, needs, wants, hopes, fears, and values. In a work situation, for example, expression of interests will yield information about whether someone is more interested in flexibility or productivity in their schedule or prefers more job security in his present job rather than more opportunity in a risk-taking venture. In a consumer relationship, expression of interests may reveal whether a person is interested in immediate independence that can be achieved through use of special equipment or eventual independence without special equipment that may be achieved by continuation of the current therapy program. Failure to explore interests or hopes of a consumer but instead promoting use of equipment, because you as the therapist think equipment is the best solution, or setting the schedule, because you are the boss, can lead to resistance and defensiveness. As therapist, you and the consumer are interested in the kind of independence that satisfies the consumer or, as boss and employee, in the kind of schedule or opportunity that motivates your employee. Common interests are the basis for collaborative planning.

Identification and Development of Consultation Strategies

The next step in the process is to focus on *inventing options of mutual gain* and to insist on *objective criteria*.[3] Inventing options follows the rules of brainstorming with everyone involved generating as many options for solving a problem as possible and not passing judgement during development of options. Options can consist of trying the equipment for a month and then deciding, or using the equipment only for long distances, or flexing the schedule on lower volume days, etc. When all ideas have been expressed, criteria are established for selecting the possible solutions. Criteria might include such requirements that schedules must be productive for the individual and the department or equipment must be in a reimbursement category. After matching options to criteria and eliminating some, the remaining options are eligible for final selection. Because options were developed by working together, it is not difficullt to agree on final selection. Usually, the person closest to implementing the final selection is in the best position to choose.

Implementation

Adoption of assistive technology is facilitated by a consultation process that considers both the relationship between interpersonal communication and the consultee's self-esteem and the factors that influence diffusion of innovative solutions to problems. In order to succeed, the consultant attends to the information being shared and the meaning associated with the information by clarifying relationship issues and content issues whenever they arise. The consultant also attends thoroughly to the factors of relative advantage, compatibility, complexity, trialability, and observability on a continuous basis. The situation involving the one-arm drive wheelchair would appear to have included the factors related to adoption, but, indeed, the trial period was insufficient, and the family was not advised to test the chair under all conditions before deciding to purchase. The consultant not only identifies possibilities for learning, observing, or trying but also makes sure that the learning or experience is appropriate to the decisions or selections that need to be made by the consultee.

In many instances, assistive technology services are provided by team consultation. All the concepts about communication apply to teams as well as individual providers. In fact, strategies for separating the people from the problem and establishing common interests become even more important when expertise and relationships of team members are also factors in decision making. Larson and LaFasto[6] have identified characteristics of successful teams. Some of the characteristics are particularly relevant to assistive technology teams and are known as the four "Cs". Teams with a *clear and elevating goal* for providing consumer-centered services have experienced more successful outcomes. A clear goal might be to provide the most effective and efficient consumer-responsive driven assistive technology services in a community. Consultants are often asked to work with teams to identify their goal. Time spent clarifying and developing commitment to the goal provides the foundation for team communication. Teams with *competent* members whose areas of competency are well known to other members and consumers have more successfully established team roles and reduced uncertainty over who does what during a team assessment. *Commitment* to excellence in service and satisfaction with team process means the team can focus on consumer concerns rather than team process concerns. The result is increased consumer responsiveness and improved collaborative decision-making. Finally, a *collaborative* climate among team members establishes a culture of joint decision-making with respect for all team member contributions. Working together collaboratively as a team carries over to working collaboratively with consumers of assistive technology services as members, and in some situations, leaders of their own team. Consultation on team building by focusing on team communication, collaboration with each other and with consumers, and resolution of differences by establishing mutual interests strengthens both technology delivery and interpersonal competence.

Evaluation

Evaluation of the individual or team process and the recommendations emanating from consultation can be accomplished by measures of satisfaction in both the process and the outcome. Is the consultee satisfied with quality of life? Has function or independence improved through use of technology? Does technology operate efficiently and effectively? Does outcome match goals for lifestyle? Did the consultation process empower the person by providing opportunities for collaboration and choice? Ultimately, only the consumer's actions and words provide valid evaluation. A wheelchair with no signs of wear, a communication device used on special occasions, a computer that isolates rather than promotes inclusion are signs that the consultation process did not succeed in promoting adoption of technology. A person fully included in family life, work, school, and play, with the technological adaptations transparent and person and abilities obvious, represents successful adoption of technology.

Potential for Future Involvement

Available technology continues to change rapidly. As an individual's abilities with technology increase, there will be more possibilities for adding technology-supported functions to the person's repertoire. Opportunities exist to build on technology skills of both consumers and providers of services by periodic re-evaluation of status and continual development of expertise as a consultant in a rapidly changing environment.

CONCLUSION

Communication serves to link people together in relationships, including consultative relationships. Communication provides opportunities to share information and meaning associated with information. Recognizing that people invest themselves in the ideas and feelings they share provides insight into importance of verbal and non-verbal communication in promoting acceptance of new ideas and resolution of differences. In both acceptance and resolution, such basic concepts as developing ideas together, communicating clearly to reduce uncertainty and complexity, relating new ideas to familiar ways of working or functioning, and creating opportunities for observation and trial can strengthen a consultative relationship. The advent of more complex and effective assistive technology for persons with differing abilities has increased the need for consultants who can facilitate adoption of technology by both producers and consumers of technology services. Consultants' ability to apply basic principles of communication and of diffusion of innovation are particularly relevant for promoting adoption of advanced assistive technology.

REFERENCES

1. Dance F, Larson C: *The Function of Human Communication*. New York, Holt, Rinehart and Winston, 1976.
2. Fisher R, Ury W: *Getting to Yes*. Boston, Houghton Mifflin, 1981.
3. Fisher R, Brown S: *Getting Together:* Boston, Houghton Mifflin, 1988.
4. Folger J, Poole M: *Working Through Conflict*. Dallas, Scott, Foresman and Company, 1984.
5. Grady A: Adapting computer technology: A challenge for occupational therapy, in *Technology Review '90*. Rockville, American Occupational Therapy Association, 1990.
6. Larson C, La Fasto F: *Team Work*. Newbury Park, Sage Publications, 1989.
7. Murphy J: *Managing Hope*. Houston, Healthcare Rehabilitation Center, 1989.
8. Rogers E: *Diffusion of Innovations*. New York, The Free Press, 1983.
9. Vanderheiden G: Service delivery mechanism in rehabilitation technology. *Am J Occup Ther* 1987; 41:703–710.

PART III

The Potential for Occupational Therapy Consultation

The interactive and diverse nature of consultation creates unique and challenging situations. The knowledgeable consultant recognizes that as an informed consumer, she must utilize key resources and concepts to support her decision making.

Kornblau, addressing legal issues, and Hansen, discussing ethical considerations, alert us to many issues confronting consultants. Closely intertwined, legal and ethical concerns arise when we consider aspects of contract negotiation, service delivery, employment, regulatory issues, and expected competency in the performance of a consultant role, to name just a few.

In today's litigious society, the consultant must make sure that her consultation business relationships are established in a forthright and legally acceptable manner and her business behaviors meet established professional codes. The consultant, Kornblau advises, would be well served to obtain legal counsel when starting a business and developing contracts.

She points out many regulatory subtleties that can impact the consultant's critical decision-making process. Starting a business requires familiarity with innumerable laws and regulations. The wrong decision can make the difference between a business's success or failure. An attorney who is knowledgeable in business matters and aware of liability issues should be a resource for the consultant.

Ethical parameters affecting the consultant and consultation process include the issues of professional competency, compliance with laws and regulations, truthfulness, and appropriate behavior. Hansen discusses the importance of ethical conduct and presents ethical dilemmas that could arise in the course of consultation.

The occupational therapist's code of ethics (see Appendix C) includes reference to the consultant's role. As a resource and guideline for conduct, it helps shape the consultant's thinking. It does not, as Hansen points out, provide resolution for a specific ethical dilemma. In this chapter, you are challenged to consider several consultation dilemmas, weigh possible solutions and their consequences, and then choose the action that would be most appropriate.

Potential and practicing consultants should utilize the information presented in these chapters. The authors combine expertise in their specialized field along with an understanding of the consultation process, thus providing a comprehensive and informative picture of the legal and ethical issues in consultation.

SECTION A

Legal and Ethical Issues in Occupational Therapy Consultation

CHAPTER 38

Legal Issues in Occupational Therapy Consultation

Barbara L. Kornblau, J.D., O.T.R., C.I.R.S.

OVERVIEW

Suppose the risk manager of a major airline, Wings, contacted you, an occupational therapist, to help him solve a problem. You recently treated a Wings reservations clerk for carpal tunnel syndrome. Your visit to her job site showed you that the computer keyboards forced the reservations clerks to work with their wrists positioned in static hyperextension.

The job site report you prepared found its way onto the risk manager's desk. It seems that Wings Airlines spends an overwhelming majority of its workers' compensation claims on carpal tunnel syndrome injuries. Your report focused on the cause of the problem. The risk manager wants you to provide consultation services to Wings Airlines to develop some strategies to help the company cut down on the incidence of carpal tunnel syndrome among its employees.

This hypothetical situation raises many legal questions for the occupational therapy consultant. How should the agreement between Wings Airlines and you, the consultant, be structured? Should you present the airlines with a written contract? What if problems develop over your performance and the airline sues you?

If the job is too big and you need to hire other therapists to help, can they be independent contractors? How should you structure the contracts with the other therapists?

Do you need an attorney? Is it possible that as a result of your consultation you might be asked to testify in court about the airline's efforts pursuant to the reasonable accommodations provision of the Americans With Disabilities Act (ADA)?[26]

Will you increase your exposure to malpractice by taking on this project? Are you liable if the airline fails to follow your advice and its employees continue to get carpal tunnel syndrome? Should you keep your communications with the airline confidential?

594

The author attempts to answer some of these questions and to steer the occupational therapy consultant along the path to competent legal assistance. This chapter familiarizes the occupational therapy consultant with some of the legal issues affecting occupational therapy consultation practice. The author does not intend that this chapter substitute for competent legal counsel. In fact, the author encourages readers to contact an attorney with any questions that they may have about the issues presented.

This chapter is not intended to advise occupational therapists about legal issues concerning occupational therapy direct patient care. Rather, the author addresses issues raised specifically by the various models of consultation.

For the purpose of this chapter, the author assumes that the consultant advises the consultee about programs but does not implement them. The author further assumes that the occupational therapy consultant makes recommendations to the consultee and the consultee is free to decide to accept them and follow the recommendations or reject the recommendations.

Since the consultant does not provide direct patient care services, the author has omitted certain topics that sometimes arise as a result of direct patient care such as the intentional torts and assault and battery.

LAW AND ETHICS

As already mentioned, this chapter discusses legal issues affecting occupational therapy consultation. Following this review of legal implications is a discussion of ethical considerations for the occupational therapy consultant. However, the subject of legal issues is not complete without some mention of the relationships between legal and ethical conduct.

In addition to the legal considerations that govern the professional conduct of the occupational therapist, the occupational therapy code of ethics also guides the conduct of the occupational therapy consultant.[2] Professional ethical standards tend to cover areas of practice that are deemed undesirable or unacceptable by the profession although they are not expressly prohibited by law.

There are situations, however, where the courts will look at the ethical standards of a profession. In the absence of any clear legal authority governing the conduct of an occupational therapy consultant, the courts may need to find a standard of care to govern the occupational therapy consultant's conduct. The courts may look to the standard of care of a similarly situated professional or the court may look to the profession's self-imposed standards to determine potential liability.[13]

While no court has yet interpreted the occupational therapy code of ethics as a basis for determining the conduct of an occupational therapy consultant, the possibility remains for its future use by a court of law. Courts have already interpreted ethical guidelines and standards of care belonging to the medical, legal, and accounting professions. It is likely that the courts would do the same with the occupational therapy code of ethics and standards of practice, should the situation arise. Thus the occupational therapy consultant would be protecting herself from potential legal liability by following the code of ethics and standards of practice promulgated by the American Occupational Therapy Association.

THE ATTORNEY'S ROLE WITH THE OCCUPATIONAL THERAPY CONSULTANT

Consultation practice involves weaving through and around a web of regulatory and legal red tape. The occupational therapy consultant is not expected to go through this legal maze unassisted. Numerous questions arise regarding various statutes, regulations, and rules that affect the occupational therapy consultant from both a day-to-day business aspect and a practice issue aspect.

As the occupational therapy consultant faces this plethora of questions and decisions, the attorney enters the picture. A good business attorney plays the part of tour guide from development of an idea through the reality of its purpose, from start to finish.

Developing a consultation practice in occupational therapy forces the consultant to decide exactly how to structure her practice legally. The law classifies business entities into three forms—the sole proprietorship, the partnership, and the corporation. In choosing the entity, the consultant must consider whether someone else will share in the ownership of the practice. The consultant must consider which entity will require payment of the least amount of taxes. The consultant may also want to look at which form is the simplest and least expensive to establish and maintain.

On a practical level, the attorney addresses the basic consultation practice needs. The attorney answers the consultant's questions regarding choice of entity. He helps the consultant decide whether the practice should be designed in the form of a sole practice, partnership, or corporation. The attorney drafts and files any documents that may be necessary to start the consultation practice, such as articles of incorporation and partnership agreements. He assures that the consultant procures the necessary licenses, insurance coverages, and permits. He assists the occupational therapy consultant in formally obtaining a name for her practice.

Before the occupational therapy consultant meets with an attorney, she should make a list of her questions and concerns. At the first meeting, the consultant should feel free to ask the attorney questions about his experience with similar consulting and health care related businesses.

Fee arrangements should be discussed openly. Attorneys usually charge for their services by time. They usually divide an hour into ten segments and charge a minimum of 1/10 of an hour for every task. Attorneys may require a retainer or a lump sum amount of money up front from which they will deduct their fees as they expend the time. Some attorneys may charge a set fee for preparation of a specific document, such as a contract. Others may charge a set fee for setting up a corporation. An attorney may charge a specific amount for a specific task, such as reviewing a lease. Remember that most attorneys charge for photocopies and for time spent on the telephone and reviewing letters.

Contracts and the Occupational Therapy Consultant

Since an occupational therapy consultant is in the business of selling her advice to various facilities, programs, and agencies, the attorney advises the consultant about her entry into the consultation system and her relationships with clients. The occupational therapy consultant faces complex dealings with employees, contracting agencies, and facilities. Working with potential employees and contracting agencies or facilities forces the therapist to acquire a basic working knowledge of contracts and the elements usually found in an occupational therapy consultation contract.

Laypeople often attach a sort of mystical connotation to the term *contract*. One conjures up notions of a lengthy formal document, written on parchment, in advanced legalese, perhaps with some fancy calligraphy. In reality, a contract is merely an agreement between two or more parties, in which each party to the agreement agrees to do something or refrain from doing something in exchange for the other party's agreeing to do something or refrain from doing something.[3]

The requirement to agree to do something or refrain from doing something is called *consideration*.[3] This is an essential element of the contract—no consideration, no contract. Examples of consideration include salary paid to an employee in exchange for work performed, or payment made in exchange for consultation services.

A contract may be oral or written. For example, in certain situations a consultant may form a contract by verbally agreeing to do something and shaking hands on it. A simple verbal contract is formed when two playmates agree, "You give me your bubble gum and I'll give you my comic book."

Oral contracts are often suspect, since they are not all-inclusive in their terms. In some cases they are not enforceable because they may violate certain laws and legal principles. The author does not recommend oral agreements for occupational therapy consultation contracts.

Two parties may form a written contract by merely writing a letter to someone summarizing a meeting during which the parties discussed how they planned to proceed with or complete a project. A contract can be an agreement written on the back of a napkin in a restaurant. Anytime someone says, "Sign here," there is a good chance that the document in question is a contract.

The occupational therapy consultant should follow the famous rule: "Get it in writing." All agreements made between the parties should be in writing and all agreements should be expressed in the body of the contract. Should the contract end up as the basis of a lawsuit, most courts will not allow a party to present evidence that explains the terms of the contract.[8] Therefore, the language used should be as simple and unambiguous as possible.

Contract law provides that courts interpret ambiguous terms *against* the party who drafted them.[8, 10] The courts will give the words in a contract ordinary meaning unless the words are defined otherwise in the contract. The same word will be assigned the same meaning throughout the contract. When the courts attempt to determine the meaning of words, they will look at the custom in the industry. The parties' past relationship and performance will also be looked at if the court must define the contract's terms.[8, 10]

The occupational therapy consultant's contract with the consultee should include specific information about the services the consultant is to perform under the contract and the time frame during which the services will be performed. The contract should include the amount of compensation that will be paid for the services and when and how it will be paid, that is, daily, weekly, or monthly. The consultant may want to consider a late fee for payments made in excess of a specified time period or a discount for early payment. The contract should address the manner in which the parties may terminate the contract. The parties will probably want to address the issue of confidentiality, especially if the parties will be sharing confidential information with each other. Table 38–1 summarizes key points the consultant should consider when developing a contract.

The parties may want to consider a clause providing for mediation and/or arbitration should a dispute result under the contract. Litigation is very expensive and should be avoided wherever possible. Besides the expense, it probably will not look good for an occupational therapy consultant to sue a client. For example, the negative publicity from suing a small town hospital would probably discourage other potential consultees from purchasing the consultant's services. Mediation and/or arbitration save the consultant money and keep her out of the court's system.

During contract negotiations with potential consultees, the consultant should keep in mind any special regulations that may affect the area of consultation. Certain regulations may dictate that specific clauses be included in the contract. For example, certain government programs may require contractors to express that they comply with Civil Rights Acts of 1964 Title VI and do not discriminate in their hiring practices. Contracts involving Medicare consultation may require a

TABLE 38–1
Key Points to Consider in Developing Consultation Contracts

1. Services to be performed
2. Time period within which the consultant must perform the services
3. Amount of compensation for services
4. When and how compensation will be paid
5. How the parties may terminate the contract
6. Confidentiality of information
7. Mediation/arbitration
8. Compliance with federal statutes

clause agreeing to comply with the Section 952 of the Omnibus Budget Reconciliation Act of 1980 that requires the therapist to maintain patient accounting records for 4 years under certain circumstances and allows access to those records to the Secretary of Health and Human Services as well as the Comptroller of the United States.[29]

This discussion is limited to some basics of contract principles. The author highly recommends engaging the services of an experienced business attorney to draft the occupational therapy consultant's contracts. The attorney assists the occupational therapy consultant in developing contracts keeping in mind the law and her interests and practice needs or the interests of her employing hospital, agency, or other facility.

Negotiating contracts is a complicated process. How do you know if and when you need an attorney? There are several rules of thumb.
Consult an attorney if the following apply:

- You have never negotiated a contract before;
- The consultee has an attorney;
- The consultee prepares the contract;
- The contract holds particular importance to your practice;
- The contract addresses liability issues.

First, if the consultant is a novice at contractual matters and negotiating for the first time, she should consult an attorney. Second, if there is an attorney negotiating on the other side, the occupational therapy consultant should engage an attorney as soon as possible. It is difficult for a layperson to match wits with a lawyer.

Third, if the consultee has a contract prepared or hands you a standard contract, have an attorney review it before you sign it. One of the author's biggest problems as an attorney is cleaning up the mess after someone has already signed a contract. It is much easier to perform preventive measures than after the fact, especially when it comes to contracts.

Fourth, the occupational therapy consultant should seek an attorney's advice if a contract holds a particular significance or importance to her practice. The contract may hold this importance because of the amount of money it represents to the practice or to the department or perhaps it will lead to more business in the future from the same consultee or a long-term commitment. Sometimes a consultant may find herself hiring an attorney or contacting her hospital's attorney to participate in contract negotiations for a contract of minor significance to the overall practice simply because the situation is likely to repeat itself with other potential consultees. In this scenario, the attorney will draft a form contract that can be used for subsequent similar situations.

For example, suppose an occupational therapist who works in a hospital develops a program consulting to business and industry. The consultant recommends ergonomic adaptations to the workplace so businesses may comply with the reasonable accommodations requirements of the Americans With Disabilities Act. If the hospital's attorney drafts a standard form contract, the occupational therapy consultant probably will be able to use the same contract as she acquires other business clients.

Some consultants use a standard contract as a basis from which to work and make appropriate changes to fit the particular circumstances. While this may work some of the time, the occupational therapy consultant should have all changes in the standard form contracts reviewed by an attorney before she signs them.

A consultant may come across a situation where the consultee presents a standard contract insisting that the consultant sign it as is, claiming the contract cannot be negotiated because it is standard, or boilerplate. Under the law, all terms of a contract are negotiable. However, in reality, if you are a single consultant negotiating with a major company, your relative bargaining power or the company's policy may eliminate the possibility of negotiating contract terms. A judgment will have to be made on a contract-by-contract basis whether to accept the term or attempt to negotiate.[18] The consultant will probably want to contact her attorney before she signs on the dotted line if the standard terms are disproportionately not in her favor, ambiguous, or simply foreign to her.

Finally, an attorney should be consulted where contractual agreements address liability issues. Liability issues involve deciding who will bear the risks under the contract. The attorney can advise you about shifting the risk and minimizing the risk to you and your practice or your department.

Sometimes a consultant may rent space from a consultee as part of the contract arrangements. For example, if an occupational therapy consultant contracts with a nursing home to evaluate all of the residents for the home's activity program and to monitor compliance with the restraint reform regulations, the contract may include leasing office space on the grounds.

Leases come under the umbrella of contracts and as such should also be reviewed by an attorney before the consultant signs on the dotted line. Commercial leases for office space are complicated documents, the terms of which rarely resemble plain English. Interpreting commercial leases is an art that should be performed in consultation with an attorney. With the help of an attorney, commercial leases may be negotiated, especially in a financially troubled renter's market.

The occupational therapy consultant will want to confer with an attorney regarding collections matters if she has difficulty collecting her fee from a consultee.[13] The attorney can help the consultant set up a system for collecting fees, send a demand letter, or take further action. The attorney can help the consultant write her own system of demand letters so that she can do most of the legwork before proceeding to litigation.

Employment Contracts

The attorney also plays a big role in drafting and negotiating employment contracts. The relationship between employers and employees is based on a contract. A contract means that an agreement exists between the parties governing the relationship. Unless a law or regulation dictates otherwise, the parties determine the rate of pay, hours worked, job responsibilities, and other terms.

The body of law developed by judicial decisions in a particular state, called the common law, also affects the contractual relationship. For example, certain principles may have developed through the common law that create an employment contract. For example, some state courts such as Nevada, Maryland, and Michigan have held that the contents of an employee handbook imply a contract.[41–43, 45] This means that in these states the courts will look at the employee handbook as terms of a contract. Other state courts have not agreed with this assertion.[40]

Since contracts govern the employment relationship, the parties must decide if a written contract between them is necessary to clarify the relationship. In an occupational therapy consultation practice, the author advises the use of written contracts to protect the practice, the department, or the business.

For example, suppose that an occupational therapy consultant wishes to hire a therapist to consult to a countywide school system. If the position requires the employer to give the employee access to valuable consultee information such as billing rates and other confidential information, the employer will want some guarantee that the employee will not leave her position taking valuable information with her. A written contract can cover such a situation with a noncompetition clause. For example, the clause may prohibit the employee from soliciting the employer's clients and include a trade secrets provision protecting confidential business information such as billing rates.

The written contract also protects the employee. It spells out the employee's rights and responsibilities, so that the employee knows exactly what her employer expects from her.

A written contract generally covers such basic points as the position the employee holds, duties, pay, benefits, and termination of employment. Other clauses will apply, depending on the practice or department and the parties needs. It is a good idea to have an attorney draw up a standard employment contract for you, which can then be modified for individual circumstances that arise through negotiations with potential employees. Individual items in the employment contract, such as the amount of salary, vacation, and other benefits, may be changed based on agreements made with the individual employee. A written contract should protect both parties from misunderstandings.

The attorney plays a significant role in drafting contracts for independent contractor services. Here again, occupational therapy consultants often use standard form, or boilerplate independent contractor contracts that their attorneys draft and then are adapted to the specific circumstances.

Beware of the independent contractor's contracts. Contract negotiations with prospective employees should not include negotiating to designate someone an independent contractor, unless the person is in fact an independent contractor. The independent contractor is actually a private practitioner. This chapter discusses at length the differences between an employee and an independent contractor according to the standards used by the Internal Revenue Service and those developed by common law. The occupational therapy consultant must be aware of the dangers of erroneously classifying an employee as an independent contractor. A misclassification of an employee as an independent contractor can cost the consultant/ employer in taxes, 41.5% of the misclassified worker's compensation.[4]

The occupational therapy consultant should establish an ongoing relationship with the attorney so that dialogue may continue as practice needs change. If a consultant begins her practice out of the guest room in her home, new questions and problems will arise as she expands her practice, hiring employees, procuring independent contractors, acquiring office space, and perhaps eventually branching out into other cities or states. At the same time, the experienced consultant with an established practice will always find that questions arise as new clients are procured and new projects develop. With growth and change come more legal questions and the need for more advice from the business attorney.

Laws and Regulations Affecting Consultation

The occupational therapy consultant will want to consult with an attorney to familiarize herself with new laws and regulations that may affect her practice from a practical standpoint or from a practice standpoint. For example, the occupational therapy consultant may need to find out specifics of the new Americans With Disabilities Act to decide what her responsibilities are regarding employing a disabled person or to advise a client about setting up a program to make reasonable accommodations for newly hired disabled employees.

A therapist who consults to nursing homes may need additional information about the new Omnibus Budget Reconciliation Act of 1987 (OBRA) regulations so that she can advise the facilities how best to comply with its requirements.[28] Not all attorneys are qualified to answer questions about these technical health-related issues. The consultant will want to seek advice about these matters from an attorney who specializes in health care law.

Familiarity with a variety of other legal specialty areas will be necessary, depending on the area of the consultation practice. For example, an occupational therapy consultant may want to confer with a labor lawyer if her practice involves consultation regarding the development of job trial or work therapy programs. The author has seen numerous programs that give the injured worker or rehabilitation patient a job trial in a hospital or rehabilitation center. Under the Federal Fair Labor Standards Act, these "workers" must be paid minimum wage if they are providing the institution with an economic benefit.[27] Many of these, albeit well-intentioned programs, do not pay the workers for the work they do, thus violating this federal law. An occupational therapist who consults in this area should seek the advice of a labor lawyer so that she does not suggest programs that might break the law.

An occupational therapy consultant who advises facilities about developing work hardening programs will want to stay on top of any changes in the workers' compensation laws. This consultant will probably want to retain the services of an attorney who specializes in workers' compensation should the state pass a new workers' compensation law or institute new regulations.

An occupational therapy consultant who wishes to offer consulting services under the new Americans With Disabilities Act of 1990 (ADA) may want to consult with a labor lawyer to learn about the specifics of the new act's provisions concerning employment of disabled individuals. The ADA has the potential for considerable business for occupational therapy consultants.[9] Employers will be forced to rewrite all of their job descriptions so they are very specific in describing the essential function of the job in physical terms. The occupational therapy consultant is well qualified to help employers comply with this act.

Under the ADA, employers will hire occupational therapy consultants to help them develop reasonable accommodations to enable the disabled employee to perform a job.[15] Some employers may look to the occupational therapy consultant to develop work capacity evaluations for certain classes of employees.

These examples illustrate the importance of staying on top of new laws, changing regulations, and trends affecting health care. New laws or changes in old laws can expand or eliminate an area of your consultation practice. For example, when the Diagnostic Related Groups (DRG) system became a reality in hospitals, occupational therapy consultants advised occupational therapy departments how to expand into DRG exempt programs. The departments that were prepared for DRGs expanded into numerous new program areas and felt little effect from the change. Many private insurance companies have followed Medicare's lead by also linking the diagnosis with the number of covered days of care. Thus changing laws and regulations affect trends in health care and have a significant effect on the occupational therapy consultant. See Chapter 1 for a more detailed discussion on the affect of changing trends in health care.

Locating an Attorney

One of the best ways to find an attorney is often by word of mouth. Perhaps you know a colleague who has had a good experience with an attorney who is knowledgeable about a particular specialty area.

As an alternative way to locate attorneys in the various specialty areas, the occupational therapy consultant may want to inquire whether the state bar provides a designation or certification for attorneys in specialty areas. If the bar provides the certification, then you will know that the attorney has met minimum competency requirements in the specialty area. For example, Florida provides certification for attorneys in workers' compensation and provides designation for attorneys in corporation and business law.

The National Health Lawyers Association is a good resource for locating attorneys who specialize in health law.[19] Other organizations are available for other legal specialty areas as labor, workers' compensation, and business attorneys.

Facing Litigation

The occupational therapy consultant will want to engage the services of an attorney in the event that she is sued by someone or if she finds it necessary to sue someone else. There are several situations in which the occupational therapy consultant may find herself facing litigation. Malpractice is a possible cause of action that might be filed against the occupational therapy consultant. If the consultant is sued for malpractice, she should immediately call her malpractice insurance carrier. The malpractice insurance carrier will provide an attorney to defend against the malpractice action. Malpractice is discussed in detail later in this chapter.

The occupational therapy consultant may become involved in an action for breach of contract. A breach occurs when one of the parties to a contract does not keep up its end of the bargain. The consultant might be sued, for example, if she fails to complete a particular project on time. On the other hand, a consultant might sue a consultee for breach of contract if the consultee failed to pay her. Another breach of contract action can arise if there is a dispute in the consultant's lease arrangements—either a lease for equipment or for office space.

There also may be situations where the occupational therapy consultant may be sued for a variety of civil actions, such as breach of confidentiality, invasion of privacy, defamation, and assault and battery. However, since the occupational therapy consultant usually does not provide direct patient care services, some of these civil actions are not very likely.

LIABILITY, MALPRACTICE, AND DOCUMENTATION

As an advice giver, the occupational therapy consultant holds herself out to the client as an expert in her field. The consultee relies on the consultant for accurate, up-to-date, complete, and appropriate information. Failure to provide the proper information to the consultee, in the proper manner, may render the occupational therapy consultant liable for malpractice. Since the consultant makes suggestions about programs but does not implement them, she can open herself up for malpractice by exercising poor judgment if she gives advice about something of which she lacks adequate knowledge.

Malpractice is a negligent tort perpetrated by a professional occupational therapist that causes damages.[3] In the case of an occupational therapy consultant, the damage could be to a patient in a case consultation situation where the occupational therapy consultant advised a consultee to do something that caused damages to a patient. The damage may be to a consultee, where the consultant's incorrect advice caused the client to lose accreditation.

Malpractice may occur in several other contexts. For example, if a consultee follows the consultant's advice and during the process harms someone, the consultant may be liable for malpractice. An occupational therapy consultant may find herself liable for malpractice if she fails to stay on top of the latest changes in laws and regulations and provides a consultee with incorrect information, resulting in some harm.

In other situations, liability for malpractice may arise because the consultant omitted some relevant information. For example, suppose an occupational therapy consultant is hired to assist a facility in obtaining Commission on Accreditation of Rehabilitation Facilities (CARF) accreditation. The consultant fails to inform the facility about the requirements for program evaluation. As a result, the facility fails to obtain CARF accreditation and loses its ability to bill third-party payors.

The consultant may find herself facing malpractice litigation where harm resulted to the consultee because the consultant failed to ask the consultee the right questions. In another scenario, the occupational therapy consultant may take on the consultee's liability where harm resulted to a third party by the consultant's failure to ask the right questions. For example, if an occupational therapist who consulted to private industry about ergonomic adaptations to the workplace failed to ask appropriate questions about the specific operations of a particular piece of equipment, she could take on the liability if an employee was injured operating the machine with the adaptation she suggested in place.

In plain English, malpractice is negligent performance by a professional. A malpractice action may be brought against any professional, including health care professionals, lawyers, and accountants.

To sustain a case of liability for malpractice, the plaintiff must prove four elements:[21]

- A duty to act
- Conduct below the standard of care
- Damages
- Actual cause

TABLE 38–2
Limiting Liability for Malpractice

---

1. Keep current on laws, regulations, and practice techniques.
2. Spell out specific details of consultation task in writing.
3. Carry malpractice insurance.
4. Keep appropriate business records.
5. Refer to other professionals where appropriate.
6. Provide proper supervision.
7. Document all recommendations to consultees.

First, there must be a relationship between the parties that created a duty to act in a particular way.[7] Second, the plaintiff must prove that the occupational therapy consultant's conduct fell below the professionally reasonable standard of care, thereby breaching that duty to act in a particular way. Third, there must be proof that the plaintiff suffered real damages. Finally, the plaintiff must prove that the occupational therapy consultant's breach of duty was the actual cause of the damages suffered.[5, 7, 21, 23, 24]

A Duty to Act in a Particular Way

The occupational therapy consultant owes a duty to those with whom she establishes a relationship. Thus the occupational therapy consultant owes a duty of care to the consultee and probably any reasonably foreseeable patient and/or client that will be treated following the consultant's advice.[21] This will also include the patient about whom the consultant provides case consultation. The duty owed applies to acts of omission and acts of commission. This means that the occupational therapy consultant can be liable for damages caused by things she did as well as things she failed to do.[5]

The occupational therapy consultant's duty compels her to exercise the reasonable care and skills expected of an occupational therapy consultant. The courts will inquire as to whether a reasonably prudent occupational therapy consultant would have acted in a similar manner, given the same set of circumstances.[5, 14]

Most consultees hire a consultant because they need some advice in an area in which they have no knowledge or expertise. These clients rely on the consultant's expertise when they hire her. They consider the consultant an expert as opposed to an average occupational therapist.

Since the occupational therapy consultant holds herself out as an expert, the consultant must understand the limits of her expertise and know when to refer the buyer of her services to someone else with greater knowledge and skills. The occupational therapy consultant should be aware of her credentials and her limitations.[14] A particular consultation situation may demand someone with more specialized or just different credentials. For example, in the industrial consultation previously cited, it may have been appropriate for the occupational therapy consultant to have referred to the company to an engineer or an ergonomist if the adaptations were too technical for her.

In another example, where a facility contracts with an occupational therapy consultant to advise the facility about becoming a certified rehabilitation agency under Medicare, it would be prudent for the occupational therapy consultant to refer the facility to an accountant who specialized in health care to learn more about the cost reporting requirements. Failure to refer a consultee who requires more expertise than the consultant possesses could constitute malpractice. The consultant should make sure that the professional to whom she refers the consultee is competent and has appropriate credentials.[14] If despite her efforts she is sued by the client, her defense will be strengthened by the fact that she referred her client to another competent professional.

If the consultant holds herself out as an expert in a particular area, the consultant must meet the standard of an expert in that area. The courts will look at the standard of care or the level of proficiency against which the consultant's conduct will be measured. Since there is little legal precedence in defining the standard of care that the occupational therapy consultant must follow, the courts will look to the standards of practice of similar professions, the American Occupational Therapy Association standards of practice, and the American Occupational Therapy Association code of ethics.[2, 5, 14]

Breach of Duty

The second element of malpractice, breach of duty, occurs when the occupational therapy consultant's conduct falls below the applicable standard of care. Expert witness testimony will help form the basis of proof at trial for the standard of care. The expert witness, another occupational therapy consultant, will testify as to her opinion of the standard the consultant's conduct should have measured up to.

Under the doctrine of *respondeat superior,* the occupational therapy consultant may be liable for actions of her subordinates. This is a Latin term meaning "let the master answer."[3, 5] Since the employer is in the best position to supervise and direct acts of his employee within the scope of his employment, the law imputes liability to the employer under this doctrine. Since it is based on the right of control, the doctrine of *respondeat superior* does not apply to independent contractors.[5, 24]

The occupational therapy consulant may find herself liable for the actions of her subordinates under another theory. She may find herself liable for negligent supervision if, for example, she assigns others to perform consultative services that they are not qualified to perform and she fails to supervise them properly.[14, 23]

Damages

The third element required to sustain an action for malpractice is damages or actual harm.[21] The harm caused by the occupational therapy consultant may include, for example, physical harm to a patient/client, financial harm to a consultee, loss of accreditation, or failure to acquire accreditation. Even if the occupational therapy consultant acts in a clearly incompetent manner, there is no basis for a malpractice action unless actual harm can be proven.[5]

On the other hand, if the occupational therapy consultant acts in a reasonable manner and makes appropriate recommendations, but the patient's condition in a case consultation situation does not improve, the harm alone does not constitute malpractice.

For example, perhaps as a consultant you are called in on a case consultation to advise an occupational therapy department on treatment methods for reflex sympathetic dystrophy. You recommend a standard course of treatment including weight bearing and air splinting. The patient fails to respond to the standard treatment that you recommended and develops a frozen shoulder. Just because the patient responded unfavorably to the universally acceptable treatment, it does not constitute malpractice. The occupational therapy consultant acted within the acceptable standard of care expected in a similar situation.

Causation

The fourth element required to sustain a cause of action for malpractice is causation. The plaintiff must show that the occupational therapy consultant's negligent conduct was responsible for the plaintiff's injury. The standard is the "but for" test. That is, but for the occupational therapy consultant's negligence, the plaintiff's injury would not have occurred.

Preventing Malpractice

The ultimate goal for any consultant is to prevent malpractice from ever occurring. The occupational therapy consultant can take several steps to limit her liability for malpractice (see Table 38–2).

First, the consulant should always follow the American Occupational Therapy Association code of ethics, standards of practice, and the appropriate American Occupational Therapy Association roles and functions position papers. You must stay up to date regarding state and local laws and regulations that affect practice so that your advice will be current. Spell out in detail the specific task about which you have contracted to consult. The specifics should be spelled out in writing, either by contract or by letter, so that the parties are clear about the tasks to be performed.

As preventive maintenance the occupational therapy consultant should attend continuing professional education to keep current on practice techniques in the field and attend professional meetings regularly. Read professional journals to stay abreast with the latest research. To protect yourself in case a lawsuit is filed, carry malpractice insurance. You should also maintain appropriate business records.

Be aware of the need to refer a consultee to another professional. Understand the limitations of your credentials. Select competent personnel with due care and carefully define their responsibilities. Do not delegate consultation tasks to unqualified individuals. If you do delegate tasks to another occupational therapy consultant, make sure you provide the therapist with appropriate supervision if necessary. At the very least, monitor the subordinate consultant therapist's performance. Be sure to provide the subordinate therapist with enough information and enough authority so that she may perform the assigned task.

Documentation

Good documentation is the fundamental tool that the occupational therapy consultant has at her disposal to prevent malpractice. The occupational therapy consultant should maintain files on all of her consultees and case consultations. She should take notes at all meetings with consultees and write memos to the file detailing the meeting's subject, questions asked, and the suggestions offered. The occupational therapy consultant also should send a copy of the memo or a separate memo to the consultee summarizing the meeting so that both parties have the same understanding of the advice given by the consultant.

Where involved in case consultation, the occupational therapy consultant should make specific notes about the patient and/or client. The notes should include findings and recommendations. The consultant should send her findings and recommendations to the consultee as well as keeping records for her file. This will protect the consultant from liability, should injury occur to the patient if the consultee elects not to follow the consultant's advice for treatment or program management.

Telephone calls should be logged and recorded in the consultee file with a brief explanation of the subject matter, questions asked, and suggestions offered. If a problem arises, the consultant should document the steps she takes to solve it. If the consultant performs research to solve a problem, she should detail her methods and sources in a memo to the file. Always leave a paper trail that can be retraced and revisited in the future if needed to help prove that you acted within an acceptable standard of care for an occupational therapy consultant.

In all situations, the occupational therapy consultant should document termination of services. At the time of termination, the consultant should summarize the reason for the termination, the recommendations made, and to whom they were made.

CONFIDENTIALITY

Remember that this volume is about occupational therapy consultation, not direct patient treatment. This section addresses confidentiality issues for the occupational therapy consultant, not direct patient treatment confidentiality issues.

Confidentiality raises several issues for the occupational therapy consultant. Initially, the consultant confronts this issue at the contract negotiations stage. Since the consultee must share certain confidential information with the consultant, the consultee will want assurances in the contract that the information disclosed to the consultant will be confidential.

For example, suppose that a consultant is called in to assist Good Care Hospital in setting up a head trauma program. No doubt Good Care Hospital has already put together statistics, projections, and budget figures that it will have to share with the occupational therapy consultant. Obviously, Good Care Hospital does not want to share this information with a neighboring, competing facility. It will want the contract to reflect the desired confidentiality.

This element of confidentiality is also important from the occupational therapy consultant's perspective. The occupational therapy consultant will want to stress to her consultees that she keeps everything confidential to enable the consultees to share vital information more easily. Confidentiality falls under the necessary prerequisites to establish trust within the consultation relationship. See Chapter 6 for a discussion about establishment of trust with the consultee. For example, an internal consultant consulting from one department to another in a hospital will be able to accomplish her project more effectively if the staff know they may trust her to keep all communication confidential and not report them to the supervisor or to the administration. As a consultant, your policy should be to treat every communication with the consultee as confidential.

If the consultant participates in case consultation, she must be aware that professional licensing and other state laws, Medicare/Medicaid and other federal laws,[30] Joint Commission on Accreditation of Health Care Organizations, (JCAHO),[16] Commission on Accreditation of Rehabilitation Facilities (CARF),[6] and the occupational therapy code of ethics require occupational therapy consultants to keep patient information confidential. Some courts may allow recovery for damages for failure to maintain the confidentiality of patient records under various theories, including constitutional right to privacy, breach of an implied contract with the patient, breach of the duty of confidentiality, and defamation through written or oral communications.[5, 7, 14, 18, 23, 24]

There are several exceptions to the confidentiality requirements. Most states now have child abuse reporting laws that require health professionals, teachers, and others to report suspected child abuse.[11, 14, 23, 44] If an occupational therapy consultant is retained to do case consultation in a facility for severely retarded children and she has reason to believe that one of the children is being abused, despite confidentiality of patient records she is required by law to report it. Usually this report is made by telephone to a central registry.

The occupational therapy consultant is under no duty to keep information about illegal activities confidential.[2, 14, 23] For example, if a facility/consultee tells the consultant about a referral scheme that violates Medicare's fraud and abuse provisions, the consultant has no duty to keep that confidential. In fact, the consultant should consult an attorney to be sure that she protects herself from accusations of participating as a conspirator in the scheme, since she advised the facility about Medicare and she had knowledge of the illegal plan.

An occupational therapy consultant can disclose confidential information with the consent of the patient/client. It is good practice to get the consent in writing.

In certain circumstances, the consultant may be compelled to disclose otherwise confidential information without the patient's consent. For example, the patient usually waives confidentiality by filing a workers' compensation claim or filing a lawsuit. The duty to maintain patient confidentiality ends when the consultant receives a subpoena to testify in court. Under subpoena, the occupational therapy consultant must answer questions about information that the consultant would otherwise consider confidential.

During the discovery process prior to trial, the parties to these claims have the right to obtain medical records. If the consultant performed case consultation, chances are that her records will be subpoenaed. If the consultant is served with a subpoena *duces tecum*, then the consultant must provide copies of her records.

FRAUD AND ABUSE

Health care practitioners who work with Medicare and/or Medicaid will find themselves amid the complex regulatory requirements that accompany these federal programs.[30] An occupational therapy consultant who deals with Medicare and/or Medicaid must understand some basics of the fraud and abuse provisions. Many states have similar fraud and abuse provisions in their laws. Unfamiliarity with these provisions could leave the occupational therapy consultant open to civil and criminal charges resulting in termination of provider agreements, payment of restitution, severe fines, and a maximum of 5 years in federal prison.[31-34]

The Medicare-Medicaid Laws specify prohibited acts (see Table 38–3). Under these federal programs, one is prohibited from submitting false claims for payment, making false statements in a request for payment, illegal remuneration including kickbacks in return for goods or services paid for in whole or in part by Medicare/Medicaid, and solicitation, receipt, or an offer or payment to another person for the referral of an individual to a person of any item or service for in whole or in part by Medicare/Medicaid.[35-38]

Since this volume concerns occupational therapy consultation and not direct patient care services, the fraud and abuse provisions concerning claims for payment should not affect the consultant. The consultant should have limited contact with direct care services that would result in Medicare/Medicaid billing. Hertfelder

TABLE 38–3
Prohibited Acts Under Medicare and Medicaid

1. Making false claims for payment
2. Making false statements for payment
3. Paying kickbacks for goods or services
4. Soliciting, making an offer for payment, or accepting payment for patient referrals

and Crispen provide a discussion about Medicare's fraud and abuse provisions and billing practices.[13]

The occupational therapy consultant who provides case consultation will want to be aware of the remaining provisions concerning illegal remuneration including kickbacks in return for referrals for goods or services from other practitioners. For example, an occupational therapy consultant provides case consultation for a nursing home to determine the need for adaptive equipment. She recently heard a rumor from a reliable source that the ABC Durable Medical Equipment Company would give referring therapists 20% of the purchase price as a commission for any referral made. She will probably violate the fraud and abuse provisions of Medicare if she tells the patient to purchase the equipment from this company.

Similarly, a nursing home consultant performing needs assessments for a feeding program refers patients to her partner, a speech therapist, for a dysphagia work-up. She will probably find herself violating the fraud and abuse provisions of Medicare, since the partnership agreement provides that the occupational therapy consultant gets one third of the fees for all patients that she brings into the partnership.

Subcontractor vs. Employee

The author has repeatedly encountered occupational therapists who erroneously refer to themselves as independent contractors. The average occupational therapist possesses the notion that merely because one is self-employed, employed part time, or paid on an hourly basis, she is an independent contractor. To dispel this myth, one must understand the nature of the employment relationship and the basics of law surrounding this relationship.

The occupational therapy consultant plays a role in the employment relationship as either employer, employee, independent contractor consultant, or self-employed consultant. A self-employed consultant can also be considered an independent contractor if she provides services to a facility or corporation, for example. Her relationship to the consultee facility or corporation is as an independent contractor.

Federal, state, and local laws impose various rights, obligations, and duties on employers and employees. Whether or not a particular federal law affects an employer usually depends on the number of employees he or she has or various other factors, such as whether the employer receives federal assistance. For example, a business is subject to the Fair Labor Standards Act[27] if the business employs two or more employees.

State and local laws affecting employers and employees depend on the location of one's practice, and, therefore, will vary from place to place. For example, if an occupational therapist opens a consulting practice in Florida, state law requires that all of the occupational therapists she employs be licensed.[12] However, an occupational therapy consultant seeking to hire other therapists in a nonlicensure state will not be affected at all by licensure unless or until the law changes.

It is impossible for the author to address all of the laws governing employers, since they vary so much from place to place. This discussion presents some basic information, but employers and employees will have to seek additional information from an attorney, the Senior Core of Business Executives (SCORE), or Small Business Administration workshops in order to cover all the bases.

As previously discussed, the relationship between an employer and his employees is based on a contract. The terms *employer* and *employee* come from the former terminology "master and servant." Master and servant indicates that a relationship exists where one person who employs another has control over the manner in which the work is performed. The employer is the master over the work of the servant, the employee.[10]

In plain English, an employer can tell the employee precisely how he or she wants the job done. The employer can tell the employee what time to report to work, how to perform the job, when to perform the job, and to what standards. An employer also may terminate the employee if he or she fails to perform as ordered.

An occupational therapy consultant may be an employee of either a facility, such as a hospital or school system, or a private practice. For example, a school system may employ an occupational therapy consultant to train teacher aides in the proper feeding of severely handicapped children. A hospital may employ a consultant who performs functional capacity assessments and makes recommendations to prospective employers. A consultant may be employed by a private practice to teach and train new staff members or advise contracting facilities about restraint reform strategies under the new Omnibus Budget Reconciliation Act of 1987 (OBRA) regulations. This text has other examples of employees who function as consultants (see Chapters 7 through 15).

Not all persons providing consultation services will be employees. One can structure a relationship with a therapist providing consultation services so that she may be considered an independent contractor. The independent contractor is based on a contractual relationship with another person or entity to perform a task. However, the person engaging the services of the independent contractor does not control the person or his or her performance and is only interested in the results. The difference between the employer/employee relationship and the independent contractor relationship is the right of control over the work.[1, 10] Remember that the occupational therapy independent contractor is herself a private practitioner.

The mere existence of a written contract agreeing to be an independent contractor and not to take withholding taxes does not an independent contractor make, a common myth. The author has been involved with home health agencies that hire therapists to provide direct occupational therapy home health care. The agencies call these therapists independent contractors merely because the therapists sign a contract and agree to accept payment on a per treatment basis, without any payroll taxes withheld or social security taxes or workers' compensation insurance paid by the agency. These home health agencies and nursing services are coming under very strict scrutiny from the Internal Revenue Services (IRS).[4]

The author often has heard occupational therapists say, "She's just an independent contractor" referring to someone who is, in fact, a part-time employee. One does not become an independent contractor by agreement between the prospective employer and a potential therapist-for-hire. One does not become an independent contractor by designation by the employer. While it may sound like a simple way to avoid the administrative headaches of paying payroll benefits, and social security taxes, calling someone who is really an employee an independent contractor is a dangerous game with painful consequences.

For example, suppose a private occupational therapy consultant, ABC Consultants, sends a contract occupational therapy consultant to teach a class about the use of adaptive feeding devices to the staff at a nursing home. On her way to the facility, her car is hit by a drunk driver, causing serious physical injuries. If workers' compensation declares that she is an employee for workers' compensation purposes, the state may look to the ABC Consultant's pocketbook to pay for the care and other expenses, if, they determine, years down the road, that ABC was responsible for providing workers' compensation insurance. Depending on ABC's location, the state may fine ABC for not having the proper workers' compensation insurance coverage.

In addition to all the problems ABC faces with its state workers' compensation system, ABC will also incur the wrath of the IRS, a most unpleasant experience. The IRS will come after ABC for back payroll taxes, withholdings, and social security. They will audit the records of all of ABC's other so-called independent contractors for their back payroll taxes, withholdings, and social security.

In order to avoid these headaches, the employer must be certain before she contracts with a therapist that the therapist is in fact an independent contractor. Both the IRS and the common law have developed tests for making this determination. The tests involve a set of factors that evaluate whether a person is an independent contractor.

The common law test, which is developed from decisions of previous cases, would be used by the courts if a question arose about workers' compensation coverage in the nursing home consultation/car accident example just cited. The court's goal in the common law test is to determine whether the employer has the legal right to control both the method and result of the services.

To answer this question, the common law has developed a test that includes ten factors (see Table 38–4). The courts will look at each factor and apply the facts of the particular case to the individual factors. Let us examine those factors as the court would, using the nursing home consultant as an example:

1. *The extent of control the "employer" may exercise over the details of the work under the agreement.* The court will look at the contents of the contract between the ABC consultants and the occupational therapy consultant ABC sent to teach the class. The court will be looking for evidence of control, such as the necessity to work set hours, work at specific places, follow the general policies of the employer, or ability to be terminated at will by the employer.

2. *Whether or not the employee is engaged in a distinct occupation.* The courts will probably agree that occupational therapy is a distinct occupation.

TABLE 38–4
Common Law Test for Independent Contractor Classification[1,4,39]

1. The extent of control the "employer" may exercise over the details of the work under the agreement
2. Whether or not the employee is engaged in a distinct occupation
3. The kind of occupation and whether the work is usually performed under the supervision of the employer or by a specialist without supervision
4. The skill required in the particular occupation
5. Whether the employer supplies the tools and the place of work for the worker
6. The length of time the person is employed
7. Whether payment was by time or by the job
8. Whether the work is part of the regular business of the employer
9. Whether or not the parties believe they are creating an employment relationship
10. Whether or not the principal is or is not in business

3. *The kind of occupation and whether the work is usually performed under the supervision of the employer or by a specialist without supervision.* The contract occupational therapy consultant who teaches a class to the staff in a nursing home probably does not need supervision. If, however, she does require supervision, the courts will look at this as further evidence of the employer's control over the employee.

4. *The skill required in the particular occupation.* Occupational therapy consultation requires specific training and skill.

5. *Whether the employer supplies the tools and the place of work for the worker.* In the example we are discussing, the court will look at whether the employer supplied the contracting consultant with the handouts, charts, and sample eating devices for the in-service. If ABC consultants gave the "contract" consultant an office to work in to prepare for the in-services, the court will look at that as further evidence of control, the key element to prove an employer/employee relationship. However, the fact that the services are performed off the premises of ABC consultants may be evidence that the consultant is an independent contractor.

6. *The length of time the person is employed.* The courts will look at whether the therapy consultant is employed for a specific period of time, by the job, or until terminated by the employer. If the contract therapist's commitment is for a limited period of time, this will support ABC's position that the consultant is merely an independent contractor.

7. *Whether payment was by time or by the job.* The courts will look at whether the contracting consultant is paid by the hour, the week, by the consultation assignment, or the job. In other words, is the employer paying the contracting therapist for teaching classes at the nursing home or for 3 hours of work, 5 days per week?

If the consultant were paid for teaching classes, this would support the position that the consultant is an independent contractor. Payment for teaching classes is payment by the job. If the consultant were paid for working 3 hours, 5 days per week to teach classes, this would tend to show that the contracting consultant was a part-time employee, since she is paid by the hour not the job.

8. *Whether the work is part of the regular business of the employer.* The court will examine whether providing consultative services is part of ABC Consultants' regular business. If it is, then this will tip the scale toward an employer/employee relationship. However, an argument could be made to tip the scales back toward the independent contractor relationship if, for example, ABC Consultants limits its consultation services to pediatrics and contracted with this therapist to provide geriatric consulting, which ABC normally does not do.

9. *Whether or not the parties believe they are creating an employment relationship.* The court will look at whether or not ABC signed a contract with the occupational therapy consultant and what kind of relationship the parties intended.

10. *Whether or not the principal is or is not in business.* In our example, the court will see that ABC Consultants is in business.[1, 39]

The IRS guidelines conduct a similar inquiry to determine whether or not a worker is an employee or an independent contractor. The IRS looks at whether the person or persons for whom the services are performed exercise sufficient control over the individual for the individual to be classified as an employee.[22] This inquiry involves 20 factors set forth by the IRS[25] (see Table 38–5).

There are several precautions that the occupational therapy consultant can take to protect her independent contractors from being deemed employees. These obviously are not definitive methods of protection but may prove helpful. Once again, the author suggests consulting an attorney for additional information concerning this matter. First, workers should perform services pursuant to written contracts for a stipulated period of time, not terminable at will. The terms of the contract must be followed.

Second, the contract should not mention anything indicating that control over performance has been retained by the person for whom services are being performed. For example, it would be contrary to an independent contractor arrangement to state that the independent contractor must follow all policies of the employer.

Further, do not put the words *employment contract* across the top of the contract. The author has seen this done on a number of occasions, especially in

TABLE 38–5
IRS Factors for Independent Contractor Classification[4,13,22,25]

1. Compliance with instructions
2. Training provided in order to perform job in a particular manner
3. Integration of services into business operations
4. Services personally rendered
5. Hiring, supervising, and paying assistants
6. Continuing relationship between worker and the person services are provided for
7. Set work hours
8. Full-time hours required
9. Work performed on employer's premises
10. Services performed in a set order of sequence
11. Required oral or written reports
12. Payment by the hour, week, or job
13. Reimbursement for business or travel expenses
14. Furnish tools and materials
15. Significant investment in the facilities used to perform services
16. Realization of profit or loss
17. Working for more than one firm at a time
18. Making services available to the general public
19. Right to discharge for reasons other than nonperformance to contract specifications
20. Right to terminate relationship without incurring liability for failure to complete job

contracts with home health agencies. As a general rule, never use the words *employee* or *employer* in a contract with an independent contractor. Always refer to the independent contractor in the contract as the *independent contractor* or the *consultant*. If you are in a position to contract with an independent contractor, resist the temptation to refer to yourself as the employer. Rather, in the contract with the independent contractor, use the term *company, corporation,* or the name of your company instead of *employer*.

The contractor must also provide that the worker may reject jobs offers without penalty. The worker must also retain the right, under the terms of the contract, to select other employment opportunities.[4]

Consulting to Attorneys

The occupational therapy consultant should find growing opportunities for consultation with attorneys. The occupational therapy consultant fills many roles in the medicolegal arena.[17] With current trends in health care, the occupational therapist will find herself filling the role of expert witness in cases dealing with the Americans With Disabilities Act (ADA), Omnibus Budget Reconciliation Act of 1987 (OBRA), and workers' compensation.

Black's Law Dictionary defines "expert witness" as "One who by reason of education or specialized experience possesses superior knowledge respecting a subject about which persons having no particular training are incapable of forming an accurate opinion or deducing correct conclusions." In order to present her opinion at a deposition or at trial, the occupational therapy consultant must qualify as an expert witness.[13a] Qualifying as an expert witness requires the occupational therapy consultant to present her credentials under oath. The consultant will be qualified by the court as an expert witness in cases where she has expertise. For example, occupational therapy consultants would be appropriate experts to testify about the reasonable accommodations provisions under the Americans With Disabilities Act or alternative to restraints under the Omnibus Budget Reconciliation Act of 1987 regulations.

Occupational therapists often ask the author, "How do you make contact with attorneys?" First, start with your own attorney. Does his or her type of practice lend itself to your areas of consultation expertise? Ask if he or she can introduce you to some colleagues in the same or in different areas of practice.

Take advantage of attorneys you may have had contact with in the past in relation to former patients/clients. Your consultees' attorneys might be interested in your consultation services. A contract often can be made through a former patient if the patient was involved in a workers' compensation claim or personal injury case while you treated him or her.

Often local service or professional organizations such as Rotary or Kiwanis allow you to meet an attorney in a quasi social context. This contact may give you a foot in the door and lead you to making contacts with other attorneys. Try making follow-up phone calls to the attorney's office at 5:05 or just after the attorney's secretary leaves for the day. Many attorneys answer their own phones at this time. Arrange a personal meeting with the attorney as a follow-up to letters or phone calls.

One problem the occupational therapy consultant will encounter in trying to develop a consultation practice with attorneys is that most attorneys do not know what occupational therapists do. The occupational therapy consultant will need to launch an education campaign as part of her marketing plan. Attorneys need to be sold specifically on how the occupational therapy consultant can assist their clients.

When approaching attorneys, dress and act professionally. At your initial meeting, the attorney will be looking to see what kind of a witness you will make and how a jury might perceive you. You must impart a feeling of self-confidence.

Before you meet with an attorney, find out about the practice. Does the attorney practice workers' compensation, labor, or personal injury? During your initial meeting, give the attorney some specific case examples about the kind of information you can provide and how you can add to his or her cases. Do not overwhelm the attorney with handouts and brochures.

If you develop a relationship with an attorney and begin to get referrals from the attorney, always ask him or her what kind of documentation is expected. Sometimes attorneys do not want written records of the services that you perform for them. Always ask the attorney what records or documents he or she wants you to bring with you should one of the parties want to take your deposition.

Sometimes your role as a consultant will not involve courtroom testimony but rather work performed behind the scenes. The occupational therapy consultant is probably one of the best health professionals to review and decipher medical records for the attorney and translate the information into functional problems that may be included in demand letters.[17] Another role the occupational therapy consultation plays behind the scenes deals with life care planning and determining future equipment needs for the catastrophically injured.[17]

SUMMARY

The practice of occupational therapy consultation is a complicated process that presents many legal issues. The occupational therapy consultant should secure competent legal assistance in such situations as developing a consultation practice, negotiating contracts, and protecting oneself from liability. The complexities of contract construction, independent contractor status, and the fraud and abuse provisions of various Medicare and Medicaid regulations all may require legal advice.

Changing laws, regulations, and trends in health care challenge the consultant to keep abreast of the latest legal issues. The attorney and the occupational therapy consultant can jointly face these and other issues that may arise in practice.

The occupational therapy consultant is an expert in her clients' eyes. As an expert, the consultant owes certain duties to her clients. Since clients rely on the consultant's expertise, the consultant must be sure to give accurate advice that falls within her area of expertise. She must know the limits of her credentials and expertise so that she may advise clients to act in the proper manner, both legally and ethically.

REFERENCES

1. 1 Restatement of Law, Agency (2nd ed.) § 220 (2).
2. American Occupational Therapy Association: Occupational therapy code of ethics. *Am J Occup Ther* 1988; 12:795.
3. *Black's law dictionary,* ed 5. St Paul, Minn, West, 1979.
4. Broad and Cassel: Re: Employee vs. Independent Contractor Status, (Memo) Miami Office, Feb 5, 1991.
5. Calloway S: *Nursing and the Law.* Eau Clare, Wisc, Professional Education Systems, 1985.

6. Commission on Accreditation of Rehabilitation Facilities: *Standards Manual for Organizations Serving People With Disabilities*. Tucson, Ariz, Commission on Accreditation of Rehabilitation Facilities, 1988.

7. Christofeffel T: *Health and the Law*. New York: Free Press, 1982.

8. Corbin on Contracts §573 et. seq. St Paul, Minn, West, 1963.

9. Earith K: ADA: A good match for OT. *Advance Occup Ther* 1991; 7:34.

10. Fla. Jur. Forms §20:2. Rochester, NY, Lawyers Cooperative, 1987.

11. Fla. Stat. §415.504.

12. Fla. Stat. §436.201 et. seq.

13. Hertfelder SD, Crispen C: *Private Practice Strategies for Success*. Rockville, Md, AOTA, 1990.

13a. Hertfelder SD, Gwin C: *Work in Progress: Occupational Therapy in Work Programs*. Rockville, Md, AOTA, 1989.

14. Hopkins R, Anderson, S: *The Counselor and the Law*. Alexandria, Va, American Association for Counseling and Development, 1990.

15. Hyde, KE: Employment discrimination under the Americans With Disabilities Act. *Florida Bar Journal* 1990; 64:47.

16. Joint Commission on Accreditation of Health Care Organizations: *Accreditation Manual for Hospitals 1988*. Chicago, Author, 1988.

17. Kornblau, BL: The role of the occupational therapist in the medicolegal arena. *Work Programs SIS Newsletter* 1988; 2:1.

18. MacDonald MG, Meyer KC, Essig B: *Health Care Law: A Practical Guide*. New York, Mathew Bender and Associates, 1985.

19. National Health Lawyers Association: 1620 Eye Street, NW, Suite 900, Washington, DC 20006, (202) 833-4784.

20. O'Leary H, Imperato G: Defending a health care provider in a criminal fraud investigation. *Florida Bar Journal* 1991; 65:90.

21. Prosser WL: *Law of Torts*. St Paul, Minn, West, 1971.

22. Rev. Rul. 87-41, CB 1987-1, 296.

23. Stromberg CD, et al: *The Psychologist's Legal Handbook*. Washington, DC, Council for the National Register of Health Service Providers in Psychology, 1988.

24. Warren DG: *Problems in Hospital Law*. Germantown, Md, Aspen, 1978.

25. Weinstein M: *Mertens: The Law of Federal Income Taxation,* Vol 13. Deerfield, Ill, Callaghan, 1991.

26. Americans With Disabilities Act PL 101-336, July 26, 1990.

27. Federal Fair Labor Standards Act, 20 USC §201 et. seq. (1978 and Supp. 1987).

28. Omnibus Budget Reconciliation Act of 1987, PL 100-203, 101 Stat. 1330 (OBRA).

29. Omnibus Budget Reconciliation Act of 1980, 42 U.S.C. § 1395x(v)(1)(I) (1982).

30. Social Security Act, 42 U.S.C. § 1395 *et. seq.*

31. 2 U.S.C. 1395cc(a)(3).

32. 18 U.S.C. §1031.

33. 31 U.S.C. §3729.

34. 42 U.S.C. 1395(b)(2).

35. 42 U.S.C. 1395nn (a–d).

36. 42 U.S.C. 1395(b)(1)(A), (b)(2)(A).

37. 42 U.S.C. 1395(b)(1)(B), (b)(2)(B).

38. 42 U.S.C. 1396h.

39. *Canter v. Cochran,* 184 So, 2d 173 (Fla. 1966).

40. *Muller v. Stromberg Carlson Corporation,* 427 So. 2d 266 (Fla. 2d DCA 1983).
41. *Pine River State Bank v. Mettille,* 333 N.W. 2d 622 (Minn. 1983).
42. *Southwest Gas Corporation v. Ahmad,* 668 P.2d 261 (Nev. 1980).
43. *Staggs v. Blue Cross of Maryland,* 486 A.2d 798 (Md. App. 1985).
44. *State ex rel. D.M. v. Hoester,* 681 S.W. 2d 449 (Mo. 1984), 44 A.L.R. 4th 643.
45. *Toussaint v. Blue Cross and Blue Shield of Michigan,* 408 Mich. 579 (1980).

CHAPTER 39

Ethical Considerations for the Consultant

Ruth A. Hansen, Ph.D., O.T.R., F.A.O.T.A.

An occupational therapist with several years of practice experience in school systems was hired by the director of an intermediate school district to evaluate the occupational therapy services provided within that system. Specifically, the therapist/consultant was asked to assist in developing guidelines to evaluate the occupational therapy staff and their service delivery model. The director indicated that this was a routine evaluation and was not initiated because of any specific concerns or problems.

On the first visit to the school, the consultant discovered that the occupational therapy staff were angry about the consultation and suspicious of the director's motives. The consultant interviewed all the staff, reviewed all records, and spent time observing therapy sessions.

After collecting these data, she spoke with the director indicating she felt that a redistribution of staff was warranted. She also mentioned that she was aware the occupational therapists in the system disagreed with her. Prior to submitting her final written report she was told that the director had cut one staff line and severely cut back on the occupational therapy services for students with neurological impairment. In pondering these unexpected consequences, the consultant identified several ethical concerns:

1. How does one assure that there are no hidden agendas? What should a consultant do when it is apparent that there are hidden agendas or disparate motives behind the request of consultation?

2. What, if any, obligation does the consultant have to the staff?

3. How should differences of opinion related to recommendations be dealt with? Is it the consultant's responsibility to clarify her position with the staff?

4. Will the final report be shared with all the staff? If not, she fears that her report will be used to justify future administrative decisions even if they are not in harmony with the actual recommendations she made.

5. How can the consultant be sure that the students who need services receive them? What, if any, responsibility does she have to them?

In other chapters in this text, techniques and procedures are described that would have alleviated some portion of the problems/conflicts described in this case. Nonetheless, even an experienced consultant can be faced with perplexing, and sometimes serious, ethical concerns.

It is apparent in this scenario that in consultation, just as in other professional roles, it is important to consider ethical dimensions. This chapter is divided into four major sections: an overview of ethical theory and terminology, a discussion of professional codes of ethics, a systematic inspection of some of the potential issues/conflicts that can occur when consulting, and the presentation of a systematic method of analysis for resolving ethical dilemmas.

OVERVIEW OF ETHICAL THEORIES

To read and understand a discussion of ethics requires some knowledge of philosophical theory and basic terminology.

A few of the more commonly used terms are as follows:

Dilemma. Situation in which one moral conviction or right action conflicts with another. It exists because there is no one clear-cut right answer.
Autonomy. Right of an individual to self-determination. Also, right of a profession to control its own practice.
Paternalism. Action taken by one person in the best interests of another without their consent.

Strong	Exercised against the competent wishes of another.
Weak	Action taken that is presumed to be according to the wishes of the person; usually done because of the individual's age or mental status.

Beneficence. Doing good for others or bringing about good for them. The duty to confer benefits on others.
Nonmaleficence. Not harming or causing harm to be done to oneself or others. The duty to ensure that no harm is done.
Rights. Specific legal, moral, and/or social claims we possess that require others to act in specific ways toward us. With all rights is the implied obligation or duty on the part of the other person (privacy, confidentiality).

Justice. Act of distributing goods and burdens among members of society.

Distributive.	Comparative treatment or allocation of benefits and burdens to groups or individuals.
Compensatory.	Making reparation for wrongs that have been done.
Procedural.	Assuring the processes are organized in a fair manner.

Beyond familiarity with terms, it is essential to understand various theoretical perspectives that are the foundation of ethical deliberations.

One of the reasons that ethical conflicts occur is because of value differences between the concerned individuals. Philosophers study the underlying rationale that individuals use when determining a right course of action. Glenn Graber[3] has organized the philosophical theories into two major groups—teleologic and deontologic. Table 39–1 illustrates some of the critical differences between these two perspectives.

In the case at the beginning of the chapter, the consultant could have weighed right action from either view. Depending on the weight or value given to various parameters of the situation, the resolution could be similar or very different. Regardless of outcome, the deontologist would consider the duties involved and deliberate what the primary duty would be, whereas the teleologist would weigh the possible consequences of various actions and aim for a resolution that provided the greatest benefit for the largest number of people (greatest good for the greatest number).

PROFESSIONAL CODES

When examining the ethical aspects of consultation, another obvious resource or reference is professional codes of ethics. A code is written as a public declaration of the values and "right" behavior for members of a profession, because society permits various professions extraordinary privileges. Examples of these privileges

TABLE 39–1
Theories of Moral Obligation

	Determine Right Action	Goal	How to Resolve Conflict
Teleology	By the consequences of the act	To do good and avoid harm	Produce the greatest good for the greatest number
Deontology	By identifying what one's duty is.	To respect others	Weigh all duties and select the primary one.

are access to confidential information and permission to touch and manipulate another person's body. Professionals are also in positions of influence, with power to make decisions and recommendations that will affect others.

The code of ethics of the American Occupational Therapy Association[1] was written to cover the multiple roles that therapists play, including that of a consultant. Major themes evident in the stated principles are autonomy, beneficence, maintaining and accurately representing one's level of competence, compliance with laws and regulations, truthfulness, and appropriate behavior with professional colleagues.

The codes of different professional groups vary and emphasize the unique aspect of a particular discipline or role. For example, the code of ethics of the American Psychological Association includes statements concerning methods of soliciting potential clients, providing services by mail, phone, or by means other than a professional relationship, how to determine rates for professional services, and such things as providing test security. It is interesting that the code of ethics of the American Association for Counseling and Development includes a specific section on consultation and admonishes the counselor to remain issue focused, to have a clear understanding/agreement about the goals of the consultation, and to limit the scope of the contact to the consultation to the specific agreement.

Professional codes are standards of ethical conduct and are usually written in general and, sometimes, abstract language. Although they are useful resources to determine general guidelines of conduct, they do not provide resolution for specific ethical dilemmas. The analysis system presented later in this chapter should prove helpful in reaching a comfortable and defensible resolution to ethical quandaries.

POTENTIAL ISSUES AND CONFLICTS IN CONSULTATION

Keeping the terminology, philosophical perspectives, and professional codes in mind, it is now time to consider some of the more frequently encountered ethical dilemmas or issues in consultation.

First of all, it is useful to examine the multiple forces and various interests involved in the context of a particular consultation. To whom does the consultant owe ultimate allegiance, the individual or facility who requested the service, one's professional colleagues, the persons who receive treatment or care in the facility, or oneself? It becomes evident that conflicts arise because different individuals and/or groups have priorities and goals that are not complementary to one another.

In order to approach this topic systematically, you may find the following set of questions helpful. They can be used to examine the concerns and values (vested interests) of all the individuals and groups who are affected by the process both prior to, during, and after the consultation.

1. The consultant
   • Does the consultant possess the requisite knowledge, skills, and attitudes to do a competent job?

- Does the consultant have any vested interests in the outcomes/recommendations of the consultation?
- Does taking on this role create conflicts with other roles the occupational therapist has assumed?
- Is the consultant aware of her own biases, which may influence the recommendations?

2. Employer (individual or agency paying for the consult)
- Is the purpose of the consultation clear?
- Are the goals of the consultation consistent with the values/beliefs of the consultant?
- How does the employer intend to use the consultant's recommendations?

3. Professional and technical staff
- How will the staff be affected by the consultant's report?
- How can needed changes be promoted with the least amount of upheaval?
- Which personnel are likely to be most in concert or in disagreement with the recommendations?
- What do the professional and technical staff perceive as the reason for the consultation?
- Will the staff have the opportunity to provide input during the consultation process? Will they be able to give feedback on the recommendations?

4. Consumers of occupational therapy services
- How might the patients/clients be affected by this consult?
- Will their best interests be served?
- How can their best interests be served?

5. Community and society
- Does this consultation have the potential to improve or distort the existing systems of distributive, compensatory, or procedural justice?

SYSTEM OF ANALYSIS

A systematic method of analysis to resolve ethical dilemmas is helpful. The method described in Table 39–2 was developed by Kyler-Hutchison and Hansen[4] and is based in part on the work of Aroskar.[2] It consist of another series of focused questions that are answered in order to weigh possible solutions and their consequences. The result is a resolution that can be explained clearly to others.

In order to understand how this system works, the following consultation dilemma will be analyzed step by step.

A consultant was asked to help restructure the activities program in a 120-bed nursing facility where a new program director with no prior experience in this type of work was hired. The program had been inconsistent and had been staffed by temporary employees for the preceding 6 months.

TABLE 39–2
System of Ethical Analysis

1. Who are the "players" in the dilemma?
2. What other facts/information do you need?
3. What are the actions that might be taken?
4. What are the consequences (ethical, medical, and/or legal) of each action?
5. Choose an action or combination of actions that you would recommend and defend it.
   Is it legal?
   Is it balanced? Fair to all concerned?
   Does it set up a win-win situation if possible?
   How does the decision make you feel about yourself?

Two years ago a certified occupational therapy assistant (COTA) was hired as the activity director. Gradually she began to provide more and more treatment to the point that she is now working full time, has a very large caseload, and no time to help guide or supervise the new activities director.

The consultant was asked to spend 2 half days a week working with the new director over a 3-month period.

In the first month, the consultant learned that the COTA took this position right after passing the national certification exam. At no time in the past 2 years did she have the benefit of close OTR supervision. In fact, the OTR supervisor meets with her only once a month. The OTR has spent the majority of the time during these monthly meetings signing the COTA's notes and evaluation reports. The OTRs felt that since the residents are elderly, all that was required was an activities of daily living (ADL) program, and the COTA was qualified to perform these evaluations.

1. *Who are the "players" in this situation?* The primary players are the nursing home administrator, the consultant, the COTA, and OTR supervisor, the new activities director, and the nursing home residents. A secondary group would include the rest of the nursing home staff, the residents' families/significant others, and agency or company paying for services. At a tertiary level are the state regulatory board, if there is one, the state and national occupational therapy organizations, and the national certification board.

2. *What other facts/information do you need?* Has the OTR supervisor ever considered providing direct supervision to the COTA to assure that she has the competency to perform the evaluation and treatment tasks for which she is now responsible? Has the COTA asked for closer supervision to assure competency? What are the state regulations regarding COTA supervision? What are the standards of the professional association regarding practice roles and supervision? Is the nursing home administrator aware of this situation?

3. *What actions might be taken by the consultant?*

    a. The consultant could ignore the situation because the stated purpose of this consult is to assist the activity director.

    b. The consultant could talk with the nursing home administrator to determine whether there is concern/support for including the COTA competency and supervision issue as part of the consultation contract.

    c. The consultant could speak with the OTR and develop a plan to provide the necessary supervision for the COTA that the OTR can present to the administrator.

    d. The consultant could speak with the COTA to determine if she feels a need for closer supervision. If she does, the consultant could help her develop a plan to obtain the supervision, preferably with financial support from the facility.

    e. The consultant could report the lack of supervision to the state regulatory board if there is one, to the national professional organization, or the national certification board.

4. *What are the consequences of these actions?*

    Action a. This is obviously a low profile approach. The consultant stays focused on the assigned task and ignores the COTA issue. Of course, if the COTA is not competent to be doing the evaluations and treatments then the best interests of the residents will continue to be ignored and payments will continue to be made for inadequate service.

    Action b. In this situation, the consultant takes the risk of upsetting the administrator. Of course, there is the chance that the administrator was unaware of the questionable practices and is willing to pay for the necessary supervision.

    Action c. Again, the consultant takes a risk. The OTR may feel the situation is none of the consultant's business and that the OTR's professional judgment and integrity are being questioned or challenged, particularly if the limiting of treatment to ADL is discussed. On the other hand, the OTR may welcome an ally in presenting a request for more supervisory time with the COTA.

    Action d. The response of the COTA is also unknown. She may feel she is being forced to take on tasks for which she has not been adequately trained. But she could just as easily feel that she is well qualified to carry on the evaluations and treatment procedures she is currently performing. If the consultant could and would observe the COTA's performance, the question of her competence could be determined.

    Action e. This is a fairly radical action and probably would be a last resort if all other strategies failed.

5. *Choose an action and defend it.*

This analysis does not include all possible actions and views of this situation. But it is a starting point for you to think about how you would try to resolve this dilemma. You can see that the final resolution is often a combination of several possible actions. Often, an important element in the resolution is the timing and sequencing of actions. Is it better to go to the administrator, the COTA, or the OTR first? This, of course, is a judgment call based on the consultant's assessment of the degree of receptivity and flexibility of each person. Also, the consultant must decide whether this issue should be addressed, since it is tangential to the purpose of the consultation. What are the consultant's professional obligations in this instance?

This case is presented to give you food for thought and to illustrate how the analysis system can be useful in sorting out the issues and possible resolutions to an ethical dilemma.

Another serious ethical concern occurs when the consultant recommends that occupational therapy services should be increased or initiated. The following scenario exemplifies a possible ethical conflict.

An occupational therapist employed by a hospital also provides pediatric consultation and treatment services on her own. Her 10-hour workdays allow her to have 1 free day a week. The hospital had recently started services to community sites, such as nursing homes and group homes, and was looking for other service sites in the community.

A local school district contacted the therapist directly. They asked her to consult with them about the types of services they would need for nine students with severe, multiple handicaps. The school system has never had an occupational therapist on staff. The consultant spent time talking with the administrator and teaching staff, met with concerned parents, and evaluated all of the students. She recommended in her final report that all nine children needed occupational therapy at least once a week. The school administrator asked that the consultant consider providing the therapy for these students and asked her to set her fee for providing these services. What should the consultant do?

In this case, the ethical conflict may not be as obvious. Let us go through the analysis process one more time.

1. *Who are the players?* The persons who are directly affected are the school staff, the students, and their parents. Beyond the immediate school environment are the other students in the school system, the members of the community who pay for school services, the hospital that employs the therapist 4 days a week, and other occupational therapists in the area.

2. *What other facts or information do you need?* The consultant would want to know why the school system has not hired an occupational therapist in the past. She would want to know if the hospital (her primary employer) was, in fact, seriously considering outreach services to school systems. Does the consultant have the time to pick up this contract with the school on her 1 free day?

3. *What actions might be taken by the consultant?*
   a. The consultant could accept the offer of a contract to provide the recommended services.
   b. The consultant could suggest that the school administrator ask for contract bids from other agencies and independent contractors.
   c. The consultant could refuse the contract.

4. *What are the consequences of these actions?*

Action a. The consultant would be providing services for students but would be restricting the accessibility of the contract to others in the area who may be equally qualified to provide the required services.

Action b. The consultant may, in fact, end up with the contract, but there is assurance that others, including her primary employer, have the opportunity to put in a bid. This action also acknowledges the relationship between the therapist and hospital and prevents a conflict of interest issue from arising.

Action c. The consultant will have assured that there is no conflict of interest. But, if the administrator does not put out a bid for the contract or is not able to contract with the hospital or a qualified therapist to provide the services, the students will not be treated.

5. *Choose an action and defend it.*

In this situation, the consultant is bound ethically to recommend that the administrator put the contract out for bid from qualified agencies or professionals in the community. The explanation provided under Action b gives the rationale for this position. Many consultants do not understand that there is a clear distinction between short-term, very time-limited consultation and the transition that occurs when they move into providing other services in the facility (direct service, supervision, or training). When other activities are being initiated as a direct result of consultative recommendations, the professional can be considered to be self-serving, and/or working under a conflict of interest unless bids for services are sought. In this case, the conflict of interest is heightened because the therapist also works for a potential competitor.

Another similar and equally confusing set of circumstances occur when the therapist attempts to fill multiple roles within the same facility. The role of consultant, when combined with that of practitioner, educator, supervisor, or manager will create ethical conflicts similar to those described in the previous case.

As a conclusion to this chapter, here is a third scenario for you to analyze independently.

An experienced consultant was hired by the administrator of a developmental center to determine which clients might be candidates for community living. In addition, she was expected to develop a program for those clients who were to receive community living training. The occupational therapy department consisted of the director, two staff occupational therapists, and two aides. All personnel were in civil service positions with detailed job descriptions. The administrator for the occupational therapy department was a nurse/rehabilitation coordinator and was the person who requested the consultant.

The consultant began by evaluating the clients who were assigned to the occupational therapy director. In all the charts, she noticed that OT evaluation reports are labeled screening when the assessment was brief. These screening reports were handwritten and were performed by the OT aides. The more detailed and comprehensive evaluations were typed and had been signed by the OT director.

In order to clarify the procedure, the consultant talked to one of the aides. The aide said that she not only performed the screenings, but also had done all of the evaluations. She stated that all the occupational therapy staff were aware of this but everyone was too afraid to say anything because the OT director made it clear that the staff's jobs would be in jeopardy if they complained.

The consultant met with the director about the community living program and, in the conversation, mentioned her concern about the practice of having aides do the evaluations. The director replied that these tasks were part of their job description and, therefore, were allowed. The consultant reviewed the elements of screening versus evaluation with the director to clarify her concern. The director refused to discuss the issue any further and admonished the consultant to stay focused on the community living program rather the inner workings of the department.

In a joint meeting with the OT director and the nursing/rehabilitation coordinator, the consultant again broached the subject. The coordinator stated her support of the OT director's decisions and asked the consultant to limit her concerns to the parameters of the consultation contract.

What should the consultant do?

SUMMARY

In this chapter, you have had the opportunity to gain some insight into the ethical parameters of consultation. First an overview of the important terminology and two major theoretical perspectives commonly utilized in ethical deliberations were presented. Next was a discussion of the purpose and scope of the occupational therapy code of ethics, followed by a brief listing of some differences in emphasis across two other professional codes. To examine the potential issues that may arise while consulting, the perspectives, needs, rights, and duties of the various parties involved in a consultation are examined. And, finally, you were introduced to an analysis system that can be used to examine and resolve ethical dilemmas.

REFERENCES

1. American Occupational Therapy Association: Occupational therapy code of ethics. *Am J Occup Ther* 1988; 12:795.

2. Aroskar MA: Anatomy of an ethical dilemma: The practice. *Am J Nurs* 1980; 4:661.
3. Graber GC: Basic theories in medical ethics, in Monagle JF, Thomasma DC (eds): *Medical Ethics: A Guide for Health Professionals*. Rockville, Md, Aspen, 1988, pp 462–475.
4. Hansen RA, Kyler-Hutchison, PL: Light at the end of the tunnel: Resolving dilemmas. Workshop, Baltimore, Md, AOTA annual conference, April 1989.

SECTION B

The Business of Occupational Therapy Consultation Practice

CHAPTER 40

Developing a Consultation Practice

Cynthia F. Epstein, M.A., O.T.R., F.A.O.T.A.

Entrepreneurship is neither a science nor an art. It is a practice.—*Peter Drucker*[3]

Establishing a consultation practice, a business, can be an exciting, challenging, and rewarding experience. Autonomy, the opportunity to practice in nontraditional environments, and a more flexible lifestyle are among the many attractions. Financial insecurity, extensive time commitments, and responsibility for all work performed are some of the risks. Considering all factors, increasing numbers of health care professionals are choosing to be in business for themselves.[4, 5]

This trend has been reflected in survey data compiled by the American Occupational Therapy Association. A dramatic 76% rise in occupational therapist self-employment was seen from 1982 to 1990. Twenty-six percent of all therapists responding to the survey in 1990 reported that they were self-employed. While specific data are not available regarding the percentage of self-employed therapists identifying consultation as a primary or secondary function, 6.5% of all those surveyed indicated consultation as their primary function, and approximately one third stated it was their secondary function.[1] The very nature of private practice lends itself to increasing opportunities for consultation. Recent literature discussing private practice supports this viewpoint.*

Experienced occupational therapy consultants who contemplate establishing a business bring important knowledge, skills, and training to this new venture. You must consider personal, professional, organizational, financial, legal, and environmental issues when contemplating a role as consultant or entrepreneur. However, the weighting and focus differ in these two roles.

---

* References 2, 6, 7, 9, 10, 12, 13, 15, and 19.

As a consultant, you view the situation from the client's perspective. The consultant analyzes the situation and then presents specific recommendations for the client's consideration. The control and decision-making power lie with the client. As entrepreneur, the consultant's client is her business. The role and focus becomes managerial in nature and the consultant is the one in control.

This chapter discusses what the consultant must consider when establishing a consultation practice. We review how to enter the world of business along with personal characteristics and professional concerns which are part of that decision. Organizing your business, including legal, financial, and environmental aspects, provides the foundation for future success. These issues and other related business concerns are addressed here.

BEGINNING

How do you begin? Many different routes exist. These may be found on the job, in the community, through colleague referral, moonlighting, advanced study, and/or the desire for change.

Initial Experience

Opportunities to utilize consulting skills as an internal and/or external consultant usually first arise while employed as a direct service provider. As the therapist's expertise and consultation abilities are recognized, invited consults outside the regular employment setting may occur. The therapist's repertoire and visibility in the health care community gradually expands. The world of private practice as a consultant has begun.

While this may be more typical, many other routes are available. Therapists interested in community or professional issues become involved in volunteer activities that require consultation skills. One quickly thinks of the local religious group needing barrier-free access for their congregants, or the family friend suddenly needing guidance in selecting a rehabilitation oriented nursing facility for a parent. The therapist responds to the need, the community's networking begins, and soon the volunteer consultant is flooded with requests. At some point, volunteer time becomes a paid consultantship.

Therapists with special expertise often share their knowledge with colleagues through writing, lectures, and informal consultation. Soon requests for paid consultation services find their way to the consultant.

For some, the need for radical change in direction may spark the move. In this instance the prospective consultant may have had very limited field consulting experience, but should have a solid background in consulting theory and principles.

The motivation to step into a full-time consultation business may evolve from the experiences we have discussed. Certainly these part-time experiences have provided positive reinforcement for the consultant/entrepreneur. Other important motivators include the desire for independence and success and the potential for increased earnings.

Personal Characteristics

Motivation must be supported by the personal characteristics needed for business success. Establishing a business means taking a risk and moving forward with confidence and determination. Realistic self-appraisal of your ability to handle the multiple demands of entrepreneurship is therefore an important first business step. Assessing and understanding your strengths and weaknesses in the context of owning and operating a business will help assure success.[7]

Entrepreneurs take calculated risks. They weigh advantages and disadvantages of given situations and choose achievable challenges. Risk taking requires creativity and innovation that must be tempered with realistic understanding to achieve a successful outcome.[22]

Many of the consultant traits we have discussed are necessary for the entrepreneur. Among others, these include self-confidence, sound judgment, and knowledge of self. McClelland[11] points out the need to be future oriented, with a high energy level and desire to assume responsibility. You must also be a self-starter, capable of realistic planning and goal-oriented leadership, and take pride in a job well done.[22]

The potential entrepreneur must carefully weigh the many advantages and disadvantages of being in business. You must be prepared to survive such trials and tribulations as irregular income, long hours, isolation, and unpredictable fluctuations in client markets. Concerns such as these must be balanced against the more positive aspects of independent practice: potentially greater income, opportunities for creative problem solving, and flexibility in lifestyle.

The consultant's personal goals have a major influence on the business. Choice of consultation models, area of expertise, family commitments, and outside interests must all be factored in. The various practice models described in this text speak eloquently to these concerns and to the professional concerns you must consider.

Professional Concerns

Clients seeking consultative services expect a high level of professional competence. The prospective consultant/entrepreneur must be able to demonstrate a high degree of professional knowledge and skill in consultation along with specialized occupational therapy expertise. As we observed earlier, this broad knowledge base applies to both the consultant and entrepreneurial hats you wear. This knowledge is not static and must be constantly updated. Greater amounts of time and money must be allocated to keep current and future oriented.

As consultant, you understand that the client is the primary focus. As entrepreneur, a balance must be achieved so that the client's needs are appropriately met while business needs are effectively addressed. This must be done in an ethical manner.

For example, you may have several different contractual agreement formats. Facilities may contract for services by the hour, day, job, on a retainer, or the client may have an open-ended agreement with the consultant. If a consultant's client roster suddenly dips, with a concurrent drop in cash flow, there may be a temptation to expand services at a site with an open-ended contract. Before going this route, the consultant should step back and assess objectively the client's need versus the consultant's financial need. This is only one example of many ethical dilemmas facing the consultant/entrepreneur.

Many interpersonal, technical, and consulting skills are needed by both the consultant and the entrepreneur. Again in each role, the view and emphasis differ. For the entrepreneur, two critial skills are communication and analysis.

Communication skills are one of the consultant's keys to success. Objective listening, observing, identifying, and reporting are the heart of a consultant's task. As entrepreneur, these same skills must be used objectively and subjectively. From a business perspective, you must be able to communicate effectively with clients, employees, and colleagues. How you use these skills is a good indicator of how successful you will be.

Similarly, the consultant is asked to diagnose a given situation for a client. These analytical skills are constantly in play in business. You must, for example, analyze the structure needed for the organization, the strength of the proposed plan, and the market to be addressed. A business succeeds when the analysis is correct.

The consultant-entrepreneur's success is linked to her ability to be creative, futuristic and realistic. (Figure 40-1) She must adeptly assess each situation in relation to her client and business environments; orchestrate an action plan that addresses immediate and future needs; and maintain a realistic approach to business management.

FIGURE 40–1

Consultant-Entrepreneur Attributes

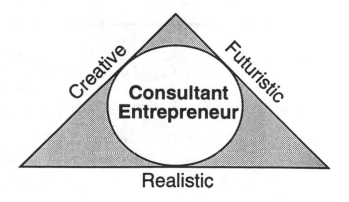

Personal and professional concerns help to shape the business and direct its focus. At the start of a consultation practice, it is important to recognize these multiple concerns and to assess yourself and your abilities critically.

PLANNING

The parallels and contracts we have drawn between consultation and entrepreneurship can be continued in the planning stage. Table 40–1 identifies basic elements needed to establish a plan from each perspective.

As is true in consultation, a plan forms the basis for decision making in business. The bottom line, or financial outcome is the critical concern. How successful the business's product (consultation) will be depends on how thoroughly the prospective entrepreneur has researched and analyzed the business plan.

Establishing a Business Plan

Market assessment provides the prospective entrepreneur with specific information about the geographic area to be served, the potential pool of clientele, and their possible consultation needs. As is true in the needs assessment phase of consultation, it is a time-consuming task that must be done carefully and completely. If funding is available, it may also be prudent to hire a marketing consultant to guide the process.

Starting with an in-depth look at the geographic area to be served, information is extrapolated from such local sources as the chamber of commerce, newspapers, health care facilities and agencies, educational programs, health-focused volunteer organizations, and colleagues. Depending on your particular consultation expertise or product, the emphasis will vary.

For example, in 1978, an initial market assessment was conducted for the proposed company, Occupational Therapy Consultants, Inc. (OTC). The initial geographic area to be served was central and northern New Jersey. The proposed

TABLE 40–1
Establishing a Plan

Consultation	Business
Needs Assessment	Market Assessment
Diagnosis	Statement of Mission and Purpose
Problem Identification	Business Concept
Goals	Goals
Implementation Strategies	Organizational Plan

product was consultation services for long-term care, most specifically nursing facilities. The assessment therefore targeted such information and referral sources as area nursing home administrators, hospitals, social service agencies, rehabilitation centers, area offices on aging, the State Department of Health section on long-term care, local libraries and chambers of commerce, occupational therapy colleagues, and colleagues in other health care professions.

The information gathered, combined with changes that had recently occurred in the licensure standards for long-term care facilities, indicated that there was a strong interest and need for both consultative and restorative occupational therapy services in area nursing facilities. During the survey process it became evident that immediate referrals were available and that a roster of clients could quickly be developed for both service models.

One of the other important findings in this assessment was the lack of competition. There were few therapists in nursing facilities, and minimal consultative and restorative services were being provided. Those involved in this market were usually working in isolation and lacked a cohesive, well-structured approach to service delivery.

Analyzing these data, in combination with the principals' prior experience as independent practitioners, provided a firm base for a decision to establish the company. It was evident that a need existed. With knowledge of the market, realistic projections could be made regarding expected financial earnings. It was then possible to define the practice further in regard to its mission and purpose.

A *mission statement* or *statement of purpose* briefly defines the purpose of the business, its clientele, location, and overall goals. While specific organizational goals change as a business develops, a general goal remains. Schrello[16] suggests that the mission and purpose statement should contain at least four elements: products, markets, uniqueness, and performance measures.

For example, In New Jersey, OTC has a twofold mission and purpose. First, the provision of comprehensive, high quality, cost-effective occupational therapy consultative and restorative services for health care clientele in New Jersey requiring such services to improve, develop, and/or expand their functional capacities within given environments. Second, to provide a supportive and enriched working environment for consultants and therapists in the practice. This statement has guided the practice's development, creating a two-pronged approach that has supported the overarching concern, excellence in consultation services.

Once a mission statement has been developed, it should serve as a guiding principle for the practice. It should meet today's needs and tomorrow's prospects.

A *business concept* logically follows the development of a mission or statement of purpose. Here you define the where, what, and when of the business.

Going back to our example, the initial business concept looked at service in central and northern New Jersey. The location of organization's headquarters was another question. The choice was central New Jersey, which was important in terms of future growth. While the areas of consultation and restorative treatment had been identified, the types of occupational therapy consultation had not been specified. Program development, educational, clinical, collegial, systems, and organizational development models were identified. It was expected that consultation would occur at all levels.

Since this company had decided to start out as a small, part-time operation, the "when" was dictated by the time available. Initially, services at client sites were limited to approximately 20 hours per week. This did not take into account the many hours needed for planning, marketing, and general business operations, done at the company office or the principal's home.

The overriding *business goal* is straightforward—to be financially solvent. When starting out, this may mean just breaking even and covering all business costs, including a small salary for the owner. Or it may mean receiving at least the same financial remuneration you received on a job, plus covering all costs. Realistically, you should consider the first year in business as a loss leader. Firmly establishing the business and a line of credit are primary objectives which, in the end, lead to a successful venture. By developing specific and realistic financial objectives for the first year of operation, a goal of financial stability can hopefully be achieved.

In our example, financial objectives included the following:

- *Minimize expenses* through use of available resources. This included sharing office space with another firm, using a typing service, purchasing moderately priced supplies, owner design and layout of business cards, stationery, brochure, and logo.
- *Obtain financial guidance* through consultation with an accountant and banker. This included determining the structure of the company, the method of bookkeeping, procedures necessary for reporting to the Internal Revenue Service and state agencies, cost-effective banking options and forecasting methodology that helped identify expected sources of income.
- *Minimize risks* through consultation with a lawyer and use of strategic planning. This included determining a form of business and developing contract formats; guidance regarding malpractice concerns; understanding federal, state, and local regulations that affected business operations.
- *Develop a consultant roster* of therapists to be on call as independent contractors when business needs exceeded the time available from the principals of the organization. This roster was made up of highly experienced professionals whose standards of practice matched those of the organization and who agreed to reimbursement under the organization's fee structure.

These and other goals and objectives help to set the stage for an organizational plan. When complete, the business plan will be an essential tool that will help to guide the business.

An *organizational plan* describes the structure of the business, its personnel business form, and financial management plan.[7]

Most businesses begin as small operations, and the number of personnel involved are usually limited. In addition to professional staff, you should, at a minimum, have some general office help to perform such tasks as reception, typing, filing, and bookkeeping/billing. The temptation to save money by performing these tasks yourself is great. However, time spent in these activities could be spent producing revenue. Since time is money, you need to use it judiciously.

Delegating work to other personnel should also include the engagement of outside consultants. These include on-call consultants and such important financial consultants as an accountant and lawyer.

- *On-call consultants* acts as a pressure valve, helping meet unexpected demands.
- The *accountant or business adviser* helps to organize the business's financial structure, select the form of business, evaluate the tax consequences of various decisions, structure the accounting and bookkeeping methodology, and assist in requests for loans.
- Consultation with a *lawyer* provides important guidance in selecting a form of business, developing contractual agreements, leasing space, understanding liability issues, meeting regulations, and collecting debts.[7]

When selecting legal and business advisers, it is helpful to establish general criteria to make an informed decision. Here are some points to consider:

- Does the adviser have expertise in health-related areas?
- Have colleagues recommended using this adviser?
- What is the availability of the adviser?
- Does the adviser have experience working with consulting firms?
- What options are available regarding fees?
- Are reports generated in a timely fashion?
- What is the range of services that can be provided?

These and other specific concerns should be kept in mind when selecting these advisers. By establishing comfortable and open working relationships with your advisers, an important part of the business support system is in place.

The form your business should take is also a critical decision. Using the expertise of chosen advisers and reviewing all data gathered for the business plan will contribute significantly to this part of the decision-making process.

Forms of Business

There are three basic types of business organizational forms: sole proprietorship, partnership, and corporation. Each has its own advantages and disadvantages. Determining which form is best depends very much on individual circumstances. A basic understanding of each will help in deliberations, and will allow for more in-depth discussions with your lawyer and business adviser.

Sole proprietorship is the most common route taken by those who choose to become a consultant/entrepreneur. It is the least complex from a legal and accounting standpoint. As an outright business owner, you must assume all the risks and will, ultimately reap all the rewards.

The owner may hire or subcontract with other consultants to provide services to clients. When considering employees or independent contractors who are sub-contractors, you must understand important tax and legal ramifications (see Chapter 38). Detailed records must be kept of all income and expenses, and the consultant/entrepreneur is responsible for paying required taxes in a timely manner.

A sole proprietorship allows the consultant to maintain freedom and control over all aspects of business. Its major drawbacks are those of liability and responsibility for the performance of all business obligations. Given the litigious nature of our society, you must be concerned with potential liability issues. Should a suit occur, the owner's personal assets are at risk.[8] When the owner is sick or on vacation, no one may be available to cover. Clients may cancel contracts, thereby causing a financial drain on the practice. Pursuing this form of business means that the consultant must plan carefully to develop backup strategies that will help minimize these problems.[14] Information available through the Small Business Administration[20] will be a helpful guide.

The author, for example, first started business as a consultant using the sole proprietorship form. The consultation practice was a part-time business, allowing time for important roles as wife, mother, and community volunteer. Over a period of 12 years, the business expanded and gradually began to occupy more time. With the growth, it became necessary to hire other therapists and office personnel. When that juncture was reached, a change in business form was considered. Partnership and a corporate status were both options.

A *partnership* joins two or more persons in a business venture. Each partner contributes assets to the business, is liable for debts, and is eligible to receive a specific percentage of the earned income, as established in the partnership agreement. Should there be business losses, each partner is personally responsible to cover the loss.

Forming a partnership is not an expensive proposition and should be done with the assistance of an attorney. In the interests of all concerned, each partner should be represented by his or her own attorney. The agreement should also provide options for dissolution.

In a consultation practice, partnership has some distinct advantages in the areas of support, resource access, backup personnel, expanded visibility, and the diverse expertise of each partner. Partnerships require an interactive relationship that is mutually supportive. Similar to a marriage, they require close and harmonious work. When there is a mutual fit, the group benefits extensively and the practice matures exponentially.

When there is disharmony, the practice's creative abilities are threatened and productivity is thwarted. Disagreements or negative perceptions on the part of one partner can affect the practice as a whole, causing deterioration of its major asset, the partner's synergistic working relationship.[17]

To consider this business form, consultants should know each other well and have had experience working together. A successful occupational therapy partnership in Canada started in this manner, and has continued to expand since inception.[6] This can be a professionally rewarding relationship and offers distinct advantages to both the client with multifaceted needs and the consultant seeking a supportive business relationship.

A *corporation* is viewed by law as a legal entity. This means that the organization has the power to execute contracts, incur indebtedness, own property, and perform business as if it were a person.[21] The corporation is liable for its business debts, but the owner and/or any employees are not. The consultant may own stock and/or assume a position as an officer in the corporation. The corporation can employ the consultant/owner, as well as others.

The costs of establishing and maintaining a corporation are much greater than that required for the other forms of business. Decisions regarding advantages of incorporation require in-depth assessment and guidance from a legal and tax viewpoint. Issues to consider in addition to that of liability include tax and legal reporting requirements, ability to control the corporation, and nonprofit versus for-profit incorporation.

While a corporation is a legal entity, and it takes responsibility if a client sues, the need for professional liability coverage for consultant employees still exists. The corporation is responsible for purchasing this liability malpractice insurance. Corporations can also provide expanded pension, health insurance, and continuing education benefits to their employees in addition to reimbursable business expenses. In a partnership or sole proprietorship, these benefits would appear as a deduction to income on the partner or owner's tax form.[4]

For example, when OTC was incorporated in New Jersey, extensive meetings were held with the company's legal and tax advisers prior to final determination of the business form. Projections were made regarding potential earnings and the need for employees. The financial status of the corporate owners was reviewed to determine their best business interests. A financial plan was suggested for the corporation and the owners. Based on this in-depth analysis, a decision was made to incorporate rather than form a partnership. The corporation's continued growth and development since 1979 is a positive endorsement of this initial planning strategy.

The financial management part of the plan requires looking at sources of financing and the projected income and expenses for the first 2 years of operation. This is a brief but concise budget statement that is a series of assumptions until the business is actually organized and operational.

Expenses are broken down into three major types: fixed, variable, and capital. Fixed expenses are costs that stay constant and are payable at a fixed time. They include such major areas as rent, wages, insurance, and taxes. Variable expenses fluctuate but are always part of the package. They include such items as telephone, postage, travel, entertainment, printing, independent contractor fees, and utilities. Capital expenses are included as part of the start-up costs. They are usually onetime expenses. Included in this category are deposits for the rent and telephone, and purchase of furniture, computers, and other office equipment.

Forecasting income is usually more difficult than estimating expenses. You can look at the projected bottom line expenses, and try to use this figure in forecasting. Prior consulting experience, knowledge of the going rate for consultation services, and the response noted as part of the market assessment all contribute to the income projection developed.

The business plan can also be used as a loan proposal, and it must be as accurate as possible. A start-up loan may make the difference between success and failure. Undercapitalization is the primary cause of failure for a new business. The first 3 years are the critical, as this is when the business is most vulnerable. While being conservative in your business can be seen as a virtue, being too conservative in terms of necessary funding can lead to failure.

When seeking a start-up loan, be prepared to provide the lender with information on personal assets and liabilities. Banks and the Small Business Administration are two sources for business loans. If you qualify, it is possible to apply for special business loans that target minorities or other special populations.

A comprehensive business plan is the road map used to organize your trip into entrepreneurship.[14] Successful completion of the first year in business will depend on how well you orchestrate the organizational plan.

ORGANIZING

Necessary consultant skills and abilities have been discussed at length in this text. Utilizing key consulting concepts and theories will facilitate the development of a responsive organization. Occupational therapy skill and expertise, combined with the various consulting models and levels and related areas (including system theory and strategic planning) form the base. Business skill and ability are the critical issue. With an organizational plan in place, specific business aspects of the practice can be addressed.

In the occupational therapy community, many consulting practices operate as solo enterprises. Partnerships and corporations are less common. While there are differences in the organizational design of each business form, a common thread is evident. Using the mission and purpose statement as a guide, the organization's leader establishes basic structures to integrate necessary business functions, critical client service components, and the practice's human resources.

Business Functions

The consultant/entrepreneur must bring business knowledge and skill to her new enterprise, along with occupational therapy consultation expertise. Comprehensive business knowledge and skill may not be part of the consultant's repertoire. Should such be the case, the skilled leader will delegate aspects of business management to others. Managing the business's finances, the bottom line issue is a primary concern.

Financial management controls expenses and income, plans and implements the structure needed for this control, strategically plans future needs, and assures that the business adheres to required regulations governing the financial aspects of business.

An *accounting method* should be identified for the business. This can be either a cash or an accrual method. Using the cash method, all income paid to the business and expenses paid out in a given year are reported in that year, except for certain expenses that need to be depreciated over time. The accrual method requires that you report all income billed out in a given year, even when the income is not received and all expenses incurred and even if the payment has not been sent.

Various *bookkeeping systems* are commercially available for use in a small business.[7, 20] These can be purchased through business supply firms in both computer and paper formats. Guidance from a business adviser will help assure correct choices. By establishing the right accounting and bookkeeping practices at the start of business, you save countless hours and obtain important future planning information.

Regulatory requirements, such as an employer identification number, special state permits, quarterly tax payments, reports to federal and state agencies, and timely payment of tax obligations must be part of financial management. Many businesses rely on their accountant or business adviser to prepare these papers. Helpful booklets and information sheets are also available from the Internal Revenue Service (IRS) and state tax offices.

Organizing finances at the start of a business usually means that the owner must be prepared to support the business, and herself, with personal funds or with an outside loan. When using personal funds, those targeted for the business must be placed in the business's account. Mixing personal and business funds clouds financial management and raises potential problems with the IRS.

For instance, when OTC was formed, the principals in the corporation each put a set amount of their own personal money into the business account. They decided not to draw a salary for the first 3 months. During this time, the operating expenses were from the start-up monies provided. As income began to trickle in, the bookkeeping reports clearly indicated that salaries again needed to be postponed. This strategy was feasible because prior planning had been done, and the owners were prepared for a lengthy wait before drawing a salary.

The *fee structure* set for a new consulting business should be based on labor costs, overhead, the area's going rate for services, and what is considered a reasonable profit. The fees established should assure a year end break-even point for the practice.

When establishing fees, the consultant/entrepreneur should look at what the consultant would earn if employed by an established practice or organization. This annual salary must then be broken down to a daily hourly rate.

For example, Mary Jones, OTR, earned $52,000 a year at XYZ Hospital. She is now establishing a consultation practice and wants to maintain that level of compensation. On her job, Mary was paid for 261 workdays. To obtain her daily rate, she divided her salary by 261 days, which equated to $199.23, or $200 a day. Figuring an 8-hour workday, she was paid $25 per hour.

To determine her charges as a consultant/entrepreneur, Mary now must factor in the business's overhead, which includes fixed, variable, and capital expenses. On a monthly basis, this comes to $4,800. Another overhead cost is the 5 days a month Mary must devote to marketing and professional development. Therefore, her business only has 15 days a month to earn its fees. The overhead cost of $4,800 is divided by 15 days, giving a $320 cost per day for overhead. The total costs for the new consultation business are $520 without including a profit margin. With a 20% profit margin, equaling $104, the business's daily rate for consultation services should be $625 per day.[17] Checking rates charged by other consultation practices in the area, Mary determines that the $625 figure is competitive.

Organizing an effective and efficient financial management approach will pay immediate dividends. It provides the entrepreneur with a realistic performance appraisal in a timely fashion and helps to establish a forecasting mechanism for future planning. It identifies problem and growth areas. It is an important entrepreneurial tool.

Client Service Components

Many of the critical client service components you must consider fall under marketing. While this important area will be fully addressed in Chapter 41, particular aspects of marketing should be considered when organizing a business. Business location, naming the practice, and essential introductory business materials are primary considerations.[17]

The name and location of the business are visible public information. Conveying the right message regarding who you are and where you can be found are part of important first impressions.

The name you choose for your firm is your introduction—indeed it is a prominent part of your business apparatus—along with your logo, or symbol, if you choose to use one.

Those consultants who are solo practitioners usually maintain the business in their name. Partnerships or corporations, however, may wish to establish a distinct name for the practice. The name chosen has important marketing considerations.[18] It can help sell the service and also may determine your market. Occupational Therapy Consultants, Inc., for instance, identifies the business's focus but does not limit the target population the way that Pediatric Occupational Therapy Consultants would.

The location of a consulting business has more flexibility than that of a private practitioner engaged in direct treatment services. Since most consulting time is spent at client sites, the business office should be central to the geographic area targeted for services. In the case of a solo part-time practice, the location often will be a home office. When an office in the home is used, carefully review all tax implications and necessary requirements with an accountant or tax specialist.

In the case of a partnership or corporation, where more than one consultant requires office space and support services, you should consider routing from the office to major highways when you choose the location. Travel time is a major cost and easy access to major roads will cut driving time to client sites. The office site should also allow room for growth.

Remaining in an initial location for several years helps to generate informal and network-related referrals. These clients may locate the business through various sources, including local groups that may have misplaced your card, but remember the street where your office is located. At a minimum, if the office site moves, the telephone number should remain intact if possible. When rent and support service costs are very high, the entrepreneur may want to consider sharing space with another group to cut down overhead.

OTC, for example, started out in shared office space. The other firm was a company of tax specialists, whose seasonal business required year-round space and some year-round staff. This arrangement allowed the consulting group to share not only space expenses, but also important support services and equipment. Reception, bookkeeping, duplicating, typing, and computer services were shared. During the peak tax season, the consulting group was able to arrange for extra help so that important business functions were not lost in this time of stress.

As both companies grew, the need for larger quarters became imperative. The shared location had proved beneficial to all concerned, and therefore a space was found that was adaptable for both groups. By keeping the office in the same general area, the telephone numbers remained the same, and informal business referrals continued.

Essential introductory business materials such as stationery, business cards, a logo, and brochure will provide the new business with tangible professional symbols of the company. Visual and sensory impressions are conveyed through the graphic design, layout, and quality of paper you use. The brochure should provide a concise statement of the consultants' capabilities. Prospective clients want to know about the consultant product they are buying. The brochure should be graphically interesting and professionally presented. Used in combination with a business card, individualized letters, and an initial visit, the brochure reinforces the consultants' abilities and maximizes visibility. The brochure, business card, logo, name, and location are also part of a larger marketing plan. This important area is discussed in greater detail in Chapter 41.

Human Resources

Staff employed or contracted to the practice are the hub of a service-oriented business. Most consultation businesses start as sole proprietorships, and staffing concerns do not arise as a major issue during the first year. The consultant/owner usually performs all roles and sets policies to suit given needs.

In group or corporate practice, there is a need for both professional and support personnel. At the professional level, you may hire employees, subcontract with independent contractors, or both. If an employer decides to use independent contractors, there are many legal and financial concerns. The detailed discussion on the use of independent contractors, found in Chapter 38, should be reviewed when this strategy is considered.

Employees are a significant business responsibility. Multiple state and federal laws mandate the establishment of specific policies and procedures to protect the employee. Fair labor standards must be considered, workers' compensation insurance provided, and compliance with various labor and revenue service procedures assured. Because of the many nuances in laws regulating employment, it is wise to obtain legal counsel when setting up personnel policies and procedures.

Another important issue, especially for consultation practices, is employee competition. A consultant employee may develop a close relationship with one of the company's major clients and then leave. The former employee may then solicit the client.

Realizing that such scenarios are possible, the consultant/entrepreneur should consider using a restrictive clause when hiring new employees. Often termed a noncompete clause, this offers the employer some protection. If you consider this option, legal counsel is important. Chapter 38 discusses this issue at some length.

Gaining and retaining employees are important considerations. The professionals in the practice have been selected for their skill and expertise. The owner should encourage a participatory management approach that will allow these skilled personnel to contribute to a workable and fair employee benefit program. Involving them in personnel committees, planning of continuing education programs, and/or good and welfare committees are some examples.

Organizing a business is a complex, time-consuming, and challenging task. It is important for the consultant/entrepreneur to delineate the structure to be used. The business will operate smoothly when there is a clear plan for financial management, complemented by client service components that support both client and consultant needs. In addition, there must be employee recognition and support to help form a cohesive and harmonious organization.

SUMMARY

A rapidly expanding consultation marketplace beckons the experienced therapist. Opportunities exist to operate as a single entity or as part of a group or organization. Establishing a consultation practice requires business skills in addition to those of a consultant. Careful planning, use of appropriate resources, and expertise valued by clientele, will help the consultant develop a successful business.

Occupational therapy consultation is provided to diverse healthcare client systems, who require high quality services, delivered in a cost effective manner. The consultant achieves this through careful planning, development, and monitoring of her business. Important interrelationships between consultation, business planning and marketing must be recognized and used judiciously to develop a responsive and capable organization. This requires the consultant-entrepreneur to be creative, futuristic and realistic. Using these attributes in combination with business skills will help her move effectively into new markets and confidently assume new challenges.

REFERENCES

1. American Occupational Therapy Association: *1990 Member Data Survey*. Rockville, Md, Author, 1991.
2. Christenson MA: The occupational therapist as consultant. *AOTA Administration and Management SIS Newsletter* 1990; 6:3.
3. Drucker PF: *Innovation and Entrepreneurship: Practice and Principles*. New York, Harper & Row, 1986.
4. Epstein CF: Consultation: Communicating and facilitating, in Bair J, Gray M (eds): *The Occupational Therapy Manager*, rev. ed. Rockville, Md, AOTA, 1992.
5. For the Record. *OT Week*. April 18, 1991; 6:14.
6. Goldenberg K, Quinn B: Community Occupational Therapy Associates: A model of private practice for community occupational therapy, in Cromwell FS (ed): *Occup Ther Health Care* 1985; 2:2.
7. Hertfelder SD, Crispen C (eds): *Private Practice: Strategies for Success*. Rockville, Md, AOTA, 1990.
8. Holtz H: *How to Succeed as an Independent Consultant*, ed 2. New York, Wiley, 1988.
9. Hurff JM, Lowe HE, Ho BJ, et al: Networking: A successful linkage for community occupational therapists. *Am J Occup Ther* 1990; 44:424–430.
10. Jacobson SL: Group consultation—a private practice model for the 1990s. *AOTA Administration and Management SIS Newsletter* 1988; 4:1.
11. McClelland DC: *The Achieving Society*. New York, Free Press, 1967.
12. Olin DW: Evolution of a private practice. *AOTA Administration and Management SIS Newsletter* 1990; 6:3.
13. Quinn B: Private practice—a challenging alternative. *WFOT Bulletin*, 1989; 19:28–33.
14. Ryan MC: Getting started in private practice. *AOTA Administration and Management SIS Newsletter*. 1988; 4:2.
15. Schaaf RC, Gitlen LN: Early intervention: New directions for occupational therapists, in Johnson JA, Ethridge DA (eds): *Occup Ther Health Care* 1989; 6:3.
16. Schrello DM: *The Complete Marketing Handbook for Consultants*, vol I. San Diego, Univ Assoc, 1990.
17. Shenson HL: *Complete Guide to Consulting Success*. Wilmington, Del, Enterprise, 1987.
18. Shenson HL: *Shenson on Consulting*. New York, Wiley, 1990.
19. Shriver DJ: A new arena for occupational therapy: Workers' compensation and person injury, in Cromwell FS (ed): *Occup Ther Health Care* 1985; 2:2.
20. Small Business Administration. *The Small Business Directory, Form 115A*. Denver, SBA Publications, 1990.
21. Sullivan CA: Business and management aspects of private practice in speech-language pathology and audiology, in Butler KG (ed): *Prospering in Private Practice: A Handbook for Speech-Language Pathology and Audiology*. Rockville, Md, Aspen, 1986, pp 149–165.
22. Woody RH: *Business Success in Mental Health Practice*. San Francisco, Jossey-Bass, 1989.

CHAPTER 41

Marketing: A Continuous Process

Cynthia F. Epstein, M.A., O.T.R., F.A.O.T.A.

> Until a consulting practice learns to market consistently it is not in control of its destiny.[22]—*Don Schrello*

Marketing is a critical factor in the successful operation of an occupational therapy consultation practice. It will influence the proposed business plan, initial implementation phase, ongoing operations, evaluation process, forecasting considerations, and long range planning necessary for survival of the practice. When planning reimbursement strategies, it is a key consideration. Consultation, an indirect service, will not qualify for payment under direct treatment funding sources. Integrating marketing into every aspect of one's occupational therapy consultation practice is therefore not a consideration—it is a priority!

Often, marketing is equated with selling or public relations. The concept of marketing is, however, much broader in scope. As a business function, the consultant uses marketing to identify client needs and wants. Marketing analysis helps the consultant pinpoint those clients she can best serve and indicates specific services to offer. Marketing will influence how business is conducted and the image conveyed by the consultant. A broad range of skills will therefore be needed to allow the consultant to sense, serve, and satisfy her clients.[6, 12]

Consulting practices require a distinct marketing perspective. Shenson, a well-known authority on consultation, perceives marketing professional consulting services as unique and fundamentally different from marketing products. Consultants who "master the art and science of marketing [their] professional practice [will] benefit economically and enjoy a [higher] level of personal satisfaction" than their peers.[25,pxiii–xiv] Shenson's research indicates that the distinction between the successful and not so successful consultant is not so much a function of their technical or professional expertise, but, rather, their skill in marketing and selling.[23]

650

Marketing influences all consultation activities, whether these are offered on an internal or external basis. It begins the very moment one decides to offer occupational therapy consultation and continues as an ongoing and integral practice component until the consultant permanently shuts her doors. The consultant's professional services, her product, cannot be separated from her image, expertise, personality, or philosophy. She is always "on stage" and must maintain awareness that today's actions effect tomorrow's business.

This chapter will provide prospective and current consultants with a review of marketing concepts and a comprehensive picture of consultation marketing strategies. While the needs of both internal and external consultants are addressed, emphasis is placed on the external consultant or entrepreneur. The examples provided will hopefully stimulate readers to develop their own marketing philosophy. With this in hand, the consultant will be able to develop a context for practice that supports and enhances her professional expertise while appropriately expanding successful consultation service delivery.

MARKETING CONCEPTS

Marketing is a system for organizational planning that is developed from an information base. It involves offering something of value (consultation services) for consideration by a specific group of clients (target market) who, in turn, will offer the consultant something of value, usually payment of a fee.[19] Kotler and Armstrong define marketing as "a social and managerial process by which individuals and groups obtain what they need and want through creating and exchanging products and value with others."[12, p5] A *market* is the group of individuals who have an actual or potential interest in purchasing the consultant's services.[13]

Exchange is viewed as the core marketing concept. In consultation, an exchange begins when a client with specific needs and wants approaches, or is approached by, a consultant whose services may resolve the issue at hand. For the exchange to occur, specific conditions must be met. Each party must have something of value for the other, and they must be able to communicate and negotiate in order to identify terms for an agreement.[12] When these conditions are met, the client and consultant may reach an agreement in which the exchange takes place. The consultant will provide the specific services needed and wanted. The client will pay the consultant's fee and provide other support as agreed upon (i.e., office space, computer assistance, etc.).[12, 18]

The consultant uses a marketing management approach to guide planning and strategy implementation. This will help her achieve desired exchanges with identified target markets.

Occupational therapy has a broad base and applicability to provide consultation in many different health care markets. The consultant's task is to define specific market segments or target markets where a client group with similar needs and interests may desire her services. Concurrently, she must maintain a posture which will allow responsiveness to other potential markets where her expertise can be utilized. For example, a consultant with a technology-focused practice may initially concentrate on a target market where the need is specialized seating and wheeled mobility. This naturally leads the consultant to expand her knowledge base, which then may include barrier free issues and architectural design concerns. Given current mandates for inclusion of the disabled in all aspects of community life, a new target market could then emerge, focused on issues of accessibility.

Marketing is not just a management function. It is a total organizational philosophy and orientation.[13] In developing a philosophy to guide marketing efforts, the consultant must consider the interests of her practice (external consultant) or organization (internal consultant), her clients, and society. At times these interests may conflict.[12]

Societal Marketing Concept

The *societal marketing concept* is a recently developed marketing management philosophy. This concept expands the traditional marketing concept, where the consultant's task is to research the needs and the wants of a specifically defined target market and to deliver the desired services. It incorporates a more humanistic component, the consideration of client and society's well-being.[12, 13]

Today's ecological problems, political upheavals, economic crises, and social welfare concerns affect marketing and its role in society. Marketing should, therefore, not only consider immediate client wants; it should also consider long-range client welfare, which may additionally affect society's well-being.

In our technology example, the consultant must maintain a state-of-the-art knowledge base and be current regarding implications for funding. State agencies, such as Medicaid, constantly seek methods to stretch their limited budgets. Often, this restricts the specialized equipment they will purchase for populations they are mandated to serve. Thus, a case-centered collegial consultation may be requested by a client colleague regarding a patient's need for a new wheelchair seating system. The client and patient want a total replacement of the old chair. This would include a new wheelchair frame and customized seating insert. Funding will be sought through Medicaid.

The consultant's task is to provide expertise regarding the system's design and facilitate the development of a justification report to fund the new chair. She is aware that Medicaid has a pool of used wheelchair frames, in excellent working order. The style required for the patient in question is in the pool. Use of such equipment helps extend limited Medicaid monies, thereby allowing a greater number of patients to receive needed equipment. Part of the consultant's societal marketing task will be to educate her client and channel the decision making process, so that the justification requests a pool wheelchair frame, rather than new equipment.

A consultant practice (internal and external) which reflects a societal marketing concept may be characterized as having:

- *A specific client philosophy.* The practice's plans and organization reflect understanding of the important role played by target markets, client needs and wants, and their relationship to societal well-being.
- *An integrated marketing perspective.* The practice incorporates market analysis, planning, implementation, and control into its ongoing routine.
- *A broad information base.* The practice receives information from many interrelated resources, thus obtaining the multilevel information that is required when considering target market clients and the societal issues affecting them.
- *A strategic orientation.* The practice is future-oriented and generates strategies and plans which address long-range marketing goals.
- *An efficient operation.* Marketing activities are continuously monitored to assure cost effectiveness.[12, 13]

Consultants who utilize this approach in their practice will develop "an organization that is highly responsive, adaptive, and entrepreneurial in a rapidly changing environment."[13, p37]

Strategic Planning

To develop a dynamic marketing program that subscribes to a societal marketing philosophy, the consultant must consider client needs and wants in concert with a concern for societal well-being. This must first be reflected through a strategic planning process. Strategic planning "provides a springboard for systematic thinking that launches creative and intuitive ideas." This process allows the consultant to "look ahead, anticipate problems and plan alternative responses when they are necessary."[20, p30]

Kotler and Clarke suggest that health care organizations must be adaptive to respond to important environmental changes. An adaptive organization is able to "revise its mission, objectives, strategies, organization, and systems to align with its opportunities." In this era of rapid change, the consultant is confronted with multiple environmental forces, such as "changing demographics, increased competition, increased government regulation, altered reimbursement policies, changing social behavior and values, and new technologies. . . ."[13, p81] To survive successfully, the consultant/entrepreneur must have a clearly defined mission statement and long-range plan. (See Chapter 40.) This forms the basis for strategy development and implementation. A future-oriented perspective must also guide the consultant's thinking as she anticipates crucial risk-taking moves.

To develop a strategic plan, the consultant analyzes the positive and negative forces which will affect her practice. She considers the composition of her current client base; what she projects it will be if she maintains her present course of action; and what it could or should be if strategic changes were introduced.[3] Ostrow points out that occupational therapists can utilize their problem-solving skills, honed in clinical environments, and apply them to strategic planning.[21] Basic steps in a strategic planning system as discussed in Chapter 3 should include:

- Environment/situation analysis.
- Decision making.
- Identification of strategic issues.
- Development of general objectives.
- Development of specific program objectives.
- Formulation of strategic plan.
- Formulation of operational plan.
- Development of evaluation, monitoring, and tracking systems.

When results do not meet expectations, the consultant must review the process and return to her analysis and decision making phases. This is a natural task for consultants, as it is analogous to the consultative process itself. Strategic planning thus becomes an organizing tool for the consultation practice and for its marketing plan. Figure 41–1 illustrates the combining of important marketing elements to achieve a consultation marketing philosophy.

An occupational therapy consultation practice that subscribes to a societal marketing philosophy, utilizing a strategic planning system, will develop a broad and effective base for market planning. This sets the stage for, and may be concurrent with, an in-depth analysis of the client market.

MARKET ANALYSIS

The Marketing Environment

A key part of the marketing management process is the analysis of marketing opportunities. This analysis is based on information gathered through environmental assessments.

FIGURE 41–1

Building a Consultation Marketing Philosophy.

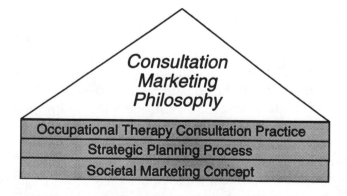

POTENTIAL CONSULTATION ENVIRONMENTS

Occupational therapists analyze environmental forces that affect their patients, in order to plan appropriate and effective intervention strategies. The occupational therapy consultant must follow the same course when considering her target markets. "The marketing environment consists of all the actors and forces that affect the [consultant's] ability to transact effectively with [her] target market."[12, p79] This environment is viewed from two perspectives, the microenvironment and the macroenvironment.[12]

Microenvironmental Analysis

Success within a given target market is the product of many different interactions. The microenvironment consisting of forces close to the consultant, will have the most direct effect. This includes four elements:

1. The consultant's internal business structure.
2. The identified client markets she proposes to serve.
3. The consultant's potential competitors.
4. The publics that have an interest in or impact on the consultant's ability to provide services.

The *consultant's business* must be critically analyzed to assure that market planning has taken the organization's strengths and weaknesses into consideration. A marketing perspective cannot start and end with the consultant alone. It must be reflected by everyone in the organization who interacts with external sources. The receptionist, typist, bookkeeper, and others in a small organization must be aware of, and sensitive to, the needs of the business' client group(s). In larger organizations, this must be reflected through various department heads and their respective staffs.

The consultant's *client markets* are viewed from the perspective of consultation levels. Most consultant practices will provide service at all three levels. Therefore, the consultant must understand the needs and wants of specific clients who require case-centered consultation; colleagues who require educational consultation; or larger systems which require program and/or administrative consultation. (See Chapter 2.)

The consultant's *competitors* must be analyzed in detail. Their approach to service delivery, ability to serve the market effectively, potential for collaborative involvement, cost effectiveness of their services, and their long- and short-range planning are all important concerns. To gain strategic market advantages, the consultant must effectively position her services against those of her competitors in the minds of potential clients.[9, 12]

The consultant's microenvironment also includes various publics. Kotler and Armstrong define a public as "any group that has an actual or potential interest in or impact on an organization's ability to achieve its objectives."[12, p60] They perceive seven types of publics which influence organizational functioning: financial, media, governmental, citizen-action, local, general, and internal publics. From a consultative perspective, these publics would influence the organization and its marketing strategies as follows:

- *Financial publics*. These are the consultation practice's funding sources, i.e., banks, investors, stockholders. The consultant seeks their good-will and continued support, so that her financial base is secure.
- *Media publics*. The consultant continuously seeks visibility through various media.
- *Government publics*. Health care consultation requires continuous monitoring of regulations and possible review with legal advisors.
- *Citizen-action publics*. Consumer groups can provide the consultant with important information and support, particularly when working with Level 3 client systems.
- *Local and general publics*. Expanded visibility and a broader client base may be achieved through involvement in local and community wide programs and organizations. This may include making donations of time and/or money.
- *Internal publics*. In larger consultation organizations and internal consultation settings, the management and staff of the total organization must be informed and motivated to support a positive marketing perspective.

Market planning must consider the consultation practice's publics, as well as the client market to be served. This dual perspective will provide the consultant with a broad base of support for her services.[12, 13]

Macroenvironmental Analysis

The larger macroenvironment considers forces that impact potential opportunities and/or threats to the consultation practice. An analysis of this environment should include review of demographic, economic, natural, technological, political, and cultural forces.

For example, a consultant considers the establishment of a consultation practice focused on the injured worker. She plans to locate in north central New Jersey, but could also extend her market into metropolitan New York City.

Demographics provide her with information on the size, density, location, age, sex, and race of injured workers, nationally and regionally. She learns that an increasing number of mid-life women are becoming injured, and that these numbers are rising more rapidly in central New Jersey. Employment sites for many of these women are the production lines and research centers of pharmaceutical companies.

Economically, she notes that the number of female injured worker compensation cases has grown 30% in the pharmaceutical field within the last 2 years. The central New Jersey corridor has a heavy concentration of pharmaceutical corporations. This industry is experiencing rapid growth and has shown a steady rise in profits. Since worker injury is costly, these employers will be motivated to prevent such problems.

Natural forces may have played a role in this unexpected rise. The ban on certain propellants, previously used by some of these companies, combined with concerns regarding chemical pollutants and non-biodegradable containers created a need to revise production protocols on a variety of products. One pharmaceutical company, in particular, reported a rise in hand injuries, which occurred on their newly revised production line.

Technologically, multiple new products were being contemplated by pharmaceutical companies in the region. Biotechnology was a major focus. From an injured worker perspective, the consultant observed that there were accidents in the research laboratories which might require closer scrutiny.

Political forces were supportive to the consultant's interests. New and expanded regulations emanating from federal and state departments of labor mandated closer monitoring of injuries and development of prevention strategies.

The *cultural environment,* which is concerned with the forces that affect society's basic values, perceptions, preferences and behavior, favored the growth of prevention and wellness programs for workers in the region. The consultant had already been involved in a local county health fair. She highlighted benefits achieved through worksite modification and special exercise for those prone to back injury. Her presentation drew many requests for information and elicited extensive comments from several pharmaceutical employees who felt this area was not being adequately addressed by their employers.

The consultant's macroenvironmental analysis led her to conclude that her identified injured worker focus was appropriate. Her target market picture was much more specific by virtue of her analysis. The location was changed to central New Jersey, and New York City was no longer considered. Since demographics indicated a larger midlife female population, she would need to adapt her training materials with this in mind.

Her initial focus would be the numerous pharmaceutical corporations located in this region. Information gathered during macroenvironmental analysis would become the foundation for marketing strategies. She also recognized that big-picture marketing strategies must have support from within.

The consultant and her organization must utilize microenvironmental analysis data to educate and prepare themselves for entry into this market. This required an intensive review of the internal organization's readiness to work with this industry. Knowledge of the pharmaceutical industry's specialized language, equipment and environments; product development emphasis; injured worker costs; and current prevention programs were important concerns. The consultant had had prior experience with injured workers from one pharmaceutical company, while working as a specialist in hand injuries. This provided her with immediate resources.

Expectations were that all three levels of consultation would be provided. Beginning with case consultation, the consultant planned to work through both the employee health and human resources departments.

Potential competitors had to be considered. These included private practice therapy groups who treated injured workers and consultants marketing their services as ergonomic engineers. The consultant knew she needed to have more extensive information regarding her competition, and published materials which would support use of her services rather than those of her competition.

Since she expected this planning process to take major funding, she needed to secure additional monies through her backers. She also built visibility through a well-orchestrated plan addressing the media, employee unions, regional and local community groups. Membership in national and state occupational therapy organizations, as well as other rehabilitation organizations, provided important networking opportunities and relevant current information. She would keep abreast of work related issues, legislative changes, and continuing education opportunities through these organizations and their publications.

Target Market

Environmental analysis used by the consultant helped segment her identified market, the injured worker, into a more specific target market. She was now able to plan and implement a marketing process targeted to at risk and injured pharmaceutical workers, located in a specific geographical region.

Research also provided her with a competitive edge. The industry's growing population of injured female workers had not been identified by others offering similar consultation services. Their promotional materials and training programs emphasized male workers with back injuries. Clearly, part of the consultant's target market strategy should be to point out the many women in this industry who were at risk for, or currently had, work-related hand injuries. This smaller segment of the target market is often referred to as a market niche.

Market Niche

In this case example, the consultant had taken her environmental analysis down another step and identified a specific segment of the injured worker population—a market niche—the injured female worker. As a small company, new to the industry, she must utilize creative methods to effectively position her services. This niche strategy will allow her to address the needs of a select but important group of people.

Niche marketing will provide a unique approach and different perspective from that of her competitors. Training and promotional materials can be uniquely designed; workplace assessments can address ergonomic differences between male and female workers; and the psychosocial environmental concerns of female workers can also be highlighted.

Using this niche marketing strategy, the consultant should find quick acceptance for her proposal and an invited entry to address the need. A continual environmental analysis would then allow the consultant to pinpoint other related needs in this industry, which she could effectively address at a later time.

This case example has discussed the important analysis of multiple factors and forces to consider as one plans entry in a given market. Figure 41–2 illustrates this process.

Multifaceted environmental concerns form a part of the consultant's market analysis. Broad-based environmental analysis is critical to planning. Using this information base, the consultant moves forward, making decisions which address today's needs and tomorrow's potential.

FIGURE 41–2

Analyzing the Consultation Market

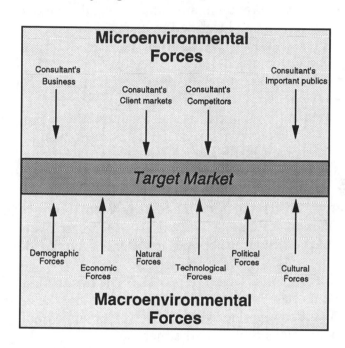

MARKETING STRATEGIES

Marketing occupational therapy consultation services requires an understanding of basic marketing concepts and their key elements, using a particular perspective. Marketing concepts were originally developed to sell physical products. Successful marketing makes the difference in your purchase of a Coke™ versus a 7-UP™ or a Ford™ versus a Nissan™. Services, however, are intangible; you cannot touch, taste, or smell the offered product. Thus, the consultant must recognize that not only are her services intangible, but that they are inseparably connected to her image and that of her business or organization. This perspective must be kept in mind as she develops her marketing mix.

Marketing Mix

The *marketing mix* consists of strategies which can be used to influence the demand for services in a target market. These are known as the controllable marketing variables of product, price, place, and promotion—often termed the "four Ps."[9, 11, 12, 19] The consultant studies her target market's needs and wants, and then designs appropriate services (her products) using effective pricing, location, and communication to inform and motivate potential clients to purchase her services.

Product

The product, occupational therapy consultation services, may have multiple "product lines" developed for a given market. The injured worker case, previously discussed, is an example. The product line developed around hand injuries occurring in a specific industry, predominantly among female workers. This segment of the industrial marketplace was identified by the consultant as her most promising target market. Later products may address such areas as back injuries, stress management, or job accommodation.

From an internal consultant perspective, consider the occupational therapist working in a long-term care facility. In this setting, she might see the need for a wheelchair management system that would assure better maintenance and use of facility equipment and, more appropriate, consistent positioning of patients.[5] Using environmental analysis, the consultant develops a proposal for this product. Her proposal calls for the development of a system that would be cost effective, provide greater equipment efficiency and more functional patient performance, and would address new regulatory mandates. With this in hand, the internal consultant would then present the proposal to her employer. She would seek approval to provide consultation services in order to facilitate development of this product.

Consultation, as we have seen, is a process. The occupational therapy consultant's product has its base in both technical expertise and the consultant's knowledge and skills. This combination allows the development of multiple product lines and a quick response to emerging market needs.

Consultation, as a *service product,* can be characterized as being intangible, inseparable, variable, and perishable.[12] While we have acknowledged the intangible nature of consultation, we should consider other characteristics of a service product.

Inseparability.—The consultant, her business or organization, and her client or client system are intimately connected. The client is present when the service is produced. Both consultant and client contribute to the consultation process and effect the service outcome.

Variability.—Consultation services can vary in accordance with the consultant's perspective, her interactions with the client, and the energy level and frame of mind of both parties at the time of interaction. Office employees can also contribute to the consultation encounter. Inconsistent behaviors and communications with clients lead to variable perceptions. The quality of all services must constantly be monitored as the consultation progresses.

Perishability.—Occupational therapy consultation services are perishable when a limited or fluctuating need exists. A consultant with a school-based target market does not have access to clients when school is not in session. A consultant whose target market includes state institutions must obtain contracts in these facilities when their budgets are first approved. As the fiscal year draws to a close, monies for optional projects are difficult or impossible to obtain.

A target market plan should consider these factors in consultation product design, along with a concern for the functional quality of the services delivered. Product quality depends on both the consultant's specific expertise and the way in which the services were delivered.[12] To establish and maintain a market, the consultant must provide a quality product.

Price

Price is another important component in the consultant's marketing mix. Many internal and external factors must be taken into consideration. Internal factors include the practice's overall goals and objectives and those related to the target market; costs directly and indirectly related to the provision of the specific consultation product; and the perspective and judgement of those responsible for setting the price, be it the consultant and/or another individual in the organization.

If, for instance, the consultant has just started to provide services in a specific target market, her pricing may be highly competitive, with very little profit margin. This may be done to get a "foot in the door" which hopefully leads to other referrals. Later contracts can then be priced allowing a better profit margin.

As was noted in Chapter 40, the entrepreneur consultant may be able to establish a fee for services based on what her expected salary would have been as an employee. Using a specific formula, she incorporates productive and non-productive time along with her overhead, which includes such business costs as rent, utilities, telephone, and support services. A significant non-productive cost to include is time spent in marketing. Well-known consultants suggest devoting the equivalent of one day a week to marketing activities and allocating at least 20% of the budget to this important business component.[1, 8, 23, 24, 25] This then yields a base for determining an hourly or daily fee for services. Along with this, the consultant must consider a profit margin and the rates competitors are charging for similar services. The total package is then analyzed in order to arrive at the actual fee for service.

External factors which affect pricing include type of market, level of competition, current economic situation, and legislation influencing client needs. For instance, when the Americans With Disabilities Act was passed, many firms learned they were not in compliance with new regulations.[10] Consultants with backgrounds in engineering, occupational health, vocational counseling, and occupational therapy began to compete for this market. Concurrently, there was a recession which limited funding for consultation. Occupational therapy consultants had to take these factors into account as they considered establishing competitive fees.

Management consulting firms usually figure their fees by dividing costs into thirds. These represent cost of the job, non-marketing overhead, and marketing overhead. To include a profit margin, which may range from 10 to 20%, they shade allocations for each cost center, according to the proposal they are costing out.[24]

Occupational therapy consultation is labor intensive and therefore personnel costs are greater. Figure 41–3 illustrates projected allocations for the case example consultation proposal. Note that the profit margin is minimal, since this consultant is interested in gaining entry to a target market. She might, in fact, work at cost without profit, if this was necessary to gain a foothold in the identified market.

The consultant must keep in mind that, while her special expertise is an important component in obtaining business, her clients frame their needs and wants within their business constraints. Good marketing and business practices include realistic fee setting that is profitable for the consultant and realistic for the client.

Various consulting experts differ on how to set fees. They agree, however, that a thorough assessment of all related costs is necessary in order to determine the most advantageous payment method. One can charge for consultation services by the hour, by the day, by establishing a fixed price per consultation, or on a retainer basis. Each method has its supporters.

Schrello[22] recommends an *hourly* fee, since it is difficult to define "a day." He points out that some clients take advantage of the consultant's flexibility, and turn 8 hour days into 18 hour days! An hourly rate will assure payment for days which extend into nights. For the benefit of both parties, their agreement should delineate the minimum to maximum range of hours expected to complete the consultation.

FIGURE 41–3

Allocation of Costs for Fee Setting When Entering a New Target Market

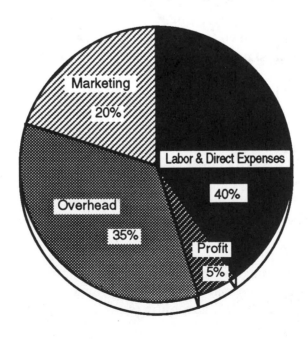

Payment by the hour is more common when the amount of consultation time required is not clear. This may be the case when performing a preliminary needs assessment. With in-depth information, a more specific time frame and fee can be identified for the comprehensive consultation.

Many consultants use a *daily fee* structure. They define the number of work hours in their consultation day when the contract is written. A day rate makes record keeping easier and billing less cumbersome.[8] Consultants billing either by the hour or day may also negotiate payment for such costs as travel, parking, hotels, meals, typing, telephone, and copying. The exact package of add-on costs varies with each agreement. Consultant and client may agree that no add-on costs will be included; they may identify a select few; or they may identify an extensive list that is acceptable to both parties.

Shenson[24] considers the most efficient and financially rewarding method to be *fixed-price* contracts. Surveys conducted by his organization indicate that consultants using this method earn more money than their peers. From a cost effective and quality assurance perspective, this pricing strategy holds up well.

A fixed-price contract requires careful determination of the client's needs to accurately set a fee. The consultant must determine:

- Time required to address client needs.
- Time cost, including labor, overhead, and profit.
- Site specific cost, i.e., travel, expenses, outside specialists.

When a client purchases services at a fixed fee, there are no "cost over-runs" and specific time parameters are established. It is the consultant's responsibility to cost out the service so that adequate time and personnel and overhead costs are included. If the consultant finishes early, and runs an efficient operation, her profit is larger; if she is late, runs into greater overhead expenses, or needs to call in extra help, she may end up losing money. In either case, the client is assured of services at a specific cost. The responsibility for efficient service delivery and greater profit rests with the consultant.

Retainers are also commonly used when contracting services. In some cases, the consultant requests "a retainer" as the initial payment for services when the preliminary consultation phase has begun. This may serve as reimbursement for the needs assessment phase. It can be followed by a more definitive contract, using an hourly, daily, or fixed price configuration. Retainer agreements are also used for clients who need periodic services. These agreements usually establish a minimum level of service to be provided. Beyond this minimum, additional fees are required.

Setting the appropriate fee, using a methodology which best serves the client and consultant, will lead to greater satisfaction for both parties. The value of the consultant's service is, in the end, decided by her clients. When prices are too high for the perceived value of service, the client will not make further purchases. Consultation services rely heavily on referral; a well-priced, well-received product will grow quickly in the identified target market.

Place

Consultation services are most commonly delivered at the client site. The consultant must determine how to place her services so that they are customized for each client in her target market. She must place them with her client efficiently and effectively. This is accomplished with an alternate "P," the *proposal*.

When clients seek services they frequently request a consultation proposal. Some proposals are given verbally, when the consultant and client meet to discuss a particular project. Most often, however, the proposal is carefully and clearly written by the consultant after she has thoroughly reviewed the consultation request. This document serves to identify the consultant's expertise and multi-faceted abilities that she will use to address client needs. In some cases, the proposal and contract can be the same document. More commonly, the proposal is a preliminary document, serving as a business and marketing tool.

A well-written proposal is the hallmark of a professional consultant. It demonstrates a professional attitude and sets the tone for future interactions. A good proposal is the "placing" marketing tool that convinces the client to retain your services.

Proposals may be written or verbal. As a written document, the format may be a multi-page proposal with appendices, a letter proposal, letter of agreement, or a contract. Some consultants recommend a less formal approach and prefer to work with verbal rather than written agreements.[1] However, all agree that some confirming documentation must exist. This should outline the responsibilities of both parties and specify the task(s) to be carried out by the consultant to reach agreed upon goals. Sample proposals and contracts are included in the Appendix.

The proposal provides the consultant with an opportunity to define the client's problem clearly and sketch a creative solution without disclosing key approaches planned for use. It whets the client's appetite and shapes his ideas and opinions about the project. The work demonstrates thought and research on the part of the consultant, while making the client aware that actual work on specific needs will be delivered during the consultation.

Fee setting, the price component, is also addressed. It describes the job to be performed by the consultant and states the cost for this service. The professionally presented proposal speaks well for the consultant; it indicates that she is, indeed, worth the money she is asking.

The consultant's proposal also provides an opportunity to demonstrate business acumen. It is written in the language of her target market, which enables a potential client to quickly become immersed in the material presented. The concluding section of the proposal is the budget.

This comprehensive document may set the stage for contract negotiations or serve as the contract itself. By placing a well-organized and convincing proposal in the client's hands, the consultant sets the stage for the consultation relationship. When several consultants are vying for the same client, the professional quality of your proposal will place it above that of your competitors.

Promotion

Promotion is the most familiar of the marketing mix concepts. It is the method used to communicate information regarding consultation services to specific markets. Promotional activities extoll the merits of the services and persuade clients to purchase them. The main promotional tools are advertising, sales promotion, public relations, and personal selling.[9, 12] Personal selling requires careful planning and a consultant who stays continuously alert for spontaneous opportunities to promote herself and her product(s). Mass marketing requires a more studied and structured approach, which need not rely as heavily on the consultant's skills alone.

Advertising utilizes paid media to inform and remind prospective clients of the consultant's services. Typical promotional strategies include telephone directory ads; brochures and other direct mail pieces describing the consultant's skills, abilities, and accomplishments; and business cards which create an image while giving important primary information.

Each target market presents opportunities for advertising. Industry publications, conference booklets, calendars, and fund-raising journals seek advertisers. The consultant may purchase a line, page, or part of a page to highlight her services. Advertising can also take the form of "give aways". Imprinted pens, magnets, coffee cups, key rings, note pads, and portfolio covers are just a few of the many items available. The end of the year also presents advertising opportunities. Holiday greetings and calendars are two commonly used communication and advertising tools.

Consultants frequently publish newsletters which discuss common problems faced by target market clients. This medium gives them an opportunity to highlight their expertise, educate potential clients who may not realize they have a need for services, and heighten client awareness to the consultant's availability.

The pharmaceutical industry consultant might, for example, prepare a newsletter discussing workplace design and its relationship to upper extremity cumulative trauma disorders. A case highlight could illustrate her success in redesigning workspace for a production line, which resulted in dramatic reduction of carpal tunnel syndrome. Copies of the newsletter can then be mailed to managers in the human resource and employee health departments of her target market. This strategy will alert potential clients and peak their interest.

Shenson notes that not only are newsletters excellent avenues to entice purchase of consultation services, but that they can also be packaged to elicit subscriptions in select markets. His survey of consultants showed that those with the highest incomes frequently used this technique.[23]

Sales promotion, where the consultant offers an incentive to potential clients who may need her service, is a less common technique. One strategy suggested is to offer free advice. Using an ad or flier, the consultant highlights a particular area of concern to a target market. The potential client is encouraged to contact the consultant in regard to this specific area to obtain free advice.

For instance, when the Americans With Disabilities Act(ADA) was implemented, many new regulations were promulgated. Among them were requirements to review job descriptions and provide job accommodations so that more disabled persons qualify for work.[2, 10] A consultant seeking this type of consultation task might highlight the issue in a flier or ad. She would offer to send those contacting her further information. The information sent could consist of a bibliography, recent interpretive guidelines, and a brief summary of some salient points from the regulations. Of course, she would simultaneously provide information about her services and follow up with a telephone contact.

The idea in sales promotion is to entice your client, provide a "taste" of the product, and encourage a desire for further contact. The client has received something small of value, at no cost, and is now ready to consider purchase.

Public relations is the mass marketing promotional tool that, from a consultation perspective, is closest to personal selling. Favorable publicity, a favorable personal and company image are public relations goals. In the case of consultation, a service, marketing should address image building. An effective public relations campaign will make the consultant's services appear more tangible and will create a positive image, tying the consultant, her expertise and that of her practice into one package.

The public relations process used for political campaigning provides an example of image building, or "person marketing."[12] While consultants may not have a public relations officer to create "photo opportunities" or to put a "spin" on their latest case, the press and other media can and should be accessed.

News releases, highlighting recent achievements or lectures, can be developed. A study or survey, conducted by the consultant, form the basis for a radio or TV interview. Articles published in magazines or journals which cater to the consultant's target market are effective testimonials to expertise. Lectures, given at meetings attended by potential clients, or those in a position to refer clients, bring visibility and referrals.

As we noted in the pharmaceutical case example, the consultant had participated in a community health fair. This public relations activity is keyed to the societal marketing concept, as it's focus is prevention and wellness through education of the general public. However, from a business perspective, image building and high visibility opportunities also make this a valuable public relations promotional activity.

Corporate identity materials also play an important role in recognition of the consultant and her practice. Attractive, distinctive and memorable logos, well designed business cards, stationery, and brochures; proposal formats and presentation covers which are well thought out and effectively packaged, are a part of an effective public relations plan.*

The consultant herself may volunteer time and contribute money to public service activities which relate to her target market(s). A consultant working within the developmentally disabled marketplace, may become involved in Special Olym-

---

* References 4,5,8,12,14,22,23

pics or wheelchair athletic organizations. Should mental health be her area of interest, she may seek appointment to a local board which oversees mental health programming in her county. If accessibility for the disabled is her area, involvement in the local parks and recreation commission may be appropriate. These activities provide the community organization with needed volunteer expertise and give the consultant a broader information base plus greater visibility.

Personal selling, the consultant's core promotional tool, is energized by the mass marketing tools of advertising, sale-promotion and public relations. Consultation is not a tangible product that has unlimited mass marketing opportunities. It does, however, have unlimited opportunities for creative personal selling, the consultant's key promotional strategy.

Selling may conjure up a negative picture if one views it from the perspective of "sales" and/or "sales pitch" promotions we have all experienced. From a consultation perspective, it is viewed as a personal interaction between two or more people, where communication, astute observation, and the ability to make quick adjustments are critical factors.[12]

A viable consultation practice must incorporate personal selling. "Marketing makes the task of selling easier; it sets expectations, it informs, it educates."[25, p6] Both marketing and selling are vital for success. Successful marketing prepares the client for the sales transaction. Marketing activities establish the consultant's image and reputation and increase the potential client's awareness of her availability to provide services. Selling provides the consultant with an opportunity to personally inform the client of her knowledge and skills and to relate these to the prospective client's specific needs and wants.[25]

Consultation experts agree that the most effective sales strategy is a personal referral. Shenson's study of successful consultants indicated that over 69% used client referrals as the basis for their marketing promotion.[25] McFarren points out another important factor to remember in regard to referrals. "Someone . . . pleased with [consultation] services will tell, on average, three other people. Someone who is displeased will tell eleven."[14, p18-2]

Presenting oneself to prospective clients requires planning and thoughtful preparation on a personal level. The consultant considers such areas as dress, presentation materials, presentation style, timing, and communication strategies. Her environmental analysis will also have provided key client information, which she will have integrated into her presentation plan. If she has already had a brief preliminary meeting with the client, this may influence such choices as her style of dress (tailored suit versus more casual outfit), method of presentation (informal versus video and slides to augment handouts) and her communication strategies (reflective versus directive.) Refer to Chapter 5 for further discussion on this topic.

Personal selling is an ongoing process. One never knows where or when the next referral source or potential client may arise. A very successful consultation was initiated by a consultant while she was a passenger on an airplane. Seated next to a man who was busy pouring over architectural drawings, she noted that he occasionally referred to photographs of people in wheelchairs. When the dinner break occurred, she initiated a conversation and casually informed her seatmate of her consultative experiences, including designing of specialized apartments for the disabled. This led to a discussion of the plans her seatmate was reviewing and their eventual use, a design for a group home for physically disabled young adults. The resultant consultation involved helping this client, an architect, plan the facility. The architect, in turn, referred the consultant to the agency who commissioned the plan. Work with the agency then centered on program development and implementation.

This case example illustrates the need for continuous preparation, so that one can "seize the moment!" While it is evident that personal selling is the consultant's most important tool, it is the unique blending of all marketing strategies which forms the ideal marketing plan for a given practice. Figure 41–4 illustrates this concept.

Marketing is an inherent part of any consultation practice. Utilizing theory and principles, the consultant entrepreneur selectively applies marketing strategies that promote her services in given environments. Recognizing that this is an ongoing process, she must develop a philosophy for practice which includes continuous marketing.

WORKING THE MARKET

Successful consultants possess the necessary attitudes and attributes to be successful marketers. These abilities must be energized through a marketing plan and

---

FIGURE 41–4

Promotional Marketing

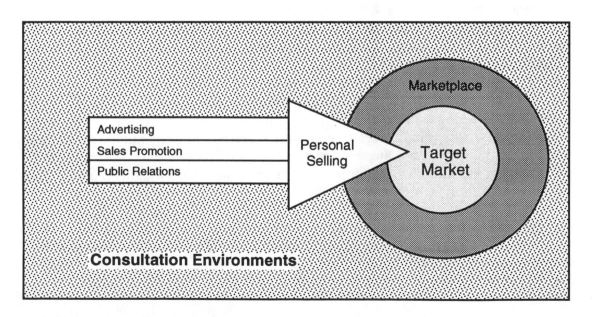

applied effectively using selective strategies. Consultation, a service product, therefore requires skillful marketing and selling and consistent dedication of time, energy, and money to the process.

Marketing is an ongoing activity. As we have noted, the consultant and her practice are always on stage. Her services cannot be separated from her image or reputation. Nor can the need for marketing be separated from the consultant's business expenses, professional consultation activities, or continued development of expertise. Marketing must be treated with the same regard that one uses in treating valued clients. Working the market means integrating consistent and meaningful marketing into consultation practice management.

This chapter has discussed various strategies necessary to integrate marketing into a practice. Two areas, indirect and referral marketing, are of particular importance to the consultant. They are marketing threads which should be woven into the fabric of the consultant's daily routine.

Indirect Marketing

The best reflection of effective marketing is when prospective clients seek the consultant. To achieve this goal, the consultant must enhance her professional stature and reputation through a form of personal selling, indirect marketing. Strategies should increase visibility and indirectly promote services. There are many indirect strategies to consider. Those used more frequently include networking; speaking and conducting workshops; authoring articles and books; and developing and marketing information products.

Networking serves as an excellent referral source. Networking opportunities arise frequently within one's profession, and in identified target markets. The consultant should consider becoming active in local, state, and national occupational therapy organizations and groups; membership in other professional organizations related to identified target markets; and involvement in local community agencies, boards or groups.[4, 15]

Networking can also provide opportunities for societal marketing. In California, for example, occupational therapy consultants helped form a coalition of agencies to advocate, coordinate and provide opportunities for persons with disabilities. Through this group, they have helped the community disabled access transportation, increase their recreational opportunities, and sustain jobs. Interprofessional connections fostered through this networking process also helped expand the consultants' advocacy activities for disabled persons. Outcomes have included an annual art show for persons with disabilities, expansion of public library services to meet the needs of those with developmental disabilities, and the inclusion of an occupational therapist position in a grant which provided services for disabled students.[7]

To use the networking process most effectively, the consultant must not sit idly within the group(s) she joins. It is through active involvement and assumption of leadership roles that visibility is attained and referrals are facilitated. Membership in a group is the starting point. Leadership not only helps obtain business, it also provides the consultant with further growth opportunities. Resource information is expanded, problem solving skills are enhanced, and consultation skills are honed. Through this process, the consultant's professional abilities are extended and strengthened.

Speaking at and conducting workshops provide opportunities to demonstrate expertise, problem solving abilities, organizational skills, and dynamic communication. Invitations to speak and educate other peer professionals and potential clients should be sought. Community service organizations are eager to have a new voice and presence at their meetings. Trade and professional associations want relevant, meaningful speakers who will present something of interest and value to members.

Seminars are equally important opportunities. The consultant may choose to organize and sponsor her own seminar or find an external sponsor. Today's information-based society and rapidly evolving technology require a knowledgeable workforce. Seminars are a particularly attractive method of quickly obtaining relevant information. Developing and presenting seminars of interest will facilitate the consultant's exposure to those who are in a position to use her services, or initiate a referral.[1, 4, 16, 17, 25]

While *authoring articles and books* may seem a foreboding task, it can be a valuable and consistent source of referral. Many professional groups generate weekly or monthly publications. Invariably, there is a need for new material that presents a fresh perspective on topics of concern. Their editors are more than willing to assist a novice author's article preparation. As the consultant's writing skills expand, she may seek publication in more prestigious journals or books. This free exposure not only keeps the consultant's name and organization in front of her market, it also provides concrete substantiation of her expertise.[1, 23, 25]

A client proposal that contains an addendum with a copy of a relevant article authored by the consultant, reinforces an expert image. Well-written, informative articles are passed on to decision makers at various levels in the corporate world. The ripple effect of this indirect marketing strategy is continuous.

Developing and marketing information products is not a common strategy for occupational therapy consultants. It usually evolves from market needs that the consultant has observed in the course of business. Bachner and Cunninghis describe the development of information products within their consultation practices in Chapters 9 and 11. The author, in her practice, also published and marketed a monograph that provided expanded visibility and increased referrals in the long-term care marketplace.[5]

Leading consultants strongly recommend publication of a newsletter as a marketing information product. The newsletter is viewed as a promotional tool for prospective and current clients. The newsletter should be narrowly focused, thus increasing the likelihood of target market readership. A well written, professionally presented newsletter familiarizes prospects with the consultant's expertise and her services. A newsletter with items of interest will also be shared, thus increasing visibility and potential referrals.[8, 22, 23, 25]

Indirect marketing presents varied opportunities to help the consultant subtly differentiate her services from those of competitors. Her active involvement in professional and community organizations creates a presence that is recognized, respected, and appreciated. Lectures, seminars and, publications acknowledge expertise, maintain visibility, and create a basis for quick recall when consultation services are considered. These marketing strategies flow naturally into a referral marketing approach.

Referral Marketing

Based on surveys of successful consultation practices, a well-managed occupational therapy consultation practice should be able to generate 80% of its business through referral.[25] Referrals and recommendations pave the way to an open door. The quality and effectiveness of your services have been promoted to a potential client by someone else. This is the most cost-effective marketing method.

Referral marketing focuses on the satisfied client who has used the consultant's services and the strategies used to encourage these clients to make referrals. It must consider creating network referrals; establishing a quality reputation; and maintaining the image of a dedicated professional.

To create *network referrals* the consultant must encourage referral sources to contact the potential client, rather than doing so herself. If the first call is made by the consultant, it is viewed as soliciting business. Therefore, the consultant must facilitate referral by using supportive strategies. A luncheon meeting with the consultant, potential client, and referral source may be one avenue. Other strategies may include:

1. Obtain in-depth data regarding the potential client's information needs on a topic. Suggest that the referral source mail this information to the potential client, indicating the consultant as the source. If the consultant must mail to the prospective client directly, it should be done with a cover letter that indicates the material is sent at the suggestion of the referral source. Indicate availability, should more information be required.

2. Advise referral sources that you don't solicit business. Suggest that the potential client be advised of your abilities and availability.

3. Use your knowledge regarding the referral source and the potential client to identify other innovative ways for the referral to be made without your taking the first step.[25]

It is critical for the consultant to maintain visibility and communication with her referral sources. Periodic telephone follow-up calls or a brief note to advise that the referred client's problems are being addressed helps generate continuing referrals.

Establishing a *quality reputation* requires faithful adherance to practice standards and ethics and a consultation philosophy that reflects concern for clients and society. Clients must value the consultant's expertise, perspectives, and approaches. These perceptions must be corroborated by professional activities, publications, and service to the community. Referrals are generated when the referring party is confident that the consultant's services will benefit the client. The concern is for the client, not the consultant. To support this image, the consultant must work diligently to assure that her behavior, business dealings, and practice are carried out in a professional and ethical manner.

It is also advantageous to have potential clients learn of the consultant's services through several referral sources. With expanded visibility and a broader reputation, the consultant is able to utilize multiple clients and/or colleagues as part of her referral network.

Maintaining *an image of hard-working consultant* is usually not difficult. Consultation requires a great deal of time and effort. There may, however, be times when all the hard work does not produce paying clientele. At that point, it is tempting to aggressively seek new business at the slightest hint of a potential client. Such a strategy portrays exactly the wrong image, that of someone hungry for work, who is not sought after for her services. Potential clients and referral sources must perceive the consultant as busy, successful, and in demand. The stance must indicate that, while she is interested in new referrals, she always has enough work to keep her well occupied.[1, 25]

Referral marketing requires an intuitive understanding of how and when to let potential referral sources know that you value and appreciate receiving their referrals. This marketing strategy can prove most lucrative and professionally rewarding. It is, therefore, important for the consultant to learn, practice, and perfect strategies that expand her referral market.[25]

CONCLUSION

A successful consultation practice must incorporate marketing into every aspect of business. Consultation is a service product and therefore is intimately related to the image, expertise, personality and philosophy of the consultant. Marketing consultation services requires astute identification of a client market, their needs and wants, in order to offer appropriate and desirable services.

Marketing concepts influence organizational philosophy and orientation. Through the use of a societal marketing concept the occupational therapy consultant expands the traditional marketing views to incorporate a more humanistic approach, which considers the well-being of both client and society. This concept is congruent with occupational therapy philosophy, and recognizes the environment's important role in planning and achieving identified goals. The consultant must also use strategic planning, in conjunction with a societal marketing philosophy, to assure a broad base for marketing management.

While many perceive marketing as advertising and selling, marketing's true value lies in its use as a diagnostic tool which helps determine who, what, when, and where to deliver consultation services. A key element in marketing management is analysis of macroenvironmental and microenvironmental forces, which provides necessary data to identify, confirm, and plan for services to specific target markets.

To develop need-satisfying services for specific clients, the consultant must price her offerings attractively; present a consultation proposal or agreement which places her services above those of competitors; design service products to meet client demands; and promote these services with an emphasis on indirect marketing techniques. A broad range of skills is therefore needed to sense, serve and satisfy any client market. Successful consultants must continuously dedicate time, energy, and money to this business component.

Today's occupational therapy consultant marketplace has expanded far beyond the walls of hospitals and institutions. Skyrocketing costs have created demands for alternative, cost effective approaches to health care, with a greater emphasis on prevention. This marketplace presents golden opportunities for knowledgeable, creative, and intuitive occupational therapy consultants to expand their services using a marketing philosophy and approach which is congruent with their practice beliefs.

REFERENCES

1. Bellman GM: *The Consultant's Calling*. San Francisco, Jossey-Bass, 1990.
2. Bowman OJ: Managers to play an important role in implementing the Americans with Disabilities Act. *AOTA Admin and Mgmt Sp Int Sec Newsltr* 1991; 7:3.
3. Drucker P: *Management: Tasks, Responsibilities, Practices*. New York, Harper and Row, 1973.
4. Epstein CF: Consultation: communicating and facilitating. in Bair J, Gray M (eds): *The Occupational Therapy Manager*, rev. ed. Rockville, MD, AOTA, 1992.
5. Epstein CF: *Wheelchair Management Guidelines*. Somerville, NJ, Occupational Therapy Consultants, 1981.
6. Gilkeson GE: Occupational therapy leadership potential can be developed through marketing techniques. *Occup Ther in Health Care* 1985; 2:4.
7. Hurff JM, Lowe HE, Ho BJ, et al: Networking: a successful linkage for community occupational therapists. *Am J Occup Ther* 1990; 44:424–430.
8. Holtz H: *How to Succeed as an Independent Consultant*, ed 2. New York, John Wiley & Sons, 1988.
9. Jacobs K: Marketing occupational therapy. *Am J Occup Ther,* 1987; 41:315–320.
10. Jurk JK: The Americans with Disabilities Act. *AOTA Phys Dis Sp Int Sec Newsltr* 1991; 14:3.
11. Kautzmann LN: Marketing occupational therapy services, in Cromwell FS (ed): *Private Practice in Occupational Therapy*. New York, Haworth Press, 1985.
12. Kotler P, Armstrong G: *Principles of Marketing,* ed 5. Englewood Cliffs, NJ, Prentice-Hall, 1991.
13. Kotler P, Clarke RN: *Marketing for Health Care Organizations*. Englewood Cliffs, NJ, Prentice-Hall, 1987.
14. McFarren SS: Marketing and public relations, in Hertfelder SD, Crispen C (eds): *Private Practice: Strategies for Success*. Rockville, MD, AOTA, 1990.

15. Micheals PS: Role of networking in managerial development. *AOTA Admin and Mgmt Sp Int Sec Newsltr* 1986; 2:3.
16. Miyake S, Kraml-Angle D: From hospital to community—the health care challenge of the 1980's, in Johnson JA, Jaffe E (eds): *Occupational Therapy: Program Development for Health Promotion and Preventive Services*. New York, Haworth Press, 1989.
17. Miyake S, Lucas-Miyake M: Health promotion: a marketing tool for industry, in Johnson JA, Jaffe E (eds): *Health Promotion and Preventive Programs: Models of Occupation Therapy Practice*. New York, Haworth Press, 1989.
18. Olson TS: Health care marketing, in Hopkins HL, Smith HD (eds): *Willard and Spackman's Occupational Therapy,* ed 6. Philadelphia, Lippincott, 1983.
19. Olson TS, Urban C: Marketing, in Bair J, Gray M (eds): *The Occupational Therapy Manager*. Rockville, MD, AOTA, 1985.
20. Ostrow P: Strategic planning, in Bair J, Gray M (eds): *The Occupational Therapy Manager,* Rockville, MD, AOTA, 1985.
21. Ostrow P: Strategic Planning. *AOTA Admin and Mgmt Sp Int Sec Newsltr* 1987; 3:4.
22. Schrello DM: *The Complete Marketing Handbook for Consultants*, 2 vols. San Diego, CA, University Association, 1990.
23. Shenson HL: *Complete Guide to Consulting Success*. Wilmington, DE, Enterprise Publishing, 1987.
24. Shenson HL: *The Contract and Fee-Setting Guide for Consultants and Professionals*. New York, John Wiley & Sons, 1989.
25. Shenson HL: *Shenson on Consulting*. New York, John Wiley & Sons, 1990.

SECTION C

Rationale for the Development of an Occupational Therapy Theory of Consultation

CHAPTER 42

Toward a Theoretical Model of Occupational Therapy Consultation

Evelyn G. Jaffe, M.P.H., O.T.R., F.A.O.T.A.
Cynthia F. Epstein, M.A., O.T.R., F.A.O.T.A.

"If occupational therapy is to experience significant growth in the next
25 years, it must be via development of its potential for providing health
consultation. . . ."—*Wilma West*

INTRODUCTION

Overview of a Theoretical Model of Occupational Therapy Consultation

The goal of this chapter is to examine the basis and present a rationale for the
development of a theoretical model of occupational therapy consultation. Such a
model will provide a base of knowledge to strengthen practice, and it will validate
the premise that consultation is an inherent part of the occupational therapy
process. The proposed model is a synthesis of the theoretical bases from which the
process of consultation and the principles of occupational therapy are derived, and
it provides a framework for occupational therapy consultation practice.

The nature of occupational therapy practice fosters an environment of mutual
cooperation between the dysfunctional patient and the therapist. An inherent goal
is to enable disabled individuals, through improved occupational performance, to
function in daily life and take charge of their lives.[70] Similarly, the nature of
consultation requires an environment of mutual cooperation and collaboration
between the client system and the consultant. Enabling the client, through improved performance, to create positive change and increase the organization's
functional performance is the consultation goal.

Underlying both processes is a strong foundation in systems theory, which, by
definition, acknowledges the integral part played by the environment. The environ-

ment can have both a direct and indirect influence on the occupational performance of a given patient/client. Therefore, occupational therapists must be skilled in the therapeutic use of the environment. As therapists identify environmental implications, utilizing direct therapeutic intervention, a role shift may occur that requires a consultative approach. This shift does not preclude the therapist's continued treatment role, rather it imposes a duality of roles within the environmental context. While not always acknowledged as an important component of practice, occupational therapy clinicians, educators, and researchers use consultation principles routinely in their professional activities. Further development of consultation skills will enhance the therapist/consultant's effectiveness in facilitating patient, and/or client achievement of improved function.

The proposed occupational therapy consultation model is based on human ecology with a foundation in systems theory and recognizes the dynamic quality of the patient/client environment and therapist/consultant environment interactions. Ecology, the study of the relationship between organisms and their environments, recognizes the dynamic state existent between the various components of the ecosystem. These components are continuously altered by the interplay of natural and human influences. Using extensive and intensive analysis of the environment, the therapist, as consultant, applies the principles of occupational therapy and the process of consultation to facilitate and enhance function for the client system. Working within the client's natural setting, the consultant seeks to preserve the supportive and nurturing aspects of the environment, while encouraging adaptation and change to further the goal of improved function. With a perspective that emphasizes important concepts of prevention, the consultant aims to help the client prevent future problems.

This occupational therapy model of consultation and the generic process of consultation are derived from many of the same scientific theories. A fundamental aspect of this model is the incorporation of basic occupational therapy principles; philosophical assumptions, including man's interrelationship to his environment; and the theoretical premises by which the profession is identified. This model, developed from a synthesis and integration of these bases, provides a theoretical framework and guide to occupational therapy consultation practice.

Using an occupational therapy frame of reference, the therapist, as a health consultant, can create an environment for change. Applying occupational therapy concepts, principles, and practice approaches, the consultant is able to transfer these abilities into an effective consultation model. This chapter examines the concepts underlying the synergetic relationship between occupational therapy, human ecology, and consultation.

CONSULTATION: AN INTEGRAL COMPONENT OF OCCUPATIONAL THERAPY PRACTICE

Evolution into Consultation

Occupational therapy clinical practice requires specific knowledge and skills and the ability to assume various roles. As discussed earlier, therapists in clinical settings often are required to assume both clinical and consultative roles. For clarity, many discussions compartmentalize these functions into direct and indirect services. The inference is that they always should be discrete entities. In practice, however, the therapist moves naturally from one role into the other, often within the space of a single client session.

The clinical decision-making process requires that the therapist maintain awareness of many factors which contribute to the problem being treated, as well as of the environmental context required to support desired functional outcomes. Control, a key determinant in treatment, may shift from therapist to client to caregiver as the need to address environmental issues arises.

The total environment is an important concern for the clinician as well as the consultant/therapist. In both roles, he or she must recognize interactive environmental dynamics that influence the outcome of planned interventions. The environment is viewed from human and non-human, or physical, perspectives. The physical environment—space, objects, sensory cues, and their relationships—are critical concerns. A cognitively impaired older person, for example, will respond more appropriately in a low stimulus environment where familiar furnishings, glare free light, and mild temperature provide a calming and supportive setting. The human environment—health professionals, family members, caregivers, and friends surrounding and supporting this person—also must understand and respond appropriately to behaviors that may appear aberrant to an uneducated eye. Without this human and non-human environmental support, the patient/client's improved function cannot be sustained.

The therapist may assume the role of "environmental manager,"[55] facilitating social or cultural change within the human environment to support the treatment goals established. Concurrently, she may assume the role of "environmental engineer"[52, 55] to address physical/architectural environmental barriers. The human environment must demonstrate motivation for change. Change, then, can be facilitated through a collaborative and/or educational consultation approach. Thus, the therapist's role shifts to a consultative perspective within the larger treatment context, and consultation becomes part of the service delivery model.

Using the treatment setting as her invited, planned, or opportunistic entry point, the therapist/consultant seeks sanction for her consultation role with the client/caregiver or support system. This takes place within or in relation to the natural environment and acknowledges the environment's important role in achieving the client's long-term goal. Familiarity with the initial presenting problem facilitates the development of a diagnostic base for the consultation. The therapeutic relationship with the client has allowed the building of trust, essential to the consultation process. The locus of control is the most critical part of the shift. Many therapeutic relationships foster dependency, therefore the client and caregiver may expect to be led rather than to have to participate in solving the problem and controlling the final decision. While most occupational therapy interventions inherently involve the patient and caregiver in the collaborative development of the treatment plan, the final decision making power usually rests with the therapist.

Successful transition to a consultation model, therefore, requires that the therapist/consultant accurately assess patient/client and caregiver readiness and motivation, so client and caregiver can assume a more directive role in decision making and implementation.

The use of both the direct treatment model and the indirect consultative model allows the therapist/consultant to orchestrate the gradual transfer of control to the client and caregiver through an educational process. As the emphasis on consultation builds, the therapist/consultant also may be required to assume an advocacy role and to address issues that will have an impact on the client's natural environment. These often include issues related to the health care system in general and to the social support system, and issues that may have legal implications for the client's welfare.

This natural evolution from therapist to consultant and the fluidity of role shifts within the treatment context provides the therapist/consultant and her patient or client with a flexible, goal-directed plan and process. The use of consultation enhances and reinforces the chances of maintaining achieved functional outcomes. The client will have a stronger commitment to sustaining the positive change, with the secure knowledge that the therapist/consultant is open to renegotiation should the need arise.

In their own practice evolution, the principle authors have analyzed the development of their therapist/consultant roles. Throughout their professional careers, occupational therapy principles have guided their activities. Additional training in the theory, process, and basic concepts of consultation enhanced their knowledge and skills. The following vignettes are shared to help the reader view the rhythmical flow of consultation principles and the environmental and systems influences that supported their clinical judgments and guided the evolution of their consultative practice model.

The Therapist/Consultant in an Acute Care Community Hospital

Acute-care settings require adherence to a medical model structure and an understanding of the fiscal constraints governing patient length of stay. As a relatively new occupational therapy graduate, Cynthia Epstein worked in a community hospital which served a culturally diverse population in a large urban community. Her primary caseload consisted of older persons with diagnoses of cerebral vascular accidents (CVA), lower and upper extremity fractures, and congestive obstructive pulmonary disease.

Treatment interventions were time-limited, due to length of stay constraints and minimal staff availability. In this medically focused environment, Epstein was required to generate specific measurable objectives for her treatment and relate them to functional outcomes. Her interventions mandated adherence to treatment strategies which were focused in a biomechanical frame of reference, where the emphasis was on range of motion, muscle strength, motor planning, coordination, and self-care activities of daily living. Yet she felt the patient population required a more holistic approach to achieve the identified functional goals. The acute-care environment had the potential to support this concern, given the relatively consistent presence and proximity of the patients' community caregivers.

Hospital-based caregivers, less consistent and more stressed by productivity demands, could not be counted on to provide ongoing environmental support. Within the staff pool, however, select caregivers had responded positively to Epstein's educational programs regarding carry-over of treatment gains to the daily care routine. Assuming a consultant role, she worked with the medical and nursing staff to help plan a rehabilitation unit within the hospital. Motivated staff caregivers then could be trained and assigned to the unit. An environment was planned to allow for a more holistic team approach to treatment.

In this changed environment, Epstein, in her role as therapist/consultant, then would be able to utilize both direct treatment and indirect consultative strategies as the need arose with given patients, staff, and caregivers. Financial implications and length of stay were constraints placed on the therapist/consultant and the team, forcing increased emphasis on consultation. As she used a more collegial and educational approach, the therapist/consultant's influence was extended into the community settings. Here she consulted with community caregivers and community-based professionals, who were to assume supportive and/or treatment roles with each patient.

Working extensively in the patients' natural environments, inside and outside the hospital, helped Epstein expand her consultation skills. Increasingly, she became aware of the synergistic relationship between the natural environment, the patient, and the patient's human support system. The dynamic interplay between the individuals involved, their cultural heritage, social interactions, and multiple system needs, led to an increased awareness of the potentially important role that occupational therapy consultants could play.

Further study of consultation theory, process, and principles followed and Epstein expanded her practice, using both clinical treatment and consultation models. Sparse and often minimally utilized occupational therapy services in long-term care presented a challenge. Convinced that a combined treatment and consultative approach could strengthen occupational therapy services, improve patient function, and expand team involvement, she organized a group practice based on this belief. The utilization of collegial consultation and mentorship for the therapists/consultants in the group has been an equally important concern.

Schools, developmental centers, adult–day-care centers, nursing homes and home settings are now common sites for the group's clinical and consultative services. The practice philosophy, mentioned above, has helped therapists in the group develop and expand their consultative skills. Through this expanded emphasis on consultation; administrators, managers, and staff in institutional and community programs, as well as individual patients/clients in these settings, have developed and enhanced their functional abilities.

The Therapist/Consultant in a University Medical Center and Teaching Hospital

Transition from traditional occupational therapy practice in institutional settings to a broader concept of the delivery of services, in a variety of environments, usually occurs over time. Evelyn Jaffe became interested in the concepts of consultation as part of her occupational therapy activities during the late 1960s, while on the staff of the Children's Psychiatric Hospital at the Neuropsychiatric Institute, University of Michigan Medical Center. Many of the leaders in social research cited in this text, including Ronald Lippitt and Floyd Mann, were working at the University of Michigan's Institute for Social Research and Survey Research Center during this time. Their views on social behavior, systems theory, change theory, organizational development, and consultation concepts were of particular interest to this therapist. As an early student of Ronald Lippitt, during her undergraduate education, Jaffe became aware of the need to understand human behavior and to learn how to develop change strategies if one was to work with individuals or groups in any capacity.

Health professionals involved in the community mental-health movement in Ann Arbor were allied with Research Center scientists, some of whom also served as clinical faculty for the Neuropsychiatric Institute (NPI). Their collaboration and interchange of ideas provided stimulating and provocative discussion for the university hospital staff. Jaffe, as a member of an NPI staff development committee, became involved in the development of a psychiatric staff consultation training program, primarily for psychiatrists in residency.

Participation on this committee provided Jaffe with an opportunity to receive comprehensive training in the skills and process of consultation, establish outreach services to community agencies, and, eventually, develop a community fieldwork program for occupational therapy students. Although sanctioned by hospital executive administrators, there was little approval, support, or encouragement from the department of occupational therapy to venture into the community. This was a novel idea, considered by many department staff to be outside both the function and role of the occupational therapists in the institution.

At this time, there were very few, if any, community field placements for affiliating occupational therapy students. Jaffe presented a proposal, with clearly stated goals and educational objectives, to convince supervisory occupational therapy staff to allow students release time from their clinical duties, once a week, to participate in an *experimental* community placement. Influenced by Lippitt's concepts of planned change,[39] the therapist attempted to convey change-theory ideas to the staff, recognized their initial resistance to untraditional therapist and student roles, and proposed a trial period, with continual monitoring and evaluation of the program.

The community field placement project was created because of Jaffe's conviction that occupational therapists needed to have greater understanding of normal behavior and functional performance, and standard growth and development in order to understand the pathology and dysfunction they were expected to treat in the clinic or institution. Additionally, it was felt that occupational therapy concepts and knowledge could be applied to services to the community that currently were not being utilized. Resources for community fieldwork placements were identified and contacts were made to various agencies prior to the development of a program for occupational therapy students.

This community involvement also led to the realization that prevention of dysfunction should be part of the training of occupational therapists. Although concepts of disease prevention and health promotion were not acknowledged widely at this time, several occupational therapy leaders, as mentioned in Chapter 7,[21, 64, 67] had expressed the need for members of the profession to expand their practice into the community and adopt preventive approaches to the delivery of their services. Consultation in the community was an opportunity for occupational therapists to be involved in changes in the delivery of services that included expansion beyond traditional health care practices.

Community student placements emphasized the role of the occupational therapist as a change agent regarding the lifestyle and behavior of individual participants in community agencies or programs, and the organizational structure and program planning of the agencies themselves. Jaffe, in her roles as consultant to community agencies and student fieldwork supervisor, established the networks necessary for students to conduct community recreational programs; public school tutoring for pupils with special needs; programs at group settlement homes for disadvantaged children; and other special community activities. These included activity and music programs in community preschools and homes for older adults and support groups for children with learning disabilities, shutins, stroke patients, and developmentally delayed young people. The students had an opportunity to observe normal patterns of life stages and learn how occupational therapy concepts could be applied to settings outside the traditional medical institution, while providing preventive health services at all levels of prevention intervention. Additionally, the therapist/consultant improved her own consultative skills and strengthened her personal convictions of the role of occupational therapists in community health, disease prevention, and health promotion.

These early consultation experiences and the community field placement program for occupational therapy students were the forerunners of a career as a private community consultant. Jaffe has expanded her initial consultations, while maintaining traditional occupational therapy concepts and the basic principles of a holistic, ecological approach to occupational therapy service delivery. Further development of a consultation practice has emphasized concepts of disease prevention and health promotion throughout the consultative activities. These activities have included consultations to teenage-parent programs and community-wide maternal and child health programs for high-risk populations; identification of children at risk; public school organizational development; and development of family life education and parenting skills programs in public schools. In addition, consultations have been provided for program development in community agencies, identification of community mental health priorities, and health education in the workplace to a number of facilities and corporate industries. Although the consultations are varied, requiring a full repetoire of roles and functions, all are based on basic models of consultation theory and the model of occupational therapy consultation proposed in this chapter.

Relationship Between Treatment and Consultation

These vignettes illustrate familiar practice concerns, reframed to help the reader focus on the reciprocal relationship between treatment and consultation roles. As therapists, the authors found that their patient/client interventions required ongoing awareness of the larger environment or community systems. To assure the desired functional outcomes, a consultative role was integrated into their practice model. This natural evolution did not separate the clinical or direct treatment model artifically from the consultative or indirect model. The underlying goal was to provide help for the patient or client and the system or environment. Plans were developed to meet their needs. It was clear to the authors that the consultative aspects of planning were critical components in the overall intervention strategies.

The similarity between the occupational therapy treatment process and the basic process and phases of consultation is evident. It demonstrates that a mutually supportive and synergistic relationship can exist between direct treatment roles and indirect consultative approaches. Understanding and effectively utilizing these approaches help reinforce the important role of the environment for both therapist/ consultant and patient/client. Thus, the occupational therapy treatment/ consultation interaction bonds these processes together.

The transference of occupational therapy treatment planning skills to consultation planning appears to be a natural transition, easily following the progression of a practice. Figure 42–1 illustrates the similarity between these two processes, while acknowledging their unique differences.

Working within the client's natural environment, the occupational therapist may utilize each process independently or concurrently as a *process within a process*. This symbiotic relationship enhances the therapist/consultant's knowledge in each realm and her performance on behalf of the patient/client. Similarities in steps are evident as one proceeds through the various phases and looks at parallel tasks.

After the diagnostic phase (step 3), monitoring, modification, and refinement of plans, strategies, and interventions occur continually. During steps 4 through 7, the therapist/consultant constantly reassesses patient/client response. A fluidity exists which allows the therapist/consultant, in concert with the patient/client, to modulate the focus and interaction of the intervention plan. Ongoing refinement during these phases in either the treatment or consultation process assures a dynamic and responsive intervention approach. The end steps of termination and follow-up/renegotiation in each process bring the intervention to a close, with options for future involvement.

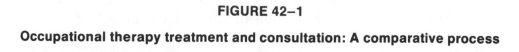

FIGURE 42–1

Occupational therapy treatment and consultation: A comparative process

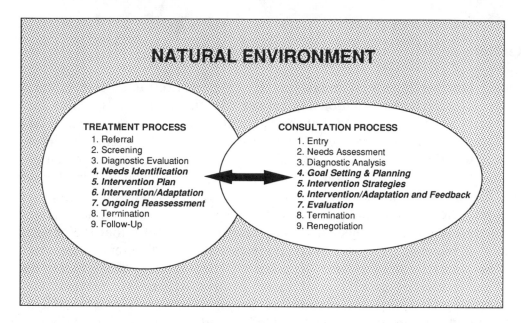

OCCUPATIONAL THERAPY CONCEPTS: A FOUNDATION FOR CONSULTATION PRACTICE

Current occupational therapy clinical practice has roots in a variety of philosophies and theoretical approaches. Concepts inherent in many of these have led the principal authors toward development of a model of occupational therapy consultation practice. In addition to occupational therapy theoretical constructs, humanistic, systems, and ecological concepts must be considered in the occupational therapy consultation process.

The theoretical constructs and frames of reference derived from occupational therapy philosophy incorporate perspectives and concepts from various schools of thought. Major themes relating to occupational therapy and consultation practice include humanistic roots and a preventive perspective. Theories and models that view the environment and concepts of adaptation as central to the therapeutic process are also important in consultation. A review of selected premises in each of these areas will identify concepts that influence and support the use of consultation in the delivery of services.

Humanistic Roots

Adolph Meyer, considered by many to be the founder of a philosophy of occupational therapy, conceived of man as interacting with his environment and living in harmony with his own nature and the nature that surrounds him. He described occupation as the way in which human behavior was organized. Health was considered the balance of work, rest, play, and sleep.[47] This holistic, humanistic approach of Meyer formed the theoretical framework of early models of occupational therapy practice.

Slagle, building on Meyer's philosophy, expanded these concepts through her focus on habit training by which mentally ill patients were provided with meaningful occupation to overcome and/or modify negative behaviors (habits) and develop positive ones.[27, 55] She instituted graded activities to nurture the development of balanced life rhythms. The patient then could carry over these new habits from the institutional environment to a natural environment in the community. In its developing years, the profession gradually established a presence in various hospital settings.

Bing, describing the "second generation" of occupational therapists, which emerged in the late 1920s and 1930s, commented on their further expansion of services within a humanistic framework. Through the efforts of this dedicated group, the definition of occupational therapy was modified to include key concepts from the social and behavioral sciences and the role played by the developmental process. At that time, occupational therapists, working in hospital-based physical and psychiatric rehabilitation programs, also assumed advocacy roles to help develop community support groups for former patients and to expand federal legislation for vocational rehabilitation services.[8]

In the middle of the 20th century, the humanistic perspective of occupational therapy was subsumed by a "scientific" medical model and a mechanistic approach, which precipitated a crisis in the practice of occupational therapy. Shannon, in his landmark treatise "The Derailment of Occupational Therapy," examines the circumstances leading to this practice crisis.[57] By allying itself with the rehabilitation movement, an outgrowth of the medical model, and by the devaluation of the traditional use of arts and crafts, occupational therapy assumed a reductionist perspective. Shannon defines reductionism, in concert with Reilly, as "the process of reducing complex phenomena into simplistic constructions of reality."[57, p232] He suggests that adherence to Reilly's broader hypothesis that "man through the use of his hands as they are energized by mind and will, can influence the state of his own health,"[51, p2] would bring the occupational therapy profession back to its humanistic roots.[57]

Kielhofner and Burke, writing concurrently with Shannon, reviewed the first 60 years of occupational therapy. They, too, noted that the humanistic roots of occupational practice had been overshadowed by dominant treatment models which reflected a reductionist approach. Meyer's model was exchanged for more tangible treatment technology, which paved the way for the development of measurable outcomes. This exchange narrowed the scope of occupational therapy practice. Kielhofner and Burke observed that a theoretical framework, if it is to encourage the advancement of the profession, must go beyond reductionism, and aim for an understanding of the principles of human adaptation. This, they proposed, could be achieved through the occupational behavior perspective.[34]

The occupational behavior perspective, initially proposed by Reilly, is a generic frame of reference.[53] Rogers states that it is "based on the occupational nature of humans and the dynamics of occupation for facilitating health and wellbeing."[55, p94] This perspective is a multidimensional concept and has a scientific knowledge base. Knowledge of occupational behavior is organized in a developmental and systems framework.

Preventive Approach

Paralleling the concerns and perspectives of Reilly and her associates, West,[64] Mazur,[46] Llorens,[40] Wiemer,[67] and Finn[21] spoke eloquently about humanistic approaches to occupational therapy practice, which could be achieved through prevention and consultation. These authors challenged practitioners to focus on the needs of individuals in the community, in addition to those in the hospital. Supporting a humanistic perspective, West proposed the role of health agent for occupational therapists. She observed that such a step would place the profession within the larger health arena, rather than remaining solely within the confines of medicine. This, she asserted, was "in keeping with our traditional concern for the person rather than just his disability."[64, p14]

Mazur, in her discussion of the occupational therapist as a consultant, supported a public health approach, or "action model," which emphasized being a helper or enabling leader for the community. This, she suggested, would provide occupational therapists with a unique opportunity" to stand for man's need for wholeness and his need for experiences to support and nurture that wholeness."[46, p421]

Llorens described and advocated a developmental approach as therapists began expanding preventive services into the community. Viewing the client from a developmental continuum perspective would allow the therapist "to support appropriate [client] growth and development and to facilitate the process of enculturation," meaning "the ability of the individual to adjust to a society's patterns of culture."[40, p338] In Llorens's humanistic view, culture can play a key role in helping the individual cope with the external environment. It has broad implications for the achievement of success across the developmental continuum of desired life roles.

Wiemer, in her discussion of prevention, observed the compatability between preventive health care concepts and occupational therapy principles. She asserted that the profession "has an obligation to make significant contributions to the promotion of society's health." Prevention, she indicated, could "be the realization of the profession's unique and real value to mankind."[67, p9]

The accelerated pace of change occurring in the early 1970s triggered Finn's concern and focus on prevention. Occupational therapists must refocus their attention to maintaining health, she stated, thus helping stem the growing tide of human suffering. Harking back to early roots, she indicated that occupational therapists must "devote [their] attention to the social disorders which not only affect the physical life of the individual but also have social, psychological and economic ramifications for the individual, his family and the society at large."[21, p61]

As occupational therapy moved into the last decades of the 20th century, these humanistic values and perspectives, which encompassed an emphasis on disease prevention; a broader understanding of systems theory; and a growing body of knowledge, indicated the profession's readiness for more extensive theory building. Theories were presented to help therapists develop a rational basis from which to make decisions.

Development of Occupational Therapy Theoretical Constructs

For many years occupational therapists seemed to practice on intuitive, basic instincts of what was good for their patients. Little thought was given to any theoretical basis for their actions, and the only common frame of reference appeared to be the professional focus on activity and activity analysis. It appeared sufficient to many therapists that validation of their practice came in the form of support from physicians, psychologists, and other respected professionals who promoted the value of occupational therapy.[42] As other allied health disciplines emerged and began struggling for identity, occupational therapists began identifying theoretical frames of reference specific to occupational therapy practice. Various conceptualizations of occupational therapy theory have evolved since. Additionally, the development of a professional theory base was considered imperative in order to articulate and validate the value of occupational therapy practice to others, including the health consumer, professional colleagues, administrators, and legislators.

The occupational therapy literature of recent years abounds with discussions of the need to articulate a professional theory, either as one unifying conceptual framework ("monism"), or as a multiplicity of constructs that contribute to a pluralistic approach to practice.[49] Also presented in the literature are definitions of theoretical terminology, descriptions of differing or complementary theoretical concepts and frames of reference, and the necessity of documenting practice methodology and validating these theories with clinical outcome studies and empirical research.* Argyris and Schon suggest that theories are important guides to professional practice, as they assist the actions of the practitioner and help explain, control, and predict behaviors.[5]

All point to professional development and maturation, and an evolving basis for practice in the search for a distinctive identity in a changing, competitive world. This evolution should be viewed as a positive force that helps create an ever-renewing discipline. Gardner supports the premise that the process of maturation

---

* References 6,12–14,23,35,49,51,55,68,71.

should not be stopped. When a profession, organization, or individual freezes change by simply acquiring established ways of doing things, they are certainly "headed for the graveyard." "In the ever-renewing society what matures is a system or framework within which continuous innovation, renewal, and rebirth can occur."[22, p5]

It is not the intent of this text to detail all the conceptualizations of occupational therapy. However, a brief review is given of some concepts that are essential as a foundation for the on-going development and maturation of a model of consultation practice. As discussed in the previous section, strong and consistent themes identified by early founders and reaffirmed by more recent theorists, are the recognition of humankind's need to engage in meaningful occupation within natural environments and the importance of adaptation and the environment as organizing factors.*

Occupation within Natural Environments

Building on the humanistic concepts established by their founders, occupational therapists proposing theoretical constructs in the latter half of the 20th century† also emphasize the importance of the environment in relation to occupational therapy practice. The dynamic interaction between the individual and the environment is viewed in relation to purposeful activity or occupation. The process of adaptation, necessary for humans to cope successfully in their environment, is reinforced as central to the occupational therapy treatment process. Occupational performance and occupational behavior frames of reference emerge, which draw on these concepts and further expand relationships to biological, behavioral, and sociocultural theories.

The occupational performance frame of reference is concerned with the accomplishment of life tasks related to self-care, play, leisure, work and learning. Performance components underlying these areas include sensory, motor, psychological, social, cognitive functions, and self-care, work and leisure.[41] It involves integration of the bio-psychosocial dimensions of man.[54] The environment, Llorens observes, demands that individuals successfully perform life tasks in order to assume social or life roles. Such roles as worker, parent, mate, and peer must also "be consistent with cultural requirements at specific ages and stages across the life span." [43, p46]

In the occupational behavior perspective, Reilly emphasizes play and work as part of a continuum in which mastery of the environment and attainment of health are achieved through occupation.[53] The environment (human and non-human) is viewed as a critical factor in shaping behavior. Human occupation (behavior) develops from "an innate urge to explore and master the environment."[34, p573]

---

* References 12,13,35,47,51,52,54,66,70.

† References 7,11,13,35,41,51,55,71.

There is a dynamic interaction between man (the system) and the environment, which produces occupational behavior. This behavior may be functional or dysfunctional, dependent upon the information received from the system. Rogers indicates that therapists "must understand the environment and how it influences occupation" if they are to facilitate human adaptation and elicit occupational behavior."[55, p105] As Reilly originally postulated, "human adaptation falters when meaning cannot be derived from environmental interactions."[53, p15]

Yerxa discusses the unique blend of values which support occupational therapy practice. She points to occupational therapy's belief in the right to a quality of life, supporting healthy behaviors, enabling patient autonomy, fostering mutual cooperation between therapist and patient, and recognition of the healthfulness of a balanced participation in activities. Occupational therapy, she asserts, must create a climate of caring in a world increasingly filled with persons with chronic disease. The skills of occupational therapists, especially in regard to environmental adaptation, are critical if we are to help prevent the institutionalization of such persons.[69, 70]

Recognizing the multiple factors influencing occupational performance, Christiansen and Baum suggest that occupational therapists use a person-environment-performance framework as their organizing concept for practice. This framework emphasizes the important role of the environment in relation to the individual's ability to perform occupations, and the role of the therapist in facilitating adaptation within the environment when performance deficits are noted.[12]

Supporting the use of environment, adaptation, and systems theory, Howe and Briggs describe an ecological systems model for occupational therapy clinical practice. They view humans and their environment as interactive, influencing each other's development. The patient is described as an open system, "surrounded by interacting environmental layers." Function and dysfunction are determined by the patient's effectiveness in achieving goals as they interact within the environment.[29]

These selected viewpoints reiterate the importance of meaningful occupation within natural environments. Successful performance of occupation also requires ongoing collaboration, leading to adaptation, between the individual and the environmental demands.

Occupation through Collaboration

A basic tenet of occupational therapy is the belief that mind-body-environment relationships are activated through occupation.[16, 66] Inherent in this concept is recognition of the patient/client as an active participant in the treatment process, who collaborates with the therapist in development of the treatment plan. Through the use of purposeful activity (occupation) uniquely tuned to the needs of the patient/client, appropriate challenges are identified, presented, and attempted. The collaborative base, which establishes the specific activity, contributes to a successful outcome. Successful performance promotes feelings of competence and provides opportunities for individuals to achieve mastery of their environments.[20]

Dunning notes that the "key to planned change is the participation of the client system in the change process."[19, p296] Advocating the role of change agent for the therapist and the involvement of the client system and/or patient, she emphasizes their collaborative relationship. The patient and client system become active participants in decisions regarding change and in the change process itself.[19]

Competence in occupational performance involves integration of the bio-psychosocial dimensions of man. The patient/client actively participates in meaningful physical, mental, and or social activities. The term "active" implies and reflects the need for a collaborative approach to the treatment process. Treatment of dysfunction, from an occupational performance perspective, takes multiple and multidimensional causes into consideration and is governed by the client's values.[54]

Through use of a collaborative treatment approach, the therapist builds patient/client self-esteem, creates an atmosphere which promotes mutual cooperation and team work; and assures therapeutic activity, which energizes the patient/client's resolution of identified problems and achievement of desired goals. Within this collaborative process, patient/client and therapist utilize an adaptive approach, supporting change that is necessary for goal achievement.

Adaptive Approach

Promotion of a healthier society cannot come about without considering adaptive approaches to lifestyle changes and environment changes. Adaptation, as discussed in the concepts associated with the process of consultation, is also a basic tenet of occupational therapy practice. The "Philosophical Base of Occupational Therapy," adopted by the American Occupational Therapy Association in 1979, states that "human life includes a process of continuous adaptation." Adaptation is viewed as "a change in function that promotes survival and self-actualization."[4]

Gilfoyle, Grady, and Moore have written extensively about the affects of the adaptation process on human development.[23, 24] Their theory of spatio-temporal adaptation is based on the concept of a spiraling continuum in which transactions with the environment occur through space and time. The development of skills is a result of the individual's transactions between himself and his environment, during which adaptation to change results in the further acquisition and unfolding of performance skills. "Throughout the progressions of development, environmental interaction provides experiences necessary to develop strategies . . . adapted to purposeful behaviors."[23, p47] Spatio-temporal adaptation utilizes basic concepts of adaptation, which include *assimilation, accommodation, association,* and *differentiation.* The continuous, ongoing process of development involves the integration of sensory input from the environment, or *assimilation;* motor output, or *accommodation;* and sensory feedback, or the process of *association;* and *differentiation.*

King views adaptation as a key tool in the occupational therapy process. It is an active response evoked through specific environmental demands. The response is organized at a subcortical level, allowing the individual to direct attention to purposeful activities. Successful adaptation is self-reinforcing, thus allowing the individual to move to more complex environmental challenges. In our increasingly complex society, the ability to adaptively respond to stress is a major concern. Therefore, King asserts, occupational therapists must focus on stress adaptation as part of their role in health maintenance and disease prevention.[36]

The use of an adaptive response and incorporation of the adaptation process as an integral part of practice is strongly supported in the occupational therapy literature. This focus is found also in the consultation literature, where it is framed in the language of "change." The consultant's role, as a change agent, must include the most efficient methodology for eliciting change. This occurs through the process of adaptation. Thus, the therapist's expertise in regard to the adaptation process will facilitate her success as consultant.

The influence of the environment, systems, and ecological concepts on occupational therapy practice and their implications for a model of occupational therapy consultation are discussed in the next section.

ECOLOGY: AN INTEGRATING FORCE

The humanistic philosophy of Meyer may be considered an ecological approach to the study of the behavior of the human organism. This conception of man's interaction with his environment is similar to that of the biological and social scientists who studied the open systems theory. From their study evolved the ecological principles of living in harmony with nature.[32, 38, 47, 63] *We propose that the theoretical foundation of an occupational therapy model of consultation should be based on Meyer's early humanistic and holistic concepts and an ecological approach to consultation practice.*

The concepts of ecology are viewed as an integrating force between the various occupational therapy postulates which guide practice and the basic consultation theoretical models presented earlier. (See Chapter 2.) In the following discussion, we consider the principles of human ecology and their relationship to the enhancement of human potential through occupational performance. The integration of a person's internal sensory awareness with his perceptions and relationships of the external world are seen as the driving force toward the attainment of wholeness and health. The influences of environmental interactions on human behavior affect performance and the development of roles and skills. These concepts form the basis for a theoretical model of occupational therapy consultation.

Systems Approach

General systems theory, developed by von Bertalanffy, emphasizes the feedback relationships among whole units and their parts or subsystems.[63] As discussed in Chapters 2 and 3, general systems theory laid the groundwork for studying the relationships of things to each other, based on the analysis of the interdependency of living organisms to their environments. Closed and open systems are characterized. The closed system does not admit external matter to penetrate the system, nor does it relate to its environment.[1] The social analogy to this type of system may be viewed in the closed social environments of totalitarian states, where outside political and social factors are not allowed to influence their basic ideology. However, as seen in the dramatic political developments in Eastern Europe in the summer of 1991, rarely can external factors be prevented forever from influencing man's reaction to powerful environmental forces. The changing map of Europe and the rapidity of the economic and political upheavals witnessed that year are evidence to this fact. These events support von Bertalanffy's and other system theorists' postulates that living organisms are open systems. Therefore, they are affected directly by external influences and interact extensively with their environment.

In the 1970s, the open system approach was embraced by a number of scientific disciplines. It was used to help analyze the effects of societal and environmental changes, which were occurring rapidly at that time. Recognizing the complex nature of occupation and its effect on the practice of occupational therapy, the occupational therapy theorists emerging at that time also used general systems theory, and the open system concept in particular, as one of their theoretical constructs.

Rogers, discussing occupational behavior, comments "occupation cannot be understood by dealing with humans as disassembled musculo-skeletal, perceptual motor or intrapsychic functions. To explain the occupational nature of humans requires that persons be viewed as wholes . . . a thinking method [general systems theory] . . . encompass[ing] the multiple dimensions of human beings" is required.[55, p115] The model of human occupation perceives the system (man) and its environment as a dynamic network of inseparable relationships.[34] Christiansen acknowledges the importance of systems theory in helping to "organize and facilitate an understanding of the complexities underlying occupational performance."[12, p38]

General systems theory and its subsequent open system approach led to the rise of the "environmentalists" and "ecologists" of the 1970s, who advocated the study of the "web of nature [or] the interrelatedness of species, and the wholeness of ecosystems."[60, p318] Rather than limit themselves to the study of selected systems or systems problems, these scientists explored the relationships of all systems of organized energy in a heuristic, analogical quest for isomorphisms. The integration of the basic postulates of the open systems approach with those of the theories of ecology provide the foundation for holistic concepts of health.

Ecological Concepts

The word *ecology* is derived from the Greek word for house *oikas* or dwelling, *oikia*. The *ecosystem* is an ecological community that together with its physical environment, forms a unit. Therefore, ecology is defined as "the science of the relationships between organisms and their environments.''[2] The study of a community of living organisms implies that there is a dynamic state between the various components of the ecosystem, which is continuously altered by the interplay of natural and human influences. Ecologists study patterns of interrelationships among subsystems and subfields of knowledge. This emphasis facilitates development of a balanced and responsive environment.

The ecological image of mankind recognizes that there is an intimate interdependence between human beings and their total environment.[18] Using an ecological perspective, the individual is viewed as part of a total system, and his health and development are dependent on many subtle factors, external and internal. The totality of development is influenced by behaviors of key individuals, cultural environment, patterns of communication, social interactions, and available support systems. Other significant factors include the impact of institutions, type and extent of cognitive enrichment, and dynamic interrelationships between all aspects of the environment.[10, 31, 32]

Human Ecology

Human ecology is described in terms of the roles of people and institutions and their interdependency. Lewin postulated that the interdependence of person and environment is a major determinent of an individual's behavior. He stated that the person is a function of the environment and the environment a function of the person. His concept of "life space," or the individual's perception of the environment, the behavior of the individual, and his ecological surroundings are factors which must be studied to understand the variations in human behavior.[38]

Human ecology aims to preserve the dynamic, action-oriented, open-ended, holistic, and value-conscious nature of the individual or system. By optimizing these synergistic interactions, the individual or system can grow and adapt to the environment.

The process of feedback, characteristic of all ecological systems, is inherent in the definition of human ecology. For example, human societies create cultural environments that in turn influence the course of social evolution.[18] Throughout the ecological process, the dynamic changes that occur during feedback require the organism or individual to adapt to these changes in order to maintain effective and successful development and survival. This was never more evident than in the dynamic changes noted above in Europe in 1991. As stated by Hinkle, "life implies a constant interaction between organism and environment,''[25, p11] and an individual's health "is intimately bound up with the adaptive demands placed on him by the environment.''[58, p334]

Bertillon wrote in the 1870s that there are only two ways of modifying man, either by modifying his ancestry (possible for future generations but difficult to apply now) or by modifying the natural or social environment.[44] An ecological approach to the enrichment or enhancement of human development and the environment would reinforce this century-old concept. Man, in his environment, can modify his own behavior and cope with changes by developing new skills and modifying environmental systems to adapt to the changes.

Ecological principles, including study and assessment of the environment, can be used to extend knowledge of human behavior by analyzing various levels of environmental settings and their interdependence.[45] Certain predictable individual or institutional behavior patterns are characteristic of social situations. The individual or institution may change behavior in new or modified social settings.[32]

A human ecological approach to occupational therapy consultation allows the consultant to develop a system-specific, interactive service delivery model that addresses these predictable behaviors. In order to use this ecological perspective effectively, one must first explore this approach in greater depth.

Ecological Conceptual Framework

Using the ecological approach, Kelly developed a conceptual framework to examine settings and behavior; increase understanding of both maintenance and change processes in the specific environment; study adaptive behavior; and develop intervention strategies to enhance adaptation to changes.[31, 45] He suggests that the interrelationships of human systems may be analyzed and studied in three ways:

- The relationship between social or organizational systems and the impact of changes in one system on another.
- The relationship between the physical environment and individual behavior.
- The relationship of the individual to his immediate social environment.[31, 32]

Four basic principles are considered in human ecological concepts:

1. The principle of *interdependence* is based on the ecosystem principle in biological ecology, which states that units within the ecosystem are interdependent. Any change in one component of the ecosystem effects changes in the relationships of the other components of the system. This principle recognizes three types of interdependence:

- Between living and nonliving parts of the environment.
- Among living elements.
- Between the structure and function of the system.[31]

In the human ecological approach, the principle of interdependence refers to how persons are linked to roles in their environment. It provides the basis for understanding the social structure of the system and subsystems.[45]

2. The principle of *cycling resources* is related to utilization of the talent and resources of an institution, organization, or community that shape its character and determine the adaptive styles of its members. This principle emphasizes the importance of analyzing past history of the system to identify how previous abilities and talents have been used before attempting to develop strategies for change.

3. The principle of *adaptation* is derived from basic ecological concepts that suggest that the specific environment shapes adaptive behaviors. Adaptation is relative to the particular environment. What is considered adaptive behavior in one environment may not be adaptive in another.

In human ecology, environments with a high rate of population change may have different social structures, interaction patterns, risks and opportunities than relatively stable settings with little population turnover. The principle of adaptation refers to the direct affect a specific environment has on the coping styles of an individual, subsystem, organization, or community, and to the patterns of social interaction within the system.

4. The principle of *succession* is based on ecological concepts and general systems theory regarding the interrelationship of the organism with its environment. The system exists in dynamic equilibrium with its environment. In order to survive, it is forced to make changes to accommodate varying demands.

This principle refers to environmental events that create forces for change in individual behavior or institutional structures. The effects of long- and short-range change processes in the environment must be examined to predict new roles, new social structures, new resources, and new or modified adaptive styles. The principle of succession provides the basis for planned change and intervention strategies.[31, 32, 33, 61]

These ecological principles are conceptualized as the natural, evolutionary processes that affect an ecosystem, community, or individual.[32] However, man and his development and behavior must not be seen as passive products of these environmental forces. Each human develops his own identity, integrating the various component parts into a coherent structure. Given genetic and environmental determinants, the individual uniquely selects, stores, and assimilates information from the environment. Each person creates patterns of behavior and responses that make up his personality and individuality. Throughout life, individual decisions, made in response to environmental influences, shape further development of roles, attitudes, and attributes.[17]

Ecological Approach to Occupational Therapy Consultation

Occupational therapy clinical practice and consultation share a common core of concern, which includes ecological and systems concepts. The basic principles of human ecology have a direct relationship to occupational therapy consultative activities. During the various phases of the consultation process, we can see the application of these principles. They provide the agenda by which the plans and development of consultative intervention strategies may proceed.

The principle of *interdependence* is essential during the entry and initial diagnostic phases of consultation. The form and extent of mutual need, cooperation, and conflict within the system should be considered when analyzing the linkage between system structure and roles of individuals.[32, 45, 61] The consultant's initial task is to assess the degree of cooperation in the system and to begin building the mutual trust and respect essential for a cooperative relationship.

In addition, structural analysis of the system and study of the external environmental factors that affect function must be considered. Study of the interdependence of political, economic, social, and technological events will help the consultant understand the consequences of alternative interventions. For example, the occupational therapy consultant in industrial settings must be aware of how legislative guidelines, regulations, and new technology affect the workplace. She must understand how to use social advocacy to develop safe changes in the work environment and recognize the economic burden corporations may sustain to adapt their setting to a healthier, safer work environment.

Throughout the ongoing diagnostic analysis and feedback phases of consultation, the consultant should be cognizant of the principle of *cycling resources* and assess how the system defines and utilizes its resources. How the system has identified and utilized talent is important to this analysis. Assessment of cooperation or noncooperation patterns, identification of the system's problems and needs, and joint planning may serve as vehicles through which mutual involvement and cooperation will develop.[32, 45, 61]

This principle can be used to assess past utilization of the system's resources. In a stable or static situation, the system may continue to employ the same type of individual, stay with familiar skills and abilities, and seek out the same resources. In a more dynamic, or changing, environment, this ecological approach may be used to recruit new talents and encourage a diverse range of skills and knowledge. During this process and analysis, needs may be anticipated and determinations made regarding the availability of future internal and external resources. Additionally, the consultant can use this principle to generate predictions about the potential of the system to develop and enhance its structure.

For instance, a program development consultant for a community agency that is undergoing change may find the principle of cycling resources extremely helpful in assessing agency resource utilization and willingness to accept new knowledge and skills. The agency may consider implementation of a teenage parent/infant development program. Here, the occupational therapy consultant can assist the client (the agency director) to review and assess the agency's available manpower, skills, and personnel talents for initial staffing requirements. In addition, help is provided to identify external resources in the community, such as pediatricians willing to accept referrals for diagnosis and treatment of high-risk infants or children identified with developmental delays, or school counselors and psychologists who could identify potential school-age parents as program participants. Other community agencies can be identified which may provide funding or in-kind services, including volunteer members of service clubs to act as surrogate grandparents or help with acquisition of toys, supplies, and capital equipment. It will be essential for the consultant and the client to determine the community's (or ecosystem's) past involvement, current interest, and willingness to participate in new programs, and to judge which areas and individuals should be tapped to contribute to this program's development. Analysis of internal and external resources, which constitute the environmental influences on the adaptive styles of the agency staff and community members, will provide valuable information for the design of intervention strategies.

This analysis leads directly to the theoretical principle of *adaptation*. As discussed in Chapter 3, it is one of the most important related concepts in the consultation process. The environment's effect on the individual, institution, or community determines reactions to change and patterns of coping styles. A major consultant responsibility is to examine what behaviors are considered adaptive in this environment. She must understand the effects of change, how behaviors can be anticipated, and perceive the client system's ability to adapt to new situations. Another high priority task is to help the client understand characteristics in the environment which may generate a wide range of adaptive behaviors. An educational approach will help the client develop or enhance adaptive behaviors and recognize the effect on himself, other individuals in the system, and on the environment itself. The outcome may be an increase in the diversity of adaptive styles, requiring a redefinition of expected behaviors in a given setting.[45]

Knowledge of the client system's adaptive styles and the social structures within the environment that shape adaptive behavior will determine the design of intervention strategies. The application of the principle of adaptation will help the consultant predict effective/ineffective behaviors that may emerge in the system. Continual monitoring will assist redesign or modification to effect healthy, functional attitudes and adaptive behavior. During the goal setting, planning, and intervention phases of the consultation, it is imperative for the consultant to be cognizant of feedback received regarding client reaction to the plans and adaptation to the intervention strategies. Development of communication channels, participatory definition of goals and evaluation criteria, and assessment of the social, environmental, and behavioral impact of new developments can be identified from the ecological perspective of adaptation.[32, 45]

For example, an occupational therapy consultant requested to develop a new program for an adult day care center must not only understand the client system's reactions to a new or different organizational structure, but must also have a thorough grounding in the adaptation process of older adults. Her program design must be based on knowledge of the client system and developmental phases of the consultation process and must be in direct concert with her professional skills in assessing program needs and adaptive abilities of an older population. The consultant must be aware of the older individual's receptivity or resistance to such external influences as new sights, sounds, events, and ideas that impinge on his personal environment. The relevance these factors have to his internal life will directly affect the older adult's acceptance of the program.[22]

Additionally, identification of the behavioral process must encompass the reactions of staff and caregivers to this elderly population. Using a human ecology approach, with knowledge of the adaptive process the consultant can adjust the program to optimize these environmental and personal interactions and help the client system, staff and its clientele (the older adult participants) adapt to the changes proposed for the adult center.

The principle of *succession* is especially important for the consultant to consider throughout the consultation process. Natural events occurring in the external environment create forces for change in an organization's structure and in the subsystems, affecting individual and system behavior. Maintenance of mutual goal definition and awareness of these forces is a crucial, ongoing task of the consultant.

Changes also may be a result of internal events, planned change, and the intervention efforts of the consultant. As the organization's environmental conditions change, new and/or adaptive behavior is required. Criteria for assessing change should include the increase in cooperation and adaptation in the client system; enhancement of resources, individual capabilities and competencies, and services; and the ultimate success of the interventions themselves. Therefore, another aspect of the principle of succession is its use in planning strategies to predict long-term development of the system and anticipate the effects of interventions and the relationship between interventions and changes in the system.[32, 45, 61]

In a consultation involving organizational development, the consultant's understanding of this principle will assist diagnosis, ongoing analysis, and development of intervention strategies. Additionally, evaluation of the effectiveness of interventions, modification of intervention efforts, and reevaluation will be more accurate, if the consultant keeps this principle in mind. For example, consultation to assess and evaluate the organizational structure of an academic occupational therapy program must include analysis of the external factors that impact the university system. Legislation and/or regulations regarding educational guidelines and funding, political influences, extramural financial support, and other economic and demographic factors must be considered. The educational consultant who will help plan and restructure the program also must be cognizant of many internal factors within the university system and various subsystems that have an impact on the school of occupational therapy. Administrative support, financial and personnel resources, university regulations, faculty resources, and the demographics of the total student body and pool of existing and potential occupational therapy students are among factors that will influence the structure and design of the department and curriculum. Additionally, the consultant must be aware of the ability of the faculty to adapt to a new or modified organizational structure.

Figure 42–2 summarizes the relationship of the principles of ecology to the phases of the consultation process.

The consultant's role and responsibility is to facilitate implementation of these principles and to provide the client system with the knowledge, skills, and alternatives to resolve current and future problems. The extent of consultant interventions is influenced by the attitudes of the client system and its images of the future in an interactive, changing society. Increased knowledge, as a generator of possibilities, enlarges the individual's range of options and makes people and systems more receptive to new ideas, attitudes, and change in former behaviors, leading to a healthier environment.[18]

Merging ecological concepts and principles into the consultation process provides the consultant with a dynamic operational framework, compatible with

FIGURE 42–2

Relationship of ecological principles to the consultation process

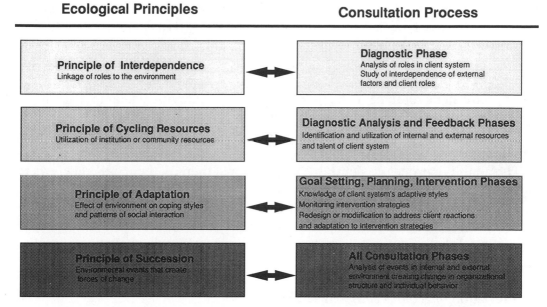

occupational therapy views. Working in varied environments, this perspective allows consultant and client to conceptualize and implement a system responsive plan which facilitates adaptation and further development of human potential.

HUMAN POTENTIAL: THE GOAL OF OCCUPATIONAL THERAPY CONSULTATION PRACTICE

We propose that there is an intrinsic relationship between selected occupational therapy concepts, ecological premises, and theoretical consultation models. Throughout the framework of these three conceptual systems, there is an emphasis on the development of human potential, which then forms the framework for occupational therapy consultation practice. To define and focus this proposed model, a broader picture of the premises underlying these conceptual systems is presented.

Occupational Therapy Concepts

The overriding philosophical tenet of occupational therapy consultation follows that of all occupational therapy practice: an emphasis on the development of the highest possible human potential through appropriate occupational performance. "Occupational therapy is based on the belief that purposeful activity (occupation), including its interpersonal and environmental components, may be used to prevent and mediate dysfunction, and to elicit maximum adaptation.''[4] Within that framework, the goal of the occupational therapy consultant is to enhance the client's ability to cope with and adapt to changes in the environment.

Adaptation

As discussed in the Change Process in Chapter 2, the adaptive reaction is triggered by *stress* in the individual's internal or external environment, which alters the system's equilibrium. Stress creates the body's orientation response, which forms the basis for the individual's adaptation and function in a changed environment.[36, 56] In the spatiotemporal adaptation theory, stress is considered a major factor in development and maturation, as the individual adapts to changes in the environment. Stress may be viewed as positive, producing higher levels of functioning and a return to equilibrium, or negative, resulting in dysfunction and maladaptive performance and behavior.[24]

The adaptive process is central to occupational therapy theory. King views this concept as a synthesizing principle for the profession. Individuals and systems use adaptation to promote survival and self-actualization. An active process, mediated by environmental demands, adaptive responses are organized most effectively at a subcortical level. Successful adaptation to environmental challenges creates a building block and a stimulus to confront the next more complex challenge.[36]

Integration of Ecological/Systems Approach

Adaptation to change in human development, organizational structure, or community environments relates to equilibrium or disequilibrium in the total ecosystem of the individual or institution. Ramo Simon, an early advocate of systems theory, stressed a total, rather than fragmentary, look at problems.[58] Foremost in the design and plan of occupational therapy consultation intervention strategies is consideration of the client in relation to his environment. The individual client or client system must be viewed as part of a total ecosystem, in which there is a dynamic interaction and interconnection with subsystems that shape the whole.

One must be able to monitor the continuously changing forces that influence behavior, whether in an individual client, an organizational system, or the whole community. The basic ecological principles of interdependence, utilization of resources, adaptation, and forces of change are natural and evolutionary processes that affect an ecosystem.[32] As environmental conditions change, due to natural evolution or intervention efforts, the consultant helps the client develop skills to manage the new and/or adaptive behavior required in the newly, changed setting.

Similar occupational therapy treatment goals may be seen within the context of an ecological approach to clinical practice. Howe and Briggs describe an ecological systems model for occupational therapy practice. They view the individual patient as an open system in the center of the ecosystem, receiving sensory information, integrating and processing this ''input,'' and responding to the environment with the ''output'' of certain behavior. The cycle is continuous and throughout the cycle feedback from environmental interchange enables the patient to monitor and modify behavior. This approach to patient care is based on the therapist's consideration of multiple aspects of the patient's environment; evaluation of the patient's degree of function or dysfunction within that environment; plan and implementation of remedial measures in the environment, whenever possible; and the design and implementation of therapeutic measures to prevent further dysfunction.[29]

Further evidence of an ecological approach to occupational therapy practice, again founded on general systems theory, is demonstrated in the proposition of occupational science as an academic discipline. Clark, et al, describe occupational science as the systematic study of humans as occupational beings. Here, again, "the person is seen as an open system in interaction with his or her environment over the entire life span, from birth to old age."[13, p302]

In this model, the human system is presented as being comprised of six sub-systems: physical, biological, information processing, sociocultural, symbolic-evaluative, and transcendental. Sociocultural influences, the person's history, and environmental challenges all provide input into the human system. Feedback from these factors to the various subsystems results in occupational behavior. Thus, "occupation" is considered the "output" of the system, which can "either facilitate or limit the capacity of the person for successful adaptation to environmental demands."[13, p302]

A major purpose of occupational science is to provide basic theoretical, scientific principles to enhance the practice of occupational therapy. The role of occupation, central to both the study of occupational science and the practice of occupational therapy, is emphasized as key to human adaptation, functioning, behavior, health, and life satisfaction. It is not viewed in isolation but as the direct result of internal and external environmental influences.

Humanism: a Holistic Approach

As systems theory became accepted and understood in the latter part of the 20th century, the philosophy that we are but the sum of our parts began to be heard in a number of fields, from economics to social studies, environmental analysis, and medicine. The term "wholism" or "holism" became a buzz word in the 1970s and 1980s. We spoke of wholistic health, the whole person, and the whole earth. As discussed earlier, occupational therapy, long before this general interest in "wholeness," was based on the theory of healing the whole person. Although this basic philosophy frequently was espoused by the profession, it was not reflected in all areas of practice. The demand to validate service delivery for reimbursement, research, and visibility resulted in overemphasis of specific modalities, technologies, or assessment instruments. The influence of the medical community to provide scientific evidence for health care practices resulted in reductionist shifts in occupational therapy to a focus on "internal muscular, intrapsychic balance, and sensorimotor problems."[35]

Recently, on a national level, there has been considerable discussion of strategies to bring back a holistic approach to practice, with a firm commitment to action.[3, 26, 69] Leaders and theorists reinforced a return to theoretical roots and the importance of the development of theory using occupational therapy concepts.

The literature dramatically expanded, and varying frames of reference emerged. Mosey discussed five philosophical assumptions, drawn from occupational therapy literature, which are derived from pragmatic, existential, and humanistic schools of thought. The key themes identified are the individual's right to a meaningful existence; the stage-specific maturation process; development of potential through personal choice; purposeful interaction with human and non-human environments to achieve potential; and the individual's inherent need for a balance of work, play, and rest.[48]

These philosophical assumptions emphasize the profession's humanistic premises and their importance to practice. Renewal of these views energized those involved in theory building during the latter part of the 20th century. Current occupational therapy concepts emphasize the effect of the environment on the quality of life and the development of the whole person. This humanistic focus is supported in the consultation process and well integrated in concepts of prevention.

Prevention

This emphasis on *holistic medicine and holistic health* has expanded the concepts of disease prevention to include health promotion and wellness. By the late 1970s, holistic thinking was not only in the realm of professional health sciences. It had spilled over to millions of individuals searching for their personal identities. The demand for some magic potion to re-integrate their personality or lead them to "higher" states of consciousness spawned a myriad of so-called therapies and religious cults under the rubric of "human potential movement," from Mind Dynamics to Silva Mind Control to the Moonies.[60]

However, the development of human potential in occupational therapy consultation practice does not rely on magic therapies, but rather focuses on the enhancement of man's ability to reach his highest potential through self-actualization, improved function, and a better life. Promotion of an individual's total well-being is a fundamental professional precept. Improvement in quality of life and the promotion of health are concepts basic to both clinical occupational therapy and consultation. Prevention of disease or dysfunction and facilitation of health and function in treatment settings, organizations, or communities are common goals. To promote a healthy environment, the therapist/consultant assists the patient/client to develop self-help skills. Generation of knowledge, self-responsibility, and positive attitudes is also a major objective in the quest for patient/client health and wellness.

The 1979 report, *Healthy People: The Surgeon General's Report on Health Promotion and Disease Prevention,* called for a second public-health revolution.[62] Modification of social environments and major changes in the government's role regarding health care were suggested. Citizens were urged to develop healthy, rather than damaging, life styles and habits. The Surgeon General emphasized the need to deal effectively with the deep social problems that destroy health. He stated that most improvement in society's health status would come about as a result of the prevention, not the treatment of, disease.

Occupational therapy consultants, trained in the principles of health, are able to provide services that support the development of well-being. An awareness of paradigms in preventive health, with a focus on health as opposed to disease and with a link to the socio-cultural, economic, political, and environmental forces that affect health, can help facilitate and achieve a healthy society.[30]

Ecological Premises

Ecology, as the study of individual organisms, their environments, and the interactions between the two, has become increasingly important to the world since concern for our endangered physical environment has grown. Health promotion and disease prevention in plants and animals, as part of that endangered environment, have come to the forefront. Human ecological principles reinforce these concerns and stress the importance of health promotion and disease prevention concepts in human life styles and professional health interventions. As described in Chapter 7, outcomes of consultation activities are related directly to levels of preventive interventions. The ultimate goal of consultation is to improve human potential through enhanced function. When considered in an ecological context, the intervention can foster the enhancement of human development and help the client system modify behavior to promote a healthier environment.

Concepts of ecological consultation include the need to understand the influences of change on the client or system. Change is often the very reason for consultation. A change may have occurred in a system or client causing pain, crisis, or problems that require help to resolve or to which one must adapt. Also, there may be a need or desire for change that results in the request for help. (This may concern change in a program or the development of new programs, or a change in life styles, workplace environment, or organizational structure.) Additionally, trends may reveal that changes will occur, and preparation for the future may require help in developing strategies to prepare for these changes.

Holmes postulates that change—not a specific change per se "but the general rate of change in a person's life—could be one of the most important environmental factors of all" (59,p328). Change requires individuals and systems to adjust their mental time maps and adapt to the effects in their own world. As Einstein postulated at the turn of the century, time is relative, not absolute. The order of events depends upon the velocity of the observer. Change, and the effects of change, may also be viewed from the individual's point of view—as in the old saying "It is in the eye of the beholder."

Gardner speaks of organizational change as "self-renewal," the reorientation of one's self or of a system in response to change.[22] This change is on-going, not a once-in-a-life-time occurrence but a continual appraisal and reappraisal of organizational life in response to the constantly accelerating rate of change in our society. Changes in organizational relationships create entirely new climates, with new sets of problems, at a faster pace than ever before.[59]

There is a direct relationship between change, whether in internal or external environments, and an individual's health.[44] The essence of the environment's relationship to the development of health and humanness is captured succinctly by the eminent biologist and social scientist Rene Dubos. Throughout his many writings, the central theme of the need to study the effects of environmental forces on society, the individual, and the future of mankind is emphasized. He has written extensively about man's need to adapt to his environment and to develop skills to cope with our fast and irregularly changing world.[17, 18] An advanced, technological society must be cognizant of all influences in the culture, including man's perception of his senses in the environment and the need for opportunities for self-expression and diversity. "Industrial civilization will have to be reformulated on the basis of human ecological principles."[17, p289]

We are moving to a more comprehensive view of progress that encompasses the human capacity for creativity, free will, and the ability to change the course of events. Consultation, based on an ecological perspective, will engender a social climate favorable to change through adaptation. A holistic view of the future envisions an environment in which there are many options. Opportunities exist for the development of human potential through effective consultation that uses these ecological premises.

Consultation Models

The various theoretical models of consultation presented earlier also emphasize development of human potential through enhancement of function and performance. Consistent in all models is the focus on improving client understanding of his system and his skill in effective system management and function. Consultant and client goals must include recognition of internal and external factors that influence change in organizational structure, individual behavior, group dynamics, processes of the system, program planning, and community action.

The models of consultation identified in this text were derived from a variety of theories, which emanated from scientific disciplines including the medical, social, biological, and behavioral sciences. These theories were reorganized to provide the basis for the development of the theoretical propositions and concepts that determined the various consultation models. The choice of consultation model used in any given situation is dependent on many variables, and one or more models may be incorporated as appropriate. The models may differ in their scope and focus, but inherent in the term *model* is the common purpose of guiding thinking to help the consultant analyze the situation, determine the intervention strategies, and develop alternatives.[12, 28, 48] The model provides a broad focus and unifying identity for the consultative activities.

The occupational therapy model of consultation we propose is based specifically on the scientific postulates of open systems theory, ecology, sociology, biological adaptation, and concepts from the behavioral sciences, including those emanating from occupational therapy theorists. This transition from theory to consultation practice requires the development of a frame of reference specific to the particular environment, needs, problems, and desired outcomes of the client system.

FRAMEWORK FOR OCCUPATIONAL THERAPY CONSULTATION PRACTICE

Determination of a specific approach to consultation is derived from the theoretical model(s) and frame(s) of reference chosen for the particular client system. As described in occupational therapy literature, the specificity of approach narrows the theoretical assumptions and forms the *frame of reference* for the practice.[12, 28, 37, 48] Frames of reference guide the initial analysis; the formulation of particular intervention strategies, goals, and sequence of activities; and the evaluation procedures most appropriate for the client system and setting. The consultant may choose more than one theoretical model or theory base to formulate the frames of reference which guide the specific consultation activities.

To provide the consultant with a basis for effective formulation of the intervention, an understanding of the development of a frame of reference is useful. Mosey suggests that a frame of reference should include:

- the information on the domain of concern
- the theories from which the frame of reference is derived
- the nature of the problem
- the behaviors indicative of the state of function or dysfunction
- the change principles upon which the intervention is based.[50]

A framework for occupational therapy consultation practice includes the basic frame of reference components that are illustrated in Figure 42–3. Using these inherent factors, a framework for occupational therapy consultation practice can be developed. The order in which these factors occur may vary with the particular client system, setting, and problem. However, utilization of a frame of reference will facilitate the consultant's planning. Particular intervention strategies, goals, sequences of activities, and evaluation procedures appropriate for each client system and setting may then be planned.

With the theoretical *model of occupational therapy consultation* as a basic guide, *frame(s) of reference* specific to the particular system are developed. Inherent in this development is thorough *information gathering* regarding the areas of concern and background for diagnosis and analysis of particular *problem(s)* encountered in the system. A study of *client system behaviors,* including attitudes and reactions to change, will indicate the system's state of function or dysfunction and will determine the plan and design of intervention strategies.

Following system diagnosis and analysis the appropriate consultative approach is chosen for the client, based on *theoretical models* of consultation, occupational therapy postulates, and other relevant theories. The consultant's critical awareness and understanding of the system's *change principles* and adaptive responses

FIGURE 42–3

Framework for occupational therapy consultation practice.

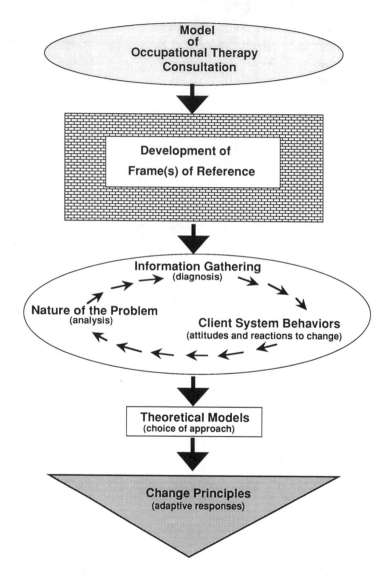

will assure development of change strategies and produce the desired outcome of improved functioning.

A THEORETICAL MODEL OF OCCUPATIONAL THERAPY CONSULTATION

Occupational therapists provide consultation services in diverse settings that require specific occupational therapy and consultative expertise. To address this diversity and the specialized knowledge base required effectively, a model of occupational therapy consultation is proposed. All occupational therapy consultative activities can then be developed from this model, which serves as a unifying concept. Inherent in the description of a model is a foundation in theory, the organization of knowledge to guide reasoning, and an identified purpose to explain and facilitate action.

Theoretical Postulates of Occupational Therapy Consultation

The proposed model of occupational therapy consultation is based on a constellation of relevant theories and principles. These are drawn from

- systems.
- ecology.
- occupational therapy, with an emphasis on humanism.
- consultation.
- health promotion perspectives.

Key concepts are the environment, human ecology, collaboration, adaptation, and enablement. The occupational therapy consultation process operationalizes these concepts to achieve improved client system function. This leads to maximizing human potential within the given environment.

The consultation *environment* serves as the mileu in which action occurs. It's pervasive influence affects all aspects of the consultation process. At varying points in time, the environment may mediate, facilitate, and/or enable adaptation and change.

Through the application of *human ecology,* based on systems theory, the consultant reinforces and facilitates an integrative relationship between client system and the environment. Thus, a dynamic balance is created, where subsystem influences are interconnected to the overall ecosystem.

The *collaboration* between consultant and client system is an interactive relationship, which assures a balanced approach to problem solving. An ongoing collaborative approach strengthens the decision making process, supports recognition of each party's unique contributions, and reinforces the concept of working together for mutual gain.

Adaptation, leading to environmental or system change, is facilitated through a collaborative approach. The consultant aids the client in identifying and implementing the appropriate plan of action, which fosters the necessary change.

Through a process of *enablement,* the client system establishes and maintains a level of environmental change, which leads to improved function. The consultant proactively supports this achievement by remaining available as resource or change agent.

Improved function leading to achievement of *human potential* is the ultimate consultation goal. Unique aspects of each consultation experience will modulate the degree of success achieved. The trajectory of any specific consultation will be influenced by ecologic and environmental forces, combined with the composition, quality, and speed of the consultative process. The targeted outcome is reached via use of a structural framework for the practice of occupational therapy consultation. Figure 42–4 presents a graphic depiction of the occupational therapy consultation model, which is founded upon the concept of achieving human potential through improved function.

   This model of occupational therapy consultation depicts the *environment* as the overall determinant of the consultation approach, surrounding the particular *frame(s) of reference* chosen for any given consultative setting. The foundation of the model is the theory of *human ecology,* which is based on general systems theory.

FIGURE 42–4

Model of occupational therapy consultation.

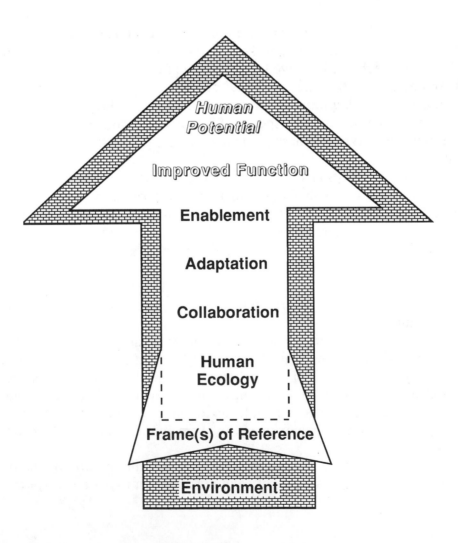

The occupational therapist, skilled in interactive patient/client relationships requiring *collaboration* and mutual cooperation, transfers her expertise and knowledge of human occupation and man's interrelationship with his environment to a consultative approach. Trained in the theory, principles, and process of consultation, the occupational therapy consultant fosters a collaborative environment within the client system. This atmosphere of shared trust and joint collaboration facilitates the consultant's ability to diagnose issues and analyze the system's adaptive ability regarding change in internal and external environments. This process culminates in a plan and procedure for *adaptation* or change.

The major responsibility of the consultant is to develop strategies which will lead to *enablement* of the client system, thus achieving the greatest possible potential. The consultation goal is to increase and enhance the client system's skills and ability to resolve present and future problems through *improved function,* thereby maximizing *human potential.*

CONCLUSIONS

"Theory without application is useless, but practice without theory is blind"—*Anonymous*

The proposed theoretical model of consultation integrates occupational therapy and consultation concepts within an ecological frame. Growing health care needs of populations experiencing occupational performance dysfunction at primary, secondary, and tertiary levels require this approach to consultation. Use of this model will enable occupational therapists to address multiple issues arising in the health care marketplace, and to provide comprehensive service to populations in need.

The development of knowledgeable, skilled occupational therapy consultants will require additional training in consultation theory and process. Educational programs must incorporate the study of health promotion and environment and systems analysis into the theoretical background of occupational therapy students and practitioners.

A broadened perspective on precursors to disease, impact of environmental factors, prevention of disability, and strategies to enhance health must occur—not only at social and political levels but in the education of health professionals. Social, economic, political, and technological changes necessitate this shift in educational focus. Static orientation of rational, familiar ideas, with an adaptation of past patterns of knowledge, must be replaced with a constantly changing, dynamic, interdependent, and complex set of concepts relevant to a rapidly changing world.

In this technotronic age, all institutions of learning spend considerable energy training highly qualified technicians who, unfortunately, may subordinate quality for quantity, and the individual to the system. It has been a basic tenet of occupational therapy that the promotion of an individual's total well-being through purposeful activity should guide practice. Therefore, occupational therapists should be trained to be more than good technicians, more than functional instruments in the process of service. They are uniquely qualified to relate their specialized skills to broader concerns about the quality of life. In addition to studying disease-related behavior, occupational therapy students and practitioners need to study the paradigms relating to human adaptation and preventive health, and the ecological concepts that focus on activities that encourage health. Practice patterns that include a consultative approach to service delivery and are based on the necessary theoretical concepts, principles, and processes of consultation should also be studied. The link to the socio-cultural, economic, political, and environmental forces that affect health should be emphasized, with a focus on the attainment of comprehensive, quality care.[30]

The occupational therapists of tomorrow must be armed with knowledge and skills that prepare them to function in a world of rapid change. They must develop practice patterns, including consultation, that provide the greatest service to their patient and client populations. If occupational therapists are to be at the leading edge of health-care delivery they "must increase [their] knowledge about and concern for *health* as well as disability, acquire the skills of *consultation* in addition to expertise in treatment, and use both in a larger-than-hospital *community*."[65] The development of a model of occupational therapy consultation will provide therapists with the essential theoretical skills and background that are necessary to facilitate this premise. It is our hope that occupational therapists can then be "specialists with universal minds,"[9] who activate, enhance, enable, and empower their clients to a maximum level of occupational performance.

REFERENCES

1. Allport G: The open system in personality theory, in Buckly W (ed): *Modern Systems Research for the Behavioral Scientist*. Chicago, Aldin Publishing Co, 1968.
2. *The American Heritage Dictionary*. New York, Houghton Mifflin, 1969.
3. American Occupational Therapy Association: Occupational Therapy: 2001. November 1978. Rockville, Author, Conference Proceeding, 1979.
4. American Occupational Therapy Association: The Philosophical Base of Occupational Therapy, Resolution 531-79. Am J Occup Ther 1979; 33:785.
5. Argyris C, Schon D: *Theory in Practice: Increasing Professional Effectiveness*. San Francisco, Josey Bass, 1984.
6. Ayres AJ: *Sensory integration and Learning Disorders*. Los Angeles, Western Psychological Services, 1972.
7. Barris R: Environmental interactions: An extension of the model of occupation. *Am J Occup Ther* 1982; 36:637.
8. Bing RK: Occupational therapy revisited: A paraphrastic journey. *Am J Occup Ther* 1981; 35:499–518.
9. Boulding K: *The Meaning of the 20th Century*. New York, Harper and Row, 1964.
10. Bronfenbrenner U: Toward an experimental ecology of human development. Am 1977; 32:513.

11. Christiansen C: Occupational therapy intervention for life performance, in Christiansen C, Baum C (eds): *Occupational Therapy: Enhancing Human Performance Deficits.* Thorofare, Slack, 1991.

12. Christiansen C, Baum, C. (eds): *Occupational Therapy: Enhancing Human Performance Deficits.* Thorofare, Slack, 1991.

13. Clark FA, Parham D, Carlson ME, et al: Occupational science: Academic innovation in the service of occupational therapy's future. *Am J Occup Ther* 1991; 45:300–310.

14. Clark PN: Human development through occupation: Theoretical frameworks in occupational therapy practice, part 1. *Am J Occup Ther* 1979; 33:505.

15. Clark PN: Human development through occupation: A philosophy and conceptual model for practice, part 2. *Am J Occup Ther* 1979; 33:577.

16. DiJoseph LM: Independence through activity: Mind, body and environment, interaction in therapy. *Am J Occup Ther* 1982; 36:740–744.

17. Dubos R: *A God Within.* New York, Charles Scribner's Sons, 1972.

18. Dubos R: *The Wooing of the Earth.* New York, Charles Scribner's Sons, 1980.

19. Dunning H: Environmental occupational therapy. *Am J Occup Ther* 1972; 26:292–298.

20. Fidler GS: From crafts to competence. *Am J Occup Ther* 1983; 35:567–573.

21. Finn GL: The occupational therapist in prevention programs. *Am J Occup Ther* 1972; 26:2.

22. Gardner JW: *Self-Renewal: The Individual and the Innovative Society.* New York, Harper & Row, 1964.

23. Gilfoyle EM, Grady AP, Moore, JC: *Children Adapt.* Thorofare, Slack, 1981.

24. Gilfoyle EM, Grady AP, Moore JC: *Children Adapt,* ed 3. Thorofare, Slack, 1990.

25. Hinkle LE: The Doctor, his Patient, and the Environment. *Am J Pub Health* 1964; p 11.

26. Hoover S: Directions for the future. *OT Week* 1990; February 19:4–5.

27. Hopkins HL: An historical perspective on occupational therapy, in Hopkins HL, Smith HD (eds): *Willard and Spackman's Occupational Therapy,* ed 6. Philadelphia, Lippincott, 1983.

28. Hopkins HL: Current basis for theory and philosophy of occupational therapy, in Hopkins, HL, Smith HD (eds): *Willard and Spackman's Occupational Therapy,* ed 7. Philadelphia, Lippincott, 1988.

29. Howe MC, Briggs AK: Ecological systems model for occupational therapy. *Am J Occup Ther* 1982; 36:322–327.

30. Jaffe EJ: Prevention: "An idea whose time has come": The role of occupational therapy in disease prevention and health promotion. *Am J Occup Ther* 1986; 40:749–752.

31. Kelly JG: Towards an ecological conception of preventive interventions, in Carter JW (ed): *Research Contributions From Psychology to Community Mental Health.* New York, Behavioral Publications, 1968.

32. Kelly JG: Ecological constraints on mental health services, in Cook PE (ed): *Community Psychology and Community Mental Health.* San Francisco, Holden-Day, 1970.

33. Kelly JG: The quest for valid preventive interventions, in Spielberger CD (ed): *Current Topics in Clinical and Community Psychology,* vol 2. New York, Academic Press, 1970.

34. Kielhofner G, Burke JP: A model of human occupation, part 1. *Am J Occup Ther* 1980; 34:572.

35. Kielhofner G, Burke JP: Occupational therapy after 60 years. *Am J Occup Ther* 1977; 31:675–698.

36. King LJ: Toward a science of adaptive responses. *Am J Occup Ther* 1978; 32:429–437.

37. Levy L: Frames of reference for occupational therapists in mental health, in Robertson SC (ed): *SCOPE: Strategies, Concepts, and Opportunities for Program Development*

and Evaluation (Application Supplement, 17–24). Rockville, American Occupational Therapy Association, 1986.

38. Lewin K: *Field Theory in Social Science.* New York, Harper & Row, 1951.
39. Lippitt G, Lippitt, R: *The Consulting Process in Action.* San Diego, Univ. Assoc., 1978.
40. Llorens LA: Occupational therapy in community child health. *Am J Occup Ther* 1971; 25:335–338.
41. Llorens LA: Changing balance: environment and individual. *Am J Occup Ther* 1984; 38:29–34.
42. Llorens LA: Theoretical conceptualizations of occupational therapy: 1960–1982, *Occup Ther Ment Hlth* 1984; 4.
43. Llorens LA: Performance tasks and rolls throughout the life span, in Christiansen C, Baum C (eds): Occupational therapy: Enhancing human performance deficits. Thorofare, Slack, 1991.
44. McLachlan G: Public health at the crossroads, in *Oxford Text of Public Health,* vol 2. New York, Oxford University Press, 1985; pp 50–62.
45. Mann PA: *Community Psychology: Concepts and Applications.* New York, Free Press, 1978.
46. Mazur JL: The occupational therapist as consultant. *Am J Occup Ther* 1969; 23:417–421.
47. Meyer A: The philosophy of occupational therapy. *Arch Occup Ther* 1922; 1:1–10.
48. Mosey AC: *Occupational Therapy: Configuration of a Profession.* New York, Raven Press, 1981.
49. Mosey AC: A monistic or pluralistic approach to professional identity. *Am J Occup Ther* 1985; 39:504–509.
50. Mosey AC: The proper focus of scientific inquiry in occupational therapy: Frames of reference. *Occ Ther Jrnl of Research* 1989; 9:195–201.
51. Reilly M: Occupational therapy can be one of the great ideas of 20th century medicine. *Am J Occup Ther* 1962; 16:1–9.
52. Reilly M: Occupational therapy—A historical perspective—The modernization of Occupational Therapy. *Am J Occup Ther* 1971; 25:5.
53. Reilly M: Play as Exploratory Learning. Los Angeles, Sage Publications, 1974.
54. Rogers JC: Order and disorder in medicine and occupational therapy. *Am J Occup Ther* 1982; 36:29–35.
55. Rogers JC: The study of human occupation, in Kielhofner G (ed): *Health Through Occupation.* Philadelphia, FA Davis, 1983, pp 93–124.
56. Selyle H: *The Stress of Life.* New York, McGraw-Hill Book, 1956.
57. Shannon PD: The derailment of occupational therapy. *Am J Occup Ther* 1977; 31:229–234.
58. Simon R: *Cure for Chaos: Fresh Solutions to Social Problems Through the Systems Approach.* New York, David McKay, 1969.
59. Toffler A: *Future Shock.* New York, Random House, 1970.
60. Toffler A: *The Third Wave.* New York, Wm. Morrow, 1980.
61. Trickett EJ, Kelly JG, Todd DM: The social environment of the high school: Guidelines for individual change and organizational development, in Golann SE, Eisdorfer C (eds): *Handbook of Community Mental Health.* New York, Appleton-Century-Crofts, 1972.
62. United States Public Health Service: *Healthy People: The Surgeon General's Report on Health Promotion and Disease Prevention.* DHEW 79-55071, Washington DC, US Government Printing Office, 1979.
63. von Bertalanffy L: *General System Theory.* New York, Braziller, 1968.
64. West WL: Professional responsibility in times of change. *Am J Occup Ther* 1968; 22:14.

65. West WL: The principles and process of consultation, in Llorens, LA (ed): *Consultation in the Community: Occupational Therapy in Child Health*. Dubuque, IA, Kendall Hunt, 1973.

66. West WL: A reaffirmed philosophy and practice of occupational therapy for the 1980's. *Am J Occup Ther* 1984; 38:15–23.

67. Wiemer RB: Some concepts of prevention as an aspect of community health. *Am J Occup Ther* 1972; 26:1.

68. Williamson GG: A heritage of activity: Development of a theory. *Am J Occup Ther* 1982; 36:716.

69. Yerxa EJ: Occupational therapy's role in creating a future climate of caring. *Am J Occup Ther* 1980; 34:529–534.

70. Yerxa EJ: Audacious values: The energy source for occupational therapy practice, in Kielhofner G (ed): *Health Through Occupation*. Philadelphia, FA Davis, 1983.

71. Yerxa EJ, et al: An introduction of occupational science, A foundation for occupational therapy in the 21st century. *Occup Ther in Hlth Care* 1989; 6:1–17.

CHAPTER 43

Summary

Evelyn G. Jaffe, M.P.H., O.T.R., F.A.O.T.A.
Cynthia F. Epstein, M.A., O.T.R., F.A.O.T.A.

"The process of consultation is challenging, awesome, rewarding, and humbling . . . it requires the constant growth of those who practice it"—*Gordon and Ronald Lippitt*

Our continuously changing, rapidly evolving health care marketplace seeks professionals capable of responding to today's needs and tomorrow's challenges. This complex society requires greater decision-making help and generation of ideas to develop and utilize current and future resources. The role of the traditional *helper* has become that of *change agent*. Consultants, therefore, are often placed at health care's leading edge to facilitate appropriate and timely responses to market demands. Consultation is a growing field in all health professions, especially in occupational therapy, and only recently has been recognized by society as an essential resource. Additionally, there are circumstances in which consultants may represent the most cost-effective solution to manpower issues, lack of human resources, and rapid change in an agency or organization.

The recent trend of social, political, and technological change does not seem to have an end. It creates challenges for innovative strategies to address these forces. There will be a continuous need for persons to help, support, and collaborate with one another to enable problem solving to proceed effectively. In other words, the need for consultation will continue to grow.

This text provides current and future consultants with a broad base of information, which was designed to enhance consultation knowledge, skill, and practice. We hope to encourage utilization of this important process by planting seeds for growth and development of occupational therapy consultation as an important aspect of practice. As a rapidly expanding area of practice, a thorough background in the principles and process of consultation is required, and this background must be supported by commitment to continuous learning.

Within occupational therapy, a consultation model of practice, based on sound principles, theoretical models, and creative thinking, must be further developed. We have illustrated increasing and varied opportunities for consultation practice;

its importance in the health care delivery system; and the knowledge base required to conduct consultative activities. As presented in previous chapters, the text's objectives are:

- to examine basic consultation concepts.
- to provide a foundation for development of consultation skills.
- to increase awareness of the critical role that consultation plays in current health care practice.
- to emphasize the importance of occupational therapy consultation as a practice method in this rapidly changing world.
- to demonstrate the natural interrelationship between consultation concepts and occupational therapy premises.
- to validate consultation as an inherent component of occupational therapy practice.
- to strengthen occupational therapy practice through expanded use of consultation approaches.
- to present a conceptual framework to guide occupational therapy consultation practice.

We have provided an overview of the evolution of consultation as a helping profession and the development of consultation within occupational therapy in particular. Consultation has been a relatively minor aspect of occupational therapy practice until recent years. Expanded visability, legislative mandates, and continuing personnel shortages increased the need and demand for consultation. The broader expertise required for consultative activities reaches beyond basic technical skills. To help other colleagues and work with entire systems, the occupational therapist must possess specific consultation knowledge and comprehensive experience. Professional training does not always include preparation for the new roles and concept applications demanded in consultation practice arenas.

The overview of fundamental consultation premises and theoretical concepts presented in this text forms a basis for study. Consultation may take many forms and follow one or several different theoretical models, as it progresses from one level of consultation to another. A complex process, consultation activities and strategies develop in relation to the complexity of the client system and the targeted population. Interwoven into the consultation fabric are such dominant concerns as the nature of the system being addressed, the consultation goal(s); the consultation model(s) best suited to address identified need(s); the relationship between the consultation intervention and the three stages of prevention; and, finally, the expected impact or outcome on the system.

Consultation levels build from case-centered consultation (Level I) to educational consultation (Level II) and peak at program/administration consultation (Level III). Within each level, one or more consultation models are chosen as means to implement the desired change. Relating change to prevention concepts helps consultant and client maintain a proactive stance, thus encouraging client empowerment and self-responsibility. Managing change requires an in-depth understanding of contributing forces and of the methods required for analyzing them.

Utilizing an open systems approach helps the consultant develop effective strategies and a plan of action which is responsive to client needs.

The consultation focus also varies, dependent upon the situation. Whether the consultant is a member of the system, functioning internally, or is brought in from outside, as an external consultant, certain basic characteristics apply. Most critical is the consultant's understanding and awareness of various approaches and possible roles required to meet specific needs of the client system.

Preparation for consultation practice includes development of necessary knowledge, skills, attitudes, and attributes. We have presented various educational avenues by which potential and practicing consultants may enhance their knowledge and skills. To achieve success, the consultant must be self-directed, highly motivated, and have a clearly defined value system. It is important to establish a reputation as a credible, mature professional, who is capable of maintaining open communications and positive client relationships.

Before embarking on a career as a consultant, the eight basic steps in the process of consultation must be understood. They are entry, contract negotiation, diagnostic analysis, goal setting and planning, intervention, evaluation, termination, and possible renegotiation. Each consultation experience requires critical analysis and judgment to ascertain the most effective approach and strategies.

The consultant must be aware of the "four Ps" of consultation: power, politics, problems, and pitfalls, and make them part of her internal monitoring system. Regulatory, legal, and ethical issues also are important and are intimately linked to the operation of the consultant's business or that of her employer.

The development of a consultation practice, a business, requires skillful blending of consultation knowledge and abilities with those of entrepeneurship. For some, who are internal consultants, the task is less awesome, since these consultants are employees of a larger organization. However, both internal and external consultants must have a keen sense of business in order to develop consultation opportunities in the most effective and efficient manner. The external consultant, or entrepreneur, establishes her business using careful planning and analysis and judicious allocation of time and money. A key aspect of her business plan is marketing.

Marketing is a continuous process that flows into all aspects of consultation. Consultation business success is intimately related to successful marketing. Using a marketing perspective, the consultant performs an in-depth analysis of both the market she has targeted and the ability of her business to respond to its needs. Establishing an effective marketing mix, the consultant identifies a needed consultation service (her product) in a particular market; prices these services competitively; provides a persuasive proposal to her potential client; and utilizes creative promotional strategies to build her referral base. Recognizing the value of marketing, the consultant dedicates time, energy, and money to this aspect of business.

CONSULTATION: A PROCESS

More than any other descriptive word, "consultation" describes a process. Components of the occupational therapy consultation process include:

- Consultation as a *helping process,* involving planning, education, and recommendations.
- Consultation as an *interactive process,* involving a sharing atmosphere and an egalitarian relationship based on mutual respect.
- Consultation as a *problem solving process,* involving issue identification, analysis, and facilitation/problem resolution.
- Consultation as a *resource identification process,* involving both available and potential internal and/or external resources.
- Consultation as a *systems process,* requiring environmental analysis, interactive communication, prevention, and enablement.

Figure 43–1 depicts this process in a graphic representation.

FIGURE 43–1

Consultation: a facilitory process.

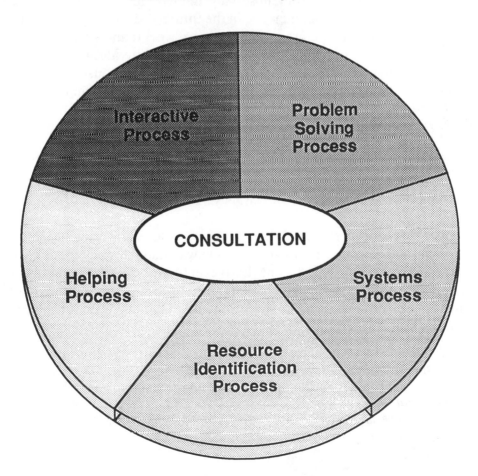

FUTURE DIRECTIONS FOR CONSULTATION

The future role of occupational therapy consultation in our health care system is related to the multiple changes and upheavals taking place nationally and internationally. To forecast this role, one must consider economic, political, legislative, technological, industrial, social, and biomedical forces. A model of occupational therapy consultation therefore has been proposed that recognizes these forces and seeks accommodation for them in the occupational therapy consultation process.

Study of social trends, as emphasized in Chapter 3, are essential in forecasting the future role of consultation in the health care delivery system. Today, demographic shifts involving many ethnic groups, have exacerbated issue of employment, acculturation, access to, and comprehension of the health care system. This large group of minorities has expanded to include older adults and disabled individuals who have benefitted from biomedical technological advances and enactment of landmark legislation. These groups provide a ready pool of manpower and resources that is underutilized and underdeveloped. This potential workforce of elderly, disabled, and ethnic minorities provides challenges to organizations and communities and expands the need and opportunities for professional consultants.

The need for help has accelerated faster than the preparation of professional helpers. Professional consultants are in constant demand and the need for individuals trained in the process of problem solving and with interactive skills necessary for successful consultation will increase in the future. Consulting has emerged as a major force in the health care arena, the business world, and society in general.

Increasing numbers of health care consumers and providers now seek a collaborative approach to service delivery. This change is in response to the increasing costs of health care, workers' compensation cases, consumer demands, and federally mandated legislation. Quality-of-life issues and health promotion needs also are receiving increased attention at state and national levels and in the private sector.

DEFINITION OF OCCUPATIONAL THERAPY CONSULTATION

Knowledgeable consumers, shrinking health care dollars, and ongoing shortages of occupational therapists contribute to the growing demand for occupational therapy consultation. Therapists using consultative activities in their practice require greater sophistication, knowledge, and intervention strategies to utilize an interactive consultation process. The model of occupational therapy consultation proposed in this text, is therefore defined as follows.

Occupational therapy consultation utilizes open systems and ecological theories; occupational therapy principles with an emphasis in humanism; and, consultation and health promotion perspectives. The occupational therapy consultation process is governed by environmental forces, human ecology, collaboration, adaptation, and enablement, in order to achieve improved client system function and to maximize human potential within a given environment.

EMPHASIS ON PREVENTION

Underlying this model is the concept of prevention and preventive outcomes. The occupational therapy consultant addresses prevention at primary, secondary, and tertiary levels. In each case, she expands the client's appreciation and understanding of important prevention strategies, thus empowering the system to remain alert, responsive, and pro-active.

The goal of all consultative activities is to enhance the client's skills and knowledge, preventing further and/or future problems. This goal is achieved by identifying the problem, analyzing the system, increasing knowledge and skills, and devising activities and intervention strategies in collaboration with the client. By encouraging and promoting a healthy environment, future unstable or dysfunctional conditions will be prevented.

CHANGES IN EDUCATIONAL APPROACH

In order to further the development of an occupational therapy consultation model, students must be provided with an expanded theoretical background and the educational support required for the study of consultation. Global influences on health and development, the prevention of disease and disability, and the promotion of a healthy society are issues which must be included in greater depth in academic and continuing education programs. Occupational therapy professional schools must help individuals to develop the ability to think creatively, hypothesize, identify patterns, and to develop and evaluate programs to enhance health in our rapidly changing and stressful society.

During the 1960s and 1970s much of the formal education of the occupational therapist focused on specific techniques for remediation, restoration, and treatment. There was a proliferation of formal assessment instruments and specific techniques or modalities to address mandates for evaluation and documentation of outcomes. This focus on proficiency in techniques led to reductionist approaches to practice, which superseded and narrowed a perspective of health care which previously had emphasized total well-being. The pressure to develop a scientific rationale for practice caused some therapists to abandon the profession's original epistemology of a dynamic, humanistic, open system approach. The narrower perspective of the medical model was embraced, emphasizing the homeostatic principle of reductionism and focusing on pathology and the reduction of symptoms. Our goal should be to balance reductionist science, with its very focused study and analysis of components, with a more holistic view, in order to develop a synthesis that can lead us to greater knowledge.

CONCLUSIONS

Futurists, predicting health care issues and trends in the 21st century, identify a broad range of consumer needs. Shifting population demographics, economic upheavals, technological advances, and epidemiological trends are among the powerful forces mandating a broadened base of practice. Community environments, which address primary, secondary, and tertiary health care needs, encourage a holistic approach to care. Occupational therapists must address these issues through varied approaches, including the expansion of consultation as a major practice component.

While multiple factors contribute to occupational therapy consultation outcomes, the environment is recognized as the primary influence in shaping adaptive behavior that leads to improved function. The consultation process and occupational therapy treatment process share this perspective. Drawing from this similar-

---

FIGURE 43–2

Factors influencing occupational therapy outcomes

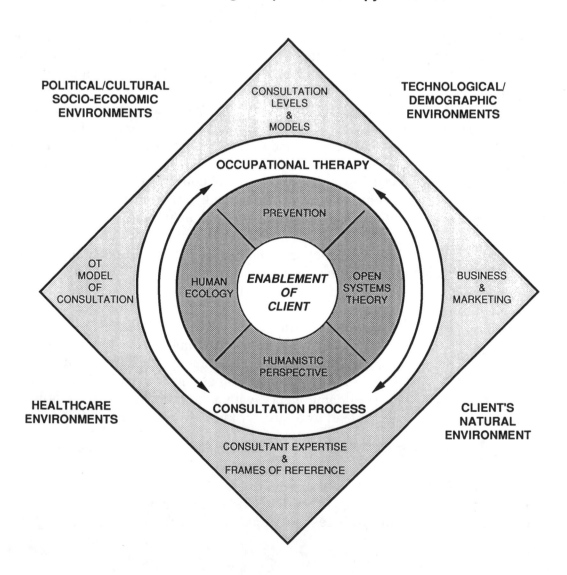

ity, the occupational therapy consultant is able to merge important concepts and develop new knowledge and skills that enable effective collaboration with clients. The consultant who recognizes and skillfully handles these many factors will achieve the consultation goal, enablement of the client. Figure 43–2 illustrates these factors.

Recent theory development within the profession has reinforced and expanded the basic consultation premise we have emphasized—the consultant should activate, enhance, enable, and empower the client and client systems to achieve maximum functional independence. While a biomechanical service delivery perspective, driven by third party payors, may still be a prevalent part of practice, new vistas have emerged that beckon the occupational therapy consultant. To address these new vistas, tomorrow's therapists must be armed with the knowledge and skills that prepare them to function in a world of rapid change. They must develop practice patterns, including consultation, that will provide the greatest service to patient and client populations.

The art and practice of consultation must become a major component of occupational therapy practice in health, education, and social service settings. It will enhance service provision, increase professional visibility, and create a dynamic position for occupational therapy in the future health care delivery.

Appendix A

Glossary

The terminology for this text is defined in terms of its use in the consultation process. In some cases, generic definitions apply, in others, the terms are specific to consultative activities.

Adaptation: the dynamic, organized process of modifying and adjusting human behavior and/or organizational structure to accommodate to new or changed environmental experiences and situations.

Advocacy: the process of active support for a specific cause, which includes the individual client and/or the client system's particular interests to improve quality of life or enhance organizational structure.

Attitudes: the expressions of behavior or disposition assumed by the consultant and/or client and the manner in which the consultant or client conveys his or her feelings and thoughts about the consultative activities.

Behavioral consultation: a case-centered or focus-specific model of consultation which utilizes strategies to modify behavior of the consultee/client system.

Business plan: an organizational tool used to guide the development of a consultation practice.

Case-centered consultation: *See* Levels of Consultation (Level I).

Change: the condition or process by which environmental influences or forces alter or transform situations, organizations, communities, and individuals; often requiring coping, modification, and adaptation.

Client: the individual, organization, or part of an organization seeking help with defining or solving a current or potential problem; the recipient of the consultant's services.

Client-centered consultation: *See* Levels of Consultation (Level II).

Clientele: the recipient or consumer of consultee or client services; for example, the patient of the "client therapist", the school children of teachers receiving collegial consultation, the residents of a nursing home undergoing consultation for staff training, program planning, organizational restructuring.

Client system: the organization or system seeking help with defining or solving a current or potential problem affecting the entire system.

Clinical consultation: a traditional patient-focused, case-specific consultation model, based on diagnosis by the expert consultant, with an emphasis on remediation and treatment.

Collaboration: the act of consultant and client working together to identify, diagnose, analyze, determine intervention strategies, and plan implementation of an agreed upon approach to problem resolution.

Collegial consultation: a peer consultation model, characterized by egalitarian mutual problem solving, in which diagnosis, analysis, and intervention strategies are determined jointly by professional colleagues, one the consultant, the other the client; the focus is usually case-specific.

Communication: the interactive method in the consultation process of linking information by coming together to discuss, deliberate, and plan a course of action to resolve a problem; one of the most important aspects of successful consultation.

Competence: the professional knowledge, skills, and abilities that convey an attitude of assurance by the consultant to the client.

Concept: the fundamental idea from which theories are formulated.

Confidentiality: the condition under which information is entrusted to the consultant and remains a confidential communication; consultative activities proceed in an atmosphere of trust, with implied confidentiality.

Conflict of interest: a situation when either the consultant or client has a hidden agenda or other interests which conflict or are inconsistent with the goals, objectives, and strategies of the consultative activities.

Confrontation intervention: provocative, active consultative strategies found most often in the social action advocacy model of consultation.

Consultant: the professional helper who has acquired a significant degree of competence in the principles and process of consultation.

Consultant roles: the consultant may assume a variety of roles to address the specific issues which include nondirective roles, where the consultant provides information; or directive roles, where the consultant assumes active leadership in training the client.

Nondirective roles may include:

- **Objective Observer/Reflector:** consultant helps client clarify the problem and gain insights.
- **Process Counselor:** consultant uses observational skills to identify, diagnose, and improve organizational relationships and processes.
- **Fact Finder:** consultant develops methodology for fact-finding and data collection.
- **Alternative Identifier/Linker:** consultant develops criteria for assessing internal and external resources and alternatives and helps client develop necessary links or networks.

Directive roles may include:

- **Joint Problem Solver:** consultant and client have a collaborative, collegial relationship for joint problem definition and decision making.

- **Trainer/Educator:** consultant plans and designs educational events and/or develops in-service training workshops.
- **Information Specialist:** consultant provides information or suggestions on specific methodology.
- **Advocate:** consultant is a persuader, provocateur, and defender of certain ideas, specific to client's needs or influences client to use certain methods of problem solving.

Consultation: the interactive process of helping others, identifying and analyzing issues, and developing problem solving strategies to prevent current and future problems.

Consultation proposal: a business tool used to market and sell services by outlining the consultant's plan for resolution of identified client problem(s).

Consultee: the individual or organization seeking help with defining or solving a current or potential problem; the recipient of the consultant's services. In this text, consultee usually refers to the specific individual, rather than group or sub-system.

Consultee-centered consultation: *See* Levels of Consultation (Level III).

Consumer: the recipient of consultee or client services.

Contract: An agreement, preferably written, between client and consultant specifying the consultation services to be provided and the responsibilities of both parties; considered a legal document.

Contract negotiation: the act of transacting a satisfactory agreement between the consultant and client regarding roles, scope of services, goals and expectations, time schedules, accountability, and fees; preferably as written contracts.

Cultural enhancement: the concept of modifying, improving, and enhancing community environments in a systems model of consultation, emphasizing the particular cultural folkways and mores of the community.

Diagnostic analysis: the act of identifying and analyzing pertinent information about the client, client system, and internal and external environmental factors influencing the system to determine goals and strategies of the consultation while maintaining confidentiality of information.

Diagnostic techniques: the methodology used to identify and determine the state of the system and the environmental influences, which may include:

- **Data analysis:** study of the information gathered; may be evaluated by formal, objective, computerized coding, or informal, observation methodology.
- **Data collection:** gathering of pertinent information may be formal or informal, such as interview, observation, surveys, questionnaires, assessments, documented reports, and records.
- **Data feedback:** the manner in which information is channeled and communicated to both consultant and client/client system; should include ongoing periodic reports.

Direct service: activities, treatment modalities, and interventions provided directly to the specific clientele; for example, therapist directed treatment procedures for a specific patient; implies implementation by person providing service.

Ecology: the science of the relationship between organisms and their environments.

Ecosystem: a unit formed by an ecological community (of living organisms) and its environment, continuously altered by the dynamic interplay of internal and external influences.

Educational consultation: an information-centered model of consultation which focuses on enhancement of client knowledge and skills; utilizing in-service training, staff development, dissemination of information.

Entrepreneur: the consultant as a business person, responsible for establishing, implementing, and operating a business as sole owner, part of a joint venture, or a major corporate stockholder.

Entry: the means by which the consultant gains access to the client or client system; through one or more of the following methods:

- **Planned entry:** consultant develops a strategy and presents a proposal.
- **Opportunistic entry:** situation arises spontaneously and consultant seizes the moment.
- **Uninvited entry:** consultant perceives need and attempts to gain entry.
- **Invited entry:** consultant is invited because of specific skills.

Environment: the complex of internal and external conditions or factors surrounding an individual or community that influences behavior and organizational structure; may consist of several different types of environment and may be viewed from micro- and macroenvironmental perspectives.

- **Human environment:** those other persons (aside from client and consultant) within the consultation setting who may influence the outcome.
- **Macroenvironment:** forces in the larger environment that impact the consultation practice, including demographic, economic, natural, technological, political, and cultural forces.
- **Microenvironment:** forces close to the consultant that affect the ability to serve specific client systems, including the consultant's business, identified markets, potential competitors, and interested or influential competitors.
- **Natural environment:** the particular client setting(s) in which the consultation occurs.
- **Physical environment:** the external factors or conditions which influence the consultation setting.

Equifinality: the principle of open systems reaching their final state or goals from a variety of alternative methods and differing conditions.

Evaluation: the process of monitoring, examining, and appraising the progress and outcome of the consultation including design and implementation of intervention strategies, development of client knowledge and skill, and efficacy of the consultation.

Exchange: A core marketing concept whereby a client obtains needed and wanted consultation services by offering something of value in return.

Expert: consultant with specific knowledge and skills in a certain subject or field.

External consultant: An independent agent, outside the organization, who is contracted by the client system to provide consultation services.

Facilitative interventions: consultative activities and strategies which help remove difficulties, initiate and direct the consultation process, and assist the client in achieving goals.

Forms of business: the type of organizational structure chosen by the consultation practice, usually with guidance from a lawyer and/or accountant; those most commonly considered:

- **Sole proprietorships:** the least complex form, where the consultant as business owner assumes all the risks and reaps all the rewards.
- **Partnership:** a separate legal entity where two or more parties contribute assets to the consultation practice, share in the profits and losses, and report gains/losses as part of their respective incomes.
- **Corporation:** a separate legal entity, with one or more stockholders, where the organization has the power to execute contracts, incur indebtedness, own property, and perform business as if it were a person.

Frame of reference: a set of concepts based on theoretical assumptions and consultation models that form the methodology and guidelines for the development of ideas, strategies, sequence of activities, direction of the consultation process, and the choice of consultant roles.

Goals: the end purpose toward which the consultative activities are directed.

Goal setting: the process of determining appropriate, realistic goals for the client through system analysis; ideally determined jointly by consultant and client.

Group dynamics: the psychological forces of group interactions and interrelationships that result in the various behaviors, roles, and interpersonal attitudes assumed in groups of people.

Helper: the individual who provides assistance, information, training, suggestions, and guidance; in this context, the *consultant*.

Heuristic approach: the consultative method that guides or furthers client investigation and discovery to enhance education and enable the client to function independently.

Holistic: constituting all the component parts and influences in a system that result in a healthy and sound approach; may refer to a social system, organization, or person. (Also considered "wholistic").

Human ecology: the concept of the interdependency of the roles of people and institutions; the influences and relationship of the environment on behavior and the dynamic, synergistic interactions of the individual or system.

Human potential: the inherent ability or capacity of the individual for growth, development, and attainment of their highest possible functioning.

Human relationships: the connections, associations, and interactions of individuals with one another.

Human resources: the individuals in an organization, agency, or community available to assist and carry out ideas, strategies, and programs.

Humanism: the philosophy and attitude that is concerned with the interests, capabilities, and achievements of human beings.

Indirect service: activities, strategies, and interventions provided by the consultant to enable the consultee or client system to address issues and/or problems; implementation of suggestions are conducted by the consultee/client system.

Internal consultant: an employee of the client system who is asked to provide consultation services within the organization.

Interventions: the helping strategies, methods, and techniques which form the basis for consultative activities.

Isomorphism: a one-to-one correspondence between elements; an analogous relationship or operation, so that the result of one activity has a corresponding affect on the result of similar activities in another.

Key individuals: persons in an organization, system, or community that have authority for decision making, have access to those with power and influence, or through whom important information can be gained and/or disseminated.

Levels of Consultation: consultation may occur on one or more levels.

- **Level I:** focused on a specific problem case utilizing a clinical perspective; considered case-centered consultation.
- **Level II:** focused on the consultee or client system, utilizing educational strategies to enhance knowledge and skills; considered educational, client or consultee-centered consultation.
- **Level III:** focused on a particular social system, utilizing strategies to strengthen administrative, management, and program planning skills; considered program and/or administrative consultation.

Locus of consultation: refers to the specific issue or problem requiring consultation, for example, the locus of the problem may be the consultee's lack of knowledge or skills, unexpected organizational changes resulting from external environmental influences, populations at risk, maldistribution of resources, etc.

Marketing: a system for organizational planning developed from an information base; a social and managerial process by which individuals and groups obtain what they need and want by creating and exchanging products and values with others.

Marketing environment: the complex of internal and external forces that affect the consultant's ability to transact effectively with a given client system or target market; viewed from macro- and microenvironmental perspectives. (*See* Environment)

Marketing mix: a set of controllable marketing variables, often referred to as the ''4 P's'' of product, price, place and promotion, that the consultant blends to achieve a particular response in an identified target market.

Methodology: the organized system of practices and procedures used in collecting data, developing consultative strategies, and evaluating the process.

Models of consultation: the various approaches to consultation based on theoretical assumptions which provides the broad focus, guidelines, and directions for consultation practice. Ten consultation models are identified in this text: (*See also* individual definitions).

Behavioral model
Clinical or treatment model
Collegial or professional model
Educational model
Occupational therapy model
Organizational development model
Process management model
Program development model
Social action model
Systems model

Monitoring: the act of continual observation and assessment of the consultation process.

Mutual cooperation: the egalitarian joint study, discussion, and deliberations that occur between consultant and client in the consultative process; essential in collegial consultation.

Mutual trust: the shared feeling of faith, respect, and confidence between consultant and client; desired in all consultations.

Networking: the process of developing communication channels for exchange of ideas and information; a means of creating feedback between consultant and client/client system.

Occupational performance: the achievement of purposeful activities that improve human function and enhance performance in areas of self-care, work, education, play, and leisure.

Occupational therapy consultation: a model of consultation based on the principles and philosophy of occupational therapy, humanism, and human ecology; an open systems, collaborative approach focusing on all aspects of client/client system environments, leading to enablement, improved client function, and maximized human potential.

Open system: a social system that receives input from all environmental forces and is characterized by the dynamic interaction of these forces on the organizational structure and functioning of the system.

Organizational development (OD): an organization-centered, management-focused model of consultation which emphasizes organizational structure, interrelationships, conflict resolution, and planned change.

Organizational diagnosis: the process of gathering information regarding the structure and operation of an organization and analyzing the data to develop intervention strategies.

Orientation response (OR): the complex, massive bodily reactions to environmental stimuli when routine, repetitive patterns are interrupted; this response provides one of the organism's key adaptive mechanisms to alterations in the environment.

Outcome: the result or consequence of the consultative activities.

Policy: a plan, based on certain principles, that influences procedures and determines decision making and action, may include:
- **Health policies:** the plans adopted by government, companies, or agencies that determine health programs, coverage, and liabilities.
- **Organizational policies:** the plans which determine the organizational structure and course of action.
- **Social policies:** those plans which affect the entire society or community and guide program development and funding.
- **System policies:** the guiding principles of a system which determines the structure, functions, and procedural operations of the system.

Postulates: a fundamental element or basic principle that is assumed as a premise or axiom and is generally accepted.

Power people: those persons who have the authority or official capacity to exert control in an organization; individuals with strong influence on decision making and implementation of policies and procedures; *See also* Key individuals.

Prevention principles: concepts which help deter, eliminate, hinder, forestall, or preclude the conditions, events, or actions that lead to problems. There are three types of prevention:
- **Primary prevention:** activities undertaken prior to the onset of the problem to avoid the occurrence of malfunction or disability in a population potentially at risk.
- **Secondary prevention:** early diagnosis, identification, and detection of populations at risk to prevent chronic dysfunction or permanent disability.
- **Tertiary prevention:** rehabilitation and remediation of a problem or illness to prevent further problems, loss, or disability.

Preventive outcomes: the result of consultation activities described in terms of their potential for social, organizational, and health preventive programming. These outcomes relate to the three levels of consultation:
- **Tertiary preventive outcomes:** modification of behavior of the specific client through maintenance at Level I: case-centered consultation.
- **Secondary preventive outcomes:** modification of behavior through skill development at Level II: educational consultation.
- **Primary preventive outcomes:** transformation, institutional, and system change through program development, management, and organizational restructuring at Level III: program and/or administrative consultation.

Problem solving: the act of resolving issues or difficulties; the ultimate goal of the consultation is to improve this ability in the client/client system.

Process management consultation: group-based model of consultation which focuses on specific management-oriented organizational processes and dynamics; intervention strategies emphasize interpersonal and intergroup process, communication patterns, group roles and functions.

Program development consultation: service-centered model of consultation based on development of new programs or modification of existing programs to improve a service delivery system.

Proposal: *See* Consultation proposal

Reframing: the process of helping the client/client system view a particular issue or strategy from a different perspective.

Roles: the function or position of the consultant and client; the characteristics or norms of behavior expected in the consultation process. *See also* Consultant roles.

Resources: available or potential supply of information, support or help used by consultant, client/client system to decrease problems and enhance solutions, for example, available capital, or financial assets, human resources (person power), data bases, and the like.

Responsibilities: the assigned or agreed upon accountable obligations and commitments of both the consultant and client.

Social action consultation: a social-reform based model of consultation focusing on social values and policies; intervention strategies are action-oriented, utilizing advocacy, and occasional confrontational approaches to effect change.

Social climate: the environment that surrounds social systems and influences functioning; includes economic, political, and cultural forces.

Social system: the organized network or set of interrelated ideas and principles of the environment or community focused on certain cultural mores, life styles, and habits of its members; the societal structure that governs policies, procedures, and the operations of the interdependent elements in a system.

Societal marketing concept: viewpoint which considers the well being of both client and society as an integral part of the marketing process.

Strategies: the consultative intervention activities designed and devised to: address specific issues, form a course of action, or implement measures to deal with client problems.

Stress: the adaptive reaction in an organism caused by certain influences, systems, forces; physiological, body chemistry, and emotional changes as a result of these influences.

Stressors: the shifts and changes in the emotional climate surrounding the organism that trigger the stress reaction; these include physical and social environmental changes, interpersonal relationships, anticipation of change, social pressures, life style modifications.

Synergistic: serving to connect or interrelate the action of two or more elements or organisms so that there is a direct correlation and interdependence of the action of one on the other.

Synthesis: the combining of separate elements or concepts to form a coherent whole, producing enhanced and/or new ideas and products.

Systems analysis: the identification and determination of the state of the system; study and evaluation of all internal and external environmental factors influencing the system to determine goals and strategies of the consultation.

Systems consultation: the model of consultation based on general systems theory focused on the mission, goals, values, and culture of a system (e.g., community, agency, school, church) or organization; utilizing planned change strategies to effect long range changes in the system.

Target market: a specific set of potential clients/client systems who share common needs or characteristics that the consultant decides to serve.

Team development: the training and skill development of a group of individuals organized to work together; utilization of process management techniques that emphasize interpersonal and intergroup process.

Technical specialist: the direct service technician with specific technical training regarding information, scientific process, application, and maintenance of particular technology; an expert service provider, not a consultant.

Technological change: the change in the environment as a result of new advances in scientific, medical, and industrial progress.

Theoretical model: the guide to consultant action, based on theoretical concepts, enabling the consultant to utilize a broad focus when analyzing client systems, choosing appropriate frame(s) of reference, and identifying procedural methodology.

Theory: systematically organized statements and assumptions derived from scientific disciplines that relate, predict, and explain concepts and behavior.

Typology: system of classification based on set of concepts.

Values: the principles and standards of an individual or organization that are held in high esteem; considered worthwhile and desirable.

Appendix B

Consultation Resources

Inclusion of information centers, organizations or publishers does not imply endorsement, nor is this intended to be a complete listing. Every effort has been made to assure accuracy, but responsibility can not be taken for errors or changes occurring since the printing.

Occupational therapy consultants must acquire a broad range of resources to maintain a current information base and expand their knowledge. This appendix is not all inclusive nor does it constitute endorsement of those listed. It is designed to provide some basic resources, and has two parts. The first section provides information sources regarding consultation, business and marketing. The second section lists resources related to consultation practice areas.

CONSULTATION, BUSINESS, AND MARKETING RESOURCES

This section identifies associations, organizations, publishers, and governmental agencies that may provide the consultant with a broad range of services and information. Many provide journals, newsletters, training programs, and data bases. Some publish texts, as well as audio and video training materials; others sponsor conferences and may also be involved in research. A query to them will bring specific information regarding their focus and the consultation resources they have available.

In addition to the sources listed, consultants who are in the process of setting up a business should check with their state's small business administration office. These offices are often able to provide free consultation, referral sources for loans, linkage to entrepreneurs engaged in a similar business, and listings of free or minimal cost training programs.

A number key appears after the name of each resource. The number indicates major services and information available through each listing. If there is a membership fee, an * appears before the numbers.

KEY FOR CONSULTATION, BUSINESS, AND
MARKETING RESOURCES

  *   Membership Fee
1. Annual Conference
2. Workshops/Seminars
3. Training Packages
4. Books and other Publications
5. Audio Tapes
6. Video Tapes
7. Journal(s)
8. Newsletter(s)
9. Data Base(s)
10. Computer Software Packages

Academy for Health Services Marketing   (*,1,2,3,4,5,6,7,8,9)
American Marketing Association
250 South Wacker Drive
Chicago, IL 60606
312-648-0536

American Health Consultants   (4,5,6,7,8,9,10)
P.O. Box 740060
Atlanta, GA 30374
800-688-2421

American Management Association   (*,2,3,4,5,6,7,8,9,10)
135 West 50th Street
New York, NY 10020
212-903-8234

American Society for Training and Development   (*,2,3,4,7,8,10)
1640 King Street, Box 1443
Alexandria, VA 22313
703-683-8100

Case Management Society of America   (*,1,2,8)
1200 17th Street
NW Suite 400
Washington, DC 20036
202-296-9200

Enterprise Publishing, Inc.   (4,10)
725 North Market Street
Wilmington, DE 19801
800-533-2665

Health Care Financing Review   (7)
Superintendent of Documents
U.S. Government Printing Office
Washington, DC 20402

Inc. Business Products   (4,5,6)
P.O. Box 1365
Wilkes Barre, PA 18703-1365
800-372-0018

U.S. Internal Revenue Service   (4)
Distribution Centers
Located in Western, Central, and Eastern U.S.A.
800-424-3676

Jeffrey Lant Associates   (2,3,4,5,6,8,9)
50 Follen
Cambridge, MA 02138
617-547-6372

Jossey-Bass Publishers   (3,4,5,6,7)
350 Sansome Street
San Francisco, CA 94104
415-433-1767

National Referral Center   (9)
Library of Congress
Washington, DC 20540
202-287-5670

Pfeiffer & Company   (2,3,4,5,6)
8517 Production Avenue
San Diego, CA 92121-2280
619-578-5900

Schrello Direct Marketing   (2,3,4,5,8)
555 Ocean Boulevard
P.O. Box 1610
Long Beach, CA 90801
213-437-2230

Shenson Consulting   (2,3,4,8)
20750 Ventura Boulevard
Woodland Hills, CA 91364
818-703-1415

University Associates, Inc.   (2,3,8)
8380 Miramar Mall, Suite 232
San Diego, CA 92121
619-552-8901

U.S. Small Business Administration
1111 18th St. NW, 6th Floor
Washington, DC 20036
202-634-1500

U.S. Small Business Administration   (4)
SBA Publications
P.O. Box 30
Denver, CO 80201-0030
800-827-5722

CONSULTATION PRACTICE RESOURCES

Every consultant should develop a list of key practice resources, to be accessed as the need arises. Given occupational therapy's broad focus, the consultant should be aware of general resources, such as federal and state agencies, national associations, organizations, centers and foundations that can provide comprehensive information from a wide information base. These can then be supplemented with other resources pertinent to the specific consultation setting. The listings provided are a small sample of resources available, and do not represent endorsement. Rather, it is hoped the reader will use these listings as a springboard to develop their own comprehensive data base. In addition to a general resource listing, resources for each consultation practice setting presented in the text are offered.

Please note that resources listed for one practice setting may also apply in others. For example, The Association for People with Severe Handicaps, listed under School Settings, may provide information relevant for consultants working in long-term care or community settings; National Clearing House for Alcohol Information, listed under Community Settings, may be helpful in industry or long-term care settings.

A resource of particular importance to the occupational therapy consultant is the American Occupational Therapy Association (AOTA). AOTA books, manuals, guidelines, Special Interest Section Newsletters, Practice Information Packets, a weekly newspaper, and a monthly journal provide important informational sources. Multi-media resources are supplemented through data bases, software packages, and access to practice experts for timely supportive information. Locally, the state occupational therapy association also should be considered a primary resource, especially from a networking perspective.

General Resources

American Association of University Affiliated Programs for Persons with
   Developmental Disabilities
8630 Fenton Street, Suite 410
Silver Springs, MD 20910
301-588-8252

American Association on Mental Retardation
1719 Kalorama Road NW
Washington, DC 20009
800-424-3688

American Council of the Blind
1155 15th Street NW, Suite 720
Washington, DC 20005
800-424-8666

American Foundation for the Blind
15 West 16th Street
New York, NY 10011
212-620-2000

American Occupational Therapy Association
1383 Piccard Drive
Rockville, MD 20850
301-948-9626

Clearinghouse on Disability Information
U.S. Department of Education
Switzer Building
330 C Street SW, Room 3132
Washington, DC 20202-2524
202-732-1723

Clearinghouse on the Handicapped
Switzer Building, Room 2319
330 C Street SW
Washington, DC 20202-2524

IBM—National Support Center for Persons with Disabilities
(Impairments: Hearing, Mobility, Learning, Speech and Vision)
P.O. Box 2150
Atlanta, GA 30055
404-364-2189

Information Center for Individuals with Disabilities
20 Park Plaza, Room 330
Boston, MA 22116
617-727-5540

National Center for Health Statistics
U.S. Department of Health & Human Services
Public Health Service
6525 Belcrest Road
Hyattsville, MD 20782
301-436-8500

National Disability Action Center
1101 15th Street NW
Washington, DC 20005
202-775-9231

National Head Injury Foundation
1140 Connecticut Avenue, Suite 812
Washington, DC 20036
202-296-6443

National Information Center on Deafness
800 Florida Avenue NE
Washington, DC 20002
202-651-5051

National Institute of Handicapped Research
Switzer Building
Washington, DC 20202
202-732-1139

National Institutes of Health
Office of Disease Prevention and Health Promotion
P.O. Box 1133
Washington, DC 20013-1133
800-336-4797

National Institute of Mental Health
5600 Fisher Lane
Rockville, MD 20852
301-443-3673

National Library of Medicine
8600 Rockville Pike
Bethesda, MD 20814
800-638-8480

National Library Service for the Blind and Physically Handicapped
Library of Congress
1291 Taylor Street NW
Washington, DC 20542
800-424-8567

National Organization on Disability
910 16th Street NW, Suite 600
Washington, DC 20006
800-248-ABLE

National Pharmaceutical Council
1894 Preston White Drive
Reston, VA 22091
703-620-6390

National Rehabilitation Information Center
8455 Calesville Road, Suite 935
Silver Springs, MD 20910-3319
800-346-2742

National Spinal Cord Injury Association
600 West Cummings Park
Woburne, MA 01801
617-935-2722

New England Index
Data Base Information on Disabilities Exchange
The Shriver Center
200 Trapelo Road
Waltham, MA 02154
617-857-1199

School Settings

Association for Children and Adults with Learning Disabilities
4156 Library Road
Pittsburgh, PA 15234
412-341-1515

The Association for People with Severe Handicaps (TASH)
7010 Roosevelt Way NE
Seattle, WA 98115
206-523-8446

Council of Exceptional Children
1920 Association Drive
Reston, VA 22091
703-620-3660

Exceptional Parent
Annual Directory of National Organizations
1170 Commonwealth Avenue
Boston, MA 02134-9942
800-247-8080

National Information Center for Children and Youth with Disabilities
P.O. Box 1492
Washington, DC 20013
800-999-5599

Long-Term Care Settings

American Association of Retired Persons
1909 K Street NW
Washington, DC 20049
202-872-4700

The Gerontological Society of America
1275 K Street NW #350
Washington, DC 20005-4006
202-842-1275

National Archive of Computerized Data on Aging
P.O. Box 1248
Ann Arbor, MI 48106
313-763-5010

National Council on the Aging
600 Maryland Avenue SW
West Wing 100
Washington, DC 20024
800-424-9046

NIA Information Center
P.O. Box 8057
Gaithersburg, MD 20898-8057
301-495-3455

Acute Settings

American Hospital Association
P.O. Box 92247
Chicago, IL 60675-2247
312-280-6000

American Medical Association
515 North State Street
Chicago, IL 60610
312-464-5000

Community Settings

Administration on Developmental Disabilities
200 Independence Avenue SW
329D Humphrey Building
Washington, DC 20201
202-245-2890

Association for Retarded Citizens of the United States
P.O. Box 6109
2501 Avenue J
Arlington, Texas 76006
817-640-0204

Bureau of Maternal and Child Health and Resources Development
Parklawn Building
5600 Fishers Lane
Room 9-11
Rockville, MD 20857
301-443-2170

National Association for Home Care
519 C Street NE
Stanton Park
Washington, DC 20002-5809
202-547-7424

National Clearinghouse for Alcohol Information
P.O. Box 2345
Rockville, MD 20852
301-468-2600

National Institute on Aging
Resource Directory for Older People
9000 Rockville Pike
Bethesda, MD 20892
301-496-1752

National Institute of Child Health and Human Development
National Institutes of Health
9000 Rockville Pike
Building 31, Room 2A03
Bethesda, MD 20892
301-496-3454

National Mental Health Association
1021 Prince Street
Arlington, VA 22314
800-969-6642

Industry Settings

American Society of Hand Therapists
1002 Vandora Springs Road, Suite 101
Garner, NC 27529
919-245-2890

Job Accommodation Network
Box 4683
Morgantown, WV 26505
800-526-7234

National Rehabilitation Association
1910 Association Drive, Suite 205
Reston, VA 22091-1052
703-715-9090

President's Committee on Employment of People with Disabilities
1331 F Street NW
Washington, DC 20004-1107
202-376-6200

Stout Vocational Rehabilitation Institute
Materials Development Center
University of Wisconsin-Stout
Menomonie, WI 54751
715-232-1342

Education Settings

American Council on Education
1 Dupont Circle NW, Suite 800
Washington, DC 20036
202-939-9300

American Association for Higher Education
1 Dupont Circle NW, Suite 600
Washington, DC 20036
202-293-6440

Association for the Study of Higher Education
Department of Educational Administration
Texas A & M University
College Station, TX 77843
409-845-0393

Regulatory Settings

Commission on Accreditation of Rehabilitation Facilities
101 North Wilmot Road, Suite 500
Tucson, AZ 85711
602-748-1212

Joint Commission on Accreditation of Healthcare Organizations
1 Renaissance Boulevard
Oak Brook Terrace, IL 60181
708-916-5600

Technology

ABLEDATA
Adaptive Equipment Center
Newington Children's Hospital
181 East Cedar Street
Newington, CT 06111
800-344-5405

Association for Educational Communication and Technology
1126 16th Street NW
Washington, DC 20036
202-347-7834

Closing the Gap
P.O. Box 68
Henderson, MN 56044
612-248-3294

National Clearinghouse on Technology & Aging
University Center on Aging
University of Massachusetts Medical Center
55 Lake Avenue North
Worcester, MA 01655
508-856-3662

RESNA
1101 Connecticut Avenue NW, Suite 700
Washington, DC 20036
202-857-1199

TRACE Research/ Development Center
Room S–151 Waisman Center
1500 Highland Avenue
Madison, WI 53705
608-262-6966

Appendix C

Codes of Ethics

OCCUPATIONAL THERAPY CODE OF ETHICS*

The American Occupational Therapy Association and its component members are committed to furthering people's ability to function fully within their total environment. To this end the occupational therapist renders service to clients in all stages of health and illness, to institutions, to other professionals and colleagues, to students, and to the general public.

In furthering this commitment, the American Occupational Therapy Association has established the Occupational Therapy Code of Ethics. This Code is intended to be used as a guide to promoting and maintaining the highest standards of ethical behavior.

This Code of Ethics shall apply to all occupational therapy personnel. The term *occupational therapy personnel* shall include individuals who are registered occupational therapists, certified occupational therapy assistants, and occupational therapy students. The roles of practitioner, educator, manager, researcher, and consultant are assumed.

Principle 1 (Beneficence/Autonomy)

Occupational therapy personnel shall demonstrate a concern for the welfare and dignity of the recipient of their services.

A. The individual is responsible for providing services without regard to race, creed, national origin, sex, age, handicap, disease entity, social status, financial status or religious affiliation.

---

* From the American Occupational Therapy Association: *Am J Occup Ther* 1988; 42:795–796. Used with permission.

B. The individual shall inform those people served of the nature and potential outcomes of treatment and shall respect the right of potential recipients of service to refuse treatment.

C. The individual shall inform subjects involved in education or research activities of the potential outcome of those activities.

D. The individual shall include those people served in the treatment planning process.

E. The individual shall maintain goal-directed and objective relationships with all people served.

F. The individual shall protect the confidential nature of information gained from educational, practice, and investigational activities unless sharing such information could be deemed necessary to protect the well-being of a third party.

G. The individual shall take all reasonable precautions to avoid harm to the recipient of services or detriment to the recipient's property.

H. The individual shall establish fees, based on cost analysis, that are commensurate with services rendered.

Principle 2 (Competence)

Occupational therapy personnel shall actively maintain high standards of professional competence.

A. The individual shall hold the appropriate credential for providing service.

B. The individual shall recognize the need for competence and shall participate in continuing professional development.

C. The individual shall function within the parameters of his or her competence and the standards of the profession.

D. The individual shall refer clients to other service providers or consult with other service providers when additional knowledge and expertise is required.

Principle 3 (Compliance with Laws and Regulations)

Occupational therapy personnel shall comply with laws and Association policies guiding the profession of occupational therapy.

A. The individual shall be acquainted with applicable local, state, federal, and institutional rules and Association policies and shall function accordingly.

B. The individual shall inform employers, employees, and colleagues about those laws and policies that apply to the profession of occupational therapy.

C. The individual shall require those whom they supervise to adhere to the Code of Ethics.

D. The individual shall accurately record and report information.

Principle 4 (Public Information)

Occupational therapy personnel shall provide accurate information concerning occupational therapy services.

A. The individual shall accurately represent his or her competence and training.

B. The individual shall not use or participate in the use of any form of communication that contains a false, fraudulent, deceptive, or unfair statement or claim.

Principle 5 (Professional Relationships)

Occupational therapy personnel shall function with discretion and integrity in relations with colleagues and other professionals, and shall be concerned with the quality of their services.

A. The individual shall report illegal, incompetent, and/or unethical practice to the appropriate authority.

B. The individual shall not disclose privileged information when participating in reviews of peers, programs, or systems.

C. The individual who employs or supervises colleagues shall provide appropriate supervision, as defined in AOTA guidelines or state laws, regulations, and institutional policies.

D. The individual shall recognize the contributions of colleagues when disseminating professional information.

Principle 6 (Professional Conduct)

Occupational therapy personnel shall not engage in any form of conduct that constitutes a conflict of interest or that adversely reflects on the profession.

Enforcement procedures are available from the Department of Professional Services, 1383 Piccard Drive, Rockville, MD 20850. Complaints should be addressed to the Standards and Ethics Chair at the same address.

Approved by the Representative Assembly, April 1988.

This document replaces the Principles of Occupational Therapy Ethics, originally approved, April 1977 and approved as revised, 1979.

CODE OF ETHICS FOR THE PROFESSIONAL CONSULTANT*

1. Responsibility

The consultant:

- Places high value on objectivity and integrity and maintains the highest standards of service; and
- Plans work in a way that minimizes the possibility that findings will be misleading.

2. Competence

The consultant:

- Maintains high standards of professional competence as a responsibility to the public and to the profession;
- Recognizes the boundaries of his or her competence and does not offer services that fail to meet professional standards;
- Assists clients in obtaining professional help for aspects of the projects that fall outside the boundaries of his or her own competence; and
- Refrains from undertaking any activity in which his or her personal problems are likely to result in inferior professional service or harm to the client.

3. Moral and Legal Standards

The consultant shows sensible regard for the social codes and moral expectations of the community in which he or she works.

4. Misrepresentation

The consultant avoids misrepresentations of his or her professional qualifications, affiliations, and purposes and those of the organization with which he or she is associated.

---

* From Lippitt G, Lippitt R: *The Consulting Process in Action,* ed 2. San Diego, Calif, University Associates, 1986. Used with permission.

5. Confidentiality

The consultant:

- Reveals information received in confidence only to the appropriate authorities;
- Maintains confidentiality of professional communications about individuals;
- Informs the client of the limits of confidentiality; and
- Maintains confidentiality in preservation and disposition of records.

6. Client Welfare

The consultant:

- Defines the nature of his or her loyalties and responsibilities in possible conflicts of interest, such as between the client and the consultant's employer, and keeps all concerned parties informed of these commitments;
- Attempts to terminate a consulting relationship when it is reasonably clear that the client is not benefiting from it; and
- Continues being responsible for the welfare of the client, in cases involving referral, until the responsibility is assumed by the professional to whom the client is referred or until the relationship with the client has been terminated by mutual agreement.

7. Announcement of Services

The consultant adheres to professional standards rather than solely economic rewards in making known his or her availability for professional services.

8. Intraprofessional and Interprofessional Relations

The consultant acts with integrity toward colleagues in consultation and in other professions.

9. Remuneration

The consultant ensures that the financial arrangements for his or her professional services are in accordance with professional standards that safeguard the best interests of the client and the profession.

10. Responsibility Toward Organization

The consultant respects the rights and reputation of the organization with which he or she is associated.

11. Promotional Activities

The consultant, when associated with the development or promotion of products offered for commercial sale, ensures that the products are presented in a factual way.

Appendix D

Proposals, Contracts, and Formats

The documents provided in this appendix have been supplied by authors of text chapters. They serve to illustrate points conveyed in these chapters and are not intended to render legal, accounting, or other professional service. If legal advice or other expert assistance is required, the services of a competent professional should be sought.

INTRODUCTION

Consultation contracts, proposals, and formats designed to gather information, are important consultant tools. As has been discussed and emphasized, prior to the development of letters of agreement or contracts, the consultant should seek legal counsel. Sample documents provided in this appendix have been used in the context of case(s) described by the respective authors of Chapters 8, 12, 13, 17, and 26.

Proposals are an important marketing tool. They provide a plan and an offer of consultation services that the client may accept or reject. The proposal may be a formal document, as in the Chapter 13 sample, or a letter, as presented in the Chapter 17 sample. Marketing handouts may also be used at preliminary meetings to briefly delineate the consulting firm's services, as shown in the Chapter 17 materials.

Agreements are set in place when consultant and client have successfully negotiated. The contract samples in this appendix range from a letter of agreement initiated by the client to the consultant (Chapter 13), to an extensive and detailed contract between a state agency and a university (Chapter 8). The case example in Chapter 17 provides both consultation and treatment. This contract was therefore formatted to accommodate the different levels of service. Less complex contract samples from Chapters 12 and 26 cover requirements identified by client and consultant in each case example.

Specific formats may be required in different consultation practice settings. They are necessary to help address data gathering and communication issues, which are key aspects of the consultant's work. Chapter 12 sample formats illustrate one consultants approach to these important concerns. In each practice environment, the consultant will find it helpful to draft formats for baseline data gathering and communication.

The sample agreements presented in this appendix are specific to the cases described. Use by others should not be considered unless further legal guidance is obtained. It is always in the consultant's best interest to work with a written contract or agreement. The document should be written clearly and be as specific as possible. Client and consultant responsibilities should be delineated. Both parties are then informed participants, and misunderstandings or disputes are less likely to occur.

Satisfied clients bring increased business. Well-written, effectively designed proposals and contracts are a professional consultant's hallmark. These important tools set the stage for a consultative relationship. Similarly, data gathering and reporting formats that support the consultation process must be effective tools for communication. A knowledgeable consultant will plan carefully, seek guidance when appropriate, and consistently monitor these tools to assure ongoing effectiveness.

CHAPTER 8
SAMPLE CONTRACT

This Agreement, made and entered into this _____ day of _____
19 __, between the State Board of Education, hereinafter referred to as the
"SBE" and the University Department of Medical Allied Health Professions,
having its principal offices at _____
_____ hereinafter referred to as the Contractor.

WITNESSETH

For and in consideration of the mutual promises to each other, hereinafter set
forth, the parties do mutually agree as follows:

A. The Contractor hereby agrees to provide professional services as follows:

1. Provide direct assistance to the Division for Exceptional Children of the
    State Department of Public Instruction in the areas of occupational therapy
    and physical therapy as part of the total effort on behalf of children with
    special needs.

    Personnel employed for the purpose of this contract will (1) meet monthly
    with Department of Public Instruction staff to provide an oral report of the
    occupational therapy needs and physical therapy needs of handicapped
    children, (2) keep abreast of changes in federal and state regulations
    that could have an impact on occupational therapy and physical therapy
    services and report the changes to the Division for Exceptional Chil-
    dren.

2. Provide assistance to the Division for Exceptional Children, and local
    school administrative units through consultative services in program plan-
    ning, development, management and evaluation in the initiation, expansion,
    and improvement of occupational therapy and physical therapy services for
    children with special needs, and in particular:

    a. Provide leadership to local school administrative units in determining
        their occupational therapy and physical therapy needs through consul-
        tant services in program planning, development, management, and eval-
        uation.

    b. Make written recommendations for the establishment and continued
        development of efficient and effective occupational therapy and physical
        therapy programs in school settings.

    c. Assist school systems through on-site consultations, telecommu-
        nications, and conferencing in planning for the employment and effec-
        tive use of occupational therapist assistants and physical therapist assis-
        tants.

    d. Provide leadership to early education for the handicapped (ages 3 & 4)
        programs in determining their occupational therapy and physical therapy
        needs through on-site consultations and technical assistance regarding
        program planning, development, management and evaluation.

    e. Develop written materials or audiovisual materials that illustrate the role of occupational therapy and physical therapy in the early education for the handicapped (3, 4, and 5 year-olds).

    f. Keep updated appropriate occupational therapy and physical therapy documents and guidelines in keeping with best professional standards.

    g. Develop and conduct staff development activities for therapists, therapist assistants, teachers, aides, and other school personnel.

    h. Develop written recommendations for retention of occupational therapists and physical therapists employed in schools.

    i. Oversee endorsement and implementation by the state agency of written recommendations for salaries, raises, professional career advancement, and personnel policies for school occupational therapists and physical therapists and occupational therapist and physical therapist assistants.

    j. Develop recruitment activities and support materials such as display board, brochures, videotapes, and national advertisements to actively recruit nationally occupational therapists and physical therapists to work in schools.

    k. Provide limited instruction to institution of high education classes and participate in other student-related activities for the purpose of recruitment and student development.

  3. Provide office space and adequate office equipment for the support of personnel employed for the purpose of this contract.

  4. Provide the state agency with documentation of the actual cost of the program at the end of each month during the contract period. The documentation will enumerate the expenditures according to the attached budget, which is made a part of this contract by reference. Invoices should be billed to _____ for approval of payment. The final invoice must be received by _____ 19 ___.

  5. Submit monthly reports to the Division for Exceptional Children, addressing the services being provided by personnel employed under this agreement. The reports will be completed and provided to the Division for Exceptional Children on or before the fifth working day of each month.

  6. Submit weekly schedules of work for personnel employed through this project as required by the Division for Exceptional Children.

B. The SBE agrees:

  1. To pay the Contractor the sum of $ _____ . Said sum to be full and complete payment for services to be rendered under contract.

  2. To monitor the planning and implementation of the services of this contract through the Division for Exceptional Children.

  3. To provide assistance to contract staff in working with the programs operated by local school administrative units and in the development of documents and materials related to these programs.

C. The dates and terms of this contract between the SBE and Contractor will be for the period of July 1, 19 ___ through June 30, 19 ___.

D. The Contractor and the SBE hereby agree to the following items and conditions:

1. That the funding and execution of the contract are contingent upon federal appropriations being made available for this purpose for fiscal year 19 __ –19 __ .
2. That salaries and wages provided for under this contract will be adjusted, either up or down, in accordance with the actual gross salaries and fringe benefits paid to these positions by the Contractor under EPA guidelines.
3. That funds cannot be transferred from one line item to another without the approval of the project coordinator.
4. That assignment of the occupational therapy and physical therapy consultants to the Division for Exceptional Children by the Contractor, as part of this agreement, will be contingent upon prior consultation with the Division for Exceptional Children.
5. That this contract is implemented to improve services to handicapped children in local school administrative units as outlined in federal and state laws.
6. That this contract may be amended only by written amendments duly executed by and between the SBE and the Contractor. However, minor modifications may be made by the SBE Project Coordinator to take advantage of unforeseen oppotunities that: (a) do not change the intent of the contract or the scope of the Contractor's performance; (b) do not increase the Contractor's total compensation; and (c) either improve the overall quality of the product or service to the State without increasing the cost, or reduce the total cost of the product or service without reducing the quantity or quality. All such minor modifications to the contract must be recorded in writing and employees or contracts with any employee of the State Board of Education or Department of Public Instruction, that fact will be immediately reported to the Contracts Officer for the Department of Public Instruction.
8. That recommendations on promotion, reappointment, and salary increases for personnel employer under this contract will be the responsibility of the Contractor after consultation with the Project Coordinator.
9. That continuation of employment for personnel employed under this contract will be based on the needs and resources of the Contractor in fulfilling the terms of this contract.

IN WITNESS THEREOF, the SBE and Contractor have executed this agreement on the day and year herein above first written.

ATTEST

FOR THE STATE BOARD OF EDUCATION

_____   _____

                                             Date

_____   _____

                                             Date

CONTRACTOR: THE UNIVERSITY

_____   _____

                                             Date

CHAPTER 12
SAMPLE CONTRACT 1

Activities Consultation Agreement

A. This Agreement is made and entered into between _____
_____, Registered Occupational Therapist (hereinafter called "Consultant"),
and _____ (hereinafter called "Home").

B. Being duly licensed and registered in _____ as an occupational therapist, Consultant agrees to provide at least four hours of consultation in the facility per month, upon the following terms and conditions.

1. Home shall retain administrative responsibility for the services rendered.
2. Consultant and Home agree to comply with all applicable laws, government regulations, and the Manual of Standards for Licensure of Long-Term Care Facilities.
3. Consultant will provide consultation to the Administrator and Activities personnel for planning and policy development regarding resident activities and reality orientation programs based on initial and ongoing evaluations.
4. Consultant will conduct in-service education as required.
5. Consultant will provide the Home with written reports and recommendations following on-site visits.
6. Home will provide space for the Consultant to properly perform her services.
7. Home will orient the Consultant as to the Home's policies, rules, and regulations.
8. For the above services and responsibilities the Consultant will be paid the sum of $ _____ per hour.
9. The terms of this Agreement will begin on _____ and will continue in effect for a period of _____ year(s), except that either party may terminate this Agreement by giving thirty (30) days notice in writing to the other party of its intention to do so.
10. This Agreement constitutes the entire understanding between Consultant and Home. This Agreement shall be construed and interpreted according to the laws of the State of _____. If any provision shall be held in violation of any law, that and only that provision shall be invalid and all other provisions of this Agreement shall remain in full force and effect.

_____   _____
Consultant   Date

_____   _____
Administrator   Date

CHAPTER 12
MONTHLY REPORT FORMAT

Activities Consultation Report

Name of Facility:

Date of Visitation:

Nature of Services:

Suggestions:

Future Plans:

Comments:

_____   _____

Consultant   Date

CHAPTER 12
SAMPLE CONTRACT 2

In-Service Consultation Agreement

This is to set forth the agreement between _____ and _____ to provide staff in-service programming. These programs will be held at monthly intervals, beginning _____ ; the topics and dates of presentation to be determined by mutual agreement with the Director of Nursing.

The fee for these sessions will be $ _____ per hour, with repeat sessions, following consecutively, billed at half that amount. The fee for all-day programs (six hours) utilizing one staff person will be $ _____ , and this may be increased according to personnel and resources utilized.

This agreement may be terminated by either party upon thirty (30) days written notice, and is renewable on an annual basis.

_____   _____
Consultant   Date

_____   _____
Administrator   Date

CHAPTER 12
EVALUATION OF GROUP LEADER

The group leader should be observed and evaluated as to his or her general skills in the following areas. (This can also be used as part of a self-evaluation process.) Please note any areas that seem to need improvement and be specific as possible in identifying the particular problems noted. Use back of form or additional sheets as needed.

NAME OF LEADER:	Always	Most of the Time	Some of the Time	Never
Meets/greets/seats residents appropriately?	___	___	___	___
Clears work areas/surfaces?	___	___	___	___
Is prepared for activity?	___	___	___	___
Displays knowledge of individual resident goals?	___	___	___	___
Makes effort to meet individual interests/needs?	___	___	___	___
Meets predetermined purpose of activity?	___	___	___	___
Has selected appropriate time length?	___	___	___	___
Has selected appropriate group size?	___	___	___	___
Is prepared with ''plan B''?	___	___	___	___
Title describes actual program?	___	___	___	___
Provides the same activity as posted?	___	___	___	___
Handles group comfortably?	___	___	___	___
Deals with problems as they arise?	___	___	___	___
Utilizes volunteers effectively?	___	___	___	___
Encourages group socialization/interactor?	___	___	___	___
Gives directions clearly?	___	___	___	___
Provides appropriate atmosphere/environment?	___	___	___	___

Specific comments/observations:

PROGRAM EVALUATION FORM

Facility name _____

Address _____

Telephone _____

Administrator _____

Other personnel who impact on activity department _____

_____

Number of residents _____

Medicare _____ Medicaid _____ VA _____ JCAHO _____

Activity director _____

   Length of service _____

   Prior experience _____

   Education _____

   Organization memberships _____

   Working hours _____

   Other responsibilities _____

Assistant(s) _____

   Length of service _____

   Prior experience _____

   Education _____

   Working hours _____

   Other responsibilities _____

Does the activity department have copies of:

   Facility organization chart _____

   Accurate job descriptions _____

   State and federal regulations _____

      Understand requirements _____

   Accurate department policies and procedures _____

   QA plan for dealing with problems _____

Are ongoing records kept of:

   Budget _____ Department input _____

   Long-range department goals and plans _____

   Minutes of meetings attended _____

   Activity breakdowns and descriptions _____

   Resources utilized/available _____

Do procedures exist for:

   Completing calendars at required times _____

   Posting calendar _____

   Other means of notifying residents of events _____

   Communicating activity schedules and needs to other departments _____

   Notifying residents of changes in location or condition _____

   Activities orientation for all new employees _____

   Monthly reports:

      Content adequacy _____

Procedure for distribution _____

Report feedback _____

Does the activity department participate in:

Care conferences _____ How often _____

Staff meetings _____ How often _____

Utilization review _____ How often _____

Discharge planning _____ How often _____

Department head meetings _____ How often _____

Inservices _____ Present _____ Attend _____

QA team _____

Surveys _____ Deficiencies _____

Recommendations/changes _____

Do other departments:

Help with transportation _____

Help with programs _____

Have awareness of scheduled activities _____

Try to avoid schedule conflicts _____

Communicate useful information _____

Cooperate with requests _____

Understand mandate of activity program _____

Does the activity program:

Base activities on identified needs _____

Base activities on interests of individual residents _____

Change as resident population changes _____

Include individual activities _____ Goals set _____

Activities for the frail/bedside _____

Activities for the cognitively impaired _____

Small group activities _____

Clubs and committees _____

Resident council _____ How often _____

Member selection _____

Staff attendance _____

Follow-up of suggestions _____

Large group activities _____

Outdoor activities _____

Provide transportation for outside trips _____

Offer weekend activities _____ PM _____

Provide materials for residents' use _____

Are staff:

Meeting number requirements _____

Utilized effectively _____

Assigned individual responsibilities _____

Using good time management techniques _____

Familiar with group dynamics _____

Effective as group leaders _____

Knowledgeable about resident population _____

Knowledgeable about individual residents _____

Tuned in to their needs/goals _____

On good terms with other departments _____

Is there dedicated space available for:

Programming _____

Equipment and supplies _____

Are other areas used _____ Outdoor areas _____

Adequate storage _____

Is there an active volunteer program _____

Recruited _____

Oriented _____

Supervised _____

Recognized _____

Retained _____

Records kept _____

Resident documentation:

Effective forms _____ Sufficient space _____

Ask right questions _____

Completed on time _____ Initial assessment _____

Updates _____

Copies kept _____ Where _____

Levels of participation indicated _____

Include physician's permission _____

How obtained _____

Is behavior described or labeled _____

Do goals address identified problems _____

Needs/interests _____

Are goals specific/measurable/observable _____

Do goals have reasonable time frames _____

Does resident participate in goal setting _____

Are needs/interests translated into activities _____

Is activities plan part of total care plan _____

Do updates include progress toward goal _____

Is there continuity in notes _____

Are there discharge plans _____

Are there discharge summaries _____

Conclusions:

Source: © Geriatric Educational Consultants, 1989.

CHAPTER 13
SAMPLE PROPOSAL

PROPOSAL FOR OCCUPATIONAL THERAPY CONSULTATION
AT

THE PARKVIEW HOME
ANYTOWN, NEW JERSEY

Submitted by:

OCCUPATIONAL THERAPY CONSULTANTS, INC.
350 GROVE STREET
BRIDGEWATER, NJ 08807

Introduction

Parkview Home, one of the earliest nursing and domiciliary facilities in this state, has an ongoing commitment to its residents in regard to the provision of quality care. Recent changes in federal and state regulations emphasize resident quality of life issues and utilization of an interdisciplinary team. In this regard, Parkview's administration is interested in determining the need for occupational therapy services at the facility.

Occupational Therapy Consultants, Inc., (OTC), is currently providing services at a sister facility in the northern part of the state and is available to provide a needs assessment for Parkview. This assessment would determine the scope of occupational therapy services needed at the facility, and would suggest a plan of action for consideration. Based on preliminary discussion with Parkview administrative staff, the following needs assessment goals are suggested:

I. Identify and rank critical occupational therapy patient service needs in the following areas:
   A. Activities of daily living (ADL)
   B. Seating and mobility (wheelchair management)
II. Identify and rank critical facility (environment) needs for specialized occupational therapy programs that utilize an interdisciplinary (systems) team approach:
   A. Human environment
   B. Nonhuman environment
   C. Systems approach via an interdisciplinary team
III. Develop recommendations for occupational therapy service implementation.

Provider History

OTC, established in 1979, has a dual mission: first, the delivery of comprehensive, high quality, cost-effective occupational therapy services to health-care consumers in New Jersey. Second, and equally important, the provision of a supportive and enriched environment for the therapists/consultants who work in the group. There are currently 40 therapists/consultants working in the practice. They are located geographically from as far north as Bergen County to as far south as Camden County.

The company has been delivering occupational therapy consultation and treatment services in community and health-care settings since 1979. Starting with services at 3 nursing homes, the sites have grown in number and diversity over the years. OTC is approved as a provider of services by the State of New Jersey Departments of Human Services, Education, and Defense.

The company is extremely proud of the diversity of skills and excellent knowledge base found among its staff. When a particular problem arises, calling for expertise in a particular area, there is usually a therapist/consultant in the group who can meet the need. The practice is highly esteemed by the occupational therapy community, and many referrals for service delivery are made by other occupational therapy practitioners in the state, as well as by satisfied consumers. The company is a designated field work site for students at the professional and technical level, from many colleges and universities in the northeast region.

Selected staff have held and/or currently hold appointments at: Kean College, Downstate Medical School, Rutgers University, Dominican College, and Columbia University. They are in demand as guest lecturers at conferences and universities, and have been peer reviewed for selection as presenters at occupational therapy conferences, and as participants in special American Occupational Therapy Association (AOTA), New Jersey Occupational Therapy Association (NJOTA), and Gerontological Society of America (GSA) Task Forces.

They are committed to professional growth and activity through participation in continuing education, professional organizations, networking, support groups, and advanced educational studies. Cynthia F. Epstein, Executive Director of the firm, is nationally recognized as a clinical master therapist and occupational therapy consultant. Her numerous articles and extensive lectures regarding consultation and services for institutionalized elderly have been widely acclaimed by rehabilitation specialists, nationally and internationally. The articles, "Seating the Institutionalized Elderly: Keys to Success" and "Specialized Seating for the Institutionalized Elderly: Prescription, Fabrication, Funding" which are attached, are examples of her concern for and expertise in positioning for long-term care residents. Given the recent OBRA mandates, this issue is of extreme importance.

OTC provides consultative and treatment services through its qualified personnel, who are certified by the American Occupational Therapy Certification Board and qualified to practice occupational therapy in the state of New Jersey. Our consultants work collaboratively with client systems to address facility needs identified initially as key concerns, as well as other concerns which may surface during the consultation process. When resident evaluation and treatment are part of our service delivery model, our therapists use a frame of reference which focuses on improving each resident's occupational performance in the areas of daily living skills, sensorimotor abilities, cognitive and psychosocial abilities, and need for adaptive aids/orthotics to enhance functional skills. The term, "occupation'' is defined as engagement in life tasks appropriate for the resident at his or her age and stage of development.

Program Proposal

The Parkview Home does not currently have occupational therapy services as a part of its team approach to resident care. Through the needs assessment process our consultants will be able to analyze facility needs and suggest a plan for development of an occupational therapy program. To facilitate communication between the consultants and facility staff, we propose the following plan for the consultation:

Time Frame:	Five days over a 3 week period.
Consultation Staff:	One senior (C. Epstein) and two junior consultant/therapists
Activities:	*Day 1*
	a. Department Head Inservice regarding occupational therapy and the consultation plan.
	b. Commence needs assessment process in Building #1, inservice unit staff as part of the process.
	Days 2, 3, 4
	a. Continue needs assessment process as described above, gradually moving into Buildings 2 and 3.
	b. Establish briefing meetings with key administrative staff, to be held each day, at a mutually agreeable time.
	Day 5
	a. Meet with administrative staff to review findings and present recommendations.
	b. Provide Department Heads with brief overview of consultation findings and recommendations, as agreed upon in earlier meeting with administration.

Within 2 weeks of completion of this process, OTC will provide Parkview with a comprehensive written report. This will specifically detail the procedures used during the consultation, the findings of the consultant team, and specific recommendations concerning implementation of an occupational therapy service at Parkview.

Consultation Process

In our view, the consultation process should foster an environment of mutual cooperation and collaboration between all participants. Enabling Parkview to consider positive change strategies, address system needs, and improve the quality of resident care is the consultation goal. The consultant's strong foundation in system theory assures a focus which considers the needs of Parkview, its residents and staff, and the environmental context in which change is being considered.

The environment is viewed from human and non-human, or physical perspectives. The physical environment considers such factors as space, objects, and sensory cues, and their relationship to resident and staff performance. Possible adaptations to the environment which support and facilitate safe and effective performance will be a consultation focus.

Continual data gathering and feedback are essential to successful consultation. Through our collaborative consultation approach, a communication network is developed. An inherent part of the network is a feedback system which facilitates review of observations, perceptions, and progress. This helps to clarify impressions, coordinate activities, and develop concurrence for suggested strategies. This will take the form of survey formats and formal and informal meetings. A final report will be prepared upon completion of the project.

Budget Proposal

OTC would be pleased to provide the services as outlined above for a fee of $_____ . This fee covers all time and expenses incurred by our consultants in regard to this project.

Start and end dates will be identified in conjunction with your needs and our availability. We trust that the information submitted is sufficient to meet your requirements. Should further information be needed, we would be pleased to submit the appropriate documents.

We look forward to the possibility of working with you on this important project.

Respectfully submitted,

Cynthia F. Epstein, M.A., O.T.R., F.A.O.T.A.

Attachments:
2 articles by C. Epstein

CHAPTER 13
SAMPLE LETTER OF AGREEMENT

**THE PARKVIEW HOME
ANYTOWN, NEW JERSEY**

July 6, 1991

Ms. Cynthia F. Epstein, M.A., O.T.R., F.A.O.T.A.
Executive Director
Occupational Therapy Consultants, Inc.
350 Grove Street
Bridgewater, New Jersey 08807

Dear Ms. Epstein,

As per your proposal and our subsequent discussion, we would like you to conduct an initial needs assessment to develop a plan for implementation of occupational therapy services at our facility.

As proposed and agreed to, the fee of $ _____ for the needs assessment has been approved. The process for payment of this fee will be handled through our Business Manager, Mr. _____. Questions regarding this matter can be handled at your first scheduled on site visit.

At your earliest contact, we will establish a timetable for the plan and also arrange for the initial orientation meeting with the deparment heads. A screen will be available for your slide presentation.

It is understood that at the completion of the assessment period, a meeting with key personnel to review the written report on the suggested implementation plan will be held and shall be the basis for discussing the proposed occupational therapy program at this facility.

We are looking forward to working with you on this most important program. Arrangements can be made through this office, Monday through Friday, 8:30 AM to 5:00 PM. If this letter meets with your approval, please sign and return the original and keep the copy for your file. Look forward to hearing from you.

Sincerely,

Deputy Chief Executive Officer

Accepted this ___ day of _____ 199 ___

By: _____
    Cynthia F. Epstein, M.A., O.T.R., F.A.O.T.A.

CHAPTER 17
SAMPLE MARKETING HANDOUT

HOSPITAL BASED
PSYCHIATRIC OCCUPATIONAL THERAPY
MANAGEMENT CONSULTATION AND TREATMENT SERVICES
provided by
COMPREHENSIVE THERAPEUTICS, LTD.

Introduction

Comprehensive Therapeutics, Ltd. (CTL) has been providing occupational therapy services to hospitals throughout the greater Chicago area for the past 16 years. Our goal is to work in harmony with clients, providing highly skilled management services, consultation, and supplemental occupational therapy services. We provide hospitals with state-of-the-art occupational therapy programs in a cost effective manner. As caseloads fluctuate, our commitment to high quality service will give your hospital a competitive edge in marketing your psychiatric program in the community.

Services

Some of the services we provide which set our company apart from others are:

- A CTL Occupational Therapy Director oversees delivery of services and is readily available to troubleshoot and provide continuous quality assurance. Our director works closely with management to determine their goals and direction and to ensure that CTL staff have the right experience and background to meet each client's requirements. Our director's services are free of charge.
- CTL pays close attention to coordination and integration of our service with other hospital services.
- Professional seminars on pertinent topics with nationally known speakers are offered 3–4 times per year. CTL clients receive one free admission per seminar as well as reduced rates for additional registrants.
- All CTL staff have up-to-date knowledge of all standards and regulations affecting hospital departments.
- CTL offers a fair and competitive price structure.

Our client relationships are viewed as a partnership, founded on a mutual desire to provide quality health care. Our clients and their patients benefit from our careful matching of their needs to the consultative and clinical abilities of our professionals. Our program goal is continual client and staff satisfaction. Client feedback is an important element in our partnership. Our objective is to build lasting relationships through attention to service and effective communication.

CHAPTER 17
SAMPLE PROPOSAL

HOSPITAL BASED PSYCHIATRIC SERVICES
MANAGEMENT CONSULTATION & TREATMENT

Dear _____ ,

After meeting with you and discussing your needs, I am confident that Comprehensive Therapeutics, Ltd. can provide you with the comprehensive occupational therapy services you require. These services will ensure successful initiation of your psychiatric occupational therapy program and to help build a solid foundation for your department. We currently have available two psychiatric occupational therapists, with the background and experience required for your program. They would be able to provide management consultation, and direct treatment services. You are welcome to interview each of them to determine which individual would best meet your needs.

The following is a partial list of duties which our consultant/therapists would be able to perform for your hospital's psychiatric unit:

1. Propose all policies and procedures for the new occupational therapy service.
2. Develop department forms related to assessment and treatment, for your consideration.
3. Draft necessary paperwork to help the hospital attain DRG exempt status for this unit.
4. Draft group protocols and a suggested occupational therapy schedule.
5. Provide inservice training to other staff regarding the role and function of occupational therapy on this unit.
6. Recommend and assist in ordering all necessary occupational therapy supplies and equipment.
7. Assist in establishing billing procedures.
8. Assist in recruitment and interview of occupational therapy employee applicants for your unit.
9. Provide occupational therapy treatment services until hospital staff can be hired.
10. Provide training and collegial consultation for newly hired occupational therapists during the initial employment phase and concurrently help establish important quality assurance mechanisms.
11. Provide ongoing consultation on an as needed basis to monitor department status, assist in development of new programs, and support and train staff.
12. Terminate service when department is functioning independently or reduce consultation hours to a minimum, based on need.

Potential Advantages of Our Service

1. Occupational therapy services can be initiated immediately.
2. Advertising costs are reduced.
3. Therapist hours are based on need and census of your unit, thus reducing cost when census is low.
4. Start-up, consultative, and administrative functions are performed by a qualified, knowledgeable, psychiatric consultant/therapist who will efficiently accomplish required tasks.
5. Assurance that a quality program will be in place quickly.
6. Effective use of manpower and expertise. Our therapist/consultant will provide efficient and highly skilled services.
7. You pay only for the hours you use; you do not pay for benefits or "down time;" i.e., unproductive time.

Potential Disadvantages of Our Service

1. **Cost.** It may appear that contractual services cost more per hour. However, a full benefit package adds at least 25–35% to an hourly rate. Additionally, the hospital must commit a certain number of hours to an employee. Using our contractual services allows the hospital to adjust therapist and consultant hours based on need for service. In actuality, *your cost may be less* through a contractual relationship.
2. **Control.** In an employee/employer relationship, the lines of control are clear. In contractual relationships where service is the product, many businesses have not been provided with clear lines of control. Our organization's consultant/therapists develop a primary relationship with our clients. They understand the uniqueness of each client relationship. Service delivery is focused on client goals and directions. To retain your business and obtain referrals once we have helped you resolve your problems, it is our job to make sure that you, our client, remain in control.

Proposed Services and Cost

During our meeting, you mentioned that you had budgeted $28,000 for an occupational therapist. With benefits, the cost to the hospital would actually be closer to $36,000. The following are three (3) models which come close to this figure at an annual cost of $34,000–$40,000. These figures are based on a contract rate of **$38.00/hour.** Billable hours are those actually provided on site by a CTL consultant/therapist.

MODEL 1

You are unable to find a qualified OTR. Utilize our service for 18 hours a week at a cost of $38.00/hour for approximately 50 weeks.   **TOTAL COST—$34,200.00**

MODEL 2

Utilize our firm as management consultants to assist you in setting up your department and to provide treatment services during your initial opening phase. We then assist you in finding an occupational therapist during the first 3 months. Once the therapist is hired, we provide ongoing consultation as needed.

Cost:

3 months of management consultation and treatment services
18 hours/week for 13 weeks at $38.00/hour	= $ 8,892.00
OTR salary for 9 months (75% of 28,000 + 25% benefits)	= 26,250.00
Approximately 4 hours/week consultation to OTR for	
9 months or 4 hours × 37 weeks × $38.00/hour.	= 5,624.00

TOTAL COST— 40,766.00*

* This is assuming the OTR's salary is $28,000 and that consultation is provided the above number of hours. Consultation could be more or less, depending on the qualifications of the OTR.

MODEL 3

Same as Model 2, except that an OTR is found after 6 months.

Cost:

6 months of management consultation and treatment
18 hours/week for 25 weeks at $38.00/hour	= $17,100.00
OTR salary for 6 months (50% of $28,000 + 25% benefits)	= 17,500.00
Approximately 4 hours/week consultation to OTR for	
25 weeks at $38.00/hour.	= 3,800.00

TOTAL COST—$38,400.00

These three models provide comparable costs. Obviously, the number of hours required will depend on census, particularly before you hire an occupational therapist. Less consultation hours may be required if you hire a more experienced occupational therapist. However, I believe by looking at these 3 models, you can see that the $34,000–$40,000 figure is a reasonable estimate of cost.

In summary, our goal is to stay within your budget and provide you with a qualified consultant/therapist. This will ensure successful initiation of your occupational therapy service by providing consultation and management direction along with treatment services. Ongoing consultation services will assist in recruiting, training, and retaining your own therapy staff, thus ensuring provision of consistent, high quality, state-of-the-art occupational therapy for your psychiatric unit.

Should you have any questions or wish to discuss any aspects of this proposal, please do not hesitate to call. I look forward to hearing from you.

Respectfully submitted,

Sandra Jacobson Lerner
Executive Director
Comprehensive Therapeutics, Ltd.

CHAPTER 17
SAMPLE AGREEMENT

PROFESSIONAL SERVICES AGREEMENT

THIS AGREEMENT is entered into _____ , 19 __ , by and between **Comprehensive Therapeutics, Ltd.,** an Illinois corporation ("CT"), 3000 Dundee Road, Suite 206, Northbrook, Illinois, 60062 and _____ , (The "Agency"), _____ _____ , _____ , _____ , _____ , **Attn:** _____ _____ , **Administrator.** Hereafter CT or the Agency may be referred to individually as a "party" or collectively as the "parties." In consideration of the premises and the mutual covenants herein contained, and for other good and valuable consideration, the receipt and sufficiency of which is hereby acknowledged, the parties hereto agree as follows:

1. Term

1.1 This Agreement shall commence the date first above written _____ , 19 __ , and shall remain in full force and effect through 11:59 p.m. on _____ , 19 __ . (the Initial Term).

1.2 This Agreement may be terminated by either party at any time, with or without cause, upon sixty (60) days prior notice in writing to the other party. Within fifteen (15) days of the date this Agreement is terminated, all manuals, equipment, and supplies belonging to a party, but in the possession of the other party, shall be returned at the cost and expense of the party in possession.

2. Services—Subject to all terms of this Agreement, the Agency hereby agreed upon for the Initial Term of this Agreement:

	DIRECT TREATMENT RATE/HOUR	CONSULTATION RATE/HOUR	MINIMUM HOURS/MONTH (Consultation only)
2.1 OCCUPATIONAL THERAPY			
___ OTR/L's			
___ COTA/L's			
2.2 PHYSICAL THERAPY			
___ Licensed PT's			
___ PTA's			
2.3 OTHER PROFESSIONAL SERVICES			
___ Ther. Recreation Specialists (CTRS)			
___ Psychosocial			
___ Social Workers (MSW)			
___ Licensed Speech/Language Pathologist			
___ Registered Nurses			
2.4 TRAVEL REIMBURSEMENT			

After the initial Term of this Agreement, services shall be rendered by CT to the Agency at CT's then customary hourly rates, as revised from time to time effective upon notice to the Agency.

3. The terms and conditions attached as EXHIBIT A to this Agreement hereof are hereby agreed to and incorporated into the Agreement by reference. Each party represents and warrants to the other party that it has read, understands, and agrees to all terms and provisions of the Agreement, its representatives are duly authorized to enter into this Agreement on its behalf, and that it has the power and authority to enter into this Agreement.

The Agency

_____

_____

By: _____

Its: _____

Date: _____

Comprehensive Therapeutics, Ltd.
  an Illinois Corporation

By: _____

Sandra Jacobson Lerner

Its: Executive Director

Date: _____

CHAPTER 17
SAMPLE AGREEMENT EXHIBIT A

ADDITIONAL TERMS AND PROVISIONS

4. Qualifications. Each therapist or other professional provided by CT pursuant to and during the term of this Agreement shall at all times be duly licensed and maintain all applicable professional requirements. Upon request CT shall furnish the Agency with a resume of the qualifications and experience of each person providing services to the Agency, together with a current copy of their license. The nature and scope of services to be rendered by CT to the Agency shall be those set forth in the CT policies and procedures manual, incorporated herein by reference, which the Agency acknowledges receipt of by its signature on this Agreement.

5. Professional Services. The Agency assumes all professional and administrative responsibility for the services rendered by CT under this Agreement. All persons rendered by CT under this Agreement shall:

5.1. Be under the general direction and supervision of the administrator or other designated facility director and will follow the ethical guidelines as set forth by their professional associations and state licenses; and

5.2. Abide by and be subject to all the Agency's policies, procedures, rules and regulations while performing services within the Agency's facilities. The Agency agrees to timely provide CT with a copy of all relevant Agency policies, procedures, rules and regulations, and all amendments thereto, as well as provide CT a copy of the medical treatment plan for each patient before treatment, and review and exchange verbal and written information related to the treatment of assigned patients among the persons involved in such treatment. The agency shall provide CT the results of any surveys of Agency patients or service providers which are designed to evaluate services of the type provided by CT under this Agreement.

6. Facilities. The Agency shall, as its sole expense, set aside and maintain within each facility within which CT personnel are to provide services under this Agreement, designated work, storage, and materials areas, materials and equipment, and reporting forms adequate for the provision of services. The Agency shall be solely responsible for all billings to and collections from patients and third party providers. CT shall provide the Agency with copies of relevant records to assist in the Agency's billing and collection efforts.

7. Medical Records. The Agency and CT acknowledge and agree that all medical records used by CT's persons under this Agreement shall be the property of the Agency. CT's personnel shall retain the right to use these records at any time for treatment purposes. CT represents that all of its personnel furnished to the Agency shall comply with all applicable state and federal laws and regulations governing the release of medical record information. CT's personnel shall provide and maintain written documentation on the individual patient charts and records of treatment, progress, and evaluations in accordance with the requirements of the Agency, federal, and state governmental agencies, and other third party reimbursement sources. CT shall make available, upon written request from the Secretary of Health and Human Services, or the Controller General of the Government Accounting Office, or from any of their duly authorized representatives, the books, documents, and records of CT necessary to verify the nature and extent of amounts invoiced by CT under this Agreement, for four (4) years after services were rendered by CT's personnel hereunder. Each party to this Agreement shall make available to the other party to this Agreement all patient information in their possession for defense of any claim.

8. Professional Liability Insurance. CT shall maintain general liability and professional liability insurance coverage for the clinical services to be rendered under this Agreement, with minimum levels of One Million Dollars ($1,000,000) per occurrence and One Million Dollars (1,000,000) aggregate per year. Upon request CT shall provide the Agency annually with a certificate of insurance upon request in such form as CT's insurance carrier may issue without additional charge to CT.

9. Billing. CT shall bill the Agency not less frequently than monthly for all charges incurred. The Agency agrees to pay for services rendered at the rates set forth herein within thirty (30) days of the date on CT's statement. The Agency may review CT's books and records within thirty (30) days of the date on CT's statement, thereafter CT's statements of balances due for that period shall be presumptively correct. In the event that CT has not received payment within thirty (30) days of the date on CT's statement, all unpaid balances shall bear interest at the rate of 1.5% per month, compounded monthly, plus all legal fees and costs of collection. CT reserves the right to discontinue thirty (30) days after notice, any or all services rendered to or on behalf of the Agency in the event any payment is not timely received, and the Agency indemnifies and holds CT harmless from and against any and all resulting damages.

10. Relationship of the Parties. CT and the Agency expressly agree that CT shall provide services hereunder as an independent contractor for all purposed, including federal tax purposes, and employees of CT shall not be entitled to any of the rights or privileges established for the employees of the Agency, including but not limited to: overtime, vacations and vacation pay, sick leave with pay, paid holidays, life, accident or health insurance, or severance pay upon termination of this Agreement. The Agency agrees that it will not withhold from any payments made to CT pursuant to this Agreement, any sums for federal, state or local income taxes, unemployment insurance, Social Security, or any other amount which is required by law to be withheld by an employer for an employee. CT agrees that all such payments that may be required by law from CT for CT's employees are CT's sole responsibility, and CT covenants and agrees to indemnify and save harmless the Agency from any and all claims as a result of CT's failure to make any such payments.

11. CT Personnel. During the term of this Agreement and for a period of two (2) years after the termination of this Agreement, the Agency agrees not to directly or indirectly hire, contract with, or otherwise solicit any person provided to the Agency by CT. The Agency hereby agrees that this restriction is reasonable and necessary to protect CT's business and does not impose any undue burden on the Agency. In the event of the Agency's breach of this provision, CT shall be entitled to an injunction stopping all prohibited conduct, in addition to damages and other actions.

12. Indemnification and Hold Harmless.

12.1. The Agency shall indemnify and hold CT harmless from and against all claims, demands, costs, expenses, liabilities, and losses (including reasonable attorney's fees) which may result against CT as a consequence of any alleged malfeasance, neglect, or medical malpractice caused or alleged to be caused by the Agency, its employees, agents, or contractors.

12.2. CT shall indemnify and hold the Agency harmless from and against all claims, demands, costs, expenses, liabilities, and losses (including reasonable attorneys' fees) which may result against or are alleged to be caused by CT, its employees, agents, or contractors, in connection with the performance of services under this Agreement.

13. Notices. All notices or other communications required or permitted to be given pursuant to this Agreement shall be considered as properly given if made in writing and either mailed from within the United States by certified or registered United States mail with postage prepaid, or by prepaid telegram and addressed to the address of each party. Any party may change its address by giving a notice in writing to all other parties stating its new address. Commencing with the giving of such notice, such newly designated address shall be such party's address for purposes of all notices or other communications required or permitted to be given pursuant to this Agreement.

14. <u>Successors.</u> This Agreement and all the terms and provisions hereof shall be binding upon and shall inure to the benefit of the parties, and their respective legal representatives, heirs, successors and assigns, except as expressly herein otherwise provided.

15. <u>Effect and Intepretation.</u> This Agreement will be executed in, and shall be construed in conformity with the laws of, the State of Illinois. In the event of any dispute between the parties, at CT's election such dispute shall be subject to binding arbitration in Chicago, Illinois, in accordance with all rules of the American Arbitration Association.

16. <u>Force Majeure.</u> In the event CT is prevented from providing services pursuant to the terms of this Agreement by forces or events beyond its control, CT's noncompliance shall be excused for the duration of such force or event.

17. <u>Severability.</u> If any provision of this Agreement, or the application of such provision to any person or circumstances, shall be held invalid by a court of competent jurisdiction, the remainder of this Agreement, and the application of such provision to persons or circumstances other than those to which it is held invalid by such court, shall not be affected thereby.

18. <u>Counterparts.</u> This Agreement may be executed in counterparts, each of which shall be an original, but all of which shall constitute one and the same instrument.

19. <u>Parties.</u> Nothing herein contained shall be construed to constitute any party being the agent of another party, except as specifically provided herein, or in any manner limiting the parties in the carrying on of their own respective business or activities.

20. <u>Pronouns.</u> As used herein, all pronouns shall include the masculine, feminine, neuter, singular and plural thereof wherever the context and facts require such construction.

21. <u>Headings.</u> The headings, titles and subtitles herein are inserted for convenience of reference only and are to be ignored in any construction of the provisions hereof.

22. <u>Entire Understanding.</u> This Agreement contains the entire understanding among the parties, supersedes any prior understandings and/or written or oral agreements among them respecting the within subject matter, and may be modified only by all parties hereto.

This contract entered into this ___ day of _____ 19___ by and between World of Work (the Agency) and Karen Jacobs, MS, OTR/L, FAOTA (the Consultant) affirms that:

WHEREAS, the AGENCY has determined that it is necessary to retain the services of a qualified consultant:

WHEREAS, the CONSULTANT is duly qualified to perform these services:

NOW, THEREFORE, the parties agree as follows:

1. The CONSULTANT shall provide any or all of the following services, as requested by the AGENCY:
   a. provide a four (4) hour in-service on marketing analysis and industrial rehabilitation;
   b. provide a four (4) hour group problem-solving session;
   c. compile a bibliography of resources on industrial rehabilitation.
2. The CONSULTANT shall provide these services to _____ (owner), _____ (owner) and _____ (clinical director).
3. The AGENCY shall obtain appropriate demographic and statistical data, program descriptions, organizational structure, public relations material, and operating budget prior to the consultancy.
4. The date the service will begin is _____ and shall extend through _____ 19 ___. The minimum number of hours contracted will be eight (8) hours.
5. The AGENCY shall provide an appropriate work space and slide projector.
6. The AGENCY shall make payments for services rendered as follows, upon receipt of statement. Fees charged will be $ _____/day including travel time at $ _____ hour plus ___ per mile for mileage and $ _____/day in childcare services. No charge will be made for office time (preparation of "follow along" market analysis).

I will fulfill the duties of CONSULTANT in accordance with all federal, state, and local regulations.

_____
Karen Jacobs, MS, OTR/L
Consultant
Occupational Therapist Registered
Licensed in Massachusetts #000000

_____
Owner or Director of World of Work

Witnesses:

_____

_____

Date _____

Future Directions: Vital Connections

Elnora M. Gilfoyle D.Sc., O.T.R., F.A.O.T.A.

While preparing these final words, I've reflected frequently on the nearly four decades of occupational therapy history I've observed firsthand. The longer I think about it, the more I am struck by the fact that occupational therapy's uniqueness is derived from a special and functional interdependency of the science of occupation and art of caring. Science and art are inherent concepts of two distinct but connected domains that are of crucial importance to the consultatory process and, in fact, to the future of occupational therapy. The first domain is the philosophy of the science of occupational therapy; the second is the philosophy of the art of therapy. Science philosophy provides a model for reasoning and methodology because science provides facts to guide our practices and assure accountability for our services. Art philosophy is the dimension that creates the conditions for science to be used. The blending of science and art provides the vital connections through which an occupational therapist links the conceptualization about a situation with chosen therapeutic actions. This connection is paramount in the therapist's caring relationship with individuals served, as the blending of science with art becomes the reasoning process that creates conditions by which the science of occupation can be used in a relationship with another person for the purpose of identifying and solving problems.[2]

Science is based on rational knowledge, because it is the discovery of general truths or the operation of laws tested through scientific methods.[5] Art is intuitive knowledge that enables us to enter into a caring relationship and apply the facts of science to the human dimensions of health. The practice of occupational therapy involves artistic application of scientific principles and concepts, rather than routine techniques and skills. Simply stated, there is a difference between knowing and doing, between knowledge and action; I believe this difference is the artistic dimension of applying the science of occupation to bring about change. Thus, the essence of occupational therapy practice is not just in its science, but in the art of applying concepts and principles of occupation to the purposefulness of selected activity for bringing about change and for maximizing an individual's performance. Huxley once stated that the great end of life is not knowledge, but action; however, as persons who provide service to others, we need to respect the words of another great philosopher who warned of taking action without the benefit of knowledge.[3]

The vital connection between rational and intuitive knowledge becomes an action process of applying scientific facts to human experiences. The connection results in a creative synthesis aimed at helping another person grow and actualize himself. Through the vital connection of science and art, the science of occupation promotes the art of human relationships and the art of purposeful activity actualizes the science of occupation. The integration of the science and art of the occupational process distinguishes our profession, but more importantly, this unique blending promotes the quality of life for the individuals we serve.

Occupational therapy is, by almost any measure, a remarkable success. Our unique blending of science and art has spawned a health promotion profession which is responsive to human behavior in an ever-changing environment. What other profession joins, so completely, the concepts of science and art to address human health and behavior? What other profession uses the daily occupations of one's life to promote healthfulness and help another gain a sense of self-esteem? What other profession bases its science on the very essence of the vital connection between humans and their "doing?" What other profession deals with a wide variety of complex dimensions of human activity? What other profession has its heritage in the essence of work? What other profession can claim its focus on the continuum of self-care, play, and work as the events that influence development, facilitate performance, and promote life satisfaction? With all its successes and growth, occupational therapy as a profession remains misunderstood by society, has not developed its own niche in the marketplace, lacks its own scientific theory base, and continues to draw its knowledge from other disciplines. Our heritage has neither defined nor limited our domain of knowledge and practice. The occupational therapy domain must be defined for us to focus our scientific efforts, avoid stagnation, and advance the realities of the occupational world.

In the quest to define occupational therapy, the authors of this text offer a theoretical model of occupational therapy consultation, a model that is based upon the nature of consultation as the mutual cooperation and collaboration between the dysfunctional client/system and the occupational therapy consultant. These authors state that the goal of consultation is to enable the consulted to create positive change through improved performance. Underlying the concepts and principles of the model presented in this text are the vital connections between science and art, consulted and consultant, person and action, system and environment. The challenge presented in this text is for occupational therapy to continue its development by providing health consultation. The focus on consultation is motivated, at least in part, by concerns for the cost of health care, the rights of all disabled persons to equal access, the varied challenges of today's health care marketplace, and a sense of the future.

Our present decade and the beginning of the upcoming century presents, at least from my perspective, the most challenging moment for occupational therapy in 40 years. This time affords us an unusual opportunity to return to our roots and consider not just direct patient-therapist services, but also the challenge to engage in an occupational therapy consultatory process that is embedded in the enduring values of facilitating a learning community for the client/system. In response to the challenge, I propose six principles to provide an effective formula for the consultatory relationship we should strive to achieve.

1. Consultation is a *purposeful* process for helping another gain self-actualization, achieve a sense of human dignity, and move toward a state of healthfulness.
2. Consultation is a *learning* process that respects the expressions of others and integrates their ideas into a mutual problem-identification and problem-solving relationship.
3. Consultation is an *open* and *just* process where individuals accept their obligations to the group and where the process guides behaviors for the common good of the individual, group, and/or system.
4. Consultation is a *caring* process where the person is honored and the well-being of each member of the process is supported, and where service to others is a process to promote self-actualization.
5. Consultation is a *celebrative* process, one in which the heritage of the profession is remembered and where the science and art of its practices affirm both tradition and change.
6. Consultation is a *community* process that values the contributions of others and the ongoing learning that occurs through the consultatory experience.

The principle of purposefulness is listed first because it is fundamental to all others. Purposefulness of the occupational process is the foundation from which the practice of occupational therapy has sustained and developed during the 20th century. Our roots are embedded in the belief that human life cannot be meaningful if it is not at the same time purposeful and directed. The purposefulness of behavior and activity gives a human life order, and it is this purposefulness that the consultatory process seeks to discover and define.

Learning as a consultation principle is carried out through reasoned discourse between two or more individuals. The free expression of ideas in a community of learning is essential for effective consultation. Each person learns through expressions of others and through valuing different perspectives. Although the therapist brings to the consultation situation certain knowledge, skills, and attitudes that reflect the profession, the consulted has ideas and perspectives that enrich the process and result in creative action to facilitate resolution.

Consultation builds community through activation of the rich resources of all members participating in the process. Consultation rejects prejudicial judgments, celebrates the diversity of ideas and perspectives, and seeks to serve the needs of all members of the group. In strengthening our practice, occupational therapists must commit themselves to building a community with clients—one that is equitable, fair, and accessible.

Although the purposefulness of consultation is the foundation for all other principles, the essence of its process is best described by the principle of caring. Occupational therapy consultation does not provide care to, nor does it take care of a person; rather, our concept of care is mutual cooperation. It is something engaged in with a person. Occupational therapy health care is a collaborative relationship geared to help another person grow and actualize. Thus, the principle of caring is a process of relationships that involve growth and development. To care for another person is to help the other grow, develop, and adapt. Caring is a process to help another gain self-actualization, achieve a state of independence, and move toward healthfulness. The caring orientation of the consultation process in occupational therapy is helping the person learn to take care of himself. Through this process, caring involves an internal receiving by the client, not an external giving by the therapist. It is through the internal receiving that occupational therapy becomes purposeful.[1]

As occupational therapists, we bring to the consultation process a rich heritage of commitment to a holistic view of humans; dedication to self-care, play, and work; a linkage between environment and health; the use of occupation or event to promote change; and the uniqueness of each individual. Each time we engage in a consultatory relationship and apply our knowledge, we celebrate these historic roots. Our profession has a unique contribution to offer persons receiving health-care services; a uniqueness that centers around a special kind of the caring relationship discussed above. Occupational therapists are not professed healers; rather, we are professed facilitators who activate our professional philosophies through a consultatory relationship with clients.

Consultation as a community process respects the values inherent in the profession. To assume our position in the consultation marketplace, we must respect both individual and interagency collaboration, as well as interdisciplinary participation, as the means by which we can best address the health and social problems of our clients. The complex problems of individuals in contemporary society are interrelated and mutually reinforcing as health, education, financial, social, employment, leisure, and legal problems surface together. As consultants, we realize that no one person or profession can serve all the needs that people have. We know that the expertise of several professions may be ultimately required; thus, interagency and interdisciplinary collaboration must be fostered in response to the complex problems of the persons we serve.

If we are to fulfill our historic mission and maintain significance in furthering the health of our society, then we must be among the vanguard in forging meaningful partnerships and alliances with our clients and with social, economic, political, and medical organizations. The need to respond to a rapidly changing environment, while also maintaining the best of the past, requires increasing communication with that environment. As our profession continues to mature and expand its services, we must avoid the tendency to develop extensive structures and unclear lines of responsibility and authority that would inhibit our response time to society's needs and demands. We must find a means to provide a common understanding of our present and predictive environments for effective occupational therapy to take place. History suggests that occupational therapy practices tend to consist of a multitude of adjustments to external demands—not adjustments based on long-range planning and reliable predictions.[4] In a new style for the profession's future, we need to look ahead and envision where we will be in 20–30 years. To do so requires an understanding of the dynamics of the external environment, a commitment to planning, development of professionals with critical thinking skills, a blending of the science and art of occupational therapy, and the proclamation of the philosophy of our profession. As we look to the future, I believe there are specific themes that are pertinent for our tomorrow. These themes are the potential of occupational therapy for the 21st century:

- Occupational therapy as a philosophy.
- The vital connection between the science of occupation and the art of human relationships.
- The ongoing interaction and mutual cooperation between client and therapist.
- Consideration of the person in context with family, environment, and organizational systems.
- Ourselves as consultants, leaders, and agents of change.
- The ethics and morals surrounding our profession.

Our potential lies in our philosophies for the significance of work, play, and self-care as occupations that contribute to the better quality of life for individuals. Through our services, we can demonstrate to society that it is possible for people to be disabled and healthy at the same time. The profession's philosophy, based upon the belief and value for humans to be engaged in meaningful activity, must be developed through scientific research, so that our science can guide our art. In our roles as agents of change or facilitators of performance, occupational therapists are transformative consultants. We have the values, philosophies, theories, attitudes, and skills to influence and empower other persons. Our major goal is to alter, diminish, or eliminate causes and effects of the environment that result in dysfunction, so people can fulfill their roles and potential.

In a few years, we will experience a new century. As we approach this new era, we must anticipate our future by identifying key trends that will shape the years ahead. The U.S. Bureau of Labor Statistics provides data on trends that are important to occupational therapy programs. The Bureau predicts that the American economy will grow at a relatively healthy pace, with service industries creating all of the new jobs and most of the new wealth. Jobs in service industries will demand much higher skill levels. In the upcoming decade, our work force will grow slowly, with the average age of the population and work force rising, together with a shrinking pool of young persons entering the work world. There will be more jobs for women and persons from disadvantaged populations, including the handicapped.

These trends have implications for occupational therapy consultants, because they create a number of important policy issues.

1. To accelerate productivity in the service industries, we must focus upon the higher education needs of tomorrow's workers.
2. Applied research must focus on solutions to maintain a dynamic aging work force and to develop programs that focus on the reconciliation of the conflicting needs of women, work, and family.
3. Educational programs, research findings, and application to occupational therapy service must provide effective means to integrate special populations fully into our economy.
4. We must improve educational preparation for all workers, focusing on alternative processes to reach individuals with special needs.

Although our services tend to focus on individuals in context with today's environment, we must not negate our obligation to society's future. Consequently, let's take a moment to think about the year 2010. Who will the occupational therapist be serving in just 20 years? It has been predicted that by the year 2010 as many as 38% of Americans under the age of 18 will belong to minority groups. Total youth population will grow faster in the Sun Belt and in states that receive large numbers of immigrants, and these states, which will be blessed with increasing populations, will be challenged by a profusion of races and cultures.

Think a moment about the children who are ten years old today. These children will be entering college by the year 2000. Of this group, 24% live below poverty level; 33% are nonwhite; 18% are born to single parents; 10% do not speak English; and 54% have mothers who work outside the home. It is also important to consider that 25% of American youth do not graduate from high school in today's society; only 59% of black children and 50% of Hispanic children graduate from high school. Also, keep in mind that 50% of today's high school graduates do not attend college. In fact, 16% of college freshmen today are enrolled in remedial courses in reading, 21% are enrolled in remedial courses in writing, and 25% in mathematics. Unfortunately, it has been identified that 50% of today's children are not equipped with the reading, writing, reasoning, and critical thinking skills that enable them to profit from rigorous higher education.

Considering these trends, the characteristics of today's youth, and predictions for tomorrow's adults, potentials for diversification of occupational therapy's role have never been greater. If we are committed to the significance of work, play, and routines of daily living in contributing to the better quality of life for all individuals, then we must expand our services from treatment-centered programs to human-centered programs—to human-centered services centered in the concepts and practices of consultation.

The future for occupational therapy, I believe, will be grounded in the theoretical concepts of normalization, social development, and primary prevention. The concept of normalization, although mutually derived from application in the field of mental retardation, has been broadly redefined to fit human management in general. Literature states that the normalization concept involves the utilization of services in which a person's life experiences can be as culturally normative as possible. Involving the natural networking of community personnel and families is inherent in the important principle of normalization. Considering a person in context with his or her environment is necessary to fully understand the person and his/her problems, and to affect meaningful change. Assessing and changing behaviors of persons and contextual systems is essential in the principles of consultation and basic to the concepts of normalization.

Social development theories are grounded in the belief that both prevention and intervention programs are most successful when a program is carried out with individuals, groups, families, or communities directly involved with the problem situation. The key component of social development is the implementation of service *with* persons in the community. An effective system of consultation must be based upon goals and strategies negotiated between local people who are responsible for implementation and those who have control over resources and legal mandates.

The theoretical concept of primary prevention is basic to occupational therapy consultation. Primary prevention involves both activities that are directed toward the elimination of potentially harmful configurations of biopsychosocial events and simultaneous promotion of beneficial configurations in any identifiable population at risk.

Occupational therapists must be educated to implement consultation programs based upon the concepts of normalization, social development, and primary prevention. We must be educated and proficient in the research skills necessary to measure the effectiveness of these programs. Our science must guide our art.

I view a future with great potential—the potential to serve humanity through the use of occupational technology and the enhancement of client-professional communication. I view a future that celebrates our heritage and connects our historic roots with the challenges to promote healthfulness. Through the vital connections of the science and art of occupational therapy, we can promote normalization, social development, and primary prevention. Our consultatory relationships will epitomize the principles of purposefulness, learning, openness, caring, celebration, and community.

REFERENCES

1. Gilfoyle, E: Caring: A philosophy for practice. *Am J Occup Ther* 1980; 34(8):519.
2. Gilfoyle, E: Creative partnerships: the profession's plan. *Am J Occup Ther* 1987; 4(12):780–81.
3. Gonzales, NL: In defense of elitism. *Science* 1981; 213:iv.
4. Gritzer, G., Arnold, A: *The Making of Rehabilitation*. Berkeley, University of California Press, 1985.
5. Webster's New Collegiate Dictionary: Springfield, MA, G. and C. Merriam, 1981.

Author Index

Subject Index